DEMCO

THERAPEUTIC HEAT AND COLD

THIRD EDITION

This volume is one of the series,
Rehabilitation Medicine Library,
Edited by John V. Basmajian.

New books and new editions published, in press or in preparation for this series:

BANERJEE: Rehabilitation Management of Amputees

BASMAJIAN: Therapeutic Exercise, third edition*

BISHOP: Behavioral Problems and the Disabled: Assessment and Management

BROWNE, KIRLIN AND WATT: Rehabilitation Services and the Social Work Role: Challenge for Change

CHYATTE: Rehabilitation in Chronic Renal Failure

EHRLICH: Rehabilitation Management of Rheumatic Conditions

HAAS ET AL.: Pulmonary Therapy and Rehabilitation: Principles and Practice

INCE: Behavioral Psychology in Rehabilitation Medicine: Clinical Applications

JOHNSON: Practical Electromyography

LONG: Prevention and Rehabilitation in Ischemic Heart Disease

REDFORD: Orthotics Etcetera, second edition*

ROGOFF: Manipulation, Traction and Massage, second edition*

ROY AND TUNKS: Chronic Pain: Psychosocial Factors in Rehabilitation

SHA'KED: Human Sexuality and Rehabilitation Medicine: Sexual Functioning Following Spinal Cord Injury

* Originally published as part of the Physical Medicine Library, edited by Sidney Licht.

Therapeutic Heat and Cold

Third Edition

Edited by

Justus F. Lehmann, M.D.

Professor and Chairman,
Department of Rehabilitation Medicine,
University of Washington,
Seattle, Washington

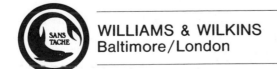

WILLIAMS & WILKINS
Baltimore/London

Copyright ©, 1982
Williams & Wilkins
428 East Preston Street
Baltimore, MD 21202, U.S.A.

Made in the United States of America

First Edition, 1958
Second Edition, 1965

Library of Congress Cataloging in Publication Data

Main entry under title:

Therapeutic heat and cold.

  (Rehabilitation medicine library)
  Includes index.
  Contents: History of therapeutic heat and cold/Sidney Licht—Thermometry/Thomas C. Cetas—Thermal science for physical medicine/K. Michael Sekins and Ashley F. Emery—[etc.]
  1. Thermotherapy—Addresses, essays, lectures. 2. Cold—Therapeutic use—Addresses, essays, lectures. I. Lehmann, Justus F. II. Series.
RM865.T46   1982   616.8′32   81-13085
ISBN 0-683-04907-0   AACR2

Composed and printed at the
Waverly Press, Inc.
Mt. Royal and Guilford Aves.
Baltimore, MD 21202, U.S.A.

Dedication

This volume is dedicated to Sidney Licht in appreciation of his great contribution to the care of the physically handicapped.

Series Editor's Foreword

This third edition of a classic work combines the erudition inherited from its former editor, Sidney Licht, with a new erudition and scientific rigor. The editor, Justus Lehmann, embodies all that I could ask for in his meticulous management of the renaissance which was needed. This volume now regains its unique place in the literature and is the ultimate authority on its subject. It deeply enriches the *Rehabilitation Medicine Library* and will expand the horizons of all who aspire to treat disabled human beings through the application of thermal energy.

The use of heat and cold in therapy remains mildly controversial. In some centers, the controversy has led to skepticism and even to rejection. Much of the problem arose in the past from lack of scientific validation. The lack of scientific rigor in past claims about the value of various methods of cooling or heating tissues was notorious.

Persuasive data have been carefully gathered and dovetailed by the outstanding authors in this book. Their efforts have been highlighted by the basic-science sections which will permit readers to evaluate carefully all therapeutic applications past, present, and future.

JOHN V. BASMAJIAN, M.D.

Preface

The review of therapeutic heat and cold in this volume extends from basic physics and physiology to clinical application and evaluation of effectiveness. The basic physics, the biophysics, the physiological response and the mechanism by which it is obtained, as well as empirical clinical indications and the available evaluation of efficacy, are reviewed for all the heating modalities and the different techniques of application of cold. This review is the outgrowth of teaching the subject matter to undergraduate and graduate students in physical therapy, to undergraduate medical students, and to residents in specialties where these modalities have been found to be useful, including training in physical medicine and rehabilitation, in orthopedics and in rheumatology. It is hoped that perusal of the text will encourage the rational use of these therapies as an adjunct to other medical and therapeutic management, and prevent its abuse both by unwarranted across-the-board rejection or overenthusiastic use. It is hoped, furthermore, that the basic understanding of these therapies will render them more effective by establishing a basis for provision and use of effective equipment and of effective techniques of application, without which these modalities are rendered useless.

JUSTUS F. LEHMANN, M.D.

Contributors

Thomas C. Cetas, Ph.D.
Assistant Professor of Radiology, Adjunct Assistant Professor of Electrical Engineering, Division of Radiation Oncology, University of Arizona, Health Sciences Center, Tucson, Arizona

Barbara J. de Lateur, M.D.
Professor, Department of Rehabilitation Medicine, University of Washington; Director of Rehabilitation Medicine, Harborview Medical Center, Seattle, Washington

Floyd Dunn, Ph.D.
Professor of Electrical Engineering, of Biophysics and Bioengineering, Chairman of Bioengineering Faculty, Director of Bioacoustics Research Laboratory, Bioacoustics Research Laboratory, University of Illinois, Urbana, Illinois

Ashley F. Emery, Ph.D.
Professor of Mechanical Engineering, Adjunct Professor in the Department of Architecture, University of Washington, Seattle, Washington

Leon A. Frizzell, Ph.D.
Assistant Professor of Electrical Engineering and Bioengineering, Bioacoustics Research Laboratory, University of Illinois, Urbana, Illinois

Eugene W. Gerner, Ph.D.
Associate Professor of Radiology, Division of Radiation Oncology, University of Arizona, Health Sciences Center, Tucson, Arizona

Arthur W. Guy, Ph.D.
Professor, Department of Rehabilitation Medicine, Adjunct Professor of Electrical Engineering, Adjunct Professor, Center for Bioengineering, University of Washington, Seattle, Washington

James D. Hardy, Ph.D.
Professor Emeritus of Epidemiology and Physiology, Fellow Emeritus of the John B. Pierce Foundation, Past Director of the John B. Pierce Foundation Laboratory, John B. Pierce Foundation Laboratory, New Haven, Connecticut

Justus F. Lehmann, M.D.
Professor and Chairman, Department of Rehabilitation Medicine, Chairman of the Commission on Rehabilitation, University of Washington, Seattle, Washington

Sidney Licht, M.D. (Deceased)
Former Curator, Physical Medicine Collections, Yale Medical Library, New Haven, Connecticut

Sol M. Michaelson, D.V.M.
Professor of Radiation Biology and Biophysics, Associate Professor of Medicine and Lab Animal Medicine, Department of Radiation Biology and Biophysics, University of Rochester, School of Medicine and Dentistry, Rochester, New York

James R. Oleson, M.D., Ph.D.
Assistant Professor of Radiology, Radiation Oncologist, Radiation Oncology Division, University of Arizona, Health Sciences Center, Tucson, Arizona

K. Michael Sekins, Ph.D.
Research Assistant, Department of Mechanical Engineering; Research Assistant, Department of Rehabilitation Medicine, University of Washington, Seattle, Washington

Contents

1

History of Therapeutic Heat and Cold

SIDNEY LICHT

Introduction

Heat has been used to appease aches and pains ever since man first experienced what the heat of the sun could do for him. Sigerist (1) called the use of heat in therapy instinctual. Of the many therapeutic agents used in ancient times, few have been used as continuously through the past into the present and, except for exercise, none has continued to be used more extensively and in more different forms than heat. Heat is generally available, relatively inexpensive and safe, and, when effective, gives almost immediate and obvious relief. In cool climates, heat has always been a comfort, and even in warm climates, the people have exposed themselves and their children to the sun. This once may have had a religious or other significance, but heat was the immediate and desired experience.

Heat has always been available where the sun shines or wherever dry sticks[1] could be rubbed together. In many parts of the world, warm to hot water springs from the ground, or there is sand, which heats only too rapidly in the sunshine. Although all these forms of heat are available free, they are not freely available, and man had to learn to make heat artificially. In so doing, he not only supplied heat for cooking and comfort, but he also burned himself. He soon learned to fear and respect the destructive as well as the comforting attributes of fire. Artificial heat was first used therapeutically to burn. The word *cautery* comes from the Greek word *to burn*.

Many primitive peoples exposed themselves to fire to drive out the demons of disease. For some, it meant applying the smoldering plant materials to the skin in tiny *bonfires* (moxa); in others it was as dramatic as walking over glowing coals (2). It was an easy step from contact with

---

[1] Since dry sticks were difficult to find in wet weather, many ancient tribes kept a fire burning at all times. According to Frazer (2), this was the probable origin of the "Eternal Flame."

1

combustion to cautery with heated metal, a procedure which has been used in some form by surgeons of all eras. Since the earlier methods of producing heat for medical applications were sometimes the same as those for cautery, and since some methods used in therapeutic heat entered medicine through the doorway of the cautery, it will be mentioned briefly.

The Cautery

Fire production was one of man's first inventions, and there was something magical about it. The open flame has remained a thing of wonder and fascination. From the beginning, it had been associated with religious ritual and the healing arts. People still "light a candle" with a prayer for improvement in health. Fire was used by many tribes to exorcise the demons of disease. Fire could be applied as a glowing coal or moxa.[2] Those tribes which learned to smelt and work iron used the red-hot iron instead of burning leaves, but in regions where metal was scarce, the moxa was used until recent times. The magic of the cautery was enhanced in ancient times by the use of special preparations. Some physicians insisted that it be made of gold or bronze, or fig wood (3).

The oldest written record of the use of the actual cautery may be found in the Edwin Smith Papyrus (4),[3] which is believed to have been written about 3000 B.C.[4] Next in antiquity to the Egyptian medical writings are

---

[2] The moxa of the last century was imported from Japan where the cottony down of the wormwood plant was rolled into a cone and placed on the skin. The tip of the cone was ignited and smoldered slowly. The burning produced a pain "which often resulted in a most salutary change in chronic illness."

Pierre-Francois Percy, Napoleon's chief military surgeon, wrote one of the most comprehensive books on cautery (Pyrotechnie Chirurgicale Pratique, Paris, 1811). He listed the many varieties of cautery which different peoples adopted according to their natural resources and prejudices. The nomads used the fatty wool of sheep, the Hindus burned the core of the rush, the Persians fired dried goat dung, the Thessalians liked dry moss, the Egyptians found cotton very suitable and Seythians heated iron. Some Greeks burned natural linen or mushrooms, others used boiling oil in which they steeped boxwood branches, asphodel root, grape vines, or laurel stems in the belief that they were adding to the benefits of heat the medical properties with which these plants were supposedly endowed. Many ancient physicians were known for the plant which they favored to carry the fire. Theophrastus preferred ground ivy, Caelius prescribed soapwort root, Paul of Egina favored birthwort and Aetius was partial to marjoram. Through repeated translations into Arabic and Italian, these beliefs became established in later times and their acceptance reached its pinnacle in the works of Marco Severino (1580–1656).

[3] "One having tumors with prominent head in his breast, and they produce cysts of pus. An ailment which I treat with the fire drill." The fire drill or fire stick was an improvement on rubbing two sticks to produce fire.

[4] At a later period, the Egyptians and others in North Africa saw a great vogue in the use of the actual cautery. A wooden handle was mounted with a steel rod which was brought to red to white heat over a coal fire. The end of the rod was rounded into one of many designs which by the end of the nineteenth century had dwindled to five: the rose, the cone, the disc, the octagen and the lancet. There were three ways of applying the cautery: the objective, in which the hot metal was brought close to the part without contact; the transcurrent, or very brief

those of Asia. The ancient Hindus regarded Charaka as the highest authority in medicine and Susruta as the highest in surgery. Susruta said that caustic is better than the knife, and the cautery[5] is better than either (6).

Asiatic medicine did not have much influence on Greek medicine, but one of the things the two did have in common was the cautery. Hippocrates was not only the best known of the ancient Greek physicians, he was also the strongest advocate of the cautery among them. He used it in many conditions, and his aphorism that fire will succeed where all other methods fail was a guide for many centuries after, especially among the Arabs. Hippocrates treated epilepsy by applying the cautery to the head. He also used it in phthisis[6] to ward off irritation in the early stages or to procure a favorable exudation in lung suppuration (3).

In ancient times, the heat most often used by physicians was the actual cautery. It was used principally for surface lesions, especially swellings which were chronic. Intense heat in the form of boiling water was also used as a vesicant. Almost every important physician of ancient times used the cautery. Thus, in 1598, when Fienus (7) of Antwerp wrote the first book on the subject, he was able to list 66 authors who had written on the cautery before him. He wrote this lengthy treatise because he considered the cautery useful although difficult and dangerous. He felt that too few physicians of his time were adequately informed on the subject. Although he used a lens[7] to cauterize a lip cancer, he insisted that "fire is the most effective and active of all cauteries."

Ancient Greek and Roman medical writings were kept from oblivion during the dark ages by the Arabs. Thus, it is no surprise that Albucasis regarded the cautery highly (10). The Arabs used it in empyema, liver abscess, rectal ulcer, fistula, and prolapse. Mohamet, the religious leader, was an amateur practitioner of medicine. His medical philosophy consisted

---

contact; and the inherent, in which the contact was more than momentary. It was used after the bite of rabid animals or poisonous snakes, in gangrenous inflammations, to stop hemorrhage, after ligating and compression had failed, and against ulcers, cancer, and other tumors (3).

[5] The actual cautery of the Hindu practitioners was applied in several forms; substances in a state of combustion, boiling fluids, heated metallic bars, or probes. Often, the metal applied to the body had fanciful shapes such as the form of the rose apple, or a serrated trident. Such instruments were used to destroy surface growth. Live charcoal was applied to the bite of a serpent (5).

[6] Celsus went much further with the cautery in phthisis. He wrote that in severe cases, an artificial ulcer should be made with the hot iron under the chin, another on the neck, two each on each breast and an equal number of the tips of the scapulae. Laforgue Sainte Rose characterized this treatment as a "cruel practice." However, it is questionable whether Celsus ever did this, since, although we have proof that he was an informed writer, we have none that he ever practiced medicine.

[7] The heat concentrating powers of the lens were known for a long time. Aristophanes wrote of burning glasses prior to 420 B.C. (8). Pliny wrote, "I have read that some physicians believe the best cautery is a crystal ball through which the rays of the sun have passed" (9).

of a trinity of treatments; honey, scarification, and the cautery. He stopped hemorrhage in one Saad ben Maaz with cauterization (11).

The actual cautery was used to stop bleeding until compressions and the ligature became more widely used after the recommendations of de Mondeville early in the fourteenth century. Although the cautery continued to be used by lay people,[8] its acceptance by physicians fluctuated. Thus, in 1751, Lafaye (13) decried the diminished use of the cautery among surgeons. Larrey and Dupuytren restored its popularity among surgeons by recommending it against poisons, tumors, and gangrene; Percy used it for rheumatic pains. Heated metal remained the most widely used form of cautery, but the burning lens[9] was not completely displaced until electricity entered the field, about 1850.

GALVANOCAUTERY

Within a very short time after Volta's description of the pile (17), interested experimenters were using it in a variety of ways. Vanquelin (18) passed the newly created current through iron wire and reported that it became red hot. Even though Davy generated great light and heat with the carbon arc a few years later, the heat potential of the electric current was not given serious consideration[10] until about the fourth decade when Recamier and Pravaz began to use it to destroy[11] uterine cancer.[12] Within a few years, it

---

[8] As late as 1856, Chrestien (12) wrote, "The use of the cautery is so widely accepted that many people apply it without consulting a physician."

[9] Baptiste Porta had favored the lens (14), but the writings of Faure (15) gave it its greatest impetus. A generation later, Bertrand (16) said that it was sometimes preferable to the moxa or hot iron, and this is readily understandable since its action was slower, thus more easily controlled and less likely to result in deep scars.

[10] In 1817, Richet (19) wrote that electricity could not be considered as a source of heat. The word *electricity* was used in the nineteenth century to refer to the static form.

[11] The first use of the galvanic current was for its caustic rather than its thermal cautery effect. Seudamore was apparently the first to note that the blood could be coagulated by electricity. In 1831, it occurred to Guérard that he could obliterate aneurysms by coagulating the blood in them, but it was not until 1846 that Pétrequin of Lyons actually succeeded in doing that. In 1837, Clavel had proposed electric coagulation of aneurysm in his doctral thesis (20).

In 1846, Crusell of Russia used galvanocautery for uretheral stricture and two years later destroyed a fungoid growth of the face with it. (He took daguerreotypes before and after the operation [April 22, 1817], certainly one of the earliest uses of clinical photography.) In 1850, John Marshall used galvanocautery to close a salivary fistula (21), and two years later Hilton and Nélaton destroyed erectile tumors with the electric cautery. Sédillot (22), claimed that he had reported on that procedure in 1849.

In 1851, Marshall proposed its use with an electrode made of a procelain olive wound with platinum wire. Middeldorpf used a platinum loop, and in 1862, Seré developed the galvanic knife which Boeckel perfected in 1873 (23).

[12] Becquerel (9) credited Fabre Palprat (24) with having first burned tissue with an electrified platinum needle in 1830 (25). Pétrequin claimed priority and admitted that the idea came to him after reading Sarlandiere's book on electropuncture published in 1823 (26).

became so widely used for that purpose that Pichard (27) called attention to its overuse.

In 1854, there appeared an article in *Lancet* in which Harding described a test on nerve pulp with the galvanic current. This set Middeldorpf of Breslau to work on the destruction of tissue with electricity, which resulted in the classic, *Die Galvankaustic*, published in 1854, which eventually led to the introduction by Paquelin (10) in 1875 of the galvanic thermocautery. An important development of this instrument was its reversion to one of the first uses of the actual cautery—hemostasis. Skene (28) adapted the hot iron cautery of Thomas Keith, which he touched to the compression clamp placed on the pedicle containing a bleeder.[13] In 1931, Jacobaeus (29) first cauterized adhesions through a thoracoscope and opened the field to cauterization of structures in closed cavities. The cautery continued for some time to be used in most conditions previously treated with the non-galvanic instrument. De Lamballe and later Velleix recommended the sweep of burning irons over the skin for the treatment of neuralgia.[14]

HIGH-FREQUENCY CAUTERY

In 1842, Joseph Henry (30) suggested that the phenomena accompanying the discharge of a Leyden jar included oscillation, a conclusion at which Helmholtz arrived in 1847 (31). In 1853, the Danish physicist Feddersen, by means of mirrors turning at great speed, showed that Henry had guessed well. Soon after, William Thomson (Lord Kelvin) established the theoretical considerations of high-frequency currents, and in 1886, Hertz[15] in Hamburg showed that an oscillating current could be produced in a sustained manner and transmitted with the speed of light (32). Within the next few years, Tesla, an engineer in America, and d'Arsonval, a physician-physiologist in France, were working with methods of producing high-frequency currents. Each suggested their use in medicine but neither for elevating tissue temperature at first.[16] In 1893, Oudin (34) modified the circuit suggested by d'Arsonval by adding a resonator, which markedly increased the voltage.

---

[13] "While thinking of an improved way to heat the clamp, my attention was drawn to the use of electricity in heating laundry smoothing irons. It then occurred to me to adapt the same heating power to surgical instruments such as the clamp and forceps." He used 10 to 35 watts of electricity.

[14] A treatment which persisted for so long that it was demonstrated to this writer when he was a senior medical student in 1930.

[15] In 1871, von Bezold published his findings on the alternating aspects of the electric discharge. In 1881, Ward and Spottiswoode produced an oscillatory current of 6000 cycles per second with a spark gap. Oliver Lodge carried out experiments similar to those of Hertz independently and at about the same time.

[16] The priority controversy was kept alive for a long time (33). D'Arsonval published his first article on the subject in February, 1891. Tesla's first article appeared on May 23, 1891. Tesla's apparatus was superior to that of d'Arsonval.

With the augmented voltage, he tried to destroy[17] the lesions of psoriasis. Rivière was the first to use the Oudin current on skin cancer in 1900, but the voltage he used was too low to destroy cells. For the rest of his life, Rivière battled for recognition of his priority[18] with de Keating-Hart, who first applied the spark to destroy tumor tissue and demonstrated the procedure at the International Congress of Electrology in Milan in 1906 (36). While the great battle of words was beginning in Paris, Finley R. Cook in New York accidentally short-circuited the current from a static electricity machine through his fingers with resultant tissue destruction. This gave him the idea of treating small tumors with the spark of static electricity, and he published his findings (37) unaware of the work begun in France.

All these applications gave relatively superficial tissue destruction, and Doyen sought a method which would give deeper penetration than the fulguration of de Keating-Hart. Doyen believed that normal cells could withstand a temperature of 60°C but that cancer cells would die at a temperature of 55°C (38). He tried to heat tissues selectively with electricity and hot water to destroy cancer cells. He believed that if he could increase the current frequency from 700 kc to 3 megacycles, he would be able to raise tissue temperatures to desired heights with greater accuracy. He asked Gaiffe, the leading manufacturer of electromedical equipment in Paris, to build such a generator, which they did with a small condenser, a resonating coil and a rotating spark gap. When the current was passed through a 2-cm disc electrode, coagulation was noted at a depth of 5 to 8 millimeters after only two minutes of contact. Thus, instead of using the Oudin resonator with the single pole electrode, he led the current into the patient through a moist pad attached to one pole of the generator with the other pole feeding the active electrode.

At about the same time (1907), Lee de Forest constructed the first radio tube high-frequency medical apparatus—the "cold cautery." With it, Neil and Sternberger made clean incisions in dogs, but American surgeons refused to try it on patients (39). De Forest offered it to physicians in Paris and Vienna, where it was soon used effectively (40,41). It was not until many years later that any American surgeon adopted this most useful invention. In 1923, Wyeth introduced an improved cutting current apparatus with controlled cutting depth. William Clark of Philadelphia altered the fulguration apparatus by increasing the amperage at the expense of the voltage, and this enabled deeper and more efficient destruction with a hotter spark. Since under the microscope the destroyed cells looked longer and shrunken,

---

[17] In 1888, Inglis Parsons tried to destroy tissue with the interrupted direct current from the secondary coil of an inductorium which delivered a 60 cycle current at 400 to 800 mA (35).

[18] The controversy between Rivière and de Keating-Hart took a strange form. Each man started a personal periodical subscribed to and written largely by his partisans. Every issue of each journal was full of self-praise and in each issue, the old priority quarrel was mentioned.

he called the process electrodesiccation when he first demonstrated it in 1910 (42).

One of the more important uses of electrosurgery is in the removal of the prostate. Edwin Beer (43) was the first to use it within the bladder through a Nitze cystoscope.[19] Collings (45) was the first to use the cutting current through a cystoscope in 1923.[20] That was the year Novak (46) destroyed tonsils with electrical coagulation. Bierman (47) devised a special clamp in 1926 which enabled him to destroy hemorrhoids without sending the current through the entire body. Kelly and Ward (39) obtained hemostasis with the high-frequency current in 1925, which allowed them to perform a breast amputation without ligatures. In the following year, Cushing (48) used electrosurgery on the brain.

Sources of Therapeutic Heat

The oldest known sources of heat are those which occur naturally. Although the heat of the sun, sun-heated sand and thermal waters are still widely used by the people to counteract real or imagined pains or illnesses, they are often self-prescribed and seasonal in use. The antiquity of these forms of therapeutic heat is too great to trace to their beginning. Medical science continues to lessen their need, but their use has not diminished much in Europe. Most forms of therapeutic heat prescribed by physicians are artificially produced and range in complexity from warmed water to ultrasound waves. Heat may be applied to the surface of the body by changes in environmental temperature (convection), by contact with warmed substances (conduction) or by radiating energy into the body.

In ancient times, conductive heat was easier to apply and was thus prescribed most often. It included the application of hot water directly or in a container, the application of heated sand, oil, grain, salt, or other solids and liquids. Radiant heat was found in the sun, the open flame, or glowing coals or metals. Until the middle of the nineteenth century, artificial heat was made only from the combustion of solids and liquids such as wood, coal, peat, oil, tallow, or alcohol. The inflammable properties of natural gas were known to the ancients, but it could be used only at the spot where it escaped from the ground. Its commercial manufacture and distribution started about the middle of the nineteenth century.[21] Electricity was not used for heating until the last decade of that century. Thus, until relatively recently, the limitations of fuel and apparatus restricted most local applications of heat to conduction, and most general applications to heated air, water, and vapor.

---

[19] Bottini of Pavia had tried galvanocautery for prostatic obstruction but faded because of uncontrollable hermorrhage (44).

[20] In 1932, J. F. McCarthy developed the electrotome which became the standard instrument.

[21] Illuminating gas was first produced by van Helmont in the early seventeenth century but was not used for illumination until 1792 by Murdoch. In 1832, Sharp used gas for cooking, but it was not until the work of Bunsen in 1855 that it became practical for heating.

In former times, home heating was expensive to install and maintain; only the wealthy few could afford it. Others who wished to experience indoor heat in the winter went to public baths[22] where there were rooms with hot dry air, hot vapor, or hot water. Although the baths were used largely for cleansing and pleasure, physicians did prescribe the various forms of available heat for hygiene and in illness. When the baths were eventually closed for moral and economic reasons, generalized applications of heat virtually disappeared during the colder months for centuries. Sweating was considered a very healthful procedure by the ancients (and by a great many people throughout the ages). It was a latter-day translation of the idea of exorcism. Sweating "carried the poisons of the body out through the pores." Reddening of the skin was also considered a desirable procedure, especially over painful areas, and heat as a rubefacient was also available at the public baths. There were many special rooms in the Roman baths. There were rooms with water or air baths at different temperatures, and these were used in varying patterns of increasing and decreasing exposure to heat and cold. The Romans used the heated bath for patients. If the patient was too weak for a full bath, he was given a partial bath. One form of bath, the *enbasis*, was a tank of hot water which Aurelianus (49) mentioned as good for sciatica. The same author mentioned swimming in warm springs for the treatment of paralysis. For the poor people it was water, for the wealthy there were baths of heated milk or oil (14).

CONDUCTIVE HEAT

The oldest form of conductive heating was contact with the waters of thermal springs and the sand heated by the sun. Almost as soon as man learned to build fires, he noted that stones in or near them maintained their heat for a long time. He soon learned to place the heated stone against a painful part. Man could not establish communities away from fresh water until he learned how to store it. Two of the earliest water containers were the bladders or skins of animals and hollow dried fruits such as gourds. Hippocrates recommended the use of small bags or bladders of warm water for sciatica and for local inflammations of the rectum. Aurelianus (49) wrote of gourds filled with hot water applied as a fomentation.[23] Hot water and vapor early became part of folk medicine and were so widely used and

---

[22] At one time, there were 800 public baths in Rome. The admission fee was very small for adults, and children were admitted free (13).

[23] Fomentations were also made by pouring warming liquids over the body or a part of the body. In *De affectionibus*, Hippocrates wrote, "When the ears become painful, bathe them and foment them abundantly with hot water (50). Warm water fomentation was recommended by many for various complaints, especially colic. Alexander of Tralles and Arctacus used it in urinary colic, and much later, Mead used it for painter's colic. Warm baths were used by Hoffman for asthenic mania, a form of treatment which persisted almost until the middle of the twentieth century, Sydenham and Boerhaave used hot baths to prevent chills.

commonplace that they were mentioned frequently in the medical literature, a status comparable to the great use and relatively infrequent mention in current literature of aspirin for headache. But as a medical prescription, heat therapy was neglected for many centuries. It was resurrected by Ambroise Paré.

Although he put an end to one form of heat (boiling oil for wounds), Paré revived interest in less drastic applications (52).[24] "Diverse fomentations are used for broken bones. When we use warm water for fomentations, we mean a temperature between hot and cold, that is, which feels lukewarm to the surgeon and patient. A fomentation of such water used for a short time moderately heats, attenuates, and prepares for resolution the humor which is in the surface of the body and draws blood to the atrophied part. It assuages pain, relaxes that which is too tight, and moderately heats the limb which has become cold as a result of tight binding or other reasons." Fallopio, a contemporary of Paré, proposed that ulcers be treated with bathing in warm water (53). "Stoving" was used frequently in the eighteenth century.

Vapor baths were resurrected in 1809 by Cochrane (54) who devised a boiler-fed bedside tent. He was able to collect signed testimonials from 70 of the most prominent physicians in London on the effectiveness of his steam tent in treating patients. La Beaume (55) found the tent soothing to the point of putting the patient to sleep.

HOT WATER

Hot water is perhaps the most widely applied agent of conductive heating, whether it be a local soak or compress or a full tub. Many variations have been used and many special containers and appliances have been tried. Water has been poured, thrown, or rubbed on the body. Pools, tanks, and other containers have been devised especially for therapeutic heat. One example was the *pediluvium*, a hot foot bath in which the leg could be

---

[24] Paré devoted an entire chapter in one of this books (51) to the construction and use of a device for treating patients with heated vapor. "Stoves may be dry or moist. In dry stoves, a hot dry exhalation is developed for application to the body making it hot and opening its pores so that sweat may pour out of them. There are many ways to develop dry heat. At Paris, and wherever there are stoves or public hot houses, they are made by fire under a vaulted furnace which heats the whole room. Also you may put hot cobblestones or bricks into a tub, having first laid the bottom with bricks or iron plates. Then place a seat in the tub were the patient will sit with a canopy drawn over him so that he may receive the heat rising from the stones and thus, have the benefit of sweating. But we must look at the patient often, for it sometimes happens that some, neglected by their keepers, otherwise engaged, become faint, and their sense failing them by dissipation of their strength, by the heat of the exhalation, have sunk down on the underlying stones and so have been carried half dead and burned into their beds. Some also take sweating in a furnace or even as soon as the bread has been removed, but of this I do not approve because the patient cannot turn around or lie down therein." The ancients produced therapeutic vapor baths by throwing red-hot stones into water (13).

immersed up to the knee. "These baths produce marvellous effects in spasmodic pains of the head, in asthenic fluxions of the eyes, in convulsive asthma, suppression of the menses, palpitations of the heart, nervous fevers and delirium" according to one author (56). The same author, Chortet, reserved his highest praise for the more universally accepted indication for heat—pain. In 1802 he wrote, "Almost all pains from the most severe to the most tolerable are more or less calmed by the application of hot water to the painful parts. . . . Heat is good in rheumatism and sciatica. . . . "

But there is something about an ordinary container of hot water which is too commonplace to be considered therapeutic by patients when they encounter it in a hospital or physician's office. When the hot water is placed in a vessel of special shape or material, it is accepted as therapy more readily by physician and patient alike. The whirlpool bath and Hubbard tank are examples. Although in each there is the element of forced air or water, we must look for the primary effect to the hot water rather than to the bubbles.

Warm to hot water has been used in musculoskeletal derangements for a long time. The ancient Romans sent their wounded soldiers to warm mineral springs for all kinds of war injuries (57).[25] Aurelianus was most explicit in his recommendations for exercising paretic muscles in *warm* springs. Thermal springs continued to be frequented for bathing and drinking, but their use in heating involved joints and muscles diminished somewhat during the latter half of the nineteenth century thanks to the efforts of Priessnitz and his followers, who extolled the virtues of the "cold water cure" (58). But the heroically unpleasant swing to cold water dimmed toward the end of the century, and warm water resumed its deserved place. In 1898, von Leyden and Goldscheider (59) recommended underwater exercise in warm water, and shortly thereafter, Preiss (60) designed the first whirlpool bath activated by an electric motor (and used primarily for gynecologic conditions). The whirled warm water bath was virtually forgotten until World War I, during which, according to Pope (61), it was used in France for military patients.[26] The apparatus was seen by Dr. Fox, who had one installed at the Walter Reed Hospital;[27] from there, the idea slowly spread throughout the United States so that by the time World War II was over, the device could be found

---

[25] During the French Revolution and for years after, heated water enjoyed a considerable vogue in the treatment of wounds. Percy, Surgeon General of the French Army, spoke highly of this treatment which Lombard had resurrected in 1786 (*Dictionnaire des Sciences Médicales*, Paris, 1814).

[26] We have made inquiries in France, especially at the library of the Val de Grâce (principal military) Hospital, and were unable to learn about the *cau couronte* which remains uncommon in the country of its origin.

[27] Captain F. A. Bardwell designed the air injector used to whirl the water (Sampson, C. M. *Physiotherapy technic*, St. Louis, 1923).

in almost every hospital with a physical therapy department. In 1928, Dr. Walter P. Blount[28] first described a much larger bath, the Hubbard tub (or tank), to which the whirl was eventually added.

Hot water has been used for a long time against chill, whether of a part or the entire body. For many years, it was the custom to administer transfusion with blood recently stored in a refrigerator. Since heart muscle is sensitive to cold, blood at low temperature reaching it may cause fibrillation. Boyan (62) passed cool blood through a plastic coil immersed in water at body temperature to avoid cold insult to the heart.

OIL AND WAX

The ancient Romans poured warmed and hot oils on the body as an embrocation especially in preparation for massage. Celsus (15) and Aetius wrote of melted wax in the treatment of styes. Arnold of Villeneuve poured melted wax on the body as therapy, and Constantin used it for ecchymosis of the eye (14). Aurelianus (49) devoted space to *ceromata*, which were animal hides soaked in oil and heated in the sun.[29] But the use of melted wax in treatment as we know it today is of recent introduction.

In 1913, Barthe de Sandfort (63) described the first paraffin bath, and in the following year, Bouet-Henry (64) brushed melted paraffin on wounds. The paraffin bath was not too widely used in France, but it received enough publicity to come to the attention of a Mr. W. L. Ingle, who owned a tannery at Cherwell in Yorkshire. He noted that some workers in his factory immersed their hands and feet in the wax vats, following which they spoke of benefits. Mr. Ingle offered the commanding officer of the nearby military hospital at Leeds, Colonel Littlewood, his wax facilities. The Colonel introduced the use of melted paraffin in his hospital in 1918 (65) whence its use spread in England as the "wax bath."[30]

---

[28] Although primarily designed for underwater exercise, the Hubbard tank was since become equally important as a method of generalized therapeutic heating, particularly in arthritis. We are indebted to Dr. Walter P. Blount for an account of the little-known details concerning its origin. The daughter of Mr. Henry Pope was severely paralyzed by poliomyelitis. He had heard about underwater gymnastics and gave his daughter exercises in an old wooden tub in the basement of his Chicago home. He asked Mr. Carl Hubbard, an engineer residing in the same city, what shape would be most suitable for such a tub. One day while Dr. Blount, Mr. Pope, and Mr. Hubbard were all at Warm Springs, Georgia, "we lay on the floor and waved our arms and legs and conceived the idea of the 'key hole' tub. One was built for Warm Springs and one for the Wisconsin General Hospital in Madison, where I was a resident." When Dr. Blount moved to Milwaukee, he had a tub installed at the Columbia Hospital, where he continued to improve upon it until it reached its present form.

[29] The patient was advised to roll back and forth in the oiled skins so that the combined heat of the oil and friction would warm his body.

[30] In 1926, Portmann (66) described an electric heating chamber for paraffin, which, when it became commercially available, greatly stimulated the use of the paraffin bath.

HEATED SOLIDS

The heating properties of sand are immediately apparent to anyone who walks on sun-baked sand with bare feet, a daily routine for many primitive peoples. There is much sand in Egypt, and Herodotus wrote of the sun baths he saw there. Oribasius (67) quoted the account of Herodotus, as did Galen, who mentioned a patient, the wife of Boethus, for whom he prescribed it (14). Dioscorides (68) recommended beach sand dried in the sun for drawing water from hydropics. The patient was covered with sand up to his neck in a sunny location. Aurelianus (49) advised this treatment in arthritis and obesity.[31]

Conductive heating was applied with all sorts of vegetable products. The favorites were hot cereals, breads, and apples. Other poultices were made with grape grounds, leaves, wood chips, eggs, animal parts, and mud (70). Sylvius used cooked apples, which he applied hot in ophthalmia. Benedict applied the same mash for hemorrhoids. Rhazes used a foment of hot masked millet to the cheek for toothache (14). The introduction of the hot water bag and the heating pad displaced the poultice which retained its place in thermotherapy into the twentieth century.

HOT WATER BOTTLE AND HEATING PAD

The idea of the hot water bottle is very old. Hippocrates used flat earthenware dishes filled with boiling water and applied them to the chest and abdomen. Rudius used a vessel filled with hot cinders for abdominal pains. Celsus wrote of *lenticulars* which were earthenware pots filled with hot oil and applied to the abdomen to provoke sweating. Vessels containing hot mixtures were applied to the soles of the feet by Hollier (14) until felt as high as the thighs in cases of sciatica.[32] Soon after the introduction of electricity as an agent for therapeutic (luminous) heat, Salaghi (71) described a heating pad he designed in 1893. In 1898, Cerutti (13), also in Italy, improved upon the thermophore by threading a light compressed cloth material with insulated wires and a temperature level regulator.

---

[31] "Sand was preferred by most writers since it remained drier than the alternative salt, but Aetius preferred the bath of heated crushed salt. He advised that the pile be at least a foot and a half high to prevent rapid dissipation of the heat (14).

Hot sand baths have continued in use throughout the ages. They were especially popular during the second half of the nineteenth century Grawitz (69) collected reports on their use from England (1872), France (1871), and Russia (1889). There are still "health stations" along the French and Italian Riviera where *psammotherapy* is practiced.

[32] This reference is made by Severin, Professor of Anatomy at Naples, the first physician (after Pare, a surgeon) to write extensively about thermotherapy. He listed all forms of heat used from the time of Hippocrates to his own in 1668.

FRICTION

Friction, rubbing, and massage[33] are no longer considered forms of therapeutic heat, but they were at one time for the obvious warming to both patient and operator.

CONVECTIVE HEAT[34]

Warmed or heated air was used for many conditions, but especially for pains in joints. Pliny (14) advised exposure in a hot air furnace[35] for arthritic joints. The hot oven was popular to induce sweating, and sweating has always been popular with a sizable proportion of the population. The Arabs used the oven frequently. When the Calif Watek-Billah was dangerously ill during an epidemic, his physicians placed him in a warm oven so often and for so long that his death was probably due to overheating (13). Gaspard Torella wrote that "the best way to cure smallpox is to make the patient sweat in a stove or warm oven for about 15 days" (13). Jean Fernel favored an even greater dosage: "The patient was placed in an oven and kept there at elevated temperatures for 20, 30, or more days." Boissier de Sauvages (73) found that heated air "relaxes our fibers which lengthen appreciably. That is why it is appropriate for the dissipation of cold tumors, painful catarrhs, to open vessels, to restore circulation to the parts which the cold deprived of movement and sensation, to increase perspiration because it dilates the pores of the vessels and the flow of liquids, to excite an intestinal movement[36] which exalts the saline and sulfurous matters, which disposes the body to a more prompt putrefaction and to move the excremental matter which stagnates."

The first scientific clinical study in thermotherapy occurred in France before 1840. It was soon all but forgotten because of local medical politics. Jules Guyot (75), a young Parisian surgeon, began in 1833 to mediate on the value of heat in wound healing. He selected some rabbits and dogs and went to his house in the country, where he set up an animal hospital and for three months devoted himself to experiments and observations on thera-

---

[33] The chief value of massage can hardly be said to be that of supplying heat. Massage as a physical agent is discussed in Volume V of *Physical Medicine Library*.

Arnold of Villeneuve Savonarola, and others used massage as a form of heat for colic (14). Guy de Chauliac wrote, "In hydropsy, the patient should be rubbed in the sun, while protecting the head and liver, for in this condition the heat of the sun is admirable" (72).

[34] The dividing line between heated air, radiant heat, and convective heat is at times tenuous. Heated air will be considered as convective heat in this survey.

[35] He described a hot-air furnace heated by the sun. Heated air, especially heated moist air, could be found at all the major public baths. Some of these were recommended by physicians for general or specific treatments.

[36] De Boissieu (74) also praised the virtues of heat in increasing motion and in lowering the viscosity of body fluids.

peutic heat. He constructed a hot air cabinet, very similar to one that Bier devised about a half-century later, heated with alcohol lamps in such a manner that he could maintain, at will, an environmental temperature anywhere between 30° and 70°C. He found that when the temperature was maintained at about 30°, the healing of wounds was more rapid. His house was near that of Magendie, whom he invited to witness his experiments. When Magendie saw the results, he insisted that the method be tried on his patients at the Hôtel Dieu. Guyot began with the treatment of ulcers, white tumor (tuberculosis), and sciatica. "Each new trial confirmed my belief that heat incubation was a powerful therapeutic agent ... but while at the hospital, I encountered many difficulties which a young man without influence or authority might experience." Eventually he was allowed to work on the kind of wound he felt could be helped most—the fresh wound following amputation. His first two trials proved so successful that he was forced to present them at the Academy of Medicine, and there, as he had suspected, he was criticized for rushing into publication with only two cases.

Guyot noted that warm baths had been used in medicine a long time. They had been given for an hour at about 30°C or with steam at 40° to 45°C. His inquisitive mind asked, "Why has not the action of heating agents been analyzed? Why has no one tried to differentiate between the effect of the gas, liquid, or solid on the one hand, and the temperature on the other? It should have been recognized that heat is the sole agent and that humidity was more a hindrance than a help." He recommended an air bath with a temperature of 36°C, which he considered the temperature of the circulating blood. Soon after his book was published, Guyot became too ill to work. "Thus, there occurred what usually happens in such circumstances; the method was not pushed and was soon forgotten by everyone" (76). And so it remained until Bier (77) began to work on tuberculosis of the extremities.[37]

When the tubercle bacillus was discovered in 1882, many workers tried to find a way to kill it without at the same time killing its human host. In little time, it was found that heat affected the bacillus adversely. Bier tried to warm the site of tubercle invasion by increasing its blood supply—hyperemia. He tried the Esmarch bandage and found it too painful. He also tried massage, exercise, electricity, and chemical rubefacients but soon came to the conclusion that "the most practical and useful agent to promote local hyperemia is heat." Since cataplasms, mud, thermophores, and compresses interfered with circulation, the hot air approach was considered the most logical. In searching for an appropriate apparatus, he was inspired by the apparatus of Quincke, who had warmed the entire body in a gas-heated chamber to promote generalized sweating. Bier devised his Bunsen burner

---

[37] In the same year, Clado (77) devised a hot air oven for heating joints in an attempt to kill the tubercle bacillus in them with heat. Thus, the great stimulus to heat therapy was an attempt to kill the tubercle bacillus.

heating hood in 1891 and reported on it in 1893. He advised the use of the alcohol lamp as the source of heat if gas were not available but predicted that "the heating apparatus of the future will be electrical."[38]

Bier developed special cabinets for each part of the body and "for the rich patients I have every individual box made to measure by a carpenter ... for hospitals the openings should have larger diameters which must be reduced with cotton as needed." Soon after the introduction of Bier's apparatus, there were many who tried to imitate or improve upon it. The Tallerman-Sheffield apparatus, first used in England (78) in 1895, found considerable favor in Europe. It was a boiler-shaped tank of copper, closed at one end and open at the other to receive an extremity. A series of gas flames beneath a closed kettle heated the air in the tank. This hot air device was much drier than that of Bier. By the end of the century, there were several manufacturers in America who were offering cylindrical and box-like cabinets heated by gas, gasoline, or electricity with valves for the interchange of air, since it was felt that the accumulation of moisture in the presence of high temperatures would result in serious skin burns (79).

As might have been expected, the new treatment with heated air was used by many in different countries with glowing reports. Hollaender found currents of hot air under pressure of value in lupus (1897); Cabitto found the warm air bath effective in relieving attacks of epilepsy (1897); and Schmeltz used thermal insufflations of the vagina in pelvic inflammations (1899). The most glowing reports were on joint disease. Sarjeant (78), using a temperature of 240°F for 40 minutes, wrote of eight cases of arthritis and sprain in which the "pain is generally not only relieved but entirely removed."

RADIANT ENERGY

Sunshine, the open fire, glowing coals and irons, and heated stones constituted the chief sources of radiant heat among the ancients. Oribasius (67) has left one of the best accounts. "Patients suffering from a chronic pain are treated with the heat from coals set up in the treatment place. The painful parts will be heated to the point at which the patient finds it difficult to continue."[39] Oribasius (67) also used the sun as a source of heat. "Exposure

---

[38] At virtually the same moment, Kellogg was using electrical luminous energy to cure joint disease in cabinets not too unlike those of Bier. In spite of Bier's prediction, nonelectrical heaters were used with Bier equipment for the next half century in Europe. Bier preferred hot air to radiant heat since air is a poor conductor, has a very limited capacity for heat, and favors the vigorous evaporation of sweat which protects the part against burns.

[39] The same book goes on to tell of another widely used form of conductive heating: "The treatment which consists in receiving heat from a heated wall produces the same effect. When the wall is moderately heated (with the built-in flue), the part to be treated is placed directly in contact with it, but if the wall is very hot, the part should be covered with heavy cloths before it makes contact with the wall."

to the sun is eminently necessary for people who need to be restored to full health and to gain weight.... Too much heat is bad for weak patients. Expose the back to the sun or the fire, for the voluntary nerves are found chiefly in that region and when they are exposed to gentle heat the body will be healthier, but remember to guard the head with some covering."

Nothing of genuine importance in radiant heat therapy occurred for many centuries because there were no new methods for producing it.[40] Artificial radiant heat was limited largely to holding heated substances near the part to be treated. In 1774, Faure (15) wrote, "It is with this application of heated bricks that one lessens rheumatic pains.... We can see with the naked eye that when heat is applied to the neighborhood of an ulcer, the surface becomes rosy in the intact places and a true flow occurs from the broken area. The improvement in circulation is demonstrated by the decreased indolence in the neighborhood of the ulcers I have treated in this way." Other forms of radiant heat included the open hearth, the flame of a candle or a glowing coal.

ELECTRICAL HEAT

Therapeutic heat did not come into its own until heating devices activated by electricity were introduced. The first attempts to generate heat electrically were incident to the search for electric light. At the beginning of the nineteenth century, Davy produced a powerful light with the carbon arc. In 1841, de Moleyne in England (82) tried to make an incandescent lamp. Four years later, Changy in France and Starr and King in Cincinnati tried again, but it was not until 1878, when Edison developed the U-shaped carbon filament in the vacuum glass envelope, that the lighting habits of the world were changed.

---

[40] The very subject of heat was not formally investigated until 1620 when Lord Bacon, in *De forma calidi*, (80) concluded that heat was motion. Boyle supposed that this motion was in small particles of heated bodies and consisted of their rapid vibration. Newton also subscribed to this view, but the French and German chemists believed that heat was a highly elastic penetrating fluid which entered the pores of bodies and made them hot. When the French chemists contrived the new Chemical Nomenclature in 1787, they thought it would be advantageous to have a distinct word for each *kind* of heat. They called the sensation heat and the state calorie.

In 1800, Herschel (81) investigated the heating effects of different parts of the visible spectrum because "it is sometimes of great use in natural philosophy to doubt things that are commonly taken for granted." He showed that red rays heat three times as much as the violet. "I likewise concluded that the full red falls still short of the maximum heat; which perhaps lies even a little beyond visible refraction. In this case, radiant heat will at least partly, if not chiefly consist, if I may be permitted the expression, of invisible light."

These rays were really *above* the red and should have been called ultra-red, whereas the rays on the other end of the visible spectrum discovered by Ritter one year later should have been called infraviolet. In 1835, Ampere showed that heat and light rays could be separated by passing them through quartz or ice.

LUMINOUS HEAT

George N. Beard must be counted among the first specialists in physical medicine in America. In 1875, J. H. Kellogg became one of his protégés (83). The new Edison light lamp[41] interested him, for to Kellogg who believed in "natural" medicine, it represented an effective substitute for sunlight. He began to work with the electric light because he believed that, since sunlight was so important to life and nutrition in plants and animals, it might be beneficial in certain illnesses. In 1891,[42] he built a rectangular cabinet with 40 lamps of 20-candle power, and interior reflectors. He had his patients sit in the cabinet completely nude, with the head outside as in the vapor baths or sweat cabinets of Quincke. He used it on many patients in the Battle Creek Sanatorium and exhibited the apparatus at the Chicago Exposition of 1893. A visitor from Germany saw the bath, visited Battle Creek to become familiar with it, and on returning to Germany began its manufacture. "The bath soon became very popular in Germany, and hundreds of Light Institutes were opened in the leading cities. King Edward of England came to Hamburg for a case of distressing gout and was relieved after a series of light baths. He ordered one installed at Windsor Castle and another at Buckingham Palace. Kaiser Wilhelm soon followed his example as did many other titled families in Europe. In time, the fame of the bath spread back to its home. A New York firm actually imported a bath from Germany as a therapeutic novelty. That bath was made from a description of it published by the author at the annual meeting of the American Electrotherapeutic Association in New York on September, 25, 1894" (84).

Light baths or heating cabinets were installed at all spas, but were also considered necessary equipment in almost all new physical therapy departments up to the time of World War II. But the more lasting result of Kellogg's work was the influence it had on the introduction of the local light bath. Smaller units were soon proposed. Lacquer designed a highly reflective nickel cabinet with six incandescent lamps to be placed over the involved area (85). Modifications of this device became the heat cradle, called by too many for too long a "baker." Marie (86) suggested that individual lamps be placed in silvered parabolic reflectors for local applications. By that time (1901), carbon filament lamps of 500 candle power were widely used in the clinic for such conditions as neuralgia and arthritis.

---

[41] The first lamp gave only a 10 candle power light and could burn for only two months. In 1903, Just used tungsten for the filament, but this did not gain commercial acceptance until 1913. Dowsing, a British engineer, invented a luminous heat lamp in 1896, which was used therapeutically by Hedley of London, but by that time Kellogg had used the Edison lamp on a great many patients.

[42] Guimbail insisted that he was the first to use the electric light bath (*Revue de Thérapeutique par les Agents Physiques*, Paris, 1896). If he did, he did nothing to further its use among physicians.

Few advances in luminous heat followed because it was so difficult to improve on so simple and effective a device as an incandescent lamp in a reflector. Lenses of various colors, materials, or construction were used to alter the light emitted. Humphris (87) suggested that the lamp be made to swing back and forth over the affected part for half an hour. The chief advance after Kellogg was the introduction of the tungsten filament lamp which emitted a smaller percentage of infrared rays and could be applied at greater energies before an uncomfortable heat sensation was experienced. Sonne (88) emphasized this in 1929 when he said, "We can absorb twice as much irradiation by visible as by invisible heat rays."[43]

One of the chief weaknesses of heat therapy has been the difficulty of measuring the amount of heat absorbed by the patient; another, of measuring or controlling the amount introduced. Thermometers were used in conjunction with light and sweat baths to record but not to control. Bierman (91) described a method of controlling the environmental temperature of the luminous heat cradle in the treatment of vascular disease in 1934.

INFRARED

At the beginning of the twentieth century, the work of Bernhard and Rollier focused attention on the use of ultraviolet rays[44] in the treatment of extrapulmonary tuberculosis. By 1910, electrically produced ultraviolet rays became commercially available, and their use increased rapidly. In 1919, when Huldschinsky proved the relationship between sunlight and rickets, the demand for apparatus increased, and the field of actinotherapy grew sufficiently large so that soon there were journals devoted to it in at least three languages. But when Hess and Steenbock showed in 1924 that the artificial light could be taken "by mouth",[45] there was a sudden diminution in the demand for ultraviolet ray equipment in the office and hospital. According to Beaumont (92), manufacturers of ultraviolet ray equipment looked for a way to continue in business. They had the stands, electrical parts, factories, and skilled workers. It had long been known that when iron is heated to a barely visible red, heat is emitted in the infrared range. It was a simple conversion from making clinical ultraviolet ray lamps to infrared burners, and soon manufacturers were promoting them as superior to luminous heat lamps. Many physicians accepted the suggestion. The infrared burner was something not commonly found in the home and, there-

---

[43] In 1820, Grotthus (89) announced a most important "law." He said, "Only the rays absorbed are effective in producing chemical changes." About a century later, Winkler (90) reminded us of its application to thermotherapy with, "There can only be an effect when the light is absorbed."

[44] A decade earlier, Palm had indicated the relationship between sunlight and rickets, and Finsen used filtered sunlight in the cure of skin tuberculosis.

[45] Irradiating the diet rather then the patient produced the vitamin D necessary to treat or prevent rickets.

fore, *more medical* than the luminous lamp which anyone could purchase at the corner shop. (It did not take too long for the infrared generator to find its way to the corner store.) Claims and counterclaims were made by the proponents of luminous and infrared sources of heat. The question of superiority remains inconclusive, and the choice of clinical apparatus has become a matter of personal conviction.

HIGH-FREQUENCY CURRENTS

The static spark was obvious to the first sandaled man who walked across a carpet in a cold, dry room. Yet it was not until 1600 that William Gilbert studied it and called it electricity. In 1672, Otto von Guericke developed a frictional machine to produce sparks, and in 1746, the Leyden jar was found to store it. It was with the frictional machine, the Leyden jar and a coil that Hertz produced high-frequency currents. In 1889, Joubert showed that, when the frequency of the current was increased beyond a certain level, the electricity would no longer cause contractions of the frog muscle. In the following year, d'Arsonval repeated Joubert's experiments and found that with frequencies above 5,000 Hz, contractions diminished and that at about 10,000 Hz they disappeared. He applied the high-frequency current to himself at an intensity of three amperes and felt only a slight sensation of warmth.[46]

By 1892, d'Arsonval was working with an apparatus capable of delivering a frequency of several hundred thousand oscillations per second (93). Until that time, electricity had been used to contract muscle or burn tissue. The idea of merely warming tissue with electricity had not been given serious consideration. Thus, d'Arsonval looked for physiologic rather than thermal effects. "I say to you that the immediate sensation produced by these currents is nil. Their passage is accompanied by physiological changes which I shall describe briefly. 1. If the current is sent through the hands covered with large electrodes, the skin becomes unfeeling for from a few minutes to a half hour." He found flushing of the skin and increased sweating and attributed these to a general vasodilating action rather than to a heat reaction. He wrote, "I believe that high frequency currents will render great service to therapeutics," but he was thinking of their effects on blood pressure and kidney output.

In 1897 (94), he added the method of autocondensation to the other manners of application previously suggested. Autocondensation, which remained popular for many years was, in effect, an unrecognized form of diathermy when first proposed. The d'Arsonval current was used by many

---

[46] A similar intensity of continuous current would have been destructive, possibly fatal. Tesla thought that the high-frequency current was not destructive because it spread over the body rather than through it. D'Arsonval said it was the speed of alternation that permitted safe penetration.

physicians in France, and their reports were as optimistic as any had been with previous forms of electricity when first introduced into therapy. Claims were made of its effectiveness in diabetes, gout, and obesity. In fact, the claims were so extravagant that many failed when they tried to repeat them. Thus, as early as 1904, Freund (95) wrote that clinical trials fell far short of what had been expected, "consequently in some quarters the whole method received unqualified condemnation." As so often happens during the early period of a new discovery in medicine, the press had its share of enthusiastic reporting. In 1899, newspapers published a sensational report that Tesla had cured pulmonary tuberculosis with the high-frequency current, whereas actually he had only suggested the possibility, based on his findings that high-frequency current which passed directly through bacilli killed them.

In that same year, von Zeyneck published a paper in which he briefly alluded to the "Durchwärmung" or heating through of his finger tips when an alternating current passed through them. He believed that the heat was produced by the passage of current through tissues just as it would when passed through any other resistance (96). According to Dark (97), he said, "The d'Arsonval oscillations may prove to be the only method to make it possible to produce an even warming of the body."[47] In September, 1907, at a medical meeting in Dresden, Franz Nagelschmidt showed the Durchwärmung possible with high-frequency currents, and at the Naturforscherkongress in Budapest in 1908, he demonstrated a more powerful machine which left no doubt about the deep heating effect of the high-frequency current. Soon after, he coined the word diathermy (98) to describe the procedure.

The first high-frequency machines were rather large and noisy. In 1900, Duddell placed a condenser across the spark gap, which changed the wave form to a more continuous type of oscillation with a musical note which came to be called the singing arc.[48] The high-frequency machine was not generally used until a few years after Nagelschmidt's demonstrations. Its chief use continued for some time to be the activation of a glass vacuum electrode with a violet brush discharge which reddened the skin and gave a

---

[47] Several writers, in an attempt to lessen the importance of later workers, have given undue prominence to this paper, for although von Zeyneck made this observation in 1899, nothing further on it came from his pen until February, 1908, when, in conjunction with von Berndt and von Preiss, he published a paper on the use of high-frequency current in joint disease. In that paper, heat penetration was mentioned as an essential part of the treatment (96), but this was two months after Nagelschmidt had given his impressive public demonstration.

[48] As the first quarter of the twentieth century was ending, a physical therapy clinic could be a rather noisy place with its static wheels spinning to make minor thunderclaps, and its spark gaps humming away. The original spark gap arced between carbons. In 1903, Poulsen improved the arc by substituting copper for the carbon (99). Later, tungsten was used. The spark gap continued to be used on diathermy machines long after electron tubes became commonplace, and even when short wave diathermy was introduced, one manufacturer insisted on using it for his earlier machines.

pleasant tingling sensation. By 1910, diathermy machines were beginning to make their appearance in supply houses.

At first, rigid metal electrodes were used, and sparking occurred where contact between them and the skin was poor. Even heavy wetting could not always prevent this. In 1911, Delherm and Laquerriere (100) introduced flexible electrodes made of fine wire screening, and soon after, Ronneaux molded tin electrodes from plaster casts of the parts to be treated. Another favorite early electrode was sponge-tin backed with chamois. The electrodes which finally came into greatest use because of their malleability were made from thin Crookes metal, which could be cut with an ordinary pair of shears into any size and shape desired.

Diathermy was soon used for many conditions. Morlet (101) treated all forms of arthritis with it in 1911. Bordier (102) used it in conjunction with X-rays to the spine for poliomyelitis, a treatment which was still considered so effective by some in Europe that in 1952 it was mentioned favorably in a paper given at the First International Congress of Physical Medicine. There was just about no organ, superficial or deep, which was not treated with diathermy. Special electrodes were devised for most of the body orifices, and it enjoyed much favor in gynecology in the treatment of pelvic disease. In 1923, Stewart wrote an entire book on the use of diathermy in pneumonia, which exhausted two editions. But it reached its greatest publicity when, in 1929, the King of England, who had worsened on ultraviolet ray treatment was improved by diathermy when given at the suggestion of Frank D. Howitt (103). At almost the same moment, across the Channel, shortwave diathermy was born.[49]

Shortwave Diathermy

Until 1929, the frequency of the current used in diathermy was approximately one megacycle.[50] In 1928, Esau, a physicist at Jena, constructed for

---

[49] Few in 1929 would have believed that the diathermy which had saved a royal life would be outlawed a quarter of a century later. In July, 1954, by international agreement, long wave diathermy could not be used unless so well shielded that its radiations did not escape from the building in which treatment was administered.

[50] When higher frequencies were introduced, the lower frequencies were called long wave or conventional diathermy. The higher frequencies were called ultrashort or shortwave diathermy. Later, when long wave diathermy was abandoned, the shortwave diathermy was called simply diathermy. An engineer named Lakhovsky (89) wrote that he began experiments in 1923 at the Salpêtrière Hospital in Paris with a *radio-cellulo oscillator* which he claimed produced waves of 2 to 10 meters. He did not state what power he used originally, and there was much secrecy about his work. In 1924, Gosset built a 2-meter apparatus with which he was able to destroy plant tumors caused by *Bacterium tumefaciens*. In the following year, Strebock produced a machine which would deliver a 38-meter wave and suggested its use in treatment. In 1926, Schereschewsky placed small animals in a condenser field of an apparatus which could deliver a 2 to 36 meter wave at 75 watts. He was able to kill flies with it, and the press responded by calling it the new "death ray" (60). In 1929, Saidman developed and used a 1.8-meter apparatus which could deliver 6 watts of energy.

Schliephake at Giessen a machine which delivered a 3-meter wave at 400 watts. Schliephake was the first to use shortwave diathermy clinically, and the first patient he treated with it was himself. In 1929, he began to work on the "selective" (that is, *specific* bactericidal) effects of shortwave, and in March "I cured myself of a furuncle on the nose in the shortest time" (105). He did much basic work on the heating[51] of animal tissues. Apparatus for the clinical application of the new form of diathermy was not placed on the market outside of Europe until 1934. In 1935, manufacturers, large and small, began to produce and sell increasing quantities of machines. At the beginning, as with the d'Arsonval current, there were many exorbitant claims. There was talk and even writing about cures of tuberculosis and cancer. The new current could light up neon tubes without contact. The glow tube was used to prove the presence of electromagnetic radiation. It was also used by a few to impress patients with the marvelous properties of short waves. In the early days, overenthusiasm and lack of precautions resulted in moderate and occasionally severe burns; but with improvement of circuit design and electrodes, burns became increasingly uncommon. The first electrodes recommended by Schliephake consisted of metal discs housed in thick glass "shoes" with considerable air spacing. In the United States, the first popular electrode was a sheet of flexible metal covered with thick layers of rubber. Although many found that the *pad* electrodes were efficient and more convenient to apply, they were condemned by organized medicine in favor of the cable electrode, first as cable wrapped around the part and later as coiled within an insulating drum.

Shortwave diathermy was promptly used in all those conditions in which long wave diathermy had been used. At first it enjoyed great use and acceptance in the treatment of paranasal sinusitis, a field well surveyed by Jouard (107). By 1937, when the first book on the subject was published in the United States (104), more than 750 articles and 18 books had been devoted to it. By 1954, when long wave diathermy had been outlawed, the shortwave apparatus had become a virtually foolproof device (as far as the infliction of burns) and was holding its own very well against the still newer form of diathermy—microwave.

Almost from its first use, there have been those who insisted that the important component of diathermy was the high-frequency energy, not the heat which resulted from its conversion. To some, this meant that a maximal effect was possible only if the heat was removed or kept to a minimum. One approach was to use doses too low to produce heat; another method was to "pulse" the energy in the belief that heat could be prevented from accumulating if repeated short bursts of energy were introduced. The therapeutic value of different forms of diathermy energy is difficult to differentiate.

---

[51] Weissenberg was the first proponent of the non thermal effects of shortwave diathermy— *low intensity treatment* (106).

Silverman (108), using bacterial infection in mice as a criterion for testing the effectiveness of interrupting the diathermy input, was unable to find any value in it.

Microwave Diathermy

Although currents of extremely high frequency were developed by the first investigators in the nineteenth century, it was not possible to produce them with sufficient power for therapeutic purposes until after the First World War.[52] Nevertheless, several investigators discussed the possibilities of and even used the radiations which came to be known as microwaves. In 1925, Stieböck (111) wrote, "Perhaps we could profit therapeutically by using wave lengths of 0.1 mm to 10 meters instead of those of 300." But this was only a speculation. Perhaps the first physician to use microwave diathermy was Denier (112).[53] He used an 80-cm wave combined with X-rays against tumor. Brunner-Ornstein and Randa (113) reported in 1937 on the use of a 60-cm-80-watt device designed by Randa, which they claimed made an X-ray refractory carcinoma disappear when treated with the combined energies of the two. It must be emphasized that the early workers were seeking not therapeutic heat but a "specific" or "selective" therapy. Microwave heating was introduced by Frank H. Krusen and his associates (114). In June, 1946, they began to heat living tissues with it and reported[54] on its thermal properties in May, 1947. They properly delayed clinical trials until the limitations of this potentially dangerous[55] radiation were estab-

---

[52] In 1920, A. W. Hull invented the magnetron which employed the principle of the magnetically controlled electron beam. In 1922, Nichols and Tear (109) experimented with radio waves of 0.2 mm and soon after Arakadieve (110), using ground metal in oil suspension claimed to reach a radiation of 8.1μ, (in the infrared range). In 1935, Heils described the principle of velocity modulation which led to the development of the klystron, another type of microwave tube. In 1940, R. T. Randall of England conceived the multicavity magnetron with which it became possible to develop microwaves of sufficient wattage to aim at a distant object and by means of reflection identify its position and general outline. The military possibilities of such a device (RADAR) were so great that the new tube was sent to the Massachusetts Institute of Technology for further development. The Institute needed a manufacturer to produce the multicavity magnetron and called on nearby Raytheon Manufacturing Company. The manufacturer saw the possibilities of the new high-frequency source in clinical medicine, and as the war ended began to produce an apparatus which delivered a 2450-megacycle current at 125 watts. Since the frequency of such a device depends upon the internal structure of the magnetron, and since tooling for different sized magnetrons is expensive, tube manufacturers have not produced equipment which will permit clinical research on other microwave frequencies.

[53] André Denier of La Tour-du-Pin, France, was one of the first clinicians anywhere (if not the first) to use microwave diathermy, ultrasound in diagnosis and treatment, and infrasound therapy.

[54] Mayo Clinic Proceedings, 22:209.

[55] Microwaves introduced into tissues at the same wattage as short waves can cause severe burns rapidly. Microwaves introduced through the cornea can produce opacities in it.

lished in animals. Later that year, microwave diathermy was "accepted",[56] and in the following months,[57] Osborne and Frederick reported on how the radiation raised temperatures in normal human subjects.

PHYSICALLY INDUCED FEVER THERAPY

Elevation of the body temperature for therapeutic purposes was an ancient idea. The presence of fever remained a clinical guess until the clinical thermometer was popularized by Wunderlich (115) in 1868. Some years later, Phillips (116) showed that fever could be induced physically with a hot bath. The body temperature was raised slightly, but not to induce fever, by the light baths of Kellogg. D'Arsonval (94) showed in 1893 that the body temperature of an animal could be elevated by placing it in a solenoid through which a high-frequency current was passing. In 1912, Rechou (111) raised the body temperature with diathermy. In 1918, Cumberbatch (117) tried to induce generalized fever with diathermy but was able to raise the temperature only one degree. In 1923, Domaggio suggested generalized diathermy for general paralysis which had been treated for some years with malaria or foreign-protein-induced fever. Clarence Neymann wanted to treat syphilis with physically induced fever as early as 1925 (118). Schamberg (119) advocated the use of physically induced fever for syphilis in 1927. Two years later, Kahler and Knollmayer (120) gave short courses of fever in a light cabinet, and Nagelschmidt (121) described a powerful autocondensation diathermy with which "we can produce fever artificially up to any desired degree." It was during that year that the General Electric Company's Orville Melland (110) noted that certain employees working near powerful shortwave generators felt feverish. The thought occurred to him that this energy might be used to raise the temperature in the treatment of syphilis. A 30-meter apparatus was given to the Western State Hospital at Bolivar, Tennessee, where J. Cash King and E. W. Cocke (122)[58] were the first to report on artificial fever produced by very-high-frequency currents.

Although the first reason for using artificial fever therapy was to treat syphilis, its greatest use was against gonorrhea in which it continued to be the only successful treatment until the advent of penicillin made the use of fever therapy in both venereal diseases obsolete by the end of World War II. Long before it was known that any disease was caused by a microorganism, Serré of Uzès (50) in 1832 proposed that gonorrhea be treated with currents of very warm water. Soon after the gonococcus had been identified

---

[56] The Council on Physical Medicine of the American Medical Association for more than a quarter of a century "accepted" new therapeutic devices if they met certain standards of performance and were advertised ethically.

[57] OSBORNE, S. L. AND FREDERICK, J. N. Microwave radiation. *J.A.M.A. 137:* 1036, 1948.

[58] In a personal communication, Dr. Cocke noted that he had began experimenting on animals with physically induced fever of high frequency origin before 1926.

by Neisser as the cause of gonorrhea, many bacteriologists determined that the gonococcus was thermosensitive.

In 1913, Santos (123) developed urethral electrodes with a central thermometer to record the heat produced by urethral diathermy. In the following year, Bromberg (124), in the belief that gonococci die when exposed to a temperature of 49.5°C for five minutes, raised the temperature of the urethra to 50°C for 15 minutes with diathermy through a urethral sound. He determined that the tissue could withstand that amount of heat for that time. He probably killed most gonococci near the sound but could not reach the deeper organisms. In 1917, Risselada (125) accepted the lethal temperature for gonococci as 42°C and placed patients in tubs of hot water until their body temperatures just exceeded that level. He had the idea, which was later crowned with success, but the entire duration of his treatment was only 40 minutes. Carpenter (126) repeated earlier experiments on the lethal temperature for spirochetes and gonococci, and they reopened the attack on venereal diseases with artifically induced fever therapy. Bierman and Horowitz (127) ensured the local rise of temperature by adding local diathermy to urethra and pelvis during generalized fever therapy. Kendall *et al.* (128) raised the cure rate to well over 90 percent by combining fever with high oral doses of sulfone drugs, with varying degrees of success claimed in arthritis, chorea, Malta fever, multiple sclerosis, and subacute bacterial endocarditis.

ULTRASOUND

Toward the end of the eighteenth century, Spallanzani (129) studied the flight of bats and noted that in spite of partial blindness they did not fly into obstacles unless their hearing was impaired. He recognized that there was a "sound" inaudible to the human ear.[59] There are many ways of producing ultrasound, but the one best suited to medical use is the reverse piezoelectric effect. The piezoelectric effect was discovered by Pierre Curie,[60] who found that a vibrating quartz crystal produced a high-frequency electric current as it was compressed and relaxed by the vibrations. In 1912, a British engineer named Richardson suggested that another "Titanic" disaster might be averted if icebergs could be detected by the echo from pulsed

---

[59] Sound is a longitudinal vibration audible to the human ear at cyclic frequencies between about 16 and 18,000 per second. Frequencies above the audible are called ultrasonic. Supersonic refers to a speed of travel greater than the speed of sound propagation through the air. Many investigators believe that ultrasound has only one effect on living tissues—that of heat. These are probably outnumbered by those who feel that the effects of ultrasound in the test tube and the human cannot all be explained as reactions to heat alone.

[60] In 1881, Lippmann reversed Curie's findings. He placed a thin layer of quartz crystal between two layers of steel and noted oscillations in the quartz when high-frequency current was applied to the steel plates. (Denier, A. *Les Ultra-Sons Appliqués à la Médecine*, Paris, 1951).

waves emitted from the approaching ship. When war broke out, an Allied Submarine Detection Investigation Committee (ASDIC)[61] was set up and in 1915, Langevin of France succeeded in producing the first piezoelectric generator for the practical use of ultrasonic waves. It was soon noted that ultrasound radiations were injurious to marine life. In 1929, Harvey and Loomis (130) showed that ultrasound at 400 kc per second was able to destroy luminous bacteria.

The first suggestion for ultrasonotherapy was made by Voss (131) in 1933 when he proposed to reduce deafness with it. Dognon and Biancani (132) gave a real stimulus to medical ultrasound when they published collected reports from the literature on the effects of ultrasound energy on tissues in 1937. Pohlman (133) and his associates at the Martin-Luther-Krankenhaus in Berlin gave the first treatment with ultrasound, as we now know it, to a woman with sciatica on June 22, 1938, after having tried it on themselves first. They used an 800 kc generator and employed mineral oil as the coupling medium between the massage head and the skin. Their report was published on the eve of World War II. High priorities on electronic equipment for war interrupted the progress in ultrasound with a few exceptions. Dussik (134) in Austria used it as a diagnostic agent during the war, and in France, Denier (135) and Dognon used it for treatment. In 1942, Pagniez (136) described the work of Gohr and Wedekind completed just prior to the war. He explained the action of ultrasound as one of micromassage. Denier used an instrument from 1941 to 1946 which delivered a 961 kc wave at 3 watts. In 65 patients, he found best results with arthritis, asthma, scleroderma, and ankylosis.

In the United States, Lynn and Putnam[62] focused ultrasound on exposed animal brain tissue and showed they could control the degree of destruction caused by it, suggesting its neurosurgical possibilities. When war ended, interest was revived in Western Europe. First to write about it was Denier. He was soon followed by Anstett (137) who, in 1948, reported good results in most of the 60 asthmatics he treated with it. In 1949, many workers had resumed or begun work in the field so that by the time of the Erlangen Conference, held on the subject in that year, 75 papers were presented on ultrasound. One of the earliest of these was again that of Pohlman (138) who reported on the value of ultrasound in neuritis, myalgia, and arthritis.[63] One of the first clinicians to give it a critical appraisal in the United States was Bierman (139), who reported good results after its use in fibrous tissue lesions.

---

[61] The information of ASDIC was generously supplied by Dr. Reginald W. Windle of Hove, England.

[62] LYNN, J. G. AND PUTNAM, T. J. Histology of lesions produced by focused ultrasound in brain tissue. *Am. J. Pathol., 20:* 637, 1944.

[63] More than 1,200 articles and books on ultrasound are listed under the section *Bibliography* by J. M. van Went in her book *Ultrasonic and Ultrashort Waves in Medicine*, New York, 1954.

The idea has occurred to several physicians to shatter abnormal mineral deposits in the human body with ultrasound. Attempts to fragment gallstones and kidney stones in vitro have been successful. Lane[64] was able to pulverize the calcific deposits of coronary arteries in postmortem specimens by introducing ultrasound into the ostium through a 1-mm waveguide.

The ideal coupling agent for ultrasound therapy is one which has an acoustic impedance approximately the geometric mean of the sound crystal and the patient. Silverman (108) found that since the acoustic impedance of water approximates that of muscle, it is best for clinical use.

MASERS AND LASERS

Fluorescence has been known for a long time; it occurs in nature. All that is required is a fluorescent mineral and a way to exclude visible light which masks the phenomenon. Fluorescence is a re-radiation of electromagnetic waves from shorter to higher wavelengths. The reflection radiates visible wavelengths in random phase and direction.

In 1951, Townes[65] advanced the idea that a phenomenon similar to fluorescence might be available with much higher (microwave) frequencies if atoms or molecules could be used as resonators. By taking the first letters of the words *microwave amplification* by the *stimulated emission* of *radiation*, he coined the word maser to describe the output. The principle was first put into operation by passing an ammonia gas beam through a microwave generator. In 1958, solids were employed and *light* rather than microwaves was amplified, giving rise to another acronym, the laser. Whereas fluorescence is a spontaneous emission, a laser is a "stimulated" emission of light in the same phase and direction. By bouncing the radiation back and forth between two parallel coaxial mirrors, there results a standing wave of "coherent" light. When a gas resonates, the resultant light is monochromatic; regardless of the medium, the emission is intense.

The first application of this extremely high energy light to medical practice was a ruby crystal synthesized from aluminum oxide and a trace of chromium oxide. When the atoms of such a crystal are "pumped" by a brilliant flash from a xenon lamp, a red laser at 6943 Å is emitted. The absorption of colored light depends upon the surface radiated; white reflects the incident beam and black absorbs most of it. Since there is much pigment in the human retina, a significant amount of light reaching it is absorbed. Inasmuch as the lens of the eye focuses light on the retina, a laser beam sent through the lens finds its target easily. The most widely used treatment for detached retina has been a coagulation of the detached tissue to "weld" it back in place. The laser affords the remarkable opportunity of selectively overheating a tiny area of the retina without compromising any other

[64] LANE, W. Z. Ultrasonic coronary endarterectomy. *Biomed. Instrument. 1:* 8, 1964.

[65] DACEY, G. C. Optical masters in science and technology. *Science, 135:* 71, 1962.

tissues. An energy of 10^{10} watts per square cm is the power density which can be transmitted for a period of as little as a millisecond.

The earliest clinical investigations of maser and lasers were in the field of *heat destruction*—"a microsurgical instrument."[66] The possibilities of additional uses in medicine and biology are as broad as the spectrum of masers and lasers—all the way from microwaves to infrared radiation.

Cold

Artificially made ice was virtually unknown before 1750, but the ancients used and enjoyed snow and natural ice. According to Monardes (140), a physician of Seville who introduced balsam of Peru and other herbs from the New World into the Old, Pliny remarked that Nero cooled drinking water and wine with snow stored in caves as did the later Roman Emperors Heliogabalus and Alexander. However, ice and snow were used long before the Roman Empire. According to Mac-Auliffe (10), Hippocrates advised cold drinks to combat fever, as did his successors Galen, Paul of Aegina, Aretacus, Celsus, Rhazes, and Avicenna. Mac-Auliffe calls attention to a sentence in the Epistles of Seneca which relates that heartburn was treated by eating snow. Galen (141), in the seventh, eighth, and ninth books of his *Methoda Medendi*, recommended cold spring water and snowcooled water for stomach and other diseases. He also noted that fish were prevented from decomposing by packing in snow.

Caelius Aurelianus (49) wrote of Themison's use of chilling plasters and cold drinks to counteract satyriasis, the origin of which was thought to be the ingestion of the satyrion, an orchid. Hemoptysis was treated by several ancient practitioners, notably Alexander of Tralles (142) by the application of cold compresses to the chest.

All kinds of lesions accompanied by burning sensations were treated with their opposite—cold. These included abscess, erysipelas, and phlebitis. Deeper inflammations such as pneumonia and meningitis were also treated with cold (13). According to Rutty (143), Oribasius bathed malignant ulcers in very cold water. Ice fragments were used for hemostasis and analgesia.

A patient with a painful sore throat was prescribed snow, to chew, by Amatus Lusitanus (140), and Savonarola cured the Duke of Ferrara of constipation by having him walk on a cold, wet, marble floor (143). In 1649, Herman van der Heyden (10) recommended immersion of the feet and legs in very cold water for arthritis, and 20 years later, Bartholin wrote that he had seen this treatment applied in Spain. Floyer (144) recommended cold baths for a variety of conditions.

In 1771, Samoilowitz (145), physician to the Czar of Russia, surrounded seriously febrile patients with snow and massaged all parts of their bodies

---

[66] GOLDMAN, L. GLENEY, D. J., FREEMOND, A. AND HORNBY, P. The biomedical aspects of lasers. *J.A.M.A., 188:* 230, 1964.

with ice, but it was probably the reports of the Curries (6,147), which told of the good results of cold baths in fever, that renewed interest in cold therapy at the turn of the eighteenth century. Many books, articles, and doctoral theses began to appear on the subject. Roubaud (148) reported on six cases of penetrating chest wounds which responded favorably to internal, local and environmental cold. Barrabé (149) wrote not only about the use of cold in disease but in hygiene. He spoke of the pleasure and comfort of iced drinks on hot summer days. Barrabé was especially impressed by the value of cold applications in inflammations of the central nervous system. He applied ice to the head routinely in patients suffering from inflammations of the head or meninges. He decried the polypharmaceutical approach to the treatment of rheumatism and recommended the use of cold to swollen joints. In 1821, Harder (150) claimed good results in virtually hopeless cases of coma with refrigeration applied to the limbs. In 1822, Frohlich (151) wrote on the reduction of fever with cold baths. He gave a detailed dosage table: for a fever of 110°F, a bath of 35°F; for 106°F, a bath at 40°F. The cold bath for typhoid fever received its greatest impetus from Ernst Brand, particularly in the latter half of the century.

Scudamore (152) packed gouty joints in ice fragments in 1823, and a year later, Tanchou (153) wrote a book on the therapeutic use of cold. Of considerable interest was the appearance in 1832 of the observations of Edwards (154) that if one hand was plunged into cold water for any length of time, the temperature of the opposite hand would also fall.

Several writers recommended the application of ice chips or very cold compresses to the skin for inflammation of wounds, and this method became quite popular about 1835 (13).

Evaporative cooling methods were introduced in 1850 by Vollemier, who cooled the skin of the forehead by evaporating ether from it. Follin tried local sprays of carbon dioxide gas for three minutes, and James Arnott of Brighton used ice as a local anesthetic[67] before surgery (13). Richard reduced the temperature of cold application further by mixing ammonium salts with the ice before applying it to the skin.

In 1850, Ribes (13) suggested ice packs to the abdomen for intestinal hemorrhage and toward the end of the century, abdominal ice packs were widely used for the treatment of appendicitis. Leduc (13) suggested the use of ice packs to the precordial region to relieve cardiac pain.

Although ice had been made artificially in very small quantities by the ancients with evaporative cooling and the aid of saltpeter, it was William Cullen of Scotland (155) who first made it mechanically in 1755 by placing a container of water over evaporating nitrous ether. The first practical

---

[67] Marco Severino, a Neapolitan surgeon who had written a book on the cautery, is credited by Fielding Garrison (History of Medicine, Philadelphia, 1929) with employing freezing mixtures in surgical anesthesia in 1646.

machine which could produce ice in commercial quantities at prices competitive with transported natural ice was invented by a Florida physician, John Gorrie (155), who obtained an English patent in 1850. He had invented apparatus for making ice and for air-conditioning rooms to make his malarial patients more comfortable. He spent his life and fortune trying to mass-produce ice. His failure to achieve this goal resulted in a progressively despondent solitude which ended in his death in 1855. It was not until about 1885 that artificial ice became commercially available in the United States.

REFERENCES

1. SIGERIST, H. E. *A History of Medicine*. New York, 1951.
2. FRAZER, J. G. *The Golden Bough*. New York, 1935.
3. LAFORGUE SAINTE ROSE, J. *Considerations sur les Propriétés Physiques du Calorique et sur les Arantages de son Application Comme Moyen Thérapeutique*. Paris, 1819.
4. BREASTED, J. H. *The Edwin Smith Surgical Papyrus*. Chicago, 1930.
5. WISE, T. A. *Review of the History of Medicine*. London, 1867.
6. JEE, B. S. *A Short History of Aryan Medical Sciences*. London, 1896.
7. FIENUS, T. *De Cauteriis Libri Quinqui*. Louvain, 1598.
8. ALLEN, C. W. *Radiotherapy and Phototherapy*. London, 1905.
9. BECQUEREL, E. *La Lumière, Ses Causes et Ses Effects*. Paris, 1867.
10. MAC-AULIFFE, L. *La Thérapeutique Physique d'Autrefois*. Paris, 1904.
11. LECLERC, L. *Histoire de la Médecine Arabe*. Paris. 1876.
12. CHRESTIEN, A. T. *Des Cautères et de Leur Valeur en Thérapeutique*. Montpellier, 1856.
13. GRASSET, H. *La Médecine Naturiste à Travers les Siècles*. Paris, 1911.
14. SEVERIN, M. A. *De la Médecine Efficace*. Geneva. 1668.
15. FAURE, J. F. Mémoire sur l'usage de la chaleur dans le traitement des ulcères. *Mem. Acad. Roy. Chirurg.*, 5: 821, 1774.
16. BERTRAND, M. *Essai Touchant l'Influence de la Lumière sur les Etres Organisés*. Paris, 1799.
17. VOLTA, A. On the electricity excited by the mere contact of conducting substances. *Philos. Trans.*, 1800.
18. AMUSSAT, A. *Mémoires sur la Galvanocaustique Thermique*. Paris, 1876.
19. RICHET, A. *De l'Emploi du Froid et de la Chaleur*. Paris, 1847.
20. BOREL, A. *L'Electrologie*. Paris, 1886.
21. MARSHALL, J. On the employment of the heat of electricity in practical surgery. *Med. Chir. Trans.*, *34:* 221, 1851.
22. SÉDILLOT, C. *Traité de Médecine Opératoire*. Paris, 1853.
23. BOECKEL, G. *Galvanocaustique Termique*. Paris, 1873.
24. FABRE-PALAPRAT, B. R. *Du Galvanisme Appliqué à la Médecine*. Paris, 1828.
25. MIDDLEDORPT, A. T. *Die Galvonokaustik, ein Beitrag zur operativen Medizin*. Breslau, 1854.
26. DUJARDIN-BEAUMETZ, G. *Dictionnaire de Thérapeutique*. Paris, 1885.
27. PICHARD, F. L. *Des Aubus de la Cautérisation*. Paris, 1846.
28. SKENE, V. J. *Electrohemostasis in Surgery*. London, 1901.
29. JACOBAEUS, H. C. The cauterization of adhesions in artificial pneumothorax. *Arch. Radio. Electro.*, 28: 96, 1913.
30. WILLIAMS, C. *High Frequency Currents in the Treatment of Some Diseases*. London, 1903.
31. BREASTED, J. H. *The Edwin Smith Surgical Papyrus*, Chicago, 1930.
32. HERTZ, H. *Electric Waves*. London, 1900.

33. BORDIER, H. Tesla or d'Arsonval? *Arch. Phys. Ther., 19:* 108, 1937.
34. OUDIN, M. Nouveau mode de transformation des courants de haute fréquence. *J. Soc. Franc. Electrothér*, 1893.
35. PARSON, I. The healing of rodent ulcer by electricity. *Trans. Gyn. Soc. Lond.*, 1888.
36. ZIMMERN, A. *La Fulguration*. Paris, 1909.
37. COOK, F. R. Cited in Kelly and Ward (39).
38. DOYEN, R. *Technique de l'Electrocoagulation dans le Traitment des Cancers*. Paris, 1917.
39. KELLY, H. A., AND WARD, G. E. *Electrosurgery*. Philadelphia, 1932.
40. CZERNY, V. Ueber Operationen mit dem elektrischen Lichtbogen. *Deut. Med. Wchnschr., 36:* 489, 1910.
41. EITNER, E. Ueber eine neue Art von Kaustik. *Wien Klin. Wchnschr., 23:* 168, 1910.
42. CLARK, W. L. Oscillatory desiccation in accessible new growths. *J.A.M.A., 55:* 1224, 1910.
43. BEER, E. Removal of neoplasma of the urinary bladder. *J.A.M.A., 54:* 1768, 1910.
44. FRISCHER, J. Prostatic hypertrophy and transurethral surgery. *Arch. Phys. Ther., 12:* 217, 1930.
45. COLLINGS, C. W. Transurethral electrosurgery in prostatic obstruction. *Arch. Phys. Ther., 14:* 581, 1933.
46. NOVAK, F. J. The electrocoagulation method of treating diseased tonsils. *J.A.M.A., 80:* 1842, 1923.
47. BIERMAN, W. Surgical diathermy in the treatment of hemorrhoids. *Brit. J. Radio.*, 1926.
48. CUSHING, H. Meningiomas arising from the olfactory groove and their removal with the aid of electrosurgery. *Lancet, 1:* 1329, 1927.
49. AURELIANUS, C. *On Acute and Chronic Disease*. Translation by I. E. Drabkin, Chicago, 1950.
50. SCOUTTETEN, H. *De l'Eau ou de l'Hydrothérapie*. Paris, 1843.
51. PARÉ, A. *Oeuvres Complètes*. Paris, 1841.
52. PARÉ, A. *The Works of That Famous Chirurgeon*. London, 1678.
53. FALLOPIO, G. *Libelli Duo, Alter Ulceribus*. Venice, 1563.
54. COCHRANE, B. *An Improvement in the Mode of Administering the Vapour Bath*. London, 1809.
55. LA BEAUME, M. *Remarks on the Medical Efficacy of Electricity*. London, 1820.
56. CHORTET, J. F. *Traité sur la Propriété Fortifiante de la Chaleur et sur la Vertu Affaiblissante du Froid*. Luxembourg, 1802.
57. FREEMAN, H. W. *The Thermal Baths of Bath*. London, 1888.
58. CLARIDGE, R. T. *Hydropathy*. London, 1862.
59. VON LEYDEN, E., AND GOLDSCHEIDER, A. Ueber kineto-therapeutische Bäder. *Zschr. Diät. Physik. Ther., 1:* 112, 1898.
60. PREISS, O. Massagebäder. *Zschr. Ärztl. Electrother.*, 1901.
61. POPE, C. The physiological action and therapeutic value of general and local whirlpool baths. *Arch. Phys. Ther., 10:* 498, 1929.
62. BOYAN, C. P. *Ann. Surg., 160:* 5, 1964.
63. DE SANDFORT, B. La kerithérapie; nouvelle balnéation thermo-cireuse. *J. Méd. Int., 18:* 211, 1913.
64. BOUET-HENRY, A. Presse méd., 1914, in de Sandfort, B. Keritherapy: A new method of thermal treatment by means of paraffin. *Med. Press., 100:* 556, 1915.
65. HUMPHRIS, F. S. Melted paraffin bath. *Brit. Med. J., 2:* 397, 1920.
66. PORTMANN, U. V. *Phys. Ther., 44:* 33, 1926.
67. ORIBASIUS, *Oeuvres*. Paris, 1951.
68. MATTIOLE, P. A. *Les Commentaires de Padaicus Dioscorides*. Lyon, 1680.
69. GRAWITZ, E. Uber die Verwendung des heissen Sandes zu therapeutischen Zwecken. *Zschr. Diät. Physik. Ther., 1:* 45, 1898.

70. STOIANOFF, B. La fangotherapie. *Ann. Méd. Phys., 31:* 217, 1937.

71. SALAGHI, S. Ueber die neuen Methoden für die örtliche Anwendung der Wärme mit besonderer Berücksichtigung eines elektrischen Thermophors. *Zschr. Physik. diat. Ther., 3:* 371, 1900.

72. DE CHAULIAC, G. *La Grande Chirurgie (1363).* Paris, 1890.

73. BOISSIER DE SAUVAGES, F. *Comment l'Air Agit sur le Corps Humain.* Bordeaux, 1753.

74. DE BOISSIEU, B. C. *Mémoire sur les Méthodes Rafraîchissantes et Echauffantes.* Dijon, 1772.

75. GUYOT, J. *Traité de l'Incubation et son Influence Thérapeutique.* Paris, 1840.

76. BAUDOT, E. *Examen Critique d'Incubation Appliquée à la Thérapeutique.* Paris, 1858.

77. BIER, A. *Textbook of Hyperemia.* London, 1909.

78. SARJEANT, J. F. Cases treated with the Tallerman-Sheffield dry air bath. *Lancet, 1:* 882, 1895.

79. SKINNER, C. E. *Therapeutics of Dry Hot Air.* New York, 1903.

80. THOMSON, T. *An Outline of the Science of Heat and Electricity.* London, 1840.

81. HERSCHEL, W. *Investigation of the Powers of Prismatic Colors to Heat and Illuminate Objects.* London, 1800.

82. LE BRETON, *Histoire et Applications de l'Electricité.* Paris, 1884.

83. BIGELOW, H. R. *An International Symposium Electrotherapeutics.* London, 1902.

84. KELLOGG, J. H. *Light Therapeutics.* Battle Creek, 1910.

85. FOVEAU DE COURMELLES, J. *Année Electrique.* Paris, 1902.

86. MARIE, T. Techniques des applications médicales de la lumière électrique. *Arch. Electrol. Méd., 9:* 717, 1901.

87. HUMPHRIS, F. H. Incandescent light as a therapeutic agent. *Arch. Roentgen Rays, 16:* 176. 1911.

88. SONNE, C. Investigations on the action of luminous rays and their mode of action. *Arch. Phys. Ther., 10:* 93, 1929.

89. HUMPHRIS, F.s. H. *Artificial Sunlight and its Therapeutic Uses.* London, 1924.

90. WINKLER, F. Etudes sur la pénétration de la lumière dans la peau. *Ann. Electrobiol., 11:* 593, 1908.

91. BIERMAN, W. Thermostatically controlled heating hood in vascular diseases of the lower extremities. *Arch. Phys. Ther., 15:* 530, 1934.

92. BEUMONT, W. Personal communication.

93. D'ARSONVAL, A. Sur les effects physiologiques de l'état variable et des courants alternatifs. *Bull. Soc. Internat. Electro.,* April, 1892.

94. D'ARSONVAL, A. Action physiologique des courants alternatifs à grande fréquence. *Arch. Electrol. Med., 6:* 133, 1897.

95. FREUND, J. *Elements of General Radiotherapy.* New York, 1904.

96. CUMBERBATCH, E. P. *Essentials of Medical Electicity.* London, 1908.

97. DARK, E. P. *Diathermy in General Practice.* Sydney, 1929.

98. NAGELSCHMIDT, F. *Lehrbuch der Diathermie.* Berlin, 1913.

99. BORDIER, H. *Diathermie et Diathermothérapie.* Paris, 1922.

100. ALBERT-WEIL. Des électrodes pour la diathermie. *J. Physiothér., 9:* 299, 1911.

101. MORLET, F. Traitement des arthrites par la diathermie. *Ann. Electrobiol., 14:* 344, 1911.

102. BORDIER, H. *Arch. Electrol. Med.,* 1912.

103. Diathermy and the king. *Brit. J. Actinother. 4:* 30, 1929.

104. DE CHOKOLNY, T. *Short Wave Diathermy.* New York, 1937.

105. SCHLIEPHAKE, E. *Les Ondes Courtes en Biologie.* Paris, 1938.

106. WEISSENBERG, E. H., AND HOLZER, W. *Foundation of Short Wave Therapy.* London, 1935.

107. JOUARD, F. Rationale of short wave diathermy in acute sinusitis. *Arch. Phys. Ther., 20:* 338, 1939.

108. SILVERMAN, D. R. A comparison of the effects of continuous and pulsed short wave diathermy: Resistance to bacterial infection in mice. *Arch. Phys. Med., 45:* 491, 1964.
109. HENRARD, E. H. *Les Ondes Hertziennes Courtes et Leurs Applications en Médecine.* Bruxelles, 1934.
110. SAIDMAN, J., AND MEYER, J. *Les Ondes Courtes en Thérapeutique.* Paris, 1936.
111. SAIDMAN, J., AND CAHEN, R. *Les Ondes Hertziennes Courtes en Thérapeutique.* Paris, 1931.
112. DENIER, A. Les ondes hertziennes ultracourtes de 80 cm. *J. Radiol. Electrol., 20:* 193, 1936.
113. BRUNNER-ORNSTEIN, M., AND RANDA, K. Versuche mit einem Magnetron-Ultrakurzwellengenerator für medizinische Zwecke. *Strahlenther., 59:* 267, 1937.
114. KAUSEN, F. H. Medical applications of microwave diathermy. *Proc. Roy. Soc. Med., 43:* 641, 1950.
115. WUNDERLICH, K. *Das Verhalten der Eigenwärme in Krankheiten.* Leipzig. 1808.
116. PHILLIPS, W. H. Hydrotherapy. *Columbus Med. J., 2:* 389, 1883.
117. CUMBERBATCH, E. P. Elevation of body temperature by the diathermy current. *Arch. Radio. Electrol., 24:* 173, 1918.
118. NEYMANN, C. The present status of electropyrexia. *Arch. Phys. Ther., 13:* 749, 1932.
119. SCHAMBERG, J. F., AND TSEUG, H. W. Experiments on therapeutic value of hot baths. *Amer. J. Syph., 11:* 337, 1927.
120. KAHLER, H., AND KNOLLMAYER, F. Ueber die Anwendung von künstlicher Hyperthermie als Ersatzmittel der experimentellen Fiebertherapie. *Wein. Klin. Wchnschr., 42:* 1342, 1929.
121. NAGELSCHMIDT, F. A new method of applying heat diathermy. Proc. Second Internat. Cong. Light Heat, London, 1928.
122. KING, J. C., AND COCKE, E. W. Therapeutic fever produced by diathermy. *South Med. J., 23:* 222, 1930.
123. SANTOS, C. Sur le traitement de la blénorrhagie par la diathermie. *Arch. Electrol. Méd., 22:* 241, 1913.
124. BROMBERG, H. *Deut. Med. Wehnschr., 4:* 79, 1914.
125. RISSELADA, A. M. Die Fieberbehandlung der Gonorrhöe beim Kinde. *Zzchr. Physik. Diät. Ther., 21:* 65, 1917.
126. CARPENTER, C. M. Artificial fever. *Phys. Therap., 48:* 264, 1930.
127. BIERMAN, W., AND HOROWITZ, E. A. A new vaginal diathermy electrode. *Arch. Phys. Ther., 17:* 15, 1936.
128. KENDELL, H. W., ROSE, D. L., AND SIMPSON, W. M. Artificial fever versus combined fever-chemotherapy in gonococcal infections. *Arch. Phys. Ther., 22:* 103, 1941.
129. LIGHT, S. Ultrasound and medicine. *N.Y. Med., 6:* 28, 1950.
130. HARVEY, E. N., AND LOOMIS, A. L. The destruction of luminour bacteria by high frequency sound waves. *J. Bacteriol., 17:* 373, 1929.
131. VOSS, O. *Arch. Ohr. Nas. Kehl., 135:* 258, 1933.
132. DOGNON, A., AND BIANCANI, E. H. *Les Ultrasons en Biologie.* Paris, 1937.
133. POHLMAN, R., RICHTER, R., AND PAROW, E. Über die Ausbreitung and Absorption des Ultraschalls im menschlichen Gewebe und seine therapeutische Wirkung an Ischias und Plexusneuralgie. *Deut. Med. Wchnschr., 65:* 251, 1939.
134. DUSSIK, K. T. Ueber die Möglichkeit hochfrequente mechanische Schwingungen als diagnostische Hilfsmittel zu verwenden. *Zschr. Neurol., 174:* 153, 1942.
135. DENEIR, A. Les ultrasons. *Presse Méd., 54:* 307, 1946.
136. PAGNIEZ, P. Les ultrasons. *Presse Méd., 50:* 741, 1942.
137. ANSTETT, P. Soizante cas d'asthme traites par less ultrasons. *Presse Méd., 56:* 100, 1948.
138. POHLMAN, R. Die Ultraschalltherapie. Stuttgart. 1951.
139. BIERMAN, W. Ultrasound in the treatment of scars. *Arch Phys. Med., 35:* 209, 1954.

140. MONARDES, N. *Joyful Newes Out of the Newe Founde World.* Translated by J. Frampton in 1575, London, 1925.
141. GALEN, C. *Epitome.* Basle, 1571.
142. WALSH, J. J. *Medieval Medicine.* London, 1921.
143. RUTTY, J. A. *A Methodical Synposis of Mineral Waters.* London, 1757.
144. FLOYER, J. *The History of Cold Bathing.* London, 1702.
145. BELL, J. *A Treatise on Baths.* Philadelphia, 1850.
146. CURRIE, J. *Medical Reports, on the Effects of Water, Cold and Warm.* Liverpool, 1797.
147. CURRIE, W. A. *Observations on the Causes and Cure of Remitting or Bilious Fevers.* Philadelphia, 1798.
148. ROUBAUD, P. D. *Sur l'Utilité de l'Application du Froid dans le Traitement des Plaies Pénétrantes de la Poitrine.* Paris, 1808.
149. BARABÉ, A. J. M. Sur l'Usage Médical de la Glace. Thèse. Paris, 1817.
150. HARDER, M. *Abhandlung aus dem Gebiete der Heilkunde.* Petersburg, 1821.
151. FLEURY, L. *Traité Thérapeutique et Clinique d'Hydrothérapie.* Paris, 1866.
152. SCUDAMORE, C. *A Treatise on the Nature and Cure of Gout.* London, 1757.
153. TANCHOU, A. *Du Froid et de Son Application dans les Maladies.* Paris, 1824.
154. EDWARDS, W. F. *On the Influence of Physical Agents on Life.* London, 1832.
155. HENDERSON, A. R. JOHN GORRIE, M. D. *J.A.M.A., 185:* 330, 1963.

2

Thermometry

THOMAS C. CETAS[1]

Introduction

HISTORICAL DEVELOPMENT

Thermometry began with the development of the air thermometer in the late sixteenth or early seventeenth century by Santorio Santorre[2], a physician trained at Padua and later a contemporary of Galileo at Venice and Padua. Santorio attached a scale to the measurement of heat and cold, and went on to record seasonal changes as well as body temperatures obtained by putting the patient's mouth or hand around the air bulb of the thermometer. An early observation was that body temperature was quite stable, although it tended to rise more quickly as well as higher if the patient was not feeling well. This was because peripheral circulation is greater in febrile patients.

Later in the seventeenth century, Ferdinand II, the Grand Duke of Tuscany who established the Accademia del Cimento, constructed a sealed thermometer in which the dilatation of spirits of wine became the thermometric fluid. Thus temperature readings were no longer sensitive to barometric fluctuations. Because of the excellence of the glass-blower Mariani,

[1] Support for much of this effort and the work in the author's laboratory has come from grant CA17343. I am indebted to several persons for assistance. In particular, Mr. Bruce Herman of the Ultrasonics Branch of the Bureau of Radiological Health and Dr. Padmaker Lele of MIT assisted on the section on thermometry in ultrasonic fields. Dr. R. P. Hudson, Deputy Director, Center for Absolute Quantities, NBS, critically reviewed the manuscript. Dr. R. Nasoni provided insight on ultrasonic CT thermometry. Miss Laura Shroff and Mr. Robert Boone performed the Ga melting point studies and a great number of thermometer calibrations. Medical colleagues, patients, and students have helped me to enjoy thermometry that goes beyond a precise calibration in an aluminum block against an international standard. Any review is bound to be incomplete. The extent of a discussion on each subject is to be taken as a reflection of my interest and awareness of the subject and not as either endorsement or criticism of any device or system.
[2] Often referred to as Sanctorius (1).

thermometers with similar characteristics could be constructed. The Duke also noted that mercury did not expand as greatly as spirits of wine, and so discarded it as a thermometric medium.

Fahrenheit, early in the eighteenth century, developed the mercury-in-glass thermometer. He also established the scale to which some of us are still bound. His fixed points were the ice point and body temperature, from which he calculated the steam point at 212°F by extrapolation (1). Fahrenheit's description of a salt-water fixed point at 0°F was probably intended to obfuscate potential competitors and to impress others with his art. Fahrenheit's rather careless lack of specifying a particular salt and salt concentration in discussing the low fixed point is out of character for a man who was so meticulous in constructing reproducable and interchangeable thermometers.

Anders Celsius about 1741 at Upsala established the centigrade scale by choosing the ice point as 100° and the steam point as 0°. Shortly after Celsius' death in 1744, a faculty colleague, Linnaeus, the renowned biologist, inverted the scale to its present form. Apparently, he waited until then to avoid embarrassing his mentor. For a readable account of the history of the thermometer, Middleton's book (1) is suggested.

Three basic points can be made from this introduction: First, thermometry has been related to medicine since its beginning. Second, the development of the science of thermometry and its contribution to medicine have depended on technical advances, and the converse is just as true. Finally, practical temperature scales, as opposed to the theoretical thermodynamic scale (Kelvin), have been based from the beginning upon defined fixed temperature points and material properties. All three of these are true today. The remainder of this chapter represents an elaboration of these points in inverse order as they apply at the present.

A useful source of thermometry information, encompassing a broad spectrum from fundamental scale definition to practical problems, is the series *Temperature* (2) which appears approximately each decade (the last edition only is cited here). The fundamentals of thermometry are reviewed by Quinn and Compton (3) and more recently by Hudson (4).

TEMPERATURE SCALES

There are two distinct types of temperature scales. The first type is based on the theoretical thermodynamic concept of temperature. This was developed over several years of rigorous thermodynamic reasoning as men began to understand the nature of heat and temperature. The absolute temperature scale was established in terms of the energy and work involved when a system (heat engine) operated between two temperatures. When defined this way, temperatures are independent of material properties such as mercury or gas expansions. The fact that different materials do not expand proportionately caused perplexity to the early thermometer makers. An absolute zero exists, although it cannot be reached, it can be approached asymptotically. Also, ratios of temperatures measured on the thermodynamic scale are more significant physically than addition of temperatures. When compared to the range of temperatures that has been produced by man, from a few microdegrees above zero kelvins in certain paramagnetic systems to millions of degrees in plasmas and thermonuclear explosions, the extremely close temperature regulation of the earth and the narrow range of temperatures compatible with mammalian survival are impressive indeed.

The second type of temperature scale is the practical or working scale. Currently, the entire world, by agreement, refers all temperature measurements to the International Practical Temperature Scale of 1968 (IPTS-68) (5). This scale was established by an international committee, and was based upon careful thermodynamic experiments. It represents the current state-of-the-art as an approximation to the Kelvin thermodynamic scale. It is believed to be accurate to about 0.01 K over most of its range below 904 K. For comparison, the precision, but not necessarily the accuracy, of most fundamental thermometry standards work below the steam point is of the order of 0.1 mK. The procedure of the IPTS-68 is to define the temperature of several natural fixed points such as the triple point of water (273.16 K = 0.01°C), and to provide a protocol for interpolation and extrapolation.

A list of these is given in Table 2.1. Between these fixed points a precisely constructed platinum resistance thermometer is used for interpolation. The interpolation function for the ideal platinum thermometer involves a polynomial with 21 terms carried to 16 significant figures. A given platinum thermometer is then calibrated at the fixed points to determine the corrections necessary to make it reproduce the scale of the ideal thermometer. This is a complicated routine, but it is quite accurate. In principle, the entire scale can be set up by following rules given in the text of the IPTS-68. Calibration of one platinum thermometer against another is not necessary. In practice, only a few of the national standards laboratories in various countries have established the IPTS-68 defined fixed points and defined the scale in this way. The national laboratories have calibrated many platinum resistance thermometers against the IPTS-68 and use these to calibrate the thermometer probes sent to them.

Thermometer Probes

GENERAL PRINCIPLES

A thermometer is any instrument which measures temperature. Any temperature-dependent parameter can serve as the basis for a thermometer; the variety of thermometer types attests to this. Because of the large number of parameters which are temperature-dependent, much engineering time is devoted to eliminating temperature sensitivities from instrumentation. Here, we are concerned with the converse—that of producing maximum

TABLE 2.1. *Defining fixed points of the IPTS-68(5)[a]*

Equilibrium state	Assigned value of International Practical Temperature	
	T_{68} (K)	t_{68} (°C)
Equilibrium between the solid, liquid, and vapor phases of equilibrium hydrogen (triple point of equilibrium hydrogen)	13.81	−259.34
Equilibrium between the liquid and vapor phases of equilibrium hydrogen at a pressure of 33, 330.6 N/m^2 (25/76 standard atmosphere)	17.042	−256.108
Equilibrium between liquid and vapor phases of equilibrium hydrogen (boiling point of equilibrium hydrogen)	20.28	−252.87
Equilibrium between the liquid and vapor phases of neon (boiling point of neon)	27.102	−246.048
Equilibrium between the solid, liquid, and vapor phases of oxygen (triple point of oxygen)	54.361	−218.789
Equilibrium between the liquid and vapor phases of oxygen (boiling point of oxygen)	90.188	−182.962
Equilibrium between the solid, liquid, and vapor phases of water (triple point of water)[c]	273.16	0.01
Equilibrium between the liquid and vapor phases of water (boiling point of water)[b, c]	373.15	100.00
Equilibrium between the solid and liquid phases of zinc (freezing point of zinc)	692.73	419.58
Equilibrium between the solid and liquid phases of silver (freezing point of silver)	1235.08	961.93
Equilibrium between the solid and liquid phases of gold (freezing point of gold)	1337.58	1064.43

[a] Except for the triple points and one equilibrium hydrogen point (17.042 K) the assigned values of temperature are for equilibrium states at a pressure $p_0 = 1$ standard atmosphere (101.325 N/m^2). In the realization of the fixed points, small departures from the assigned temperatures will occur as a result of differing immersion depths of thermometers or the failure to realize the required pressure exactly. If due allowance is made for these small temperature differences, they will not affect the accuracy of realization of the Scale.

[b] The equilibrium state between the solid and liquid phases of tin (freezing point of tin) has the assigned value of $t_{68} = 231.9681$ °C and may be used as an alternative to the boiling point of water.

[c] The water used should have the isotopic composition of ocean water.

dependence upon temperature, and eliminating any dependence upon extraneous or environmental parameters. It is not a trivial task to construct a stable, accurate, and convenient instrument which measures only temperature. Consequently, we will discuss some of the sources of error of each type of thermometer.

Even if a thermometer behaves ideally, errors in measurement can arise from poor technique. If a few general concepts are kept in mind, however, these errors can usually be kept small, or at least their presence and magnitude can be noted. Probe thermometers sense their own temperature which is determined by establishing equilibrium with the medium to be measured. Consequently, the temperature sensed is an average over a finite volume which depends upon the presence of gradients, the thermal properties of the medium and those of the probe. Heat is exchanged by conduction, convection, and radiation. Each must be considered when measuring temperatures.

Conduction is described by Fourier's Law which states that heat flow is proportional to the temperature gradient, the thermal conductivity of the medium and the cross-sectional area through which heat is flowing. Temperature measurements in the presence of steep gradients lose significance because the thermometer will sense an average value. Furthermore, thermal conduction down the thermometer leads or shaft may affect the temperature sensed and may change the gradients and temperature profiles drastically. If thermal equilibrium is desired, for example, when calibrating one thermometer against another, the system should be constructed so that the paths of heat flow do not cross the region where equilibrium is desired (that is, where the thermometers are located).

Convection can induce steep thermal gradients. Major blood vessels are not necessarily in thermal equilibrium with the surrounding tissue. Similarly, if a calibration bath is filled with viscous oil, proper mixing will not occur, and the temperature will vary significantly throughout the bath. Surface temperatures are also difficult to monitor because of radiant heat exchange as well as convective and conductive exchange. Probes placed on the surface will alter all three mechanisms and will sense not only the temperature of the altered surface, but will sense a temperature influenced by the radiative, convective, and conductive exchange of the probe with the environment. Generally, radiometric techniques such as thermography are preferable for surface measurements, if the surface has an emittance close to unity. Metals characteristically have very low emittance, but in some cases paint can be applied to raise the emittance. Tissues, on the other hand, have an emittance on the order of 0.98.

Thermometers can be characterized by several features. The choice of a particular type of thermometer for a given task will depend upon the relative merits of these parameters as well as personal preferences and availability of equipment:

Sensitivity: Some parameter, such as resistance, electromotive force, or reflected light intensity, must change monotonically with temperature; and a means must be available for measuring this change with sufficient precision. In medical applications, 0.1°C is usually adequate, but a few hundredths of a degree sensitivity is often helpful for determining small temperature differences or temporal drifts.

Accuracy: The thermometer must reproduce absolute temperatures within the limits necessary for the task. In most biomedical situations, 0.1°C accuracy is sufficient, but certain biochemical studies require higher accuracy if experimenters are to compare results properly.

Stability: Most thermometers drift with age, and so must be checked periodically and recalibrated when necessary. Examples are given later.

Response Time: Thermometer readings must keep pace with the actual temperature fluctuations of interest. The response time is usually characterized by a time constant which is defined in the following way: A thermometer is subjected to a step change in temperature ΔT_0 by plunging the probe into a water bath. The indicated change in temperature ΔT will approach ΔT_0 exponentially. The time constant is the time required for the difference between ΔT and ΔT_0 to reduce to $1/e$ or 37 percent of ΔT_0. Equilibrium, a residual difference with 5 percent of ΔT_0, is assured to be reached after an interval corresponding to about three time constants.

Passivity: The thermometer should not significantly perturb the medium to be measured, either through thermal conduction or through artifactual heating. Induction heating of electrically conducting sensors and leads has been a principal limitation of thermometry in electromagnetic diathermy fields.

Size: The sensor should be small compared to the size of the object to be measured and small enough to resolve significant temperature gradients. Its heat capacity (or more properly, its thermal inertia which is the product of density, specific heat and thermal resistivity) should be low so it will not produce a cold spot. The size of the probe is tied intimately to the two preceding items and to the problem of durability.

Temperature Indication: This refers to how temperatures are obtained from the thermometric parameter. For example, on a clinical thermometer, the height of a mercury column is read against a scale etched on a glass tube. Reading may be a little difficult, but it is certainly convenient. Neither expensive electronic equipment nor calibration tables are necessary. On the other hand, electronic thermometers are generally easier to read, to automate, and to use for process control. High precision, accuracy, and stability of the order of 0.1°C, however, require individual calibration: such thermometers frequently are not direct reading in temperature units. By implication as well, one probe cannot be substituted for another and the same read-out mechanism still be used; probes are not interchangeable at this level of accuracy.

These features are not all-inclusive nor entirely independent. Several common types of thermometers are discussed later in this chapter. An attempt is made to describe their features, drawbacks, instrumentation, and sources of error. Specific references to manufacturers and detailed circuit diagrams were considered inappropriate since companies and products change.

MERCURY-IN-GLASS

The mercury-in-glass thermometer is one of the oldest thermometers. It is a remarkable instrument in that it is essentially unchanged in form and accuracy from the time of Fahrenheit (ca. 1729). Frequently, the term thermometer is taken to mean this device only, although the word is more generally used here. Mercury-in-glass thermometers are quite inexpensive, ranging from a few dollars for a clinical thermometer to something less than one hundred dollars for the best standardized laboratory thermometer. If some care is used in the choice of a supplier, laboratory quality thermometers which are accurate to about 0.1°C can be purchased for about twenty dollars. If calibrated individually, thermometers with 0.1°C divisions can be used to maintain a scale to approximately 0.02°C. Careful, well-trained technicians at national standards laboratories routinely and reproducibly read them to 0.005°C!

One additional feature of mercury-in-glass thermometers is that the mechanism for reading the temperature is etched on the glass stem. No expensive electronics are required for obtaining a reading. On the other hand, it is not convenient to automate or electronically monitor temperatures measured this way. Circuits have been designed for this purpose, although electronic thermometers generally are used instead.

Deficiencies of mercury-in-glass thermometers are related mostly to their large mass. They cannot be used for point measurements in steep thermal gradients and have very long time constants. Finally, they are easily broken, which causes hazards from both broken glass and spilled mercury.

Several sources of error exist for mercury-in-glass thermometers. First, all thermometers should be checked upon receipt for a faulty scale, for example, the omission of a number, and for quality control in manufacture. For several years, we purchased thermometers of a specific catalog number from a well-known laboratory supply house. Without notice nor change of catalog number, the supply house began to obtain their thermometers from another manufacturer. The new thermometers were made with inferior glass tubing which results in optical distortions when reading the thermometer. The only clue to the change was that the nation in which the thermometer was made, as indicated on the back, had changed.

Occasionally, the mercury column will become separated, especially during shipment. Carefully heating the thermometer to well above its range so that the mercury expands into the enlarged cavity at the top of the column and then cooling it slowly will usually correct the problem. Alternatively, the thermometer can be cooled so that all of the mercury is drawn into the bulb at the bottom. This is easily accomplished by lowering the thermometer into the neck of a flask of liquid nitrogen. The thermometer may break, however, if it contacts the liquid or is cooled or warmed too quickly.

Glass and mercury do not expand proportionately, and glass exhibits some hysteresis in its thermal properties. Consequently, it is preferable in precision work to always work with increasing temperatures unless very long equilibration times are possible. Gently tapping the thermometer before reading will help to relieve strains in the mercury column due to surface tension. It is preferable to use mercury-in-glass thermometers in a totally-immersed fashion. If this is not possible, some corrections may be necessary because the stem and column are at temperatures different from the medium under study. Glass has a tendency to flow over a period of time, which will cause a change in the bulb volume and consequently, a shift in the calibration of the thermometer. An occasional check of the reading of the thermometer at the ice point will reveal any changes that may have occurred. The shift at the ice point can be added to the entire calibration; a complete re-calibration is not necessary. If precise work with mercury-in-glass thermometers is planned, a copy of the NBS report by Wise (6) is extremely useful.

Recently, we tested at random 22 new clinical thermometers. They were all found to be accurate to ±0.15°C at 37°C. Nevertheless, Abbey et al. (7) noted that in a sample of nearly 300 thermometers, 97.7 percent were accurate to 0.1°C initially, but only 76 percent of the thermometers were accurate after 10 months. They noted, however, that one brand of the four they tested was much less reliable than the other three.

A variation of this thermometer is the spirit- or alcohol-filled thermometer. Much of the previous discussion applies here as well. The coefficient of expansion is much larger for alcohol than for mercury, so the capillary is usually larger. Unfortunately, the expansions of the two liquids are not precisely proportional. This caused some consternation in the early days of thermometry (1). Spirit thermometers are sometimes used in the presence of strong electromagnetic fields because they are non-conductive and hence, non-interactive with the fields. In general, however, their greatest appeal lies in their low cost for the consumer market.

PLATINUM RESISTANCE THERMOMETERS

In pure ideal metals, at a temperature of absolute zero, electrons originating from the outer shells of the constituent atoms are free to travel about the well-organized lattice structure without hindrance. In real metals, electron flow is impeded by impurity atoms, dislocations in the lattice, strains and so forth which leads to a finite, temperature-independent resistance. At temperatures well above absolute zero, the electrons also are scattered by collisions with vibrating atoms in the lattice structure. The higher the temperature becomes, the greater the vibrations become, consequently the greater the resistance becomes. A temperature dependent resistance results, which is quite linear within the range of room temperature.

In 1887, H. L. Callender (1) proposed the use of pure platinum wire as a means of constructing stable precision thermometers to maintain a standard temperature scale that can be compared with scales at various laboratories. The standard platinum resistance thermometer (SPRT) is now specified as the interpolating instrument on the IPTS-68 (5) for determining temperatures between the defined fixed points of 13.81 K and 903.89 K (630.74°C). Platinum thermometers to be used as SPRT's must meet strict standards of purity and must be strain-free. The ratio of the resistance at 100°C to that at 0°C gives a measure of the purity, because of the additive component to the resistance caused by the impurities. This ratio must be greater than 1.3925 for SPRT's. Standard laboratory quality platinum resistance thermometers are quite expensive and must be handled with care to preserve their calibration. Riddle *et al.* (8) have written an excellent monograph on the use of these instruments.

Most medical laboratories will find that the SPRT is more than they require. Nevertheless, many industrial grade platinum resistance thermometers (RTD's) are available commercially. They will have typically a resistance of about 100 ohms at 0°C, compared to 25.5 ohms for the usual SPRT. The temperature coefficient is just under 0.4%/°C. They exist in a variety of configurations, but cannot be made small enough practically to fit into hypodermic needles or fine catheters. They can be quite stable if handled carefully; and because they are electronic devices, they can be automated easily for data acquisition and monitoring. The nearly linear variation of resistance with temperature simplifies the design of circuitry for direct readout in temperature units. Interchangeability is possible, but for precise work the probes must be calibrated individually.

Several sources of error exist for platinum resistance thermometers, although a little care will eliminate errors for all but the most precise measurements. First of all, the probes are sensitive to shock. Strains cause resistance, thus shock can produce shifts in calibration. Heat can be conducted through the leads and affect the temperature of the sensing element. Thus the leads should be anchored to the body to be measured if possible or, if not, to another body at nearly the same temperature. The element will self-heat due to Joule losses (I^2R) from the measuring current I flowing through the element of resistance R. The magnitude of the temperature error will depend upon heat conduction from the thermometer element to the medium being measured. Measuring the resistance at two current levels permits the temperature error to be determined. Typically, a measuring current of 1 mA will produce insignificant self-heating. Thermal emf's can occur at junctions of leads or from strains in the lead wires if they pass through large temperature gradients. Their effects can be eliminated by reversing the current flow through the thermometer. The sign of the measured voltage will change, but the contribution from the contact emf will not, thus permitting its elimination by taking the average of the forward and reverse readings.

Finally, the resistance of the thermometer leads can produce an error. For precise work, two leads are attached directly to each end of the thermometer element. Separate leads are used for the current source and for measuring the potential (V). The resistance is the ratio $R = V/I$ (Ohm's law). For less precise work, including most medical applications, the lead resistance is small compared to that of the element and usually does not change much since most of the leads remain at room temperature. Consequently, the two lead configuration is quite acceptable; and the lead resistance can be incorporated into the calibration of the probe.

A variety of circuits are used to read the resistance of a platinum thermometer. The most common for precision work are the direct-current potentiometric, the direct-current bridge, and the alternating-current bridge methods. In the first case, current is supplied to the thermometer from a stable current source and the voltage across the thermometer is read with a precision voltmeter or potentiometer. The current is determined by reading the voltage across a precision standard resistor in series with the thermometer. Current reversal techniques are used as discussed previously. Bridge techniques usually involve some variation of the Wheatstone bridge, including the Mueller Bridge for thermometers with four leads. Bridges using AC techniques have been developed which are convenient to use and which can be purchased with sensitivities adequate to the needs of many specific tasks. For biomedical applications, several companies produce instruments with linearization circuits such that the readings are in temperature units (°C or °F). The probes are not precisely similar, and the linearizations are not perfect, so individual calibrations are necessary to attain an accuracy on the order of 0.1°C.

THERMISTORS

Thermistors are also resistance devices. However, unlike platinum thermometers, they are semiconductors and have different characteristics. The electrons in a semiconductor at low temperatures are bound to the atoms which make up the solid. In contrast to insulators, the energy required to excite the electrons into the conduction band and make them available to carry electrical current is on the order of thermal energies at ordinary temperatures (0.025 eV). The number of conduction electrons, and hence the conductivity σ, is determined by the Boltzman distribution function

$$\sigma = \sigma_o e^{-\Delta/kT} \qquad (1)$$

where σ_o and Δ are constants, k is the Boltzmann constant and T is the absolute temperature in kelvins. The reciprocal of this expression gives the resistivity of the semiconducting medium. Thus the conductivity increases exponentially with temperature, while the resistivity $(1/\sigma)$ decreases exponentially. Taking the natural logarithm of the expression for resistivity and writing in terms of the resistance R of a specific device, we obtain

$$\frac{1}{T} = A_0 + A_1 \ln R \qquad (2)$$

where A_0 and A_1 are constants. Finally, if we follow Steinhart (9) and allow one additional term to correct for non-ideal semiconductors we have

$$\frac{1}{T} = A_0 + A_1 \ln R + A_3 (\ln R)^3. \qquad (3)$$

Again, T is temperature in kelvins, R is resistance and A_0, A_1, and A_3 are constants to be determined from the calibration of the probe. This expression represents the temperature versus resistance characteristic for thermistors to better than $0.01°C$ from $0°C$ to $55°C$ (10). A feature of this method is that only three constants are required to characterize the thermometer. Accurate temperatures can be computed directly by this expression from the measured resistance and displayed, tabulated or used in computer analysis.

Thermistors are constructed from a variety of sintered oxides such as MgO. A common form is a small bead of green material molded about two fine platinum leads. The beads are fired and encapsulated in glass, and probes of various styles are constructed from them. They are made in a range of sizes from about 0.3 mm diameter or less to perhaps 2 mm. The fabrication of thermistors, however, is still much of an art. Their stability varies widely from probe to probe even if made from the same basic material. Glass-encapsulated beads tend to be more stable than disks and those encapsulated in epoxy.

Thermistors have several advantages. First of all, they can be made quite small. We use commercial probes mounted in 25 AWG hypodermic needles or teflon catheters. They have a high sensitivity of about $\frac{1}{R}\frac{dR}{dT} = 4\%/°C$ which is about an order of magnitude greater than for platinum resistors. They have high precision and, when calibrated, high accuracy with relatively modest instrumentation. The stability of thermistors varies, but if care is taken in selection, it can be very good (11). The standard thermistor we use has not drifted in six years within our measurement uncertainty of $\pm0.003°C$ at the ice point. Two identical needle probes with sequential serial numbers were purchased at the same time. One of them has not drifted, while the other has required recalibration several times to keep it accurate to within $0.05°C$.

The most annoying deficiency of thermistors is that they are not really interchangeable. That is, they cannot be made to have the same R versus

T characteristic to within 0.1°C. Schemes have been designed to keep them within about 0.3 to 0.5°C, especially if larger sensors are permissible and compound units can be used. Generally, a choice must be made between direct reading and small (needle) size. Electronic circuits to convert resistance measurements to direct reading temperature units are sensitive to the specific thermistor bead. (See section on calibration for an example).

Many of the problems associated with producing interchangeable probes and circuits for direct reading in temperature units can be alleviated through use of modern microprocessor systems. The coefficients A_0, A_1, and A_3 of the Steinhart equation above for a specific probe can be stored and the temperature computed from the specific resistance readings. Accuracy, small size, direct reading, and multiple probes all become possible at once.

Circuits for reading thermistors are similar in principle to those for platinum resistance thermometers but with different specific parameters, components and instruments. Generally, direct current potentiometric methods or Wheatstone bridges are used, especially in precision work. We use the former in a "four-lead" configuration for our standard thermometers. Probes used in the clinic or in biological experiments are calibrated as two-lead devices. Digital multimeters (DMM) with a resistance mode can be used, provided the measuring current can be kept low enough. Most DMM's use currents about an order of magnitude too large, causing significant self-heating on the order of 0.5 to 2°C. In our calibration laboratory, we use a standard current of 10 μA for reading thermistors of a few kilohms. In our clinic, our DMM's use a reading current of about 100 μA for a 1000 Ω thermistor. The self-heating error in a thermally conductive medium is less than 0.01°C; however, it is much greater in a thermally-resistive medium such as air.

Alternating current techniques have not been generally applied to thermistors. Circuits using AC bridge techniques, however, have been designed for germanium resistance thermometers used as temperatures below 30 K. Since the characteristics of those thermometers are similar to thermistors, the instrumentation would be suitable for use with thermistors.

Sources of error for thermistors are similar in principle to those for platinum resistance thermometers, although they tend to be less significant because of the higher sensitivity of thermistors. Self-heating problems encountered with thermistors are discussed above. Current-reversal techniques should be used for precise thermometry with desired accuracies of better than 0.01°C. Heat conduction down the shaft of a hypodermic needle probe can be troublesome. In general, the needle should be inserted more than 4 mm into thermally conductive media to insure that its reading will be accurate to within 0.1°C (12). If the medium is poorly conductive, as in a fat layer, the error will be worse. Finally, the presence of strong electromagnetic fields can cause serious errors. This is discussed in greater detail later in the chapter.

THERMOCOUPLES

In electrical conductors, some of the electrons are free to move about much as gas molecules do in air. If a temperature difference exists between the two free ends of the metal, electrons will have higher energies at the hotter end. There will be a net diffusion of these more energetic electrons toward the cooler end. The excess charge resulting from this thermal diffusion of electrons produces a weak electrical potential difference E, the temperature coefficient of which is called the absolute thermoelectric force $dE/dT = \mu$, between the hot and cold ends. Since electrical leads must be connected to the two ends of the wire to measure this potential difference, and a similar effect will occur in the leads as in the original conductor, the voltmeter will measure the potential difference between the two metals (that is the leads and the original wire). Because the electronic structures are different for different metals, (they have different concentrations of free electrons), the thermoelectric force also will be different.

A thermocouple thermometer is constructed by placing one junction of two metals at the point where the temperature T_1 is to be measured and a second junction at a reference temperature T_0, such as in an ice point cell. The potential difference is measured with a microvoltmeter. Frequently, for thermocouple readers used in clinical or industrial circumstances, the reference junction is simulated electrically and is incorporated into the reading instrument. Because the thermoelectric force dE/dT is nearly constant near ambient and mammal body temperatures, linearization circuits are relatively straightforward. Units which are capable of reading directly in temperature units are common.

Copper versus constantan (a copper-nickel alloy), also known as a type T thermocouple, is commonly used for biomedical purposes. It has a relatively high sensitivity of about 40 μV/°C; and the materials are available at high quality and low cost. This permits the construction of probes which can be interchanged with one another without affecting the reading on the instrument. Probes are constructed by joining wires of pure copper with constantan by a simple solder joint. With care, the variation from probe to probe can be maintained within 0.1°C for temperatures near ambient. For reasons discussed later, this is usually the limit on the resolution as well. A cursory survey of supplier catalogs and technical brochures will reveal a variety of other thermocouple types and their characteristics. Nevertheless, all practical types have comparable thermoelectric powers, and so require comparable instrumentation for reading. In order to attain high sensitivity (high thermoelectric power), one metal in the couple is usually a ferromagnetic alloy which can cause difficulties in some applications.

Thermocouples can be made very small—probes in 29 gauge needles are common. Several authors (13–16) have described techniques for constructing probes on the order of 10 μm diameter for special applications. Thermocouples are less sensitive than thermistors; and more sophisticated equipment and techniques are required to use them at resolutions greater than 0.1°C. For thermistors, achieving 0.01°C resolution is very easy if individual calibrations on each probe are accepted. Thermocouple systems are less suitable as secondary standards in a calibration facility.

Sources of error (17, 18) in thermocouple systems arise from anything that will add a spurious DC voltage to the reading network. Contact potentials easily can exceed 10 μV unless care is taken. Mechanical working of the wire and consequent induced strains will cause artifactual thermal voltages as will inhomogeneities in the alloying and in the purity of the wires. Typically, these last two effects can be kept below 0.1°C for measurements in biomedical environments. Electronic biases and drifting in the reading instrumentation also appear as temperature shifts. This is one reason thermocouples are less satisfactory as thermometer secondary standards. Finally, since they are electrical conductors, they will be affected by electromagnetic fields in terms of noise, self-heating, and field perturbation. Some precautions can be taken to reduce problems, such as filtering the input to the electronic reading unit, inserting probes at normal incidence to electrical fields, electrically insulating the leads from current fields and conductors, and when possible, electromagnetically shielding the thermocouples. These measures are satisfactory in some cases and not at all in others. One additional consideration for thermocouples is that since one lead is typically a ferromagnetic alloy (constant in type T thermocouples) they will tend to be significantly affected (heated) by a strong radiofrequency magnetic field. Consequently, they may be unsuitable for any measurements in the fields produced by magnetic-induction high-frequency diathermy.

OTHER ELECTRONIC DEVICES

Nearly any parameter that varies with temperature can be made into a thermometer, provided variations in that parameter due to other effects can be controlled. Circuits have been designed using both diodes and transistors as active elements in thermometer systems. Recently, integrated circuits have been developed specifically as thermometers. These are interesting in that they can be incorporated into modern electronic systems using other integrated circuit modules for control and monitoring. They appear to be quite linear, which relieves the need for complicated linearization circuits or non-linear calibration algorithms.

QUARTZ THERMOMETER

The quartz thermometer (19) relies on the temperature dependence of the resonant frequency of a quartz transducer. It is an elegant device with a direct readout of 0.1 mK, and is used in many laboratories as a secondary standard. It is subject to vibration, shock, and drift, and so its calibration must be verified periodically (20) as with all other systems described in this chapter.

BIMETALLIC STRIPS

These thermometers are mentioned only because they are so common in our environment and are frequently used for routine measurements with low accuracy requirements. They are constructed by bonding together two metals with different thermal expansion coefficients and then coiling the bimetallic strip into a flat spiral. As the strip is heated, the coil expands according to the differing expansion of the two strips. A pointer attached to the strip indicates the temperature on a scale. They are similar to liquid-in-glass thermometers in that they are cheap, quite rugged and do not necessarily require expensive electronics for reading. A deficiency is that they are more difficult to include as part of an automated monitoring and control system. Sources of error are related most closely to the large thermal mass associated with the probe and to thermal conduction down the shaft.

These devices, however, are frequently very inaccurate. In testing three units used for monitoring temperatures in premature infant incubators, two read low by 8°F and one by 2°F!

LIQUID CRYSTAL INDICATORS

Cholesteric liquid crystals show a strong color play with temperature. As the liquid crystal is heated, the twisted stack of long molecules will twist more (or will unwind). Light at wavelengths commensurate with the spacing of these layers is reflected preferentially. Consequently, the color of the liquid crystal will pass through the spectrum as it is heated and so serve as a thermometer. These indicators have had several applications in medicine. In one, they are used to replace the clinical mercury-in-glass thermometer for measuring oral or rectal temperatures (21). We tested seven of these units and found them to be accurate within $0.2 \pm 0.2°C$, in agreement with a more extensive evaluation reported by Besley and Kemp (22). In a related application, small discs were applied to infant foreheads as a convenient means for nurses to determine if children in a nursery have temperatures within the normal range (23–24). Another use of liquid crystals in thermometry has been as an alternative to infrared sensing for obtaining breast thermograms (25, 26). In a third application, they have been used with optical fibers for constructing probe thermometers (27) that can be used in strong electromagnetic fields. This is discussed in the following section.

FIBER OPTIC THERMOMETERS

The early development of thermometers relied principally upon the thermal expansion of a medium (gas, liquid, solid) as the thermometric parameter. The reading was obtained directly from a mechanically coupled indicator moving along a scale. Examples are the mercury column in a glass stem and the pointer attached to a bimetallic strip. A second major class of thermometers involves electrical measurements such as resistance of thermoelectric power. Use of these devices was spurred by developments in the fields of electrical and electronics technology and instrumentation. Electrical signals traveling along conductors were the means of transferring information. While the reading mechanism was less direct, the opportunities for miniaturization, remote monitoring and process control were much greater. Accuracy and precision are much improved also in those situations where they are necessary. In general use, especially by laymen or the public, electronic thermometers are no better and frequently less accurate than the liquid-in-glass thermometer which was developed over 300 years ago.

Recently, a new class of thermometers has been developed which uses light propagating through optical fibers as a means of transmitting information. The primary impetus has come from the necessity for determining temperatures in the presence of strong electromagnetic fields (12, 28–31), for example, in studies of biological effects or in electromagnetically induced hyperthermia for cancer therapy. They also will be useful in other applications such as surgery where they intrinsically satisfy the most stringent requirements for electrical leakage. If the design goals of the persons developing these probes are met, they will be interchangeable, disposable and competitive with current electronic thermometers.

The instrumentation required to read each type of optical thermometer is peculiar to the given probe. A source is required which sends light to the sensor. Light returning from the sensor carries the temperature-related information through a second path to a photodetector where it is converted to an electronic signal which is manipulated to display the temperature. Most systems employ microprocessors so that the signal can be read in terms of temperature units and so that several probes can be multiplexed into one reading instrument. Most use one fiber or fiber bundle to send the light to the sensor and another to carry the return signal. We proposed (32) the use of a fiber optic directional coupler (or beamsplitter) to combine the two light paths into one fiber.

Several different types of sensors have been proposed, and new ones are added frequently. Hence any list (12, 29–31, 33, 34) is bound to be a strong reflection of the author's awareness of the state of the current literature and is likely to be obsolete before publication. Nevertheless, I will list some of those that have interested me. The first probe used a liquid crystal sensor. Several investigators worked on variations of this idea, but the Utah group (27) carried its development furthest. As described previously, a cholesteric liquid crystal undergoes a color change with temperature within a certain finite range. If red light is incident on the crystal, the intensity of the reflected light will be a function of the sensor temperature. Unfortunately, liquid crystals do not appear to have the stability necessary for thermometry. They drift both in terms of color play with temperature and in terms of the magnitude of the reflectance. Furthermore, they appear to show some hysteresis effects.

The birefringence of a single crystal of $LiTaO_3$ cleaved along certain directions is temperature dependent and can be used as the sensitive element in a thermometer. This optical thermometer (35, 36) attempted to exploit the better stability of single crystal systems. A practical probe can be made by coating one side of the crystal with a dielectric mirror and the other side with a polarizing film which serves as both polarizer of the incident light and analyzer of the light transmitted both ways through the crystal. The coated crystal is attached with transparent epoxy to the end of the optical fibers. It can be fabricated with large diameter crystals and then cut into many small individual elements for mounting on probes. Crystal thickness is about 100 μm; and probes have been made less than 0.5 mm in diameter. Smaller sizes may be attempted for the sake of compatibility with fiber optic diameters. The temperature response for this thermometer is sinusoidal, but the range can be made sufficiently broad, typically from 20 to 55°C, that the thermometer is single-valued over the temperature range of interest. Difficulties with the polarizing element caused some delays in the development of the thermometer, but these have been solved. The use of an optical reference channel was introduced to remove the effects of drifting in the electronics, light source, and photodetector at the expense of some complications in construction.

One problem with many optical thermometers has been the drift in the wavelength of the emitted light with temperature of the GaAs light-emitting diode. Christensen (36) exploited this effect by recognizing that its reciprocal, absorption of light, also would be temperature dependent. He constructed a thermometer by placing a small chip of GaAs on the end of the fiber bundle. He overcame the difficulty of light losses due to spurious scattering at the end of the fiber bundle by cutting the sensor in the shape of a prism such that light from the source fibers is offset by internal reflection in the sensor and directed into the photodetector fibers. The temperature characteristic of this probe is approximately linear over a broad range (of the order of 50°C) which is determined by the characteristics of the light source and the crystal. These probes range from 0.3 to 0.6 mm in diameter. Christensen (37) has developed a sophisticated electronics system which includes a built-in calibrator for the probe.

Sholes and Small (38) recently described a thermometer which uses the decay time of the fluorescence of a ruby crystal as the temperature-sensitive parameter. The crystal is excited with white light. The decay rate is monitored by integrating the total light emitted during two fixed time intervals of the decay. The ratio of these two signals depends on the rate or decay constant, but is independent of the absolute intensity of the emitted light and hence is independent of the degree of excitation or transmission losses. No reference channel is required. At the time of this writing, this system had been tested in the laboratory with large components, but has not yet been configured as a fiber optic probe. Samulski and Shrivastava (39) recently described a probe based upon similar principles.

The peak wavelength of the Raman scattering from a ruby crystal has been used for thermometry (40) in lipid membranes. This is an excellent example of using available systems to accomplish specific needs.

Another form of fluorescent decay thermometer (34) uses the ratio of emitted light at two wavelengths of oscilloscope phosphors as the sensitive parameter. This device also would be insensitive to the absolute intensity of the light. Two optical channels are required, however, to monitor the two different wavelengths.

The dilation of a liquid contained in a small capsule also has been used in a fiber optic thermometer (41). The reflectance of light from the meniscus varies with the liquid expansion, which can be monitored in a fashion similar to other systems.

Infrared detectors have been coupled to fibers to measure the thermal radiation at the end of the fiber and hence determine the temperature (42, 43). These systems, however, appear to be more useful at temperatures higher than those of interest in biology and medicine.

The most significant characteristic of fiber optic thermometers is that they are insensitive to the strong electromagnetic fields used to warm tissues in physical medicine, in hyperthermia for cancer therapy and in research on the biological effects of these fields. They have several other features as well. Most are very small; 1 mm diameter now is considered large. Glass has a relatively low thermal conductance, so the thermometers cause little thermal perturbation and measure the temperature of a very small region near the sensor. As a consequence of their small size, they have very fast time constants. The time constants increase somewhat by using protective teflon jackets, but the jackets can be removed in special circumstances. Finally, they have been developed with modern electronic reading units, and so have convenience and accuracy features that are not necessarily available in more conventional thermometer systems.

The major difficulty with fiber optic thermometers is that they are still not readily available. This will soon change, since private corporations are beginning to recognize the size of the potential market as hyperthemia for cancer becomes accepted. A problem with this type of sensor is that handling the optical fibers during construction is tedious. Analogs to integrated circuits, switches, directional couplers, and even suitable connectors for optical systems are still under development. Consequently, the construction of these thermometers is currently quite laborious, and they are less amenable to mass production techniques.

OTHER THERMOMETERS FOR USE IN ELECTROMAGNETIC FIELDS

Another approach to constructing thermometers that can be used in the presence of strong electromagnetic fields is to modify a conventional type of thermometer so that it is less sensitive to the field. Bowman's device (44) uses a small high-resistance thermistor as the sensor. The leads are constructed from very high resistance carbon-impregnated teflon and are connected in a four lead configuration. The measuring current is carried by one pair of leads while the potential is measured across the other pair. The high resistivity reduces the dipole currents induced by the electric field; close proximity of the leads minimizes the encompassed area of the leads and so minimizes magnetically-induced loop currents; the four-terminal configuration eliminates errors associated with lead resistances. Present thermometers are less than 1 mm in diameter. Some electromagnetic losses still occur in this thermometer, but they are very small and are of the same order of magnitude as the tissue displaced by the probe.

Larsen and colleagues (45) have worked on related types of thermometers which employ microwave integrated circuit (MIC) techniques. Narda Corporation recently announced a thermometer for use in electromagnetic fields. This also uses high resistance leads and a thermistor sensor.

Olsen and Molina (46) have constructed thermocouples from high-resistivity non-metallic conductors similar to those used for radio noise suppressors in automobile spark plugs. The high resistivity reduces interference from the electric field as previously described. Further, the materials are not magnetic, so they are less sensitive to magnetically induced noise and heating.

Chen and colleagues (47) proposed the use of the viscosity of liquids as a thermometric sensor. Changes in viscosity with temperature can be observed by measuring the pressure drop across a small orifice. The leads in this case consist of small plastic capillary tubing, while the liquid transfers the information. The system can be operated in closed-loop fashion with selected, contained fluids. It also can be operated "open loop" by using the body fluids directly as the sensing medium.

THERMOGRAPHY

In recent years, scanning infrared thermographic cameras have been used for observing and measuring thermal variations across exposed surfaces. Guy and others (48, 49) initiated their use in conjunction with tissue-equivalent electromagnetic phantom materials in studies concerned with power absorption properties in biological media. The effects of antenna and subject geometries, of heterogeneous electromagnetic properties of tissues, of interfaces between electromagnetically discontinuous materials, and of the frequency of the radiation are graphically portrayed by this method. Furthermore, the thermal artifacts which can result from inserting conductive probes into samples in strong electromagnetic fields can be observed (28, 29, 45, 49). Studies such as these have added a strong impetus to the development of the probes discussed in the preceding section.

Thermography is also useful for monitoring surface temperatures of tissues subjected to electromagnetic heating when the antenna or electrode configuration leaves part of the surface exposed (12, 49, 50). Observing temperature variations across at least one section of a treatment region is often helpful, even if that section is not the ideal one. Skin temperatures in the vicinity of a tumor or temperatures of localized surgical scars are frequently the factors that restrict a diathermy treatment. In other cases, normal blood perfusion or modest forced air flow provide adequate skin cooling. Thermography can verify that the skin temperatures are safe, and permit aggressive therapy to proceed.

In many cases, quantitative temperature data are required, rather than just qualitative determinations of thermal irregularities. The radiometric characteristics of the thermographic camera should be known, such as the wavelength band to which it is sensitive, the minimum detectable temperature, the spatial resolution, the frame rate, and sources of systematic errors. For precise work, each thermographic camera must be calibrated individually. The radiometric characteristics, such as emittance and transmittance of the surface to be monitored, must also be determined. Procedures and facilities for obtaining this information along with examples are discussed in detail in an earlier paper (51) which should be consulted if quantitative thermometry is planned. The approach is described briefly here.

The response I of a thermographic camera to a temperature T is typically given in units close to °C. However, the relationship between the temperature of an object and the radiation it emits (Planck's distribution if the source is a blackbody) is non-linear, and so a linear correspondence between the camera units and actual temperatures can hold only for a narrow range of temperatures. In one thermographic system tested, the ratio of camera units to temperature units $\Delta I / \Delta T$ ranged from 0.8°C near 24°C to 1.2/°C near 37°C. In other words, if the camera response units ΔI were assumed to be reading directly in °C, 20 percent errors in temperature differences would result near room temperature or near body temperature.

The total camera response i_1 to a specific subject s_1 at temperature T_1 is the sum of the radiation emitted, reflected and transmitted by the subject:

$$i_1 = \epsilon_1 I(T_1) + \rho_1 I(T_a) + \tau_1 I(T_b) \qquad (4)$$

Here ϵ_1, ρ_1 and τ_1 are the emittance, reflectance, and transmittance characteristics of the subject and T_1, T_a, and T_b are the subject, ambient, and background temperatures. $I(T)$ represents the response of the thermographic camera to radiation which it receives from an ideal blackbody source. The laws of radiometry (52–54) apply to this function; and the characteristics of the source are treated explicitly in the formula. A second object will have a similar response i_2. The camera is frequently and most accurately used to measure temperature differences between two sources or to measure temperature gradients on a single object; thus, the difference Δi_{12} can be represented as

$$\Delta i_{12} = i_1 - i_2 = \epsilon_1 I(T_1) - \epsilon_2 I(T_2) - (\epsilon_1 - \epsilon_2) I(T_a) \qquad (5a)$$

rewriting:

$$\Delta i_{12} = \epsilon_1[I(T_1) - I(T_2)] + (\epsilon_1 - \epsilon_2)[I(T_2) - I(T_a)] \tag{5b}$$

Here the object is assumed sufficiently thick such that no radiation from behind the object is transmitted through it ($\tau_1 = \tau_2 = 0$). We have also assumed $\rho = 1 - \epsilon$. This is a familiar expression which involves both the conservation of energy for radiation and the Kirchhoff relation, which states that the absorption of incident radiation by an object equals the radiation emitted by that object (with certain restrictions). Some features of expression (5b) must be noted. Only temperature differences are given, such as $I(T_1) - I(T_2)$. Calibration of the camera in terms of absolute temperatures is not necessary, but calibration in terms of temperature differences is essential. Ambient temperature must be recorded to account for the radiation reflected from the surface. In the infrared band, skin has an emittance of 0.98 (55), so the expression becomes quite straightforward and background radiation can be ignored. This is not necessarily true, however, for phantom studies. In the derivation of equations 5a and 5b, only diffuse background radiation is permitted. No provision is made for specular reflection of radiation emitted from a nearby localized hot source. The calibration of the thermographic camera against two black bodies at T_1 and T_2 can be represented by comparing the temperature difference as indicated by the camera $I(T_1) - I(T_2)$ with the true temperature difference $T_1 - T_2$ for each temperature interval. We usually plot

$$[I(T_1) - I(T_2)]/(T_1 - T_2) = (\Delta I/\Delta T)_{T_{12}}$$

versus the average temperature of the interval $(T_1 + T_2)/2 = T_{12}$. The temperature differences are found from

$$I(T_1) - I(T_2) = \frac{\Delta i_{12}}{\epsilon_1} + \frac{(\epsilon_2 - \epsilon_1)}{\epsilon_1}[I(T_2) - I(T_a)] \tag{6a}$$

and

$$T_1 - T_2 = [I(T_1) - I(T_2)]/(\Delta I/\Delta T)_{T_{12}} \tag{6b}$$

The value Δi_{12} is the signal difference observed on the thermographic display. It is the apparent signal difference between the two objects. $I(T_1) - I(T_2)$ is the temperature difference, in camera temperature units, after correcting the signal difference Δi_{12} by Equation 6a to account for the emittances of the objects and for diffuse reflections from the environment. The emittances are determined preferably from previous measurements with the thermographic camera (51), but sometimes published values can be used. Finally, true temperature differences are determined from Equation 6b, using the plot representing the calibration of the camera.

The limiting accuracy of measurements is determined by the minimum detectable temperature difference plus the magnitude of any systematic errors that may be present. For two systems we have used, the resolvable temperature difference was approximately 0.2°C. One of these systems introduced an error of + 0.2°C for an object appearing at the edge of the field of view compared to an object of the same temperature appearing in the center. The absolute calibration of another system depended slightly on the distance from the source to the camera.

A few other sources of error must be recognized in measurements with a thermographic camera. The first can be eliminated by verifying that the source is large compared to the spatial resolution of the camera. Another can arise from viewing the source at an oblique angle. Watmough *et al.* (56) have shown that for diffusely emitting materials, the error is not significant (0.1°C) for angles less than 30° but becomes important (several °C) for angles greater than 50°. Lewis *et al.* (57) showed experimentally, however, that significant errors do not arise until the viewing angle exceeds 75°. Finally, care must be taken to ensure that the camera optics are clean and that no localized hot sources shine on the object surface. Incandescent lights, instrumentation racks, or even the observer himself can reflect specularly from the surface of the object and be detected by the camera.

Knowledge of the infrared properties of materials such as emittance, reflectance, penetration depth, and transmittance is important in determining the temperature of the object. Reflectance and emittance are related by the expression $\epsilon = 1 - \rho$ for opaque objects in the absence of specular reflections, so these parameters can be treated together. Penetration depth is a measure of the surface "thickness" of an object. The term transmittance is used in reference to the fraction of incident radiation which penetrates windows placed in front of the object to be measured.

Pyroelectric vidicon cameras are becoming available. The detection system is different from thermographic cameras, but the general thermometry principles are the same. These systems use frame rates which are compatible with conventional video systems, and so all of that technology including image analysis is directly available at competitive costs. These systems tend to be less expensive than the usual medical thermographic systems. On the other hand, they are not yet as good in terms of spatial and temperature resolution (58). This may change, of course.

Infrared spot thermometers are subject to similar considerations as thermographic cameras. In fact, thermographic cameras are spot detectors, but with scanning optics added. Noncontact, surface-reading devices avoid many of the fundamental problems of placing probes in contact with surfaces where steep temperature gradients exist. Nevertheless, they have their own set of error sources, and so care must be taken. Shiny metals have very low emittances. Consequently, very large errors can result from using infrared radiometers to measure their temperatures.

Calibration Laboratory

Accuracy to 0.1°C cannot be guaranteed in off-the-shelf thermometers without individual calibration. Small probe thermometers mounted either in flexible catheters or in hypodermic needles are not direct reading, interchangeable and stable at this level of accuracy. Thus, a calibration facility accurate to 0.02°C should be part of every laboratory or clinic in which temperatures are a significant parameter. When secondary, working thermometers are calibrated against the standard thermometer, uncertainties still should be well below the levels of biological interest. Furthermore,

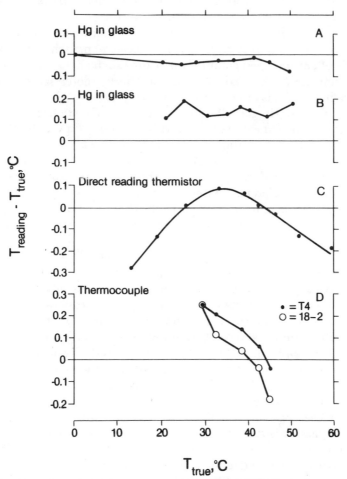

Fig. 2.1. Differences between temperatures indicated by typical direct reading thermometers and absolute temperatures as maintained by a standard thermistor. A,B: Two Hg-in-glass thermometers. C: Thermistor with an electronic read-out. D: Two copper versus constantan thermocouples read by same electronics unit (49).

calibration drifting in the secondary probes can be detected before it becomes significant. Figure 2.1 illustrates typical reading accuracies for three different types of direct-reading systems. T_{reading} is the value indicated by the thermometer, while T_{true} is the value maintained on the standard. For thermometers and thermocouples the shape of the curve depends on the electronic reader; the absolute values of temperature depend on the specific compound probe (two thermistor beads in one probe).

Two approaches to a calibration facility are possible. The first, and most common, is to maintain a standard thermometer which has a calibration that can be referred back to the IPTS-68 (5). Some type of temperature-controlled medium, such as a water bath or a copper or aluminum block, is used to maintain the unknown and standard thermometers at the same temperature for comparing readings. The other approach is to use established cells of natural fixed point temperatures such as the ice point, 0°C, or gallium point, 29.772°C, and observe the thermometer reading at these points. Each of these is discussed in this chapter.

Precision mercury-in-glass thermometers are available from a number of scientific suppliers and can be read to this accuracy, especially if a reading lens is used. Wise, of the National Bureau of Standards (NBS), has prepared a very useful manual (6) on the calibration and use of these thermometers. In addition, NBS has developed special thermometers (SRM 933 and 934) for their Standard Reference Materials program which have precise calibrations at four specific temperatures: 0°C, 25°C, 30°C, and 37°C.

We use a standard thermistor thermometer to maintain our scale. The calibration of this thermometer can be referenced back to NBS and is recorded with millidegree precision. Over the six years we have had it in our laboratory, we have not detected drifts at the ice point within our measurement uncertainty ($\sim$3 m°C). Thermistors have the advantage of high sensitivity over a selected range but require several calibration points that must be fitted to a function involving logarithms. On the other hand, industrial platinum-resistance thermometers are more linear, but require somewhat more sophisticated equipment to attain the same sensitivity. The ideal primary thermometer is the SPRT, which is the defined interpolation instrument for the IPTS-68. Unfortunately, these and the instruments required to use them are expensive. To summarize, electronic thermometry is easier to use, especially to automate and record, than that based on mercury-in-glass. It is more expensive, however, since auxillary instrumentation is necessary to obtain a reading.

A water bath with a good temperature controller and high fluid circulation is the most common apparatus used for thermometer calibration. Since thermal gradients and fluctuations can exist, care must be taken that the primary and secondary thermometers are at the same temperature when the calibration point is recorded. These effects are especially noticeable for thermometers with small thermal masses, such as thermistors or thermocouples mounted in hypodermic needles. In order to average out spatial and temporal variations on the order of 0.2°C in our bath, we constructed an aluminum calibration block inside a can which is then placed in the bath. The main heat flow is along a central aluminum rod which is the main thermal contact with the bath. When the bath stabilizes, the block comes to the average temperature of the bath, and no significant gradients can exist, so the thermometers mounted in the block are all in equilibrium at the same temperature. Tests have verified that calibrations can be transferred with m°C precision in this block. More time is required for the block to attain thermal equilibrium for each calibration point than when the bath is used alone, so calibration runs take longer. A booster heater on the block speeds the process somewhat. If only small thermometers need calibration, a block such as this can be packed in polyurethane insulation, and an electronic controller with a resistance heater can be used to maintain the temperature. It is important to consider the heat flow paths that could result in temperature gradients. Samaras and colleagues (59) have constructed a microprocessor-controlled electronic system to use for calibrations.

Two other precepts of thermometry are that no thermometer is necessarily stable and that none is indestructible. Hence, three standard-quality thermometers must be maintained to determine which one may have drifted, and all thermometers must be checked regularly, especially the standards. We have found that for various reasons, including operator carelessness, thermometer element deterioration and several unknown factors, thermometers have a finite lifetime. In our laboratory, the average lifetime is on the order of several months, except for our well-guarded standards.

Thermometric fixed points also can be used for calibration. Indeed, this is the basic philosophy behind the present world standard of thermometry, the IPTS-68. Table 2.2 shows several fixed points that are of interest to studies requiring precise thermometry between −30°C and 100°C. The most readily available is the ice point. It is easy to set up and if done properly, will reproduce much better than 0.01°C. The technique is to crush ice from distilled water, pack it into a clean vacuum flask (dewar), and add just enough distilled water to provide thermal contact. Any excess water which

TABLE 2.2. *Fixed point Temperatures of Biomedical Interest*

H_2O (F.P.)	0°C (273.15 K)	IPTS-68(5)
H_2O (T.P.)	0.01 (Exact)	IPTS-68(5)
Phenoxybenzene (T.P.)	26.87	
Ga (M.P.)	29.772	Thornton (62) and Mangum and Thornton (61) Sostman (60)
Na_2SO_4 0.10 H_2O (S.H.)	32.373	Magin et al.(64)
KF 0.2 H_2O (S.H.)	41.421	
$Na_2 HPO_4$ 0.7 H_2O (S.H.)	48.222	
H_2O (B.P.)	100.00	IPTS-68(5)

causes the ice mass to float should be siphoned off and replaced with crushed ice. The purist, of course, will instead use a triple point cell, 0.01°C = 273.16K (Table 2.3), which provides better reproducibility and is basic to the definition of the unit of temperature. These are more expensive to set up and maintain, however. The melting point of very pure (99.9999 percent pure) gallium has been shown to be very useful as a reference temperature for calibration (60–63). Complete cells ready for use can be obtained from the National Bureau of Standards and from Yellow Springs Instruments Company.

We use a gallium cell to check the stability of our thermometers after each use in the clinic. The cell is placed in a water bath at 28°C and is allowed to equilibrate. The temperature of the water bath is raised to about 30°C, or about 0.3°C above the melting point at 29.772°C. After about 30 minutes, the melting plateau is established and the temperature of the cell remains stable for several hours. Thermometers are placed in the reentrant well of the cell, one after another, and their readings are compared with the published value of the melting point. A note of caution: we found that after several months the Ga cell melting temperature became unstable and somewhat erratic. We first noticed it by observing that all newly calibrated thermistors began to show a calibration bias when compared to the Ga melting point. Intercomparisons of several stable thermistors at several temperatures indicated that the melting temperature of the cell was drifting. The shape of the melting curve at the beginning and end of the melt was consistent with an impurity in the cell (62). We then obtained another Ga cell and were able to confirm the fact that the selected thermistors were stable and that the first Ga cell was not. For perspective, however, this erratic behavior was still only of the order of 0.01°C, which is insignificant in most biomedical situations.

Magin and co-workers (64) devised a technique for using the hydration-dehydration point of certain salts in solution as temperature fixed points (see Table 2.2). In simple terms, fresh reagent grade chemicals are obtained

TABLE 2.3. *Fixed Point Temperatures Below 0.01 °C*

N_2 (B.P.)	77.348 K	−195.802 °C
Ar (T.P.)	83.798	−189.352
O_2 (B.P.)	90.188	−182.962
Kr (T.P.)	115.764	−157.386
CO_2 (S.P.)	194.674	−73.476
Hg (F.P.)	234.288	−38.862
H_2O (M.P.)	273.15	0.0
H_2O (T.P.)	273.16	0.01 (by definition)

from the local chemistry stores and are heated a few degrees above the salt hydration transition temperature. The salt is poured into a vacuum flask and is stirred mechanically. A small diameter glass tube, sealed at one end and filled with thin material or silicone oil, is inserted into the salt solution and is used as a re-entrant well to protect the thermometers from the caustic salts. The thermometers are placed in the well and are calibrated as with gallium cells. New salts are purchased for each calibration to avoid contamination. Three calibration points are adequate to determine the three coefficients that describe the thermistor resistance-temperature characteristic. Thermocouples are more linear, and three are adequate for them also. A fourth temperature point is useful as a check.

In conclusion then, calibration facilities can be set up without unreasonable capital cost, especially when compared to the overall cost of a medical or clinical program which requires accurate ($\pm 0.1°C$) thermometry. The most significant expense is perhaps that of maintaining an appropriately skilled, careful technician who can calibrate the thermometers initially and periodically check them for drift. A fully automated, microprocessor-controlled calibration unit would be helpful to laboratories that do not wish to invest time in training an individual to develop and maintain a calibration facility.

Thermometry in Therapeutic Heating Fields

STRONG ELECTROMAGNETIC FIELDS

Thermometry in the presence of strong electromagnetic fields has been recognized as difficult for many years. At the most basic level, fields emanating from the power mains are an aggravation to nearly all measurements. Precision measurements in many places are plagued by radiofrequency (RF) interference from nearby radio and television transmitters. Careful shielding and grounding of equipment, or even entire rooms, eliminates most of the problems caused by environmental RF fields.

The problem of measuring temperatures in the presence of strong electromagnetic fields is far more complex in that not only is accurate thermometry required, but it must be attained without significantly perturbing the intense applied fields. Furthermore, when these fields are used to irradiate human subjects, clinical constraints are imposed as well.

The nature and significance of the perturbing effect of thermometers in strong fields, especially in relation to electromagnetic heating, has been demonstrated graphically with a thermographic camera by Johnson and Guy (28) and by others (29). Conversely, some have claimed that their data were only minimally affected by the presence of electromagnetic fields. The discrepancy lies in the fact that many factors influence the magnitude of the perturbation. These include the field strengths, the orientation and position of the thermometer leads with respect to field orientation and phase, the degree of shielding including that due to tissue, and the geometry of the subject and the radiator. For example, in one test we performed using 3 MHz current fields to heat a man's arm, no measureable artifact appeared in temperatures monitored with a needle-mounted thermistor. However, when the same treatment was applied to an eleven-year-old girl with osteogenic sarcoma, much poorer electromagnetic coupling to the arm was achieved, and a thermometry artifact of about 1°C resulted.

The difficulty of making reliable temperature measurements in the presence of strong electromagnetic fields stems from three types of interaction between the thermometer and the field. The first is the familiar problem of electromagnetic interference (EMI) due to electromagnetic pickup by the electronic measurement system. The second is self-heating of the thermometer element from direct absorption of energy from the electromagnetic field. The third is perturbation of the electromagnetic field caused by reflection or shunting of the electric field by the thermometer or its sheath.

Several techniques can be used to reduce the magnitude of these effects. The instruments should be well-shielded and grounded, with special care taken to avoid ground loops, including those involving capacitive coupling. Radiofrequency filters in the sensing circuitry and in the power lines help as well. The thermometer leads should run perpendicular to the electric field vector and should be twisted tightly to reduce magnetic induction pickup. When possible, extraneous fields radiating from the source should be eliminated.

With respect to interference in the sensor itself, the thermometer should be isolated electrically from the electromagnetic field. For example, thermistors mounted in hypodermic needles must not be shorted to the needle or excessive RF noise will be fed to the instrumentation. Frequently, adequate temperature information can be obtained by shutting off the power periodically to read the thermometer. For some experiments, re-entrant wells can be prepared in the subject prior to heating and thermometer probes inserted immediately after the field is extinguished. The maximum temperature attained can be determined by extrapolation of the cooling curve back to the instant heating ceased. In other cases, the sensor can be inserted such that the tissues electrically shield most of the sensor leads. Practically, the magnitude of any temperature artifact is proportional to the power levels which produce the artifact.

At low frequencies below about 5 MHz, where the wavelengths are long (60 m), the leads of thermometers and of heating equipment tend to make relatively poor antennas. This reduces the problem with artifacts. At higher frequencies, these lead antennas become more efficient and the problems with noise increase. As microwave frequencies are approached, near 1 GHz, the fields can be confined better, and again noise is often less of a problem. All of these last remarks ignore, of course, the effects of the probe on the heating field. The magnitude of an artifact can sometimes be estimated by quickly switching off the field and watching the thermometer cooling rate. Presumably, a very fast change implies noise effects or cooling of a small mass confined to the probe itself and so is artifactual. A slower cooling rate suggests overall cooling of a larger tissue volume. Some investigators are using microcomputers to shut off the power and switch in the thermometers for monitoring in a regular duty cycle fashion.

These solutions are not entirely satisfactory for a number of reasons. First of all, they frequently are not adequate; significant interference remains. Shielding a sensor may reduce electromagnetic interference but also may produce a substantial reflection or shunting of the electromagnetic field. The near field of an antenna can have electric field components in all directions, and thus it may be impossible to place the leads normal to the field. The fields are especially complex in regions of curved interfaces which can focus the fields. Hot spots caused by the presence of the probe may occur somewhat removed from the probe. Thus, the common technique of momentarily switching off the field and distinguishing between the fast jump in the sensor reading which is attributed to electromagnetic interference and the slower change attributed to a real temperature change will not necessarily reveal localized tissue heating caused by the presence of the thermometer. Many situations exist for which continuous monitoring of the temperature is necessary for precise control of heating fields. Even switching the field off for a few seconds will result in a substantial temperature drop if a large blood flow rate exists in the region being heated. Finally, in a given experiment or clinical treatment, biological or physiological constraints frequently take precedence over physical considerations. Nevertheless, the above techniques must be used until the new thermometers specifically designed for use in strong electromagnetic fields become generally available.

THERAPEUTIC ULTRASOUND FIELDS

Thermometry in the presence of the intense ultrasonic fields required for therapy is, in general, less of a problem than for electromagnetic heating. This is because the ultrasonic field is confined to dense media, electromagnetic radiation does not occur, and because modern measuring and signal processing systems are electrical rather than mechanical. Hence, interference must involve electro-acoustic coupling, and so the probability of occurrence is reduced by several orders.

Nevertheless, thermometry is not free of problems peculiar to this environment. Two principal concerns are to avoid preferential heating of the thermometer probe and to avoid perturbing the ultrasonic field by the probe. Both of these are reduced by using probes with dimensions small compared to the wavelength of the sound wave. For comparison, the wavelength of a 1 MHz ultrasound wave in soft tissues or in water is about 1.5 mm. Lele (65) uses thermocouples which are 25 and 50 μm in diameter. In addition to reducing the possibility of causing scattering of the wave and reducing the area for direct absorption of energy, the small size also minimizes thermal perturbations from heat conduction down the leads. If the probes can be oriented such that the cross-sectional area exposed to the propagating wave is minimized, the interference is reduced further. Probes that have been sheathed in soft polyethylene or in any other highly absorbing material should be avoided since the ultrasonic energy absorption coefficient (in dB/cm) of soft polyethylene is approximately five times greater than that of most soft tissues (66). Bare metal has a much lower absorption than tissue.

One further source of direct probe interference arises from pulsed fields. The propagating ultrasonic wave can produce relative motion between the probe (67, 68) and the medium. This leads to viscous flow heating near the probe which would not be present if the probe were not there. This is a transient problem, however, with a short relaxation time and so is not of concern in the steady state.

The most difficult aspect of thermometry or thermal dosimetry in ultrasonic fields is common to all forms of heating by propagating energy waves. Heterogeneous tissues and the interfaces between them cause reflections, refractions, and scattering of the waves. Consequently, regions of high energy absorption (hot spots) or low field intensity resulting from shadows or wave interference are very difficult to predict. Bone/soft tissue interfaces and air/soft tissue interfaces are particularly troublesome with ultrasound. Reflections from bone will cause hot spots in the soft tissue just in front of the bone. Conversely, if the coupling to the bone becomes very good, then the high absorption of ultrasound in bone will cause the bone to heat preferentially. Measurements of the temperature at single points with a probe will not necessarily imply anything at all about the temperature of a point a few mm away.

TEMPERATURE RECONSTRUCTION

Temperature distributions in heated tissues are complicated because the heterogeneous tissue properties often lead to large variations in the specific absorption rate (SAR). In addition, variability of blood flow in different tissues leads to differential cooling. Therefore, point measurements are often inadequate. A means of obtaining a detailed temperature map in three dimensions would certainly help therapy and dosimetry. For surface measurements, thermography is a good example of detailed temperature mapping which is accomplished with straightforward analog signal processing. Computerized tomography (CT) has demonstrated that complex reconstructions of cross-sections at depth are possible. We are now faced with the task of finding a suitable, temperature-dependent parameter on which we can base such a reconstruction.

Guy introduced the use of phantom models (48) with dielectric properties similar to tissues to study power deposition. We have attempted to model crudely the effects of perfusion by forcing saline through a sponge and thermographically observing the temperature rise and steady state conditions during heating (69, 70). Sandhu *et al.* (71) have described a similar system. The results agree with surface data taken *in vivo* on a dog thigh. Nevertheless, while they are informative, phantom data still do not give accurate temperature profiles that apply to specific patients. Another approach is to measure with probes the electrical and thermal parameters of tissues for the specific patient and use these in the bioheat equation to interpolate between measured temperature points. This also requires accurate knowledge of boundary conditions. Probably this technique will be more useful in treatment planning and in retrospective thermal dose calculations than in monitoring during treatment.

A direct measurement of the temperature pattern is still necessary. Two methods for non-invasive measurements are under investigation: The first is to detect the thermal radiation emitted by tissue at microwave frequencies of the order of 1 GHz. The penetration depth of microwave radiation ranges from 1 to 10 cm in tissues. By the same token, some fraction of the radiation emitted at these depths will penetrate to the surface where it can be detected by an antenna. The net signal received represents an integrated average of the radiation emitted within the "near-field cone" of the antenna. The thermal resolution is approximately 0.1°C, and the spatial resolution, both depth and width, is of the order of one to a few centimeters. Myers *et al.* (72) and Edrich *et al.* (73) have used their radiometers to screen women for breast cancer by looking for the presence of thermal anomalies. I am not aware of any attempts yet to reconstruct the temperature patterns.

The other non-invasive approach is to measure the velocity of sound in tissue as a function of temperature. Sachs (74) discusses some ways in which thermometry may be performed, especially in a monitoring mode involving his TAST (Thermo Acoustic Sensing Technique) system. Johnson and his colleagues (75) have investigated three-dimensional reconstruction techniques for mapping velocity fields and other acoustic parameters, and have presented preliminary results of tomographic reconstructions of warm water-filled balloons in a cool water bath. The thermal resolution was of the order of 1°C; the spatial resolution was approximately 2 mm; and the scan and reconstruction times were each 5 minutes.

Bowen *et al.* (76) embarked upon a related project, but have concentrated first on characterizing the temperature dependence of the sound velocity in various tissues. Among their observations is that lipids have a negative temperature coefficient, whereas most other tissues have positive coefficients. The magnitude of the temperature coefficient depends on the amount of collagen, lipids, and other constituents present. If ultrasonic thermography is to serve as a means of temperature scanning, account must be taken of these variables. These studies have produced interesting data on the ultrasonic properties of tissues and, if thermometry proves to be infeasible, the results may lead to other benefits such as showing changes to tissues that can later be identified as consequences of therapy. The need is great, and undoubtedly other mechanisms for producing CT-type thermometry will soon be proposed and tested.

Summary

The necessity of thermometry in a clinical setting is presumed to be self-evident. Areas where it has been especially important include dosimetry in physical medicine and in clinical hyperthermia for cancer, basic studies on biological responses to thermal shocks, diagnostic procedures such as screening for breast cancer, or for observing cardiovascular circulatory problems, physiological research on the thermal responses of man and other animals, and in process control in clinical testing laboratories.

I have presented some of the philosophy of thermometry to clarify some of the basic principles and underlying assumptions of the science. Thermometry is not particularly arcane or difficult, but some care is necessary to avoid errors. In fact, it is quite easy to obtain precise results in many situations. It is also quite easy to obtain utterly nonsensical results and to do it with a flair!

Various common thermometers and a few not so common have been described. Techniques for establishing a thermometer calibration facility were discussed. Finally, some discussion was given of common problems encountered in diathermy fields of both electromagnetic and ultrasonic origin.

REFERENCES

1. MIDDLETON, W. E. K. *A History of the Thermometer*. Johns Hopkins Press, Baltimore, 1966.
2. PLUMB, H. H. (ed). *Temperature Vol. IV*. Instrument Society of America, Pittsburgh, 1972.
3. QUINN, T. J. AND COMPTON, J. P. The foundations of thermometry. *Rep. Prog. Phys. 38:* 151, 1975.
4. HUDSON, R. P. Measurement of Temperature. *Rev. Scient. Instrum. 51:* 871, 1980.
5. INTERNATIONAL PRACTICAL TEMPERATURE SCALE OF 1968. *Metrologia 5:* 35, 1969; and PRESTON-THOMAS, H. Amended edition of 1975. *Metrologia 12:* 7, 1976.
6. WISE, J. A. Liquid-in-Glass Thermometry. NBS Monograph 150, U.S. Printing Office, 1976.
7. ABBEY, J. C., ANDERSON, A. S., CLOSE, E. L., HARTWIG, E. P., SCOTT, J., SEARS, R., WILLENS, R. M., PACKER, A. G. How long is that thermometer accurate? *Am. J. Nursing, 78:* 1375, 1978.
8. RIDDLE, S. L., FURUKAWA, G. T. AND PLUMB, H. H. Platinum Resistance Thermometry. NBS Monograph 126, U.S. Government Printing Office, Washington, D.C., 1972.
9. STEINHARDT, J. S. AND HART, S. R. Calibration curves for Thermistors. *Deep Sea Res. 15:* 497, 1968.
10. TROLANDER, H. W., CASE, D. A. AND HARRUFF, R. W. Reproducibility, stability and linearization of thermistor resistance thermometers. *Temperature Vol. IV.* Instrument Society of America, Pittsburgh, 1972, p. 997.
11. WOOD, S. D., MANGUM, B. W., FILLIBEN, J. J. AND TILLETT, S. B. An investigation of the stability of thermistors. *J. Res., NBS, 83:* 247, 1978.

12. CETAS, T. C. AND CONNOR, W. G. Thermometry considerations in localized hyperthermia. *Med. Phys. 5:* 79, 1978.

13. CAIN, C. P. AND WELCH, A. J. Thin-film temperature sensors for biological measurements. *IEEE Trans. Biomed. Engin. BME-21:* 421, 1974.

14. PRIEBE, L. A., CAIN, C. P. AND WELCH, A. J. Temperature rise required for production of minimal lesions in *Macaca Mulatta* Retina. *Am. J. Ophthalmol. 79:* 405, 1975.

15. BATTIST, L., GOLDNER, F. AND TODREAS, N. Construction of a fine wire thermocouple capable of repeated insertions into and accurate positioning within a controlled environmental chamber. *Med. Biol. Engin. 7:* 445, 1969.

16. BICHER, H. I., SANDHU, T. S., VAUPEL, P., AND HETZEL, F. W. The effect of localized microwave hyperthermia on physiological responses. *Nat. Can. Inst.* (in press), 1981.

17. HOWARD, J. L. Error accumulation in thermocouple thermometry. *In: Temperature IV.* H. H. Plumb (ed). Instrument Society of America, Pittsburgh, 1972, p. 2017.

18. POWELL, R. L., HALL, W. J., HYINK, C. H., SPARKS, L. L., BURNS, G. W., SCROGER, M. G. AND PLUMB, H. H. Thermocouple reference tables based on the IPTS-68. NBS Monograph 125, U.S. Government Printing Office, 1974.

19. BENJAMINSON, A. AND ROWLAND, F. The development of the quartz resonator as a digital temperature sensor with a precision of 1×10^{-4}. *In: Temperature Vol. IV,* H. H. Plumb (ed). Instrument Society of America, Pittsburgh, 1972.

20. BENSON, B. B. AND KRAUSE, D., JR. Use of the quartz crystal thermometer for absolute temperature measurements. *Rev. Scient. Instrum. 45:* 1499, 1974.

21. BRISLEN, W., SMART, G. I. AND COLLINS, A. M. Assessment of a single use clinical thermometer. *Nursing Times, 72:* 236, 1976.

22. BESLEY, L. M. AND KEMP, R. C. *In vitro* evaluation of accuracy of a single use clinical thermometer. *Med. J. Austral. 2:* 337, 1978.

23. REISINGER, K. S., KAO, J. AND GRANT, D. M. Inaccuracy of clinitemp skin thermometer. *Pediatrics 64:* 4, 1979.

24. LEES, D. E., SCHUETTE, W., BULL, J. M., WHANG-PENG, J., ATKINSON, E. R. AND MACNAMARA, T. E. An evaluation of liquid-crystal thermometry as a screening device for intraoperative hyperthermia. *Anesth. Analg. 57:* 669, 1978.

25. DAVISON, J. D., EWING, K. L., FERGASON, J., CHAPMAN, M., CAN, A. AND VOOTHIS, C. C. Detection of breast cancer by liquid crystal thermography. *Cancer 29:* 1123, 1972.

26. LOGAN, W. W. AND LIND, B. Improved liquid cholesterol esten crystal thermography of the breast. *J. Surg. Oncol. 8:* 363, 1976.

27. ROZZELL, T. C., JOHNSON, C. C., DURNEY, C. H., LORDS, J. L. AND OLSEN, R. G. A nonperturbing temperature sensor for measurements in electromagnetic fields. *J. Microwave Power, 9:* 241–249, 1974.

28. JOHNSON, C. C. AND GUY, A. W. Nonionizing electromagnetic wave effects in biological materials and systems. *Proc. IEEE, 60:* 692, 1972.

29. CETAS, T. C. Temperature measurement in microwave diathermy fields: principles and probes. *In: Proceedings of the International Symposium on Cancer Therapy by Hyperthermia, Drugs and Radiation.* Robinson, J. E. and Wizenberg, M. J. (eds). American College of Radiology, Bethesda, MD, 1976, p. 193.

30. CETAS, T. C. Thermometry in strong electromagnetic fields. *In: The Physical Basis of Electromagnetic Interactions with Biological Systems.* Taylor, L. S. and Cheung, A. Y. (eds). University of Maryland, College Park, 1978, p. 261.

31. CHRISTENSEN, D. A. Thermal dosimetry and temperature measurements. *Cancer Res., 39:* 2325, 1979.

32. CETAS, T. C., HEFNER, R. D., SNEDAKER, C., SWINDELL, W. Further developments of the birefringent crystal optical thermometer. Abstract presented at the 1976 USNC/URSI Series on Biological Effects of Electromagnetic Waves, Amherst, MA, 1976.

33. CETAS, T. C., CONNOR, W. G. AND BOONE, M. L. M. Thermal dosimetry: some biophysical considerations. *In: Cancer Therapy by Hyperthermia and Radiation.* Streffer, C. (ed)

Urban and Schwarzenberg, Baltimore, Munich, 1978, p. 3.

34. WICKERSHEIM, K. A. AND ALVES, R. B. Recent advances in optical temperature measurement. *Indus. Res. Devel.*, *21*: 82, 1979.

35. CETAS, T. C. A birefringent crystal optical thermometer for measurements in electromagnetically induced heating. *In*: *Proceedings 1975 USNC/URSI Symposium. Johnson, C. C. and Shore, M. L. (eds). HEW Publication (FDA) 77–8011*, *11*: 338, 1976.

36. CHRISTENSEN, D. A. A new non-perturbing temperature probe using semiconductor band edge shift. *J. Bioengin.*, *1*: 541, 1977.

37. CHRISTENSEN, D. A. Experience with a four-probe non-perturbing temperature monitoring system. Presented at the Third International Symposium on Cancer Therapy by Hyperthermia, Drugs and Radiation, Fort Collins, 1980. Abstract book p. 57.

38. SHOLES, R. R. AND SMALL, J. G. FLUORESCENT DECAY THERMOMETER WITH BIOLOGICAL APPLICATIONS. *Rev. Scient. Instrum. 51*: 882, 1980.

39. SAMULSKI, T. AND SHRIVASTAVA, P. N. Photoluminescent thermometer probes: temperature measurements in microwave fields. *Science*, *208*: 193, 1980.

40. CAVATORTA, F., SCHOEN, P. E. AND SHERIDAN, J. P. An optical non-perturbing probe for temperature measurements in biological materials exposed to microwave radiation. Presented at Bioelectromagnetics Symposium, Seattle, Washington, June 1979, Abstract B-34, p. 491.

41. DEFICIS, A. AND PRIOU, A. Non-perturbing microprobes for measurement in electromagnetic fields. *Microwave J. 20:* 55, 1977.

42. DAKIN, J. P. AND KAHN, D. A. A novel fiber optics temperature probe. *Opt. Quan. Elec.*, *9:* 540, 1977.

43. HOLMES, D. E. Fiber optic probe for thermal profiling of liquids during crystal growth. *Rev. Scient. Instrum.*, *50:* 662, 1980.

44. BOWMAN, R. A probe for measuring temperature in radio-frequency heated material. *IEEE Trans. Microwave Theory Tech.*, *MTT-24:* 43, 1976.

45. LARSEN, L. E., MOORE, R. A., JACOBI, J. H., HALGAS, F. A. AND BROWN, P. V. A microwave compatible MIC temperature electrode for use in biological dielectrics. *IEEE Trans. Microwave Theory Tech.*, *MTT-27:* 673, 1979.

46. OLSEN, R. G. AND MOLINA, E. A. The non-metallic thermocouple: A differential-temperature probe for use in microwave fields. *Radio Sci. 14:* 81, 1979.

47. CAIN, C. A., CHEN, M. M., LOHLAM, K. AND MULLIN, J. The viscometric thermometer. *In*: *Physical Basis of Electromagnetic Interactions with Biological Tissues.* Taylor, L. S. and Cheung, A. Y. (eds). University of Maryland, College Park, 1978, p. 295.

48. GUY, A. W. Analysis of electromagnetic fields induced in biological tissues by thermodynamic studies on equivalent phantom models. *IEEE Trans. Microwave Theory Tech.*, *MTT-19:* 205, 1971.

49. CETAS, T. C., CONNOR, W. G. AND MANNING, M. R. Monitoring of tissue temperature during hyperthermia therapy. *Ann. NY Acad. Sci.*, *335:* 281, 1980.

50. MANNING, M. R., CETAS, T. C., MILLER, R. C., OLESON, J. R., CONNOR, W. G. AND GERNER, E. W. Clinical hyperthermia: Results of a phase I trial employing hyperthermia alone or in combination external beam or interstitial radiotherapy. *Cancer,* (in press), 1982.

51. CETAS, T. C. Practical thermometry with a thermographic camera: Calibration, transmittance and emittance measurements. *Rev. Sci. Instrum.*, *49:* 256, 1978.

52. RICHMOND, J. C. Physical standards of emittance and reflectance. *In*: *Radiative Transfer from Solid Materials.* Blau, H. and Fischer, H. (eds). Macmillan Co., New York, 1962, p. 142.

53. RICHMOND, J. C. Thermal radiation properties of ceramic materials, *In*: *Mechanical and Thermal Properties of Ceramics.* Wachtman, J. B. Jr., (ed). NBS Special Publication 303 Superintendent of Documents, U.S. Government Printing Office, Washington, D.C., 1969, p. 125.

54. WOLFE, W. L. AND NICODEMUS, F. E. Radiation theory. *In*: *Handbook of Military Infrared Technology.* Wolfe, W. L. (ed). Superintendent of Documents, U.S. Government Printing

Office, Washington, D.C. 1965, p. 3.

55. STEKETEE, J. Spectral emissivity of skin and pericardium, *Phys. Med. Biol.*, *18:* 686, 1973.
56. WATMOUGH, D. J., FOWLER, P. W. AND OLIVER, R. The thermal scanning of a curved isothermal surface: Implications for clinical thermography. *Phys. Med. Biol.*, *15:* 1, 1970.
57. LEWIS, D. W., GOLLER, H. O. AND TEATES, C. D. Apparent temperature degradation in thermograms of human anatomy viewed obliquely. *Diagnost. Radiol.*, *106:* 95, 1973.
58. VERMEIJ, G. F. The pyroelectric vidicon camera as a medical thermograph. *J. Med. Engin. Technol.*, *3:* 5, 1979.
59. SAMARAS, G. M., BLAUMANIS, O. R. AND VAN HORN H. W. Microprocessor-based thermal calibration and measurement system for thermotherapy research. (Accepted for publication) *Nat. Cancer Inst. Mono.* (in press), 1982.
60. SOSTMAN, H. E. Melting point of gallium as a temperature calibration standard. *Rev. Sci. Instrum.*, *48:* 127, 1977.
61. MANGUM, B. W. AND THORNTON, D. D. Determination of the triple point of gallium. *Metrologia 15:* 201, 1979.
62. THORNTON, D. D. The gallium melting-point standard: A determination of the liquid solid equilibrium temperature of pure gallium or the International Practical Temperature Scale of 1968. *Clin. Chem.*, *23:* 719, 1977.
63. SOSTMAN, H. E. The gallium melting-point standard: Its role in manufacture and quality control of electronic thermometers for the clinical laboratory. *Clin. Chem.*, *23:* 725, 1977.
64. MAGIN, R. L., STATLER, J. A. AND THORNTON, D. D. Inorganic salt hydrate transitions as temperature fixed points in biomedical thermometry, *J. Res. NBS, 86:* 181, 1981.
65. LELE, P. P. Induction of deep, local hyperthermia by ultrasound and electromagnetic fields. *Radiation Environ. Biophys. 17:* 205, 1980.
66. WELLS, P. N. T. *Biomedical Ultrasonics.* Academic Press, New York, 1977.
67. FRY, W. J. AND FRY, R. B. Determination of absolute sound levels and acoustic absorption coefficients by thermocouple probes—theory. *J. Acoust. Soc. Am.*, *26:* 294–310, 1954.
68. FRY, W. J. AND FRY, R. B. Determination of absolute sound levels and acoustic absorption coefficients by thermocouple probes—experiment. *J. Acoust. Soc. Am.*, *26:* 311–317, 1954.
69. STAUFFER, P. R. A magnetic induction system for inducing localized hyperthermia in brain tumors. M.S. Thesis, University of Arizona, 1979.
70. STAUFFER, P. R., CETAS, T. C. AND JONES, R. C. A system for producing localized hyperthermia in tumors through magnetic induction of ferromagnetic implants. *J. Nat. Cancer Inst.*, (Accepted).
71. SANDHU, T. S., BICHER, H. I. AND HETZEL, F. W. A realistic thermal dosimetry system. *Nat. Cancer Inst. Mono.* (in press), 1982.
72. MYERS, P. C., BARRETT, A. H. AND SADOWSKY, N. L. Microwave thermography of normal and cancerous breast tissue. *Ann. NY Acad. Sci.*, *335:* 443, 1980.
73. EDRICH, J., JOBE, W. E., CACAK, R. K., HENDEE, W. R., SMYTH, C. J., GAUTHERIE, M., GROS, C., ZIMMER, R., ROBERT, J., THOUVENOT, P., ESCANYE, J. M. AND ITTY, C. Imaging thermograms at centimeter and millimeter wavelengths. *Ann. NY Acad. Sci.*, *335:* 456, 1980.
74. SACHS, T. D. Non-invasive controlled heat deposition technique by ultrasound—a speculation. *The Proceedings of the International Symposium on Cancer Therapy by Hyperthermia and Radiation.* Robinson, J. E. and Wizenberg, M. J. (eds). American College of Radiology, Bethesda, MD, 1976, p. 209.
75. JOHNSON, S. A., GREENLEAF, J. F., RAJAGOPALAN, B., BAHN, R. C., BAXTER, B. AND CHRISTENSEN, D. High spatial resolution ultrasonic measurement techniques for characterization of static and moving tissues. *In: Ultrasonic Tissue Characterization II.* Linzer, M. (ed). NBS Spec. Publ. 525, 1979, p. 235.
76. BOWEN, T., CONNOR, W. G., NASONI, R. L., PIFER, A. E. AND SHOLES, R. R. Measurement of the temperature dependence of the velocity of ultrasound in soft tissues. *In: Ultrasonic Tissue Characterization II.* Linzer, M. (ed). NBS Spec. Publ. 525, 1979, p. 57.

3

Thermal Science for Physical Medicine[1]

K. MICHAEL SEKINS
ASHLEY F. EMERY

Nomenclature

a	radiation absorption coefficient
A	area (cross-sectional *or* surface)
Å	Angstrom (10^{-10} meters)
A_D	Dubois skin surface area
c	specific heat *or* speed of light
C	blood concentration of an arbitrary substance or entity *or* concentration of moisture (*e.g.*, on skin or in ar)
cal	calorie
d	differential symbol (*e.g.*, dT/dx)
D	diameter
$\mathscr{D}_w$	diffusion coefficient of water vapor in air
e	base of natural logarithms (2.7183)
E	energy (generalized) *or* radiative emissive power
E_b	blackbody radiative emissive power
erf	Gauss "error function"; depicted in figure 3.25
F	rate of blood flow [ml/min]
$F_{1\text{-}2}$	radiation shape factor from surface 1 to surface 2
f_b	mass-normalized rate of blood flow [ml/min $-$ 100 g]
g	local acceleration due to gravity
G	irradiation
Gr	Grashof Number
h	heat transfer coefficient
h_e	evaporative heat transfer coefficient as defined in Equation *29*
h_w	evaporative mass transfer coefficient of water vapor as defined in Equation *27b*

[1] This chapter is in part based on research supported by Research Grant #G008003029 from the National Institute of Handicapped Research, Department of Education, Washington, D.C. 20202.

h_w^*	evaporative mass transfer coefficient of water vapor as defined in Equation 27a
I	radiative intensity
J	Joule *or* radiosity
k	thermal conductivity
k_{eff}	effective thermal conductivity
L	distance *or* "characteristic" length *or* thickness
L_w	latent heat of water
ln	designates natural logarithm
m	mass *or* an exponent for forced convection in Equation 21
$\dot{M}$	rate of metabolic heat generation per unit mass
$\dot{M}_o$	basal rate of metabolic heat generation
MBF	muscle blood flow
$MM\%$	abbreviation for "ml/min − 100 g"
N	Newton (unit of force)
Nu	Nusselt Number
p	partial pressure *or* an exponent for natural convection in Equation 24
Pr	Prandtl Number
q	heat transfer rate
q''	heat flux (heat transfer rate per unit area)
q'''	internal heat generation (or dissipation) rate per unit volume
Q	thermal energy stored or gained by a system
Q_{10}	metabolic reaction rate factor defined in Equation 5a
r	radius *or* radial coordinate
R	thermal resistance
Re	Reynolds number
RH	relative humidity
R_w	Gas constant for water vapor
S	tissue content of any arbitrary substance or entity
Sc	Schmidt Number
t	time
T	temperature
T_f	"film" temperature: $(T_s + T_\infty)/2$
U	thermodynamic "internal" energy
V	volume of tissue *or* fluid stream velocity
W	Watt or thermodynamic work done by a system
x	x coordinate *or* depth position into a tissue
y	y coordinate
z	z coordinate

GREEK LETTERS

α	thermal diffusivity
α_r	radiative absorptivity
β	volume coefficient of expansion or parameter in Figure 3.22
δ	boundary layer thickness
∂	denotes partial derivative (*e.g.* $\partial T/\partial x$)
Δ	thickness (*e.g.*, Δx) *or* a change in a quantity (*e.g.* ΔT)
ϵ	radiative emissivity

γ	parameter in Figure 3.22
λ	wavelength of radiation
μ	micron (10^{-6} meters) *or* absolute viscosity
ν	fluid "kinematic" viscosity, μ/ρ
π	pi (3.1416)
ϕ	coordinate angle in spherical coordinate system (Equation *10c*) *or* shape factor angle as depicted in Figure 3.21.
ρ	density
ρ_r	radiative reflectivity
σ	Stefan-Boltzmann constant
Σ	denotes summation
θ	coordinate angle in either cylindrical (Equation *10b*) *or* spherical (Equation *10c*) coordinates
τ_r	radiative transmissivity
ω	weight fraction

SPECIAL SYMBOLS

$(\dot{\ })$	dot above a symbol indicates time rate of change of the quantity concerned
$(\bar{\ })$	bar over a symbol denotes a surface quantity which is averaged over its respective surface area

SUBSCRIPTS

a	arterial *or* denoting a substance "a"
abs	absolute (temperature)
b	blood *or* blackbody
c	convection
e	evaporation
f	denotes fluid film temperature T_f
hp	hot pack
i	initial *or* interface
m	metabolism
o	outer *or* surface
r	radiation *or* radial
s	surface *or* skin
sat	denotes saturation property (for water vapor)
seg	body segment (*e.g.*, arm or leg)
v	venous
vf	radiation view factor
w	water *or* wetted (*e.g.*, A_w)
x	x coordinate *or* depth position into a tissue
y	y coordinate
z	z coordinate
∞	denotes free stream or ambient conditions
λ	monochromatic (*i.e.*, at a specific wavelength)

Introduction

The therapeutic use of heating and cooling modalities today requires an ever-increasing sophistication on the part of the clinician. The complex thermophysiological responses of the body, when combined with an uninformed practice of thermal science, can lead on one hand to ill-founded, ineffective and even dangerous procedures, and on the other, to beneficial but poorly-understood treatment techniques which are not easily duplicated. The intent of this chapter is to provide an introduction to the basic principles and laws which describe the physical component of the body's thermal behavior, as contrasted with primarily biological phenomena such as neural and hormonal effects. The distinction between these two components is made clearer by noting that what are termed physical principles are those of thermodynamics and the science of heat transfer.

HEAT TRANSFER AND THERMODYNAMICS

Although the concept of heat (and cold, the relative absence of heat) has its roots in our basic sensory awareness and is probably among the most primordial concepts of humankind, its subtlety is such that it has only recently been understood and successfully described in a quantitative manner. In 1822, the French mathematician J.B.J. Fourier (1) published the mathematical theory which describes heat transfer by conduction. It was not until twenty or more years later that the notion of heat as a weightless, invisible fluid ("caloric") was discounted, and that heat was universally accepted to be a form of "energy." The nebulous concept of energy in the nineteenth century no doubt contributed to the mystery of heat. Here was an entity, defined by its capacity to do work, which had many varied manifestations: the potential energy of a suspended weight; the kinetic energy of the same weight in free-fall; the energy associated with pressure in a pipe or blood vessel, with the bonds of an organic molecule, with ions separated across a cell membrane, with any separation of charged particles in space, and so on. It should be made clear at the outset, however, that "heat" is not a form of energy per se, but rather is the name associated with a particular form of energy exchange.

Thermodynamics, the science dealing with the transformation of energy from one form to another and with the limits on such processes, defines two forms of energy in transit which occur without mass transfer: a. Energy exchange between two systems (bodies, masses, surfaces, etc.) which takes place only in relation to a temperature difference existing between them is said to be *heat transfer*. b. Energy exchange between such "closed" systems which is not a consequence of temperature difference is called *work*. Thus, the term "flow" when applied to heat is, strictly, incorrect since this confuses the entity exchanged with the name of the exchange process. Heat flow is colloquially accepted, however, and a convenient descriptive phrase which we shall also use. The specific entity which is exchanged during heat transfer is "thermal energy", also termed the thermodynamic "internal energy" U. This internal energy of matter is the summation of those energies whose forms tend to be randomly oriented and more or less hidden from macroscopic view. These forms of energy are associated with the kinetic and potential energies of the microscopic structural components of a substance: the molecular, atomic, nuclear, and electronic motions of translation, rotation, vibration, spin, etc., along with the various binding forces, dipole moments and such. Internal energy obviously excludes the kinetic and potential energies associated with the gross movement and position of a system as a whole and of the particles that comprise it.

By definition, the thermal energy of a system is "hidden", *i.e.*, not directly observable. The indirect observation commonly used is measurement of a system's "temperature." The concept of temperature, however, must be logically preceded by a discussion of thermal equilibrium and what is called the "zeroth law of thermodynamics." When two systems are placed together in total isolation from their environment (*i.e.*, free from all outside mechanical, electrtical, thermal, chemical, and electromagnetic influences) and all available observations and instruments (except thermometers) have determined that, after some time, changes no longer occur in either system (*e.g.*, in pressure, volume, etc.) as a consequence of their having been brought together, the systems are said to be in "thermal equilibrium" with each other. The zeroth law states the principle that if two separate systems are in thermal equilibrium with a third system, they are in thermal equilibrium with each other. Since many substances exhibit known and repeatable variations in their physical properties (*e.g.*, volume, electrical resistance or voltage, phase changes, etc.) as a function of changes in their level of internal energy, we are able to assign arbitrary scales and systems of units to these variations and to associate these units with levels of internal energy. When these "thermometric" substances (*e.g.*, mercury in glass columns, thermocouple junctions, thermistor semiconductors, liquid crystals, and so on) are placed in thermal equilibrium with systems whose internal energy we wish to quantify, we are able to assign unit values ("degrees") to their levels of internal energy, a quantity familiarly termed *temperature*. A discussion of the more practical aspects of thermometry and thermometric materials which are useful in biological temperature measurements is included in Chapter 2.

There exists a natural confusion between heat "transfer" and thermo-"dynamics" which, for the sake of semantic clarity and future discussion, should be addressed. Classical thermodynamics is not concerned with the details of an energy transformation process, but rather with the equilibrium states before and after the process and with the relationships between them. From a thermodynamic viewpoint, the amount of heat (thermal energy) ΔQ transferred during a process is simply the difference between the energy change of the system ΔE and the work done by the system ΔW. This approach considers neither the mechanism of heat exchange nor the time required for the process. It is the absence of time as a variable in thermodynamic analysis that demands a complimentary discipline, one focused on exchange rates and on the details of the physical mechanisms that influence them. Prediction of temperature, a primary coordinate in the thermodynamic description of a system, requires that the quantitative laws of energy propagation be known for the media of concern. The tools of the science of heat transfer provide such laws and the complimentary science necessary for rate quantification.

THE FIRST LAW OF THERMODYNAMICS

With the notable exception of nuclear effects ($E = mc^2$), energy is neither created nor destroyed. It is conserved and, as has been stated, may be transformed from one form to another. This universal observation is known as the first law of thermodynamics, a statement which governs all energy transformations, including those related to the human body. From this point forward, our discussion of changes in the energy state of the human thermal system will be limited to only those changes associated with the internal energy of the system, *i.e.*, $\Delta E = \Delta U$. The principle of the conservation of energy is often applied to a system or a portion thereof by forming a mathematical "energy balance." Stated in its simplest rate form for the human system,

$$\frac{dE}{dt} = \frac{dU}{dt} = \dot{Q} - \dot{W} \qquad (1)$$

where
$\dfrac{dE}{dt}$ ≡ Differential rate of internal energy increase in time t for the system (kinetic and potential energy of the body as a whole are ignored).

$\dot{Q}$ ≡ Net rate of thermal energy (heat) transferred into the body, including energy carried with incoming or outgoing mass and energy generated from heat sources within the body.

$\dot{W}$ ≡ Net rate of energy leaving the body by virtue of its doing work on its surroundings

From the standpoint of thermotherapy, the rate at which the body does external work is rarely of consequence: therefore $\dot{W} \approx 0$. Thermodynamically speaking, the human body is an "open system", meaning that material crosses its boundaries (food, drink, air, water vapor, feces, urine, and sweat) and consequently carries energy with it into and out of the body. For our purposes, however, the energy transport from all such modes of mass transfer is negligible, with the single exception of sweating; and here, only that sweat mass which evaporates is truly effective in transporting heat. More will be said of this later.

When energy is absorbed by a system, its temperature rises and we say the system "stores" thermal energy or heat. For equal temperatures, different substances store different amounts of energy E or, alternatively, require different amounts of thermal energy gain (or loss) ΔQ to undergo equal increases (or decreases) in temperature. The ability of a substance to store thermal energy is a unique characteristic (*i.e.*, "property") of that substance and is expressed as its *thermal capacitance* or *specific heat c*. Specific heat is defined by the thermal energy required to produce a unit temperature increase per unit mass, or

$$c \equiv \frac{\Delta Q}{m \cdot \Delta T} \tag{2}$$

where ΔQ is the heat required to produce a temperature change of ΔT degrees for a mass m. Expressing the internal energy change in terms of temperature change and again neglecting the external work ($\dot{W}$) done by the body, Equation *1* becomes

$$mc\frac{dT}{dt} = \dot{Q} \tag{3}$$

The value for the specific heat of a substance is normalized to that for water. A *calorie* is the quantity of heat necessary to raise the temperature of one gram of pure water one degree Celsius at 15°C (*i.e.*, from 14.5 to 15.5°C). Thus, water has a specific heat of unity in the cgs system of units.

Example 1

The "standard man" has a body mass of 68 kg, a basal metabolic heat production of about 72 kcal/hour and an averall average specific heat of 0.86 kcal/kg − °C (2). How rapidly will his body temperature rise, initially, if heat loss to the environment is precluded?

Solution

From Equation 3 we find

$$\frac{dT}{dt} = \frac{\dot{Q}}{mc} = \frac{72 \text{ kcal/hour}}{(68 \text{ kg})(0.86 \text{ kcal/kg} - °C)} = 1.23 \text{ °C/hour}$$

In the discussion and study of energy, heat transfer and thermophysiology, a number of different systems of units will be encountered, systems with which the clinician should be familiar. This is particularly true when considering that access to the literature of a variety of disciplines (medicine, physiology, engineering, etc.) spanning the last several decades may be necessary for a thorough understanding and skilled application of therapeutic heating and cooling. Table 3.1 presents the conversion equivalents for Systeme Internationale (SI), centimeter-gram-second (cgs) and Engineering units, the three sytems used most frequently in this field.

TABLE 3.1. *Conversion Factors for Units of the SI, cgs and Engineering Systems*

Quantity	Conversion Equivalents:		
	SI Units	cgs Units	Engineering Units
Length	1 meter (m) =	100 centimeter (cm) =	3.281 feet (ft)
Mass	1 kilogram (kg) =	1000 gram (g) =	2.205 pounds (1bm)
Force	1 Newton (N) =	10^5 dynes (dyne) =	0.2248 pounds (1bf)
Energy, heat	1 Joule (J) =	0.2389 calories (cal) =	9.479×10^{-4} BTU
Power, heat flow	1 Watt (W) =	$0.2389 \frac{cal}{sec}$ =	$3.412 \frac{BTU}{hr}$
Density	$1 \frac{kg}{m^3}$ =	$0.001 \frac{g}{cm^3}$ =	$0.06243 \frac{1bm}{ft^3}$
Thermal Conductivity	$1 \frac{W}{m - °C}$ =	$2.389 \times 10^{-3} \frac{cal}{sec - cm - °C}$ =	$0.5778 \frac{BTU}{hr - ft - °F}$
Specific Heat	$1 \frac{kJ}{kg - °C}$ =	$0.2389 \frac{cal}{g - °C}$ =	$0.2389 \frac{BTU}{1bm - °F}$
Viscosity (dynamic)[a]	$1 \frac{kg}{m - sec}$ =	$10 \frac{g}{cm - sec}$ =	$2419 \frac{1bm}{hr - ft}$
Thermal diffusivity (and kinematic viscosity[b])	$\frac{m^2}{sec}$ =	$10^4 \frac{cm^2}{sec}$ =	$10.76 \frac{ft^2}{sec}$
Temperature	degrees Celsius ≡ °C; Kelvin ≡ °K; Fahrenheit ≡ °F; Rankine ≡ °R		
	$°C = \frac{5}{9} (°F - 32)$; $°K = °C + 273.2$; $°R = °F + 459.7$; $°K = \frac{5}{9} °R$		

[a] The cgs unit of dynamic or absolute viscosity μ (gm/cm - sec) is defined as the "poise" (named after the French physiologist Poiseuille); 1 centipoise = 0.01 poise.

[b] Kinematic viscosity (ν) is often expressed in stokes (and centistokes). The kinematic viscosity in stokes is simply the dynamic viscosity (in poise) divided by the fluid density (in g/cm³).

THE SECOND LAW OF THERMODYNAMICS

This law has important implications with regard to the thermal behavior of the human body. As previously stated, the first law of thermodynamics states that every time energy changes form or is transferred from one system to another, the total amount of energy remains constant. The second law is based on the observation that every time energy changes form or is transferred, its potential for producing "useful" work is reduced—irreversibly and forever. Thus, energy is both conserved and degraded in quality simultaneously. The ramifications of this principle are many. At the molecular level, all spontaneous physical processes tend toward the maximum disorder consistent with the total energy of the system, the familiar entropy-maximum principle. The main form that this increase in disorder takes is an increase in random particle motions on atomic and molecular levels, *i.e.*, the production of heat. In the human body, while mechanical energy, electrical energy, and chemical free energy are readily converted to heat, the reverse does not occur. This is because the second law requires that for the efficient conversion of heat to work, a large temperature difference must exist; the body, however, is virtually an isothermal (single temperature) system. In fact, the only form of energy which animals can effectively convert to work is that inherent in specific molecular configurations of certain ingested substances, *i.e.*, the chemical free energy of food. The degradation of ingested chemical free energy is such that typically only 45 percent of the food energy intake is made available for "biologically useful" work; 55 percent is normally converted directly to heat. Of the portion available for work, a maximum of about half can be converted into "external" work (*i.e.*, skeletal muscle contraction). This means that since all "internal" biological work is indirectly converted to heat as a "waste product", at least approximately 75 percent of the chemical free energy ingested eventually appears as heat lost to the environment (3).

PHYSICAL MECHANISMS OF HEAT TRANSPORT

Most readers will be familiar with the three primary modes of heat transfer: conduction, radiation, and convection. Since only conduction and radiation transfer energy solely as a result of temperature difference, they are the only fundamental mechanisms of heat exchange in the strictest sense. Convection, which depends on mass transport as well as on temperature difference for its operation, does, however, transport thermal energy. Consequently, the use of the phrase "heat transfer by convection" has become generally accepted. The loss of water from the skin and lungs by evaporation also carries thermal energy. Thus, in the context of the body, it is convenient to treat evaporation as a fourth basic physical mechanism of heat transfer.

It has been the convention in some physical medicine circles to designate "conversion" as a fifth mechanism of heat transport, referring to the transmission of various forms of energy (*e.g.*, mechanical, electrical, or electromagnetic) into the body where they appear primarily as heat. As the name implies, this process (which includes all forms of diathermy) "converts" one form of energy into another (non-thermal into thermal), rather than transporting thermal energy from one location to another. For the purposes of our analysis, conversion methods will be treated as sources of heat within the tissue itself, as thermal energy absorbed volumetrically, and will be dealt with as such throughout the chapter.

Heat *conduction* is the mechanism of internal energy exchange between areas of different temperatures whereby the exchange of kinetic energy from particle to particle is accomplished by direct molecular collision (and by the drift of free electrons in the case of metals). This flow of energy passes from higher energy molecules (hotter regions) to lower energy ones (colder regions), as required by the second law of thermodynamics. The distinguishing feature of conduction is that it takes place within the boundaries of a body, or across the boundary of one body into another placed in contact with the first, without appreciable displacement of the matter making up the body. A short metal bar heated on one end will eventually become hot at its other end. This is a simple example of conduction. The application of hot or cold packs to the skin surface are said to be "conduction" heating or cooling modalities. The laws governing conduction can be expressed in concise mathematical terms, and often provide suitable analytical solutions to simplified problems of physiological heat transfer.

Convection is the term applied to the heat transfer mechanism which occurs in a fluid (blood, air, water, etc.) due to gross movements within the mass of the fluid. Of particular importance is the transfer of energy from the fluid to solid surfaces in contact with it. The actual process of energy transfer from one fluid particle to another, or to solid surfaces, remains one of conduction, but the energy is transported from one point in space to another primarily by the displacement of the fluid itself. If the fluid motion is due to density gradients created by temperature differences in the fluid mass, the process is termed *free convection* or *natural convection*. If the motion is due to some external means (*e.g.*, a fan or the wind) the process is called *forced convection*. Pure conduction is rarely observed in a fluid due to ease with which even small temperature differences initiate free convection currents. The mathematical description of convective heat transfer is quite complex due to the necessity of coupling the laws of fluid motion with those of heat conduction. Convection analysis is therefore usually composed of a blend of sophisticated mathematics and empirical correlations.

Thermal radiation describes the electromagnetic radiation which is emitted from the surface of a body whose surface temperature is above absolute zero. This radiation occurs primarily in the infrared (IR) band (Figure 3.1) from wavelengths of about 10^{-5} cm to 10^{-2} cm ($0.1 - 100$ μ, or $10^3 - 10^6$Å). Any radiation incident upon a surface is either: a. reflected by the surface; b. transmitted into or through it; and/or c. absorbed by it. Absorbed radiation in the thermal spectrum excites the absorbing body thermally, and thereby serves to transfer heat from the emitting surface to the absorbing surface. Unlike conduction or convection, radiant heat exchange, as for any electromagnetic radiation, does not require a medium of transport. In many instances, however, there may be a separating medium between the emitting and absorbing surfaces which (often minimally) affects the radiant exchange; such is usually the case with air. The radiant energy transfer between two radiating surfaces is one of continuous mutual emission and absorption such that the net exchange is from the hotter to the colder body. In the case of radiant thermal equilibrium, an energy exchange occurs, but with a net exchange of zero.

Evaporation, the transformation from the liquid state to the gaseous

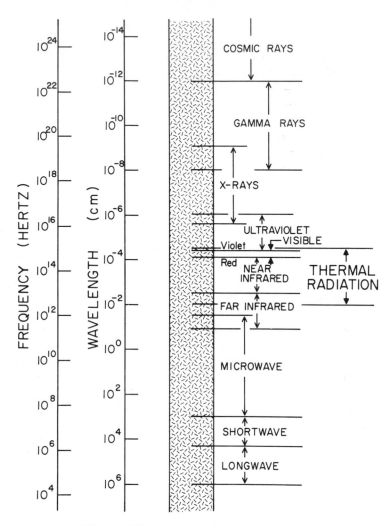

Fig. 3.1. The electromagnetic spectrum.

state, requires thermal energy for such a transition. Thus, when water vaporizes from a surface of the body, be it the skin or internal pulmonary surfaces, the heat required to produce the transition is absorbed from the surface, thereby cooling it. Some skin water loss to the environment occurs by simple passive diffusion through the skin itself; sweating, however, involves active secretion of water from specialized glands (eccrine glands). The expired air leaving the lungs is almost completely saturated with water vapor evaporated from the lining of the respiratory tract. For an individual resting in a thermally neutral (comfortable) environment, the sum of the heat loss from both transcutaneous diffusion and respiratory ventilation ("insensible" evaporation) is only about 15 percent of the total heat loss. In warm environments, however, evaporation can become the dominant mechanism of heat loss because sweat secretion greatly increases the amount of water available for evaporation at the skin surface. The sweating mechanism can also have a significant effect in applications of therapeutic heating of the body.

THERMOPHYSICAL PROPERTIES OF BIOLOGICAL TISSUES

Solution of actual thermotherapy problems requires numerical values for the physical properties of the substances under consideration. The important properties in conduction are thermal conductivity, density, and specific heat. Convection problems also depend on these properties, but due to the motion of the fluid involved, fluid viscosity also becomes important. The important properties in radiation and in both free and natural convection will be discussed in a later section; at this point it is sufficient to discuss conductive properties alone. Table 3.2 presents properties of various non-

TABLE 3.2. *Thermophysical Properties of Some Non-Biological Materials*

Material	Thermal Conductivity k		Specific Heat c		Density ρ	Thermal Diffusivity $\alpha = \frac{k}{\rho c}$
	$\frac{W}{m-°C}$	$\frac{cal}{sec-cm-°C} \times 10^3$	$\frac{kJ}{kg-°C}$	$\frac{cal}{g-°C}$	$\frac{g}{cm^3}$ (or $\frac{kg}{m^3} \times 10^{-3}$)	$\frac{cm^2}{sec} \times 10^3$ (or $\frac{m^2}{sec} \times 10^7$)
Air	0.009246	0.0221	1.01	0.240	0.00118	222.
Aluminum	204.0	487.0	0.904	0.216	2.71	890.
Brass	104.	248.0	0.385	0.092	8.52	317.
Concrete	0.934	2.23	0.837	0.200	2.31	4.90
Copper	387.	925.0	0.402	0.096	8.94	1040.0
Cotton fabric (37°C)	0.0796	0.190	≈0.167	≈0.040	≈0.160	≈1.50
Glass, plate	1.09	2.60	0.770	0.184	2.52	5.60
Ice	2.21	5.28	1.93	0.460	0.913	12.6
Paraffin	--	--	≈2.72[a]	≈0.65	≈0.90[b]	--
Paraffin oil	--	--	1.88[a]	≈0.45	--	--
Petroleum jelly	--	--	1.88[a]	≈0.45	--	--
Plexiglas	15.5	37.0	1.306	0.312	1.19	100.
Rubber	0.156	0.372	2.01	0.480	1.20	0.640
Silver	405.	966.	0.247	0.059	10.5	1560.
Steam	251	0.599	1.89	0.451	0.000596	223.
Steel, mild	45.0	107.	0.465	0.110	7.85	124.
Steel, stainless	13.8	33.0	0.465	0.110	7.91	37.9
Teflon	3.48	8.30	1.01	0.24	2.18	15.9
Water (15°C)	0.595	1.42	4.19	1.0	0.999	1.36

Unless otherwise specified all properties are at one atmosphere pressure and 25°C. Values converted from those of references 4 and 5.

[a] Specific heats from ref 20; the heat of fusion (melting heat) for paraffin is 35 kcal/kg and the melting point range is 49 - 63°C [6].

[b] Paraffin density ranges from 0.896 - 0.925 g /cm³ as a solid.

biological materials. In general, thermal conductivities of solids are about 100 times those of liquids, which in turn are about 100 times those of gases.

In employing thermal conductivity values, and other thermophysical properties as well, it is important to note the conditions of applicability (temperature, pressure, direction of heat flow relative to orientation of the material's components and fibers, etc.) of the property values. In regard to biological properties, this is especially important; indeed, it is often valuable to know the specific experimental techniques used in the property measurements. It is well known, for instance, that blood flow plays a significant role in heat transport within human tissue. Since it is difficult to separate heat exchange occurring by conduction from that of convection due to perfusion, many investigators report "effective" or "apparent" conductivity values which include a blood flow contribution. The *in vivo* thermal conductivity measurements of Reader (7) assess the effect of skin cooling on the effective thermal conductivity (k_{eff}) of superficial tissues of the lumbar region. As such, they provide a means for approximating the magnitude of this convective component in "apparent" conductivity values. Figure 3.2 displays the results from his steady state measurements of conductivity versus depth in a normal young adult male. The data indicate a progressively diminishing k_{eff} profile with decreasing skin temperature. The profiles with skin temperatures below 18.2°C show that the subcutaneous and muscle temperatures reach steady state levels which correspond to minimal blood flow rates, at which point the "effective" values approach more or less "absolute" values for the thermal conductivity of the tissue alone; specifically, $k_{eff} \rightarrow k$. Keller and Seiler (8) have mathematically modeled the effects of perfusion and metabolic heat generation on k_{eff} of superficial tissues and have shown that, under resting conditions, the metabolic influence on the apparent thermal conductivity of these tissues is minimal. They conclude that, while perfusion may vary by about two orders of magnitude, k_{eff} will not vary due to changes in perfusion by more than a factor of 4. In addition, these authors note that some of the variations in k_{eff} of peripheral tissues are due to variations in the degree to which arterial blood is pre-cooled by venous blood returning from the surface layers. (This will be discussed later as counter-current heat exchange).

Table 3.3 shows thermophysical properties for many human tissues, both excised and *in vivo* values. The conductivities reported for skin and fat are taken from perfused tissue and thus, represent effective values. For this reason, a range of values is given with the implicit assumption that the lower values reported approach the absolute tissue conductivity k.

The thermal properties of tissues are also highly affected by their relative content of fat, protein and water. Poppendiek *et al.* (9) proposed a weighted average relationship for k which takes into account a tissue's weight fractions of fat (ω_f), protein (ω_p), and water (ω_W), its respective constituent densities

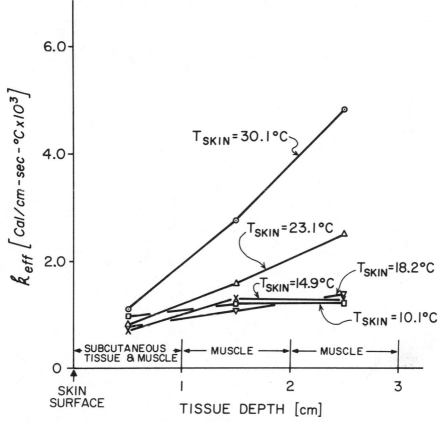

Fig. 3.2. The variation of the effective thermal conductivity k_{eff} of superficial tissues of the lumbar region during cooling, from Reader (7). The data, taken from steady state temperature versus depth profiles, are displayed as "layer values" in which the average values for each of the three tissue layers, 0–1 mm, 1–2 mm, and 2–3 mm are plotted at the midpoint of the respective layers. The outer layer is composed of skin, fat, and some muscle, while the deeper two layers are composed of muscle only.

$(\rho_f, \rho_p,$ and $\rho_w)$ and thermal conductivities (k_f, k_p, k_w). This relationship is

$$k = \rho \left[\frac{k_f \omega_w}{\rho_f} + \frac{k_p \omega_p}{\rho_p} + \frac{k_w \omega_w}{\rho_w} \right] \qquad (4)$$

where ρ is the resultant average density of the tissue. Cooper and Trezek (13) have shown that Equation 4 is in good agreement (within 5 percent) with k values measured on nearly fresh, well-preserved excised human organ tissue. The reader will note that one implication of Equation 4 is that thermal conductivity will vary with increasing or decreasing percentage of

TABLE 3.3. *Thermophysical Properties of Human Tissues and Organs* *

Tissue	Qualifications	Thermal Conductivity k $\frac{W}{m - °C}$	$\frac{cal}{sec - cm - °C}$ x 10^3	Specific Heat c $\frac{kJ}{kg - °C}$	$\frac{cal}{g - °C}$	Density ρ $\frac{g}{cm^3}$ (or $\frac{kg}{m^3}$ x 10^{-3})	Thermal Diffusivity α $\frac{cm^2}{sec}$ x 10^3 (or $\frac{m^2}{sec}$ x 1C
Skin:[a]	k_{eff} ("very warm")	2.80	6.68				
	k_{eff} ("cool")	0.545	1.30				
	k_{eff} ("upper 2 mm")	0.376	0.898	3.77[11]	0.9	1.00[11]	0.997
	k_{eff} ("cold hand")	0.335	0.800				
	k_{eff} ("normal hand")	0.960	2.29				
Subcutaneous Fat:	pure fat	0.190[13]	0.45	2.30[14]	0.55	0.85[11]	0.962
	k_{eff} (high values)	0.450[16]	0.90				
Muscle:	living muscle	0.642[16]	1.53[16]	3.75[17]	0.895[17]	1.05[11]	1.62
	excised; fresh	0.545[9]	1.30[18]	3.47[18]	.83 [18]	1.05[11]	1.49
Bone:[b]	cortical b.	2.28	5.45	1.59	0.38	1.7	8.43
	cancellous b.	0.582	1.39	1.59	0.38	1.3	2.81
	"average" b.	1.16	2.78	1.59	0.38	1.5	4.88
Blood:[c]	whole blood, Hct = 40%	0.549	1.31	3.64	0.87	1.05	1.43
	Plasma	0.599	1.43	3.93	0.94	1.03	1.48
	water (37°C)	0.628	1.50	4.19	1.00	1.00	1.50
Organs:[d]							
Kidney	excised, near fresh	0.544	1.30	3.89	0.930	1.05	1.33
Heart	excised; near fresh	0.586	1.40	3.72	0.890	1.06	1.48
Liver	excised; near fresh	0.565	1.35	3.60	0.860	1.05	1.50
Lung	excised (bovine)	0.282[9]	0.674[9]	3.72	0.888[11]	0.603[9]	1.26
Brain	excised; near fresh	0.528	1.26	3.68	0.880	1.05	1.36
Abdomen	"abdomen core"	0.544	1.30[11]	3.70	0.883[11]	1.05	1.40
Whole body (average)				3.56[2]	0.86		

* Numerical superscripts indicate the number of the reference from which the property value was taken.

[a] All skin properties from ref. 10, except as indicated by superscripts.

[b] All bone properties from ref. 11.

[c] All blood constituent properties from ref. 12.

[d] All organ properties from ref. 13, except as indicated by superscripts.

water in tissue. This influence is distinct from changes in apparent conductivity due to the convective effects of perfusion, yet it is certainly a function of blood flow. The thermal conductivities measured by Buettner (19) emphasize the need for particular care in interpreting reported thermal conductivity values of skin. By measuring the transient temperature response of the skin to a constant magnitude radiant energy (see Equation *51*), Buettner recorded conductivity variations with depth in one-dimensional conduction (perpendicular to the skin) as shown in Figure 3.3. As demonstrated, the dry, insulative surface region of the epidermis (stratum cor-

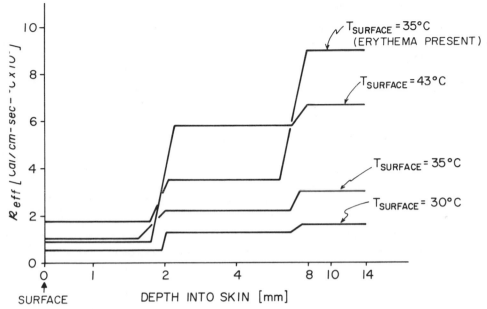

Fig. 3.3. The variation of thermal conductivity in the skin as a function of depth and steady state skin surface temperature, from Buettner (19). *Horizontal lines* indicate average values measured over the skin layer concerned. Note that the abscissa is not logarithmic from 0 to 1 mm. The surface layers show a consistent conductivity below that for water (except where erythema was present), while the deeper layers increase with water content and blood flow.

neum) has a thermal conductivity which is fairly constant, while in deeper regions within the skin, the thermal conductivity increases markedly with skin temperature, thus varying according to perfusion and water content. Vendrik and Vos (20) have proposed a thermal conductivity relationship which increases linearly with depth (to a depth of 1.3 mm) for the most superficial skin region.

SOURCES OF HEAT GENERATION WITHIN TISSUE

An energy balance applied to a tissue system requires knowing the heat generated within the tissue volume itself, as well as the rate at which energy is transferred across its boundaries. There are several processes which cause heat to be generated within the tissue volume, but from the standpoint of heat transfer analysis all such thermogenic processes may be treated identically; that is, they may be consolidated in an additive fashion into a heat source term in the tissue energy balance equation. From a physical medicine point of view, these sources may be chemical, mechanical, electrical, or electromagnetic in origin. In addition, blood flow may also be treated as a contributing source.

Chemical heat production: the only source of heat generation indigenous to the body is of course the heat produced as a by-product of *metabolism*. Because the metabolic functions of various tissues differ, some produce more heat per unit volume (q_m''') than others. In addition, because metabolism variation is one of the chief mechanisms for temperature homeostasis, metabolic heat generation can be a strong function of environmental factors. Factors such as diet, body type, age, sex, and activity level also influence metabolic heat production. Table 3.4 shows a typical range of metabolic heat generation rates for human tissues.

Metabolism, like any chemical reaction, is accelerated by an increase in temperature, provided that the higher temperature does not produce inhibitive alterations in the reactants or catalysts; the denaturing of enzymes is an example of such an inhibition in the human body. The ratio of reaction

TABLE 3.4. *Typical Metabolic Heat Generation Rates of Various Tissues and Organs*

Tissue	Anatomical Location and Qualifications	Metabolic Heat Generation		Reference No.
		$\frac{\text{Watts}}{\text{kg}}$	$\frac{\text{cal}}{\text{sec - g}} \times 10^4$	
Skin:	trunk and limbs	1.00	2.40	11
	face and neck	1.07	2.57	11
Subcutaneous Tissue	fat	0.00405	0.0097	11
	subcutaneous tissue of limbs at rest in ambient temperatures of:			
	25°C	0.380	0.91	16
	30°C	0.317	0.76	16
	35°C	0.317	0.76	16
Muscle:	resting skeletal muscle	0.67	1.6	11
	quadriceps muscle; ave. value during maximal voluntary contractions	54 ± 8.5 (S.D.)	129 ± 20.3	17
Bone:	range of metabolism in marrow of human humerus; estimated from perfusion of Table III and assumption of 4.57 ml O_2 per MM% of perfusion (see ref. 11).	0.051 to 0.103	0.123 to 0.246	21
Organs:	Brain	11.	26.4	22
	Heart	33.	79.3	22
	Kidney	20.	48.0	22
	Liver	6.7	16.1	22

rate constants for a reaction occurring at two temperatures ten degrees Celsius apart is called the "Q_{10}" of the reaction. The increase in metabolic heat production by a temperature increase of ΔT °C is quantiatively described by Van't Hoff's law:

$$\frac{\dot{M}}{\dot{M}_0} = (Q_{10})^{\Delta T/10} \qquad (5a)$$

where $\dot{M}$ is the metabolic heat generation rate at the new, elevated temperature, and $\dot{M}_0$ is that for basal metabolism within the physiological range $2.3 \leq Q_{10} \leq 2.9$ (23). This law corresponds roughly to a 10 percent increase in heat generation per degree temperature rise ΔT; consequently, a frequently used approximation to Equation 5a is

$$\frac{\dot{M}}{\dot{M}_0} = (1.1)^{\Delta T} \qquad (5b)$$

Mechanical, electrical, and electromagnetic heat production: The absorption of the various diathermic energies by tissues constitute, in effect, additional "sources" of heat generation within tissues. The detailed examination of the physical mechanisms of heat generation by such mechanical, electrical and electromagnetic means is reserved for subsequent chapters pertaining to each respective modality. For now, a few general points about diathermic heating will suffice.

The intensity of energy delivery to a tissue site by shortwave or microwave diathermy is a function of various tissue electrical characteristics; similarly, acoustic properties influence the intensity of energy deposition in an ultrasonic tissue field. The conversion of delivered power into an increase in tissue temperature, however, depends upon specific heat and density via Equation 3. A volume of fat, for example, will have approximately twice the temperature increase as an equal volume of muscle for equal amounts of absorbed energy ($1.8 \leq (\rho c_{muscle}/\rho c_{fat}) \leq 2.0$). The energy deposition or absorption patterns produced by a particular modality are usually given in terms of the spatial distribution of temperature which results from treatment, again via Equation 3, and are often expressed as "relative heating" patterns. These patterns are the temperature-depth profiles which result during "primary heating", that is, before the effects of conduction are seen. The units of relative heating are often normalized to conditions at the skin surface, i.e., $T_{skin} = 1.0$. Because of the difficulty of measuring in vivo heating without the distorting effects of conduction and blood flow response, most relative heating patterns are obtained experimentally from excised tissues, from tissue-surrogate models (phantoms), or are calculated theoretically.

BLOOD FLOW AS HEAT SOURCE/SINK

On the basis of the definitions of heat transfer already presented, it is evident that heat is primarily exchanged between blood and tissue by forced convection; this process occurs primarily on the capillary level, due to the large ratio of heat exchange surface area (capillary wall) to the volume of the convective fluid (blood). For any quantity which is exchanged between blood and a tissue volume V large enough to be assumed uniform (*i.e.*, sufficiently large to avoid excessive statistical fluctuations—Perl (24) selects a tissue volume of 0.1 mm^3 as being sufficient), a Fick principle balance for the tissue volume takes the form

$$\frac{dS}{dt} = F_a C_a - F_v C_v \tag{6}$$

This states that the rate of change of the quantity S of the substance in volume V due to perfusion equals the rate of influx of the entity (F_a = rate of arterial input blood flow; C_a = concentration of the entity in arterial blood) minus the rate of outflow (F_v and C_v being the venous, *i.e.*, exit, rate of blood flow and concentration, respectively). For the case of heat (thermal energy) storage ($S = Q$), the energy analog to concentration is $\rho_b c_b T$, where ρ_b and c_b are the density and specific heat of blood, respectively. In steady state perfusion (excluding net fluid volume shifts in the tissue such as might occur in transient edema for instance), $F_a = F_v$ and the energy balance, normalized on a unit volume basis, becomes

$$\frac{d(Q/V)}{dt} = q_b''' = f_b \rho_b c_b [T_a - T_v] \tag{7a}$$

where q_b''' is the volumetric heat absorption ($T_a > T_v$) or dissipation rate ($T_a < T_v$), and $f_b = F/V$ is the specific blood flow rate, conventionally expressed in mass-normalized units (ml blood/min-100 g tissue, or simply, MM%). Table 3.5 shows representative perfusion rates of various tissues and organs of the body under basal and a few specific hyperemic conditions. In addition, the elevated perfusion levels which may be achieved by diathermic heating of muscle tissue are shown in Figure 3.4, which displays data relating local peak muscle temperatures to the local blood flow in response to such heating occurring at the time of peak temperature.

The use of Equation *7a* permits the complex convective interaction between blood flow and tissue to be modeled simply as another source/sink term (q_b''') in the tissue energy balance (see Equation *16*). The realm of conditions under which its application is valid, however, is somewhat controversial (34, 35). The primary shortcomings of such a representation for blood flow heat transfer are that the directional characteristics of tissue perfusion are somewhat oversimplified, and the thermal effects of large and medium size vessels are ignored. Equation *7a* is predicated on two primary assumptions: first, in passing through the tissue volume, arterial blood is assumed to achieve complete thermal equilibrium with the tissue at temperature T. Second, no discernible heat exchange is assumed to occur in the

TABLE 3.5. *Typical Blood Perfusion Rates of Various Tissues and Organs*

Tissue	Anatomical Locations and Qualifications		Specific Flow Rate f_b in MM% (ml/min - 100 g)	Reference No.
Skin:	foot (dorsal surface, normal resting flow)		14.3 ± 2.6 (S.D.)	25
	calf (normal resting flow)		10.6 ± 1.3 "	"
	thigh " " "		9.8 ± 2.6 "	"
	arms " " . "		8.39	11
	hands " " "		20.07	"
	abdomen " " "		8.65	"
	thorax " " "		6.45	"
	head " " "		42.9	"
	face " " "		70.3	"
	forearm; hyperemia (reaction to ultraviolet radiation, "fully developed redness")		55.3 ± 11.2 (S.D.)	26
	forearm; reactive hyperemia ("peak value, rough approximation")		280.0	27
Subcutaneous Fat:	thigh adipose tissue; 1 subject; thickness	11 mm	5.6	28[a]
	" " " " "	20 mm	2.0	"
	" " " " "	43 mm	0.9	"
	abdomen " " ; several subjects; "	10 - 29 mm	3.04 ± 2.09 (S.D.)	"
	" " " " "	30 - 49 mm	2.15 ± 1.22 "	"
	" " " " "	> 40 mm	1.84 ± 0.71 "	"
Muscle:	anterior calf, resting flow		2.75 ± 0.65 (S.D.)	29[b]
	" thigh, " "		2.6 ± 1.0 "	30
	forearm; " " "		3.2 ± 1.4 "	27
	calf: reactive hyperemia, peak value		54.9 ± 11.6 "	29
	forearm; " " " "		50.3 ± 19.4 "	27
	anterior thigh; hyperemia in response to microwave diathermy (see fig. 4)		36.0	31
Joint:	knee, average value for skin temperature of 30°C		1.33	32
	" " " " " " " 35°C		2.92	"
Bone:	range of flow in human humerus (estimated from data of Ref. 21); flow in marrow only.		0.33 - 0.67	21
Organ:	brain		54.0	22
	heart		84.0	"
	kidney		420.0	"
	liver		57.7	"

[a] Comments in ref. 33 indicate that these fat values are possibly 20% low on the average.

[b] This is a mean value first taken from ref. 29, then increased 25% due to the systematic underestimation discussed in ref. 30.

arterial vascular tree prior to capillary level transport. Chato (36) has shown that blood flowing in capillaries equilibrates with surrounding tissue within two diameter-lengths downstream of the entrance point of the capillary. On the other hand, he finds that the blood temperature in large vessels virtually never approaches that of surrounding tissues, but that intermediate and small-artery blood approaches the surrounding tissue temperature to varying degrees. Because some heat transfer does in fact take place prior to

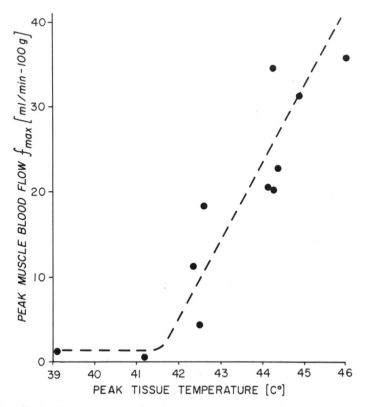

Fig. 3.4. Perfusion rates occurring in the quadriceps muscles at the time of peak temperature in response to microwave diathermy, from Sekins *et al.* (31). The elevation from basal levels of blood flow to the peak values shown occurred over about 60 to 90 seconds, in most cases, beginning after the tissue temperature exceeded threshold values corresponding to the respective peak temperature values shown.

capillary level circulation, the constant value assigned for T_a is frequently below 37.0°C, the deep core temperature, particularly for blood flow in the limbs. Pennes (37) employs $T_a = 36.25$°C for blood flow in the forearm. Incorporating these last assumptions, Equation 7a becomes

$$q_b''' = f_b \rho_b c_b (T_a - T) \qquad (7b)$$

Implicit in this development are the additional assumptions of constant thermal properties and homogeneous, isotropic tissues. The merits and shortcomings of these assumptions are discussed further elsewhere (24, 38, 39).

For most cases of heat transfer to, from and within physiological systems, such simplifications as the above, plus others, are required for a manageable analysis and clear interpretation of the role of the various parameters. In cases where the assumptions of constant properties, regular geometry, simple boundary conditions, and steady state behavior are justified, closed form, analytical solutions will often be possible and quite useful. For more complex thermotherapy situations, however, fewer assumptions can be used to simplify analysis, resulting in more complicated mathematical operations. For these cases, computer (numerical) solutions to the resulting energy equations are preferred; These approaches are presented in greater detail in Chapter 4.

The Laws of Heat Transfer

The following sections present an introduction to the basic mathematical relationships of heat transfer. For the sake of brevity, much mathematical detail has been omitted, and to reduce the level of abstraction, simplified specific examples are presented. In those circumstances where greater facility in applying the principles and a deeper understanding of the mathematics is sought, the reader is encouraged to consult the literature and the many basic texts on heat transfer (4, 5, 40, 41).

CONDUCTION

One-Dimensional Steady State Conduction

The basic relationship describing conductive heat transfer in a solid, as set down by Fourier in 1822 (1), (see Figure 3.5) states that for steady state conduction, q_x, the rate of heat transmission in the x-direction per unit cross-sectional area A, is proportional to the temperature gradient existing in the same direction, *i.e.*,

$$\frac{q_x}{A} \sim \frac{T_1 - T_2}{\Delta x} = \frac{\Delta T}{\Delta x} \tag{8a}$$

The constant of proportionality, k, is termed the *thermal conductivity* of the material. Expressed in differential form, Fourier's law, which defines k, is

$$q_x = -k\,A\,\frac{dT}{dx} \tag{8b}$$

where the negative sign is a convention adopted so that "positive" heat will flow in a direction "down" the temperature gradient, that is from a higher to a lower temperature.

Equations *8a* and *8b* are the first of many such laws encountered in energy exchange which have the general form

$$\text{Rate of Transfer} = \frac{\text{Driving Force}}{\text{Resistance}}$$

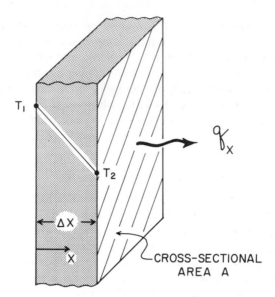

Fig. 3.5. Heat conduction in a planar slab.

or alternatively

Rate of Transfer = Conductance × Driving Force

These forms resemble Ohm's law for D.C. electrical circuits and prove themselves to be powerful tools in the solution of many heat transfer problems.

Example 2

A composite slab made of different materials a and b has surface temperatures T_1 and T_2 as shown in Figure 3.6a. The thermal conductivities are k_a and k_b, and the thicknesses Δx_a and Δx_b, respectively. Assuming that both materials are passive, *i.e.*, no internal heat generation, and that a steady state exists, let us develop an expression for the heat transfer rate per unit area, the so-called *heat flux* $q'' = q/A$, across the double-layered slab.

Solution

The Fourier Equations *8a* and *8b* cannot be used directly across the bilayered material since the thermal conductivity abruptly changes at the interface. Calling the unknown interface temperature T_i and writing Fourier's law for each layer individually,

$$q_a'' = k_a \frac{(T_1 - T_i)}{\Delta x_a} \quad \text{and} \quad q_b'' = k_b \frac{(T_i - T_2)}{\Delta x_b}$$

In the steady state, no changes in the temperature gradient occur with time;

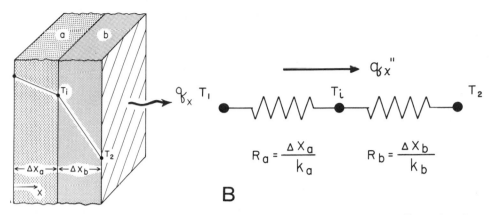

Fig. 3.6. *a*, Conduction in a composite slab; *b*, Thermal circuit for one-dimensional conduction in a bi-layered planar composite material.

and the rates of heat flux in and out of the interface are the same. Thus, $q_a'' = q_b'' = q''$; and the above equations constitute a system of two equations and two unknowns. Eliminating T_i,

$$q'' = \frac{T_1 - T_2}{\left(\dfrac{\Delta x_a}{k_a}\right) + \left(\dfrac{\Delta x_b}{k_b}\right)}$$

Note that this solution is analogous in form to Ohm's law, where q'' is the analog to current, $T_1 - T_2 = \Delta T$ may be identified with the driving potential difference, and $\Delta x_a/k_a$ and $\Delta x_b/k_b$ represent two resistances in series as shown in Figure 3.6*b*. Treating heat transfer problems as "thermal circuits" usually simplifies analysis greatly. For simple one-dimensional, steady-state conduction, the total heat flow q remains constant. The flux q'', however, will usually vary throughout the conducting material, according to geometry and the coordinate system used. While in the case of one-dimensional flow in rectangular geometry q'' remains constant, for heat flow in the radial direction in a cylinder it is the product rq'' which is constant; and for spherical coordinates r^2q'' remains constant. Figure 3.7 shows the passive, steady-state, one-dimensional heat transfer formulae, temperature profiles, and thermal resistances for the three most frequently used coordinate systems. The relationships given are for constant boundary temperatures, the simplest of analytical situations.

Example 3

It is desired to determine, *in vitro*, the thermal conductivity of various human tissues. A measurement chamber is constructed (Figure 3.8) with an inner electric heater housed in a glass cylinder which is surrounded by a

A. RECTANGULAR GEOMETRY

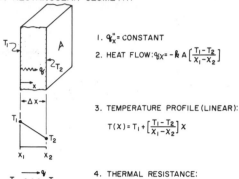

1. $q_x'' = $ CONSTANT

2. HEAT FLOW: $q_x = -k A \left[\dfrac{T_1 - T_2}{x_1 - x_2} \right]$

3. TEMPERATURE PROFILE (LINEAR):

$$T(x) = T_1 + \left[\frac{T_1 - T_2}{x_1 - x_2} \right] x$$

4. THERMAL RESISTANCE:

$$R = \frac{\Delta x}{k A}$$

B. CYLINDRICAL GEOMETRY

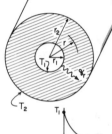

1. $r q_r'' = $ CONSTANT

2. HEAT FLOW:

$$q_r = \frac{2 \pi k L (T_1 - T_2)}{\ln(r_2/r_1)}$$

3. TEMPERATURE PROFILE (LOGARITHMIC):

$$T(r) = T_1 - \left[\frac{T_1 - T_2}{\ln(r_2/r_1)} \right] \ln(r/r_1)$$

4. THERMAL RESISTANCE:

$$R = \frac{\ln(r_2/r_1)}{2 \pi k L}$$

C. SPHERICAL GEOMETRY

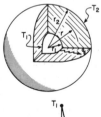

1. $r^2 q_r'' = $ CONSTANT

2. HEAT FLOW:

$$q = \frac{4 \pi k (T_1 - T_2)}{(1/r_1) - (1/r_2)}$$

3. TEMPERATURE PROFILE (GEOMETRIC):

$$T(r) = T_1 + \frac{(T_2 - T_1)[(1/r_1) - (1/r)]}{(1/r_1) - (1/r_2)}$$

4. THERMAL RESISTANCE:

$$R = \frac{[(1/r_1) - (1/r_2)]}{4 \pi k}$$

Fig. 3.7. Steady state, one-dimensional heat transfer formulae for rectangular, cylindrical, and spherical bodies without internal heat generation.

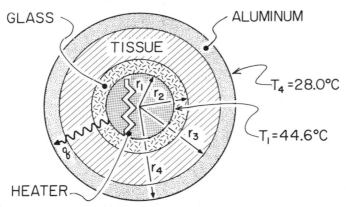

Fig. 3.8. Thermal conductivity cell of Example 3.

concentric outer aluminum cylinder. Between the glass and aluminum is an annular space to contain the tissue of interest; the ends of the annulus are kept moist to prevent tissue dehydration. The cylindrical chamber is long enough to assume that only radial conduction is significant. A sample of excised liver is placed in the chamber; and power is delivered uniformly to the heater at 25 Watts per meter of cylinder length. What is the thermal conductivity of the liver sample if the steady state temperatures measured on the inner surface of the glass and the outer surface of the aluminum (both isothermal) are 44.62°C and 28.0°C, respectively?

Solution

The heat transfer circuit for this case is

$$q = \frac{\Delta T}{\Sigma R} = \frac{(T_1 - T_4)}{R_{\text{glass}} + R_{\text{liver}} + R_{\text{aluminum}}}$$

where, per unit cylinder length ($L = 1\ m$),

$$R_{\text{glass}} = \frac{ln(r_2/r_1)}{2\pi\,k_{\text{glass}}L} = \frac{ln\left(\dfrac{1.5\ \text{cm}}{1.0\ \text{cm}}\right)}{2\pi(0.78\ W/m - °C)(1\ m)} = 0.52\,\frac{m - °C}{W},$$

$$R_{\text{alum}} = \frac{ln(r_4/r_3)}{2\pi k_{\text{alum}}L} = \frac{ln\left(\dfrac{3.0\ \text{cm}}{2.5\ \text{cm}}\right)}{2\pi(204\ W/m - °C)(1\ m)} = 0.000894\,\frac{m - °C}{W}$$

and

$$R_{\text{liver}} = \frac{ln(r_3/r_2)}{2\pi k_{\text{liver}}L} = \frac{ln\left(\dfrac{2.5\ \text{cm}}{1.5\ \text{cm}}\right)}{2\pi k_{\text{liver}}(1\ m)} = \frac{0.0813}{k_{\text{liver}}}\,\frac{m - °C}{W}$$

Thus,

$$25 \, \frac{W}{m} = \frac{(44.62 - 28.0)\,°C}{\left(.52 + \dfrac{0.0183}{k_{\text{liver}}} + 0.000894\right) \dfrac{m - °C}{W}}$$

Solving for the desired conductivity,

$$k_{\text{liver}} = 0.565 \; W/m - °C = 135 \times 10^{-5} \; cal/cm - sec - °C$$

The General Conduction Energy Equation

The conductive heat transfer rate at a point within a medium is related to the local temperature gradient by Fourier's law (Equation 8b). In many one-dimensional problems, the temperature gradient can be determined simply by inspection of the physical situation. More complex cases, especially problems which involve two- and three-dimensional heat flow, may require the use of an equation whose applicability is broader in scope than Equation 8b. On the basis of an energy balance for a differential volume (4, 5, 40, 41), the general conduction equation may be written which, in cartesian coordinates, is

$$\frac{\partial}{\partial x}\left(k_x \frac{\partial T}{\partial x}\right) + \frac{\partial}{\partial y}\left(k_y \frac{\partial T}{\partial y}\right) + \frac{\partial}{\partial z}\left(k_z \frac{\partial T}{\partial z}\right) + q''' = \rho c \frac{\partial T}{\partial t} \qquad (9)$$

where temperature T is a function of space (x, y, z) and time t; q''' is the internal heat generation rate per unit volume, and may be made up of a number of components, as previously discussed. As indicated, thermal conductivity k is generally a function of direction $(x, y, $ or $z)$, though in many cases materials may be assumed isotropic. For the assumption that thermal conductivity is uniform and constant, Equation 9 may be expressed as

$$\frac{\partial^2 T}{\partial x^2} + \frac{\partial^2 T}{\partial y^2} + \frac{\partial^2 T}{\partial z^2} + \frac{q'''}{k} = \frac{1}{\alpha} \frac{\partial T}{\partial t} \qquad (10a)$$

where $\alpha = k/\rho c$ and is termed *thermal diffusity*. Thermal energy diffuses rapidly through substances with high α and slowly through those with a low α. Further simplifications in the general energy equation are possible in certain physical situations: in steady state, for example, $\partial T/\partial t = 0$; for no internal heat generation, $q''' = 0$; for two-dimensional heat flow, only two of the partial derivatives of temperature with respect to position need be considered; for one-dimensional flow, only one need be considered, e.g., $\partial^2 T/\partial x^2$. The equivalent of equation 10a in cylindrical coordinates is

$$\frac{\partial^2 T}{\partial r^2} + \frac{1}{r} \frac{\partial T}{\partial r} + \frac{1}{r^2} \frac{\partial^2 T}{\partial \theta^2} + \frac{\partial^2 T}{\partial z^2} + \frac{q'''}{k} = \frac{1}{\alpha} \frac{\partial T}{\partial t} \qquad (10b)$$

where θ is the angle in the horizontal $(x - y)$ plane, z the vertical coordinate along the cylindrical axis, and r the radial coordinate. For a spherical coordinate system, the general conduction energy equation is

$$\frac{\partial^2 T}{\partial r^2} + \frac{2}{r}\frac{\partial T}{\partial r} + \frac{1}{r^2 \sin\theta}\frac{\partial}{\partial\theta}\left(\sin\theta\frac{\partial T}{\partial\theta}\right)$$

$$+ \frac{1}{r^2 \sin^2\theta}\left(\frac{\partial^2 T}{\partial\phi^2}\right) + \frac{q'''}{k} = \frac{1}{\alpha}\frac{\partial T}{\partial t} \quad (10c)$$

where θ is the angle between the radius r and the vertical (z) axis, and ϕ is the angle in the horizontal $(x - y)$ plane.

Conduction with Internal Heat Generation

Consider a plane slab in steady state whose surface temperatures are $T = T_1$ at $x = 0$ and $T = T_2$ at $x = 2L$, and whose mass generates heat uniformly at the rate q''' (Figure 3.9a). Assuming constant thermal conductivity and large y and z dimensions so that the temperature gradient is only significant in the x direction, Equation 10a reduces to

$$\frac{d^2 T}{\partial x^2} + \frac{q'''}{k} = 0$$

Solving this equation for surface temperatues of T_1 and T_2 results in the skewed temperature profile

$$T(x) = T_1 + \left[\frac{T_2 - T_1}{2L} + \frac{q'''}{2k}(2L - x)\right]x \quad (12)$$

Imposing equal surface temperatures, $T_1 = T_2 = T_s$, results in the symmet-

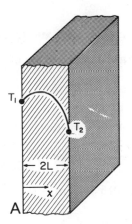
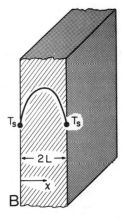

Fig. 3.9. Steady state, one-dimensional temperature profiles in a plane slab which is generating internal heat uniformly throughout its mass.

rical parabolic profile (Figure 3.9b)

$$T(x) = T_s + \frac{q'''}{2k}(2L - x)\,x \tag{13}$$

Note that to the right of the maximum temperature in the slab, dT/dx is negative (heat flows in the positive x direction), and to the left of the maximum, dT/dx is positive (heat flows negatively, out left side of the slab).

Example 4

In this example, we estimate the temperature rise in a working muscle, which is assumed to have the geometry of a cylindrical rod. Due to fiber contraction, there is an elevated metabolic generation of heat which is assumed to be uniformly distributed in the muscle. The tissue immediately surrounding the muscle is assumed isothermal at 37.0°C. Skeletal muscle typically produces basal heat generation in the neighborhood of 0.60 cal/g-hour and has a thermal conductivity of approximately 0.0015 cal/cm-sec-°C. Let us calculate the maximum temperature produced in a large muscle (e.g., the rectus femoris of the quadriceps group) which has a diameter of 5 cm and is producing heat at an order of magnitude above basal metabolism (i.e., $q_m''' = 6.0$ cal/cm³-hour, which assumes $\rho = 1$ gm/cm³).

Solution

For a cylindrical muscle (Figure 3.10) in steady state which is conducting heat radially, Equation 10b reduces to

$$\frac{\partial^2 T}{\partial r^2} + \frac{1}{r}\frac{\partial T}{\partial r} + \frac{q_m'''}{k} = 0 \tag{14}$$

where $T_0 = 37°C$ at $r = r_0$ and $\dfrac{dT}{dr} = 0$ at $r = 0$. Applying these boundary conditions and integrating twice yields the radial distribution of temperature

$$T(r) = T_0 + \frac{q_m''' r_0^2}{4k}\left[1 - \left(\frac{r}{r_0}\right)^2\right] \tag{15}$$

which yields a maximum along the centerline of the muscle ($r = 0$),

$$T_{max} = T_0 + \frac{q_m''' r_0^2}{4k} = 37°C + \frac{\left(\dfrac{6.0\ \text{cal}}{\text{hour} - \text{cm}^3}\right)(2.5\ \text{cm})^2\left(\dfrac{1\ \text{hour}}{3600\ \text{sec}}\right)}{(4)(0.0015\ \text{cal/cm} - \text{sec} - °C)}$$

$$= 37°C + 1.74°C$$

$$T_{max} = 38.74°C$$

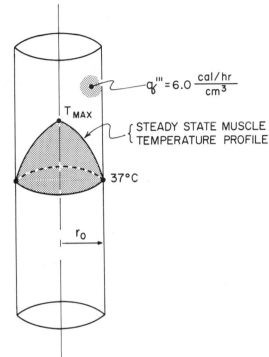

$q''' = 6.0 \dfrac{cal/hr}{cm^3}$

T_{MAX}

{ STEADY STATE MUSCLE
{ TEMPERATURE PROFILE

37°C

r_0

Fig. 3.10. The approximate temperature profile for an exercising muscle with an isothermal boundary at 37°C (Example 4).

The Bio-Heat Transfer Equation

The assumption of a uniform heat generation rate q''' in the previous example led to a greatly simplified differential equation (Equation *14*) and a simple parabolic temperature profile (Equation *15*). However, when treating blood perfusion as a heat source in tissue, the q''' term will depend on local temperature (Equation *7b*). Incorporating this term into Equation *14* yields the "bio-heat transfer equation," first presented by Pennes (37); for the condition where $\dfrac{dT}{dt} = \dfrac{dT}{d\theta} = \dfrac{dT}{dz} = 0$:

$$k\left[\frac{\partial^2 T}{\partial r^2} + \frac{1}{r}\frac{dT}{dr}\right] + q_m''' + f_b\rho_b c_b[T_a - T] = 0 \qquad (16)$$

This equation describes the steady state temperature in a cylindrical tissue segment with uniform distribution of blood flow f_b and metabolism q_m''', and constant arterial blood temperature T_a. The analytical solution to this equation involves complex mathematical relationships known as Bessel functions and is beyond the scope of this chapter. Temperature profiles predicted by this equation, as given by Pennes for a cylindrical human

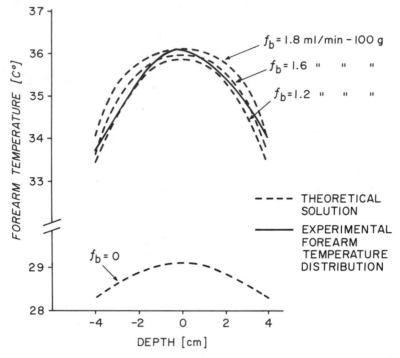

Fig. 3.11. Comparison of experimentally measured steady-state temperatures in the resting human forearm with those calculated from Equation *16* [from Pennes (37)]. The *dotted curves* are the theoretical results assuming various levels of uniformly distributed blood flow f_b, all with a uniform metabolic heat generation of $q'''_m = 1 \times 10^{-4}$ cal/sec-cm^3 and a constant arterial input temperature $T_a = 36.25°C$.

forearm in steady state under basal conditions while surrounded by air at 26.6°C, are shown in Figure 3.11. The analytical curves at three different perfusion (f_b) levels are compared with his experimentally measured forearm temperature profile. The analytical curves closely approximated the experimentally determined profile; his perfusion values correspond roughly to actual values of resting forearm blood flow (Table 3.5).

CONVECTION

Introduction

Since the solution of differential equations which describe convective heat transfer is extremely complicated, "heat transfer coefficients" are normally used. As shown in Figure 3.12, there is a temperature transition zone of thickness δ in the convecting fluid which is called the temperature boundary layer. In this layer, the fluid temperature varies from the surface temperature T_s to the fluid "free stream" temperature T_∞. "Newton's law of cooling"

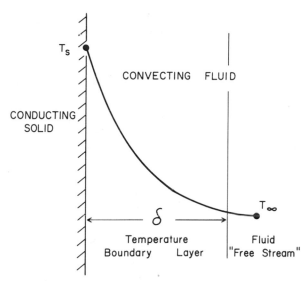

Fig. 3.12. Schematic of the "temperature boundary layer" of thickness δ occurring in the wall region of a convecting fluid. The film thickness δ is usually defined by the temperature transition zone from T_s to the fluid region which differs from T_s by 0.99 ($T_s - T_\infty$) or some other arbitrarily established percentage of $T_s - T_\infty$.

states that the heat flow q to or from the surface is proportional to the surface area A and is related to the temperature difference $T_s - T_\infty$ by a proportionality constant h_c, defined by

$$q = h_c A(T_s - T_\infty) \tag{17}$$

where the convective thermal resistance or "film resistance" between the fluid and the surface is defined as $R_c = 1/h_c A$. Clearly, the heat transfer coefficient h_c (cgs units: cal/cm^2 $-$ sec $-$ °C; SI units: Watts/m^2 $-$ °C) is a function of both the flow conditions and the properties of the fluid. It is customary, in fact, to determine h_c through experimentally derived relationships (termed "correlations") among the primary physical variables which characterize the flow situation and fluid properties. These correlations, normally expressed in terms of dimensionless parameters or "groups" of the pertinent variables, provide the most useful information about convection heat transfer as applied to thermotherapy.

Forced Convection

The *Reynolds number* (Re) is a dimensionless group which characterizes the flow, either inside or outside a duct or tube or around objects:

$$Re = \frac{V\rho L}{\mu} \tag{18}$$

where V is an appropriate characteristic fluid velocity, most frequently the free stream velocity V_∞, ρ the fluid density, μ the dynamic or absolute fluid viscosity (cgs units: poise = gm/cm-sec; SI: kg/m-sec) and L an appropriate characteristic length, such as the diameter in cases of tube flow. In general, the higher the Reynolds number, the more turbulent or chaotic the flow. For smooth-walled cylindrical tubes, the transition between orderly, "laminar" flow and turbulent flow usually occurs at $2000 \leq Re \leq 4000$. Physiological Reynolds numbers in blood vessels range from about 3400 in the aorta to 500 in a 0.4 cm diameter artery to about 0.002 in capillaries (42). Strictly speaking, the concept of a uniform fluid in laminar flow breaks down on the capillary scale, because red blood cells are approximately the same diameter as capillaries. The Reynolds number expresses the ratio of the relative magnitudes of the inertial (momentum) forces associated with the fluid motion to its viscous friction forces.

The *Prandtl number* (*Pr*) is a dimensionless group characterizing the properties of the fluid and is defined as

$$Pr = \frac{\mu c}{k} \tag{19}$$

where, again, μ is the dynamic viscosity, c the fluid specific heat, and k its thermal conductivity. Table 3.6 shows a range of typical values for fluid Prandtl numbers. The Prandtl number may be interpreted as the ratio of the ability of the fluid to transport momentum (through viscous interaction of fluid particles) to its ability to transfer heat(through conduction).

The *Nusselt number* (*Nu*) expresses the convective heat transfer coefficient in dimensionless form:

$$Nu = \frac{h_c L}{k} \tag{20}$$

where h_c is the convective coefficient of heat transfer, L a characteristic length and k the thermal conductivity of the fluid. Physically, Nu may be interpreted as the ratio of the conductive resistance of the fluid boundary layer to its convective resistance; or alternatively, as the ratio of the temperature gradient at the solid surface to the temperature gradient across the boundary layer.

Most experimental results of cross-flow forced convection heat transfer over isothermal surfaces (*i.e.*, convection over bodies immersed in the fluid with flow perpendicular to their lengthwise axes) are described by correlation equations of the form (4)

$$\overline{Nu_f} = \frac{\bar{h}_c L}{k_f} = C_1(Re_f^n \cdot Pr_f^m) \tag{21}$$

where C_1 varies according to the shape of the body's surface; n according to

TABLE 3.6. *Typical Prandtl Numbers for Various Fluids*

Fluid (all at atm. pressure)	Temperature (°C)	Prandtl No. (Pr)
air	0 - 100	0.72 [a]
steam	100°C	0.96 [a]
water	0	13.25 [b]
"	10	9.40 [b]
"	37.8	4.53 [b]
"	60	3.01 [b]
light oil	37.8	340 [a]
mercury	50	0.027 [a]
blood	37	25 [c]

[a]Ref 40, p. 636-640

[b]Ref 4, p. 501-507

[c]Ref 36, p. 2

the Reynolds number of the flow (*i.e.*, its degree of laminarity or turbulence) and *m* according to the Reynolds number and the direction of heat flow (for our purposes $m = 1/3$). It is important to note that $\overline{Nu}$ is the Nusselt number averaged over the surface of the body, and that the subscript f denotes that the fluid's thermal properties (k_f, ρ_f, c_f, and μ_f) are to be evaluated at some representative temperature in the boundary layer, usually called the "film temperature" T_f. For most situations of interest to us, $T_f = (T_{surface} + T_\infty)/2$. Table 3.7 shows values of C_1 and n which are applicable to cross-flow over cylinders of diameter D. An analogous relationship which applies to convection of gases flowing over spheres is

$$\overline{Nu}_f = 0.37\ Re_f^{0.6} \qquad (17 < Re_f < 70,000) \qquad (22)$$

Similar correlation formulae for liquids flowing over spheres, for fluid flow over a variety of shapes, for flow inside tubes and conduits of different shapes, and numerous other forced convection situations are found in most

TABLE 3.7. *Constants for use in equation 21*

$Re_f = \dfrac{\rho_f V_\infty D}{\mu_f}$	C_1 [a]	n [a]
0.4 - 4	0.989	0.330
4 - 40	0.911	0.385
40 - 4000	0.683	0.466
4000 - 40,000	0.193	0.618
40,000 - 400,000	0.0266	0.805

[a]Ref 4, p. 216

standard heat transfer texts. When applying such heat transfer correlations, it is important to understand the limits of their applicability in terms of flow regimes, geometry, temperature ranges, types of fluids (*e.g.*, gas or liquid) and the definition of the appropriate film temperature at which the fluids' properties are to be evaluated.

Example 5

It is desired to cool the skin surface of the thigh before applying microwave diathermy by blowing 5°C air over the thigh at 1 m/sec. Estimate the average coefficient of cooling around the thigh and the corresponding initial surface cooling rate of the skin.

Solution

Assuming that the cooling stream of air will suppress significant moisture losses from the thigh, the cooling problem may be modeled as simple convective heat transport from a cylindrical thigh (Fig. 3.13) of, say, a diameter $D = 15$ cm. Determining the film temperature for evaluating the fluid properties,

$$T_f = \frac{T_s + T_\infty}{2} = \frac{30 + 5}{2} = 17.5°C$$

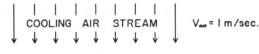

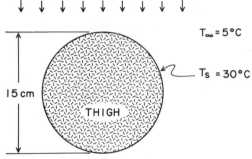

COOLING AIR STREAM $V_\infty = 1\,m/sec.$

$T_\infty = 5°C$

Fig. 3.13. Cross-flow of cold air over the cylindrical thigh of Example 5.

$T_s = 30°C$

15 cm

THIGH

For air at 17.5°C and atmospheric pressure

$\rho_f = 1.224$ kg/m³;
$\mu_f = 1.884 \times 10^{-5}$ kg/m − sec;
$k_f = 2.545 \times 10^{-2}$ W/m − °C;
$Pr_f = 0.71$;

the Reynolds number is

$$\text{Re} = \frac{V_\infty \rho_f D}{\mu_f} = \frac{(1\ \text{m/sec})(1.224\ \text{kg/m}^3)(0.15\ \text{m})}{1.884 \times 10^{-5}\ \text{kg/m} - \text{sec}} = 9746$$

From Equation 21, Table 3.7, and for $m = ⅓$,

$$\overline{Nu} = C_1\,(\text{Re}_f^n \cdot \text{Pr}_f^m) = (0.193)[(9746)^{0.618} \cdot (0.71)^{0.33}] = 50.24$$

From the definition of Nusselt number, for $L = D$, the average heat transfer coefficient is then

$$\bar{h}_c = \frac{k_f\,\overline{Nu}}{D} = \frac{(2.545 \times 10^{-2}\,\text{W/m} - °\text{C})(50.24)}{(0.15\ \text{m})}$$

$$\bar{h}_c = 8.52\ \text{W/m}^2 \text{ - } °\text{C}$$

or,

$$\bar{h}_c = 0.852\ mW/cm^2 - °C$$

The heat loss from the thigh will be maximum when the cooling is initially applied because the driving temperature difference, $\Delta T = T_s - T_\infty$, is greatest at this point:

$$\bar{q}''_{\text{initial}} = \bar{h}_c\,(T_s - T_\infty)$$

$$= \left(8.52\,\frac{\text{W}}{\text{m}^2 - °\text{C}}\right)(30 - 5°\text{C})$$

$$= 213\ \text{W/m}^2$$

$$= 21.3\ \text{mW/cm}^2$$

It is important to note that this cooling rate is the value averaged around the entire periphery of the thigh cylinder. The distribution of local values of h_c is such that the uppermost point of the thigh in Figure 3.13 would be cooled at rates higher than this average.

Free Convection

In free convection, the *Grashof number* (Gr) expresses the ratio of the buoyant forces on the fluid to the viscous forces:

$$Gr = \frac{g\beta(T_s - T_\infty)L^3}{\nu^2} \qquad (23)$$

Here the term g is the local acceleration due to gravity (m/sec^2); and β is the volume coefficient of expansion which is defined, at constant pressure, as the rate of fluid volume expansion per unit volume per degree temperature increase. Under most ambient conditions relevant to thermotherapy, air behaves as an ideal gas for which $\beta = 1/T_{abs}$ (T_{abs} = absolute temperature). L is, again, a characteristic length (meters), and ν is the ratio μ/ρ, termed the "kinematic viscosity", which like α has units of m^2/sec and represents the relative ability of viscous forces or interactions to "diffuse" through a fluid. Natural convection from isothermal surfaces is most frequently described by correlations of the form

$$\overline{Nu_f} = C_2(Gr_f \cdot Pr_f)^p \qquad (24)$$

where C_2 is a function of the surface geometry of the convecting body, and p depends on the flow regime (a common rule of thumb holds that $p = 0.25$ for laminar flow and $p = 0.333$ in turbulence). For natural convection in air over the physiological temperature range $0 \leq T_\infty \leq 50°$ and $0 \leq T_s - T_\infty \leq 15°C$, the numerical values of $\overline{Nu}$ vary from approximately 20 to 80, and the values of Gr from 2×10^6 to 1×10^9 (44). For Grashof numbers exceeding 1×10^9, the free convection flow is considered turbulent. As before, fluid properties are usually determined at the film temperature, $T_f = (T_s + T_\infty)/2$. Several values for the constants used in equation 24 for various geometries are presented in Table 3.8. In addition, the following empirical equation for free convection to or from spheres is also recommended (4):

$$\overline{Nu} = \frac{\bar{h}_c D}{k_f} = 2 + 0.43(Gr_f \cdot Pr_f)^{1/4} \qquad (25)$$

As with forced convection, many other correlations which pertain to a wide variety of geometries, fluids and natural convective flow situations may be found in the heat transfer literature.

In many cases, a driving temperature difference (ΔT) for free convection will be present along with ambient fluid motion (V_∞), conditions which lead to a combination of forced and natural convective mechanisms. The ratio

TABLE 3.8. *Constants for Use with Free Convection Correlation*

$$\overline{Nu}_f = C_2 \, (Gr_f \, Pr_f)^p$$

Geometry	$Gr_f \, Pr_f$	C_2	p	Characteristic Length, L
Vertical planes and cylinders	$10^4 - 10^9$	0.59	1/4	vertical length L
	$10^9 - 10^{13}$	0.10	1/3	
Horizontal cylinders	$10^4 - 10^9$	0.53	1/4	diameter D
	$10^9 - 10^{12}$	0.13	1/3	
Horizontal Plates:				
a) heated surface up (or cooled surface down)	$10^5 - 2 \times 10^7$	0.54	1/4	arithmetic average of plate sides $L = (L_1 + L_2)/2$
b) heated surface up (or cooled surface down)	$2 \times 10^7 - 3 \times 10^{10}$	0.14	1/3	"
c) heated surface down (or cooled surface up)	$3 \times 15^5 - 3 \times 10^{10}$	0.27	1/4	"
Spheres, short cylinders or blocks	$10^4 - 10^9$	0.60	1/4	$1/L = 1/L_v + 1/L_h$ where L_v and L_h are the vertical are horizontal dimensions respectively

Inclined flat surfaces:
  Multiply Groshof number by cos θ, where θ is the angle of inclination from the vertical, and use vertical plate constants. This approach is only valid for small θ.

Gr/Re^2 gives a qualitative indication of the influence of buoyancy on forced convection such that when the Grashof number is of the same order of magnitude or larger than the square of the Reynolds number, free convection effects cannot be ignored in comparison with forced convection. Similarly, in a natural convection process, the influence of forced convection becomes significant when the square of the Reynolds number is of the same order of magnitude as the Grashof number. Rapp (44) concludes that for problems of physiological heat transfer, whenever the driving temperature $1 \leq \Delta T \leq 10°C$ and $V_\infty \leq 0.5$ m/sec, free convection dominates to such an extent that the whole-body average convection coefficient is adequately expressed by a pure free convection coefficient.

Example 6

Calculate the rate of convective heat transfer from the surface of the thigh to surrounding stagnant air which is at 45°C if the skin surface is elevated at 35°C. Assume a cylindrical thigh, $D = 16$ cm.

Solution

The stagnant air ($V_\infty = 0$) indicates that natural convection will be the mechanism for heat flow from the thigh surface. For air at film temperature

$$T_f = (35 + 45)/2 = 40°C$$

$$\beta_f = \frac{1}{T_{abs}} = \frac{1}{313.2°K} = 3.193 \times 10^{-3}°K^{-1}$$

$$k_f = 0.027 \text{ W/m} - °C \qquad Pr_f = 0.72$$

$$\nu_f = 17 \times 10^{-6} m^2/\text{sec} \qquad g = 9.815 \text{ m/sec}^2$$

From these values,

$$Gr_f = \frac{g\beta_f \Delta T D^3}{\nu_f^2} = \frac{(9.815 \text{ m/sec}^2)(3.193 \times 10^{-3}°K^{-1})(10°K)(0.16m)^3}{(17 \times 10^{-6}m^2/\text{sec})^2}$$

$$= 1.417 \times 10^7$$

and

$$Gr_f \cdot Pr_f = (1.417 \times 10^7)(0.72) = 1.02 \times 10^7$$

(from Table 3.8, $p = \frac{1}{4}$ and $C_2 = 0.53$)

Thus

$$\overline{Nu}_f = C_2(Gr_f \, Pr_f)^P = 0.53(1.02 \times 10^7)^{0.25} = 30 \qquad (24)$$

The coefficient of convection is therefore

$$\bar{h}_c = \frac{k_f}{D} \overline{Nu} = \frac{(0.027 \text{ W/m} - °C)(30)}{(0.16 \text{ m})} = 5 \text{W/m}^2 - °C$$

The surface heat flux rate is

$$\overline{q_c''} = \bar{h}_c(T_s - T_\infty)$$

$$= (5 \text{ W/m}^2 - °C)(35 - 45°C)$$

$$= -50 \text{ Watts/m}^2 = -5 \text{ mW/cm}^2$$

The negative flow of heat denotes a net transfer of energy *into* the thigh.

Counter-Current Heat Exchange

The juxtaposition of arterial and venous vessels in limbs and other tissue regions is often justified, teleologically, on the basis of the heat exchange which takes place between these vessels. Consider, for example, the distal portion of the arm and hand as depicted in Figure 3.14. When the arterial blood entering this portion of the limb is at T_a and the venous return is at T_v, the steady state heat loss to the limb from the blood (flowing at a mass flow rate $\dot{m}_b$) will be

$$q = \dot{m}_b c_b(T_a - T_v) \qquad (26)$$

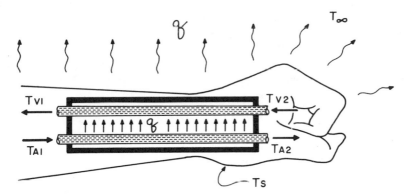

Fig. 3.14. Counter-current heat exchanger of the distal forearm and hand segment.

where c_b is the specific heat of blood. In steady state conditions, the heat loss of Equation 26 is the same, neglecting metabolism, as the heat loss to the environment from the limb, $q = h_c A_{\text{limb}}(T_s - T_\infty)$. The proximity of the two vessels provides what is called an internal "counter-flow heat exchanger" whereby the returning venous blood is warmed by heat loss from the artery, which in turn serves to cool the incoming arterial flow. The effect of this exchange is a) to lower the distal skin temperature, which reduces heat loss from the limb, and b) to conserve heat in proximal portions of the limb by heating the venous blood returning to it. The magnitude of such counter-current exchange is modulated by physiological controls which can modify the degree of shunting of blood toward the skin surface, and thus away from the "exchanger vessels", and also by vasoconstrictor responses which can alter total-limb perfusion rates, thus affecting the time of residence of blood in the exchange segment of the limb. Mitchell and Myers (45) have mathematically modeled the counterflow system of the human forearm and have found that the mechanism can produce, at most, a 5 percent decrease in forearm heat loss to cool surroundings. Seagraves (2) states that in the hand, however, heat loss reductions on the order of 50 percent may be possible. Keller and Seiler (8) estimate that counter-flow exchange in blood moving perpendicular to the skin in the superficial surface tissue of limbs may precool arterial blood on the way to the skin to such an extent that reductions in the apparent thermal conductivity of this region on the order of 50 percent may be feasible.

EVAPORATION

The driving force for the loss of moisture from the body's surface by diffusion is the difference in water concentration existing between that on the surface and that in the surrounding ambient atmosphere. This being the case, the rate of water loss $\dot{m}_w$ can be described by a relationship analogous to Equation 17 for convection,

$$\dot{m}_w = h_w^* A_w (C_{w,s} - C_{w,\infty}) \tag{27a}$$

where the evaporative mass transfer coefficient h_w^* is similar to h_c, A_w is the wetted surface area, and the moisture concentrations at the surface and in the free stream positions are $C_{w,s}$ and $C_{w,\infty}$, respectively. The concentrations are most often related to the equivalent partial pressures of water vapor, $p_{w,s}$ and $p_{w,\infty}$, by the perfect gas law such that the equation becomes

$$\dot{m}_w = \frac{h_w A_w}{R_w T_{f,abs}} [p_{w,s} - p_{w,\infty}] \qquad (27b)$$

Here a new mass transfer coefficient h_w replaces the h_w^* used with concentration differences; R_w is the gas constant for water vapor (3.47 mm Hg-m^3/kg − °K); and $T_{f,abs}$ is the absolute film temperature, $T_{f,abs} = (T_{s,abs} + T_{\infty,abs})/2$.

The absorption of energy by a unit mass of evaporating water is related to its *latent heat* of evaporation, L_w, by

$$q_e = \dot{m}_w L_w \qquad (28)$$

where $L_w = 579$ kcal/kg at 25°C and 576 kcal/kg at 37°C. Equations *27b* and *28* may be combined to yield a Newton's law type relationship for evaporative heat transfer,

$$q_e = h_e A_w [p_{w,s} - p_{w,\infty}] \qquad (29)$$

where $h_e = h_w L_w / R_w T_{f,abs}$. As is the case for the convective heat transfer coefficient h_c, local values and variations in h_e are difficult both to measure and to predict theoretically for the complex shapes and movements associated with the human body. In addition, the fractions of the surface areas of skin which are moist and their respective degrees of wettedness are often difficult to determine. Certain idealized limiting cases for evaporative heat loss, however, provide a valuable basis for predictions of actual heat loss. From the alliance of heat and mass transfer, an analytical result known as the Chilton-Colburn analogy (46) is derived that states, for the diffusion of water in air,

$$\frac{\bar{h}_w}{\bar{h}_c} = \frac{(Pr/Sc)^{2/3}}{(\rho c)_{air}} \qquad (30)$$

where Sc is the *Schmidt number*, $Sc = \nu/\mathscr{D}_w$, which is the ratio of kinematic viscosity ν of air to the diffusion coefficient $\mathscr{D}_w$ of water vapor in air; this is essentially the ratio of the relative abilities of momentum (through viscous action) and water mass to propagate or diffuse through air. Note that for air in the temperature range of physiological interest ($0 \leq T_\infty \leq 50$°C) the Prandtl number is fairly constant at $Pr \simeq 0.72$ as is the corresponding Schmidt number, here $Sc \cong 0.60$. Assuming that the $(\rho c)_{air}$ products for moist and dry air are the same, Equation *30* may be combined with either equation *21* or *24* to yield a general relationship between the average evaporative coefficient of heat transfer $\bar{h}_e$ and the average convective

Nusselt number in either forced or natural convection, which is

$$\bar{h}_e = 3508 \, \nu \overline{Nu}/L \qquad (31)$$

where ν is in m²/sec, L, the characteristic dimension, is in meters, and $\bar{h}_e$ is in Watts/m²-mm Hg.

Figure 3.15 describes the trend of $\bar{h}_e$ (here in units of kcal/hr-m²-mm Hg) for the entirely wet human body, in both forced and free convection. The body has been modeled by so-called "man-equivalent" isothermal cylinders, flat plates or spheres, where each was proportioned to have surface areas equal to the Dubois skin areas (A_D) of the human subjects who were tested for evaporative heat loss. The theoretical points are from evaporation measurements performed on the man-equivalent shapes in cross-flow air at

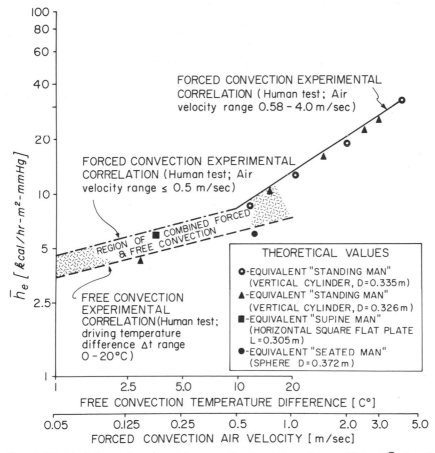

Fig. 3.15. Variation of average evaporative heat transfer coefficient $\bar{h}_e$ for the completely wet human body in both forced and free convection flow regimes. Theoretical points are calculated from Equation 31 applied to the various "man-equivalent" regular geometrical shapes. All curves and points are taken from the literature by Rapp (44).

40 to 60°C. These points show good agreement with the experimental curves resulting from the measurements on completely wet, nude human subjects under the same conditions. Rapp (44) points out that the agreement between $\bar{h}_e$, as measured from human subjects, and that of the man-equivalent shapes is typically within 10 percent.

The evaporative heat losses which occur locally, for example from a body segment such as an arm or leg, are more pertinent to thermotherapy situations than are whole-body values. One obvious approach to predicting such local evaporation is to employ segment-equivalent shapes, such as cylinders for arm, legs or thighs, and to apply Equation 31 along with the appropriate forms of Equations 21 or 24. Alternatively, Rapp relates the ratio of segmental evaporative loss to the whole-body values of Figure 3.15 (in which $A_w = A_D$) in laminar forced convection as (44)

$$\frac{\bar{h}_{e,\text{segment}}}{\bar{h}_{e,\text{body}}} = (L_{\text{seg}})^{n-1} \tag{32}$$

where L_{seg} is the segmental characteristic length (diameter or radius) expressed in feet, and "n" is the exponent of the Reynolds number used in Equation 21 (see Table 3.7). The characteristic lengths of the body segments

TABLE 3.9. *Characteristic Dimensions for "Man-Equivalent" Body Segment Shapes*[a]

Body Segment	Characteristic Dimension L_{seg}	Ratio of Wetted Segment Surface Area to Whole-Body Area A_w/A_D [%]
Trunk	D = 1 ft (30.5 cm)	35
Thighs	D = 0.52 ft (15.85 cm)	19
Lower Legs	D = 0.32 ft (9.75 cm)	13
Arms	D = 0.28 ft (8.53 cm)	14
Head	R = 0.30 ft (9.14 cm)	7

[a] As reported by Santschi in ref 44 (note that all segments are cylindrical with the exception of a spherical head)

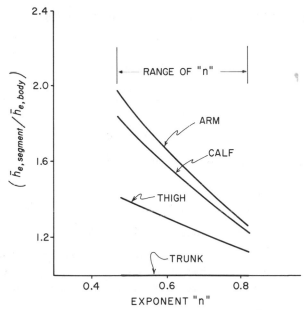

Fig. 3.16. Average evaporative heat transfer coefficient $\bar{h}_{e,seg}$ for various body segments, here expressed in ratio with the average values for a completely wet whole body $\bar{h}_{e,body}$ (Figure 3.15). These curves are based on Equation *32* as given by Rapp (44).

of an average man, along with their respective surface area percentages (relative to A_D), are given in Table 3.9. As shown in Figure 3.16, the local (*i.e.*, segmental) complete-wettedness evaporative losses always exceed whole body average values, often by a considerable degree, depending upon the segment diameter. These curves qualitatively point out the danger of using local convective coefficient values for whole-body averages and vice versa.

Example 7

Calculate the evaporative heat exchange between the thigh of example 6 and its environment if the relative humidity (RH) of the ambient air is 30 percent.

Solution

On the basis of the Chilton-Colburn analogy and Equation *31*, the coefficient of evaporative heat loss is

$$\bar{h}_e = \frac{3508\nu\overline{Nu}}{D}$$

$$= \frac{3508(17 \times 10^{-6})(30)}{(0.16)}$$

$$= 11.18 \text{ Watts/m}^2\text{-mm Hg}$$

(31)

The partial pressure of water vapor in the air is (see Figure 3.17)

$$p_{w,\infty} = RH \cdot p_{w,\text{sat}}$$
$$= (0.3)(73.3)$$
$$= 22.0 \text{ mm Hg}$$

On the skin, the water vapor is saturated at 35°C, thus

$$p_{w,s} = 42 \text{ mm Hg}$$

The evaporative heat loss from the thigh is then

$$\bar{q}_e{}'' = \bar{h}_e \Delta p_w$$
$$= (11.18 \text{ W/m}^2\text{-mm Hg})(42 - 22 \text{ mm Hg})$$
$$= 223.6 \text{ Watts/m}^2 = 22.36 \text{ mW/cm}^2$$

The significnce of heat loss via sweating is dramatized by comparing the evaporation heat loss with that of convection. From Example 6, the magnitude of $q_c{}''$ is 5 mW/cm^2; thus for this free convection regime $\bar{q}_e{}''/\bar{q}_c{}'' > 4$!

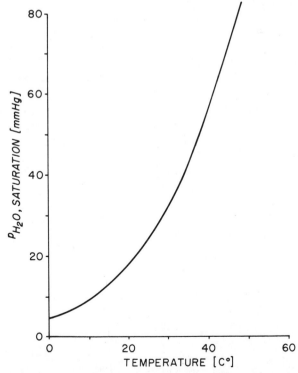

Fig. 3.17. Maximum partial pressure of water vapor (saturation value corresponding to 100 percent relative humidity) in air at atmospheric pressure as a function of temperature.

Example 8

For air blowing over the thigh of Example 5 ($V_\infty = 1$ m/sec, $T_\infty = 5°C$), let us estimate the evaporative heat loss at an instant where the thigh is completely wet and has a uniform skin temperature of 30°C, and the air stream is at 30 percent relative humidity. We can then compare evaporative heat loss to that by forced convection.

Solution

For the whole body approximated as a 1 ft diameter cylinder (44) ($L = D = 1$ ft $= 0.304$ m). The Reynolds number in this airstream is

$$\text{Re} = \frac{V_\infty D}{\nu} = \frac{(1 \text{ m/sec})(0.304 \text{ m})}{(13 \times 10^{-6} \text{ m}^2/\text{sec})}$$

$$= 2.339 \times 10^4$$

Therefore, from Table 3.7, $n = 0.618$ and $n - 1 = -0.382$. For the thigh $L_{\text{seg}} = D = 0.52$ ft. Thus

$$\frac{\bar{h}_{e,\text{seg}}}{\bar{h}_{e,\text{body}}} = (0.52)^{-0.382} = 1.284$$

For $V_\infty = 1$ m/sec from Figure 3.15, $\bar{h}_{e,\text{body}} = 12.5$ kcal/hour $- $ m^2 $-$ mm Hg and

$$\bar{h}_{e,\text{seg}} = (1.284)(12.5 \text{ kcal/hour} - \text{m}^2 - \text{mm Hg})$$

$$= 16.05 \text{ kcal/hour} - \text{m}^2 - \text{mm Hg}$$

$$= 18.66 \text{ Watts/m}^2 - \text{mm Hg}$$

For $T_\infty = 5°C$, $\quad p_{w,\infty} = (0.3)(6.5 \text{ mm Hg})$

$$= 1.95 \text{ mm Hg}$$

and at the skin surface ($T_s = 30°C$)

$$p_{w,s} = 31.5 \text{ mm Hg}$$

Thus, the evaporative heat loss, assuming complete wettedness, is

$$\bar{q}_e'' = \bar{h}_e(p_{w,s} - p_{w,\infty})$$

$$= (18.66 \text{ W/m}^2 - \text{mm Hg})(31.5 - 1.95 \text{ mm Hg})$$

$$= 551 \text{ Watts/m}^2 = 55.1 \text{ mW/cm}^2$$

From Example 5, the convective loss for comparison was $\bar{q}_c'' = 21.3$ mW/cm^2. Thus, the ratio of evaporative to convective loss in this condition of forced convection is $\bar{q}_e''/\bar{q}_c'' > 2$!

Examples 5 through 8 demonstrate the importance of the flow regime for both convective and evaporative heat transfer. In these problems, a forced movement of air at only 1 m/sec over the thigh doubled the evaporative heat loss over that occurring in a stagnant air environment, while the convective heat transfer was quadrupled!

THERMAL RADIATION

The rate at which a surface at absolute temperature T_{abs} emits radiant energy per unit surface area is termed its *total emissive power E*, and is of primary importance in quantifying radiant energy exchanges. In general, E is a complicated function of surface temperature, type, and condition of the surface, and the wavelength of the radiation of concern. There is a class of theoretically-ideal surfaces called "black" surfaces or *blackbodies* which emit and absorb all incident radiant energy at the theoretically-maximum rates at any given temperature. The rate at which a blackbody emits radiant energy per unit area at T_{abs} is

$$E_b = \sigma T_{abs}^4$$

which is known as the *Stefan-Bolzmann law*. The proportionality factor σ is a universal constant: $\sigma = 5.669 \times 10^{-8}$ W/m^2 - °K^4. A non-black surface emits radiant energy at a lower rate than a blackbody at the same temperature. The degree to which non-black emissive power falls short of ideal behavior is expressed by the *emissivity* ϵ, where

$$E = \epsilon E_b = \epsilon \sigma T_{abs}^4 \tag{34}$$

Clearly a blackbody emits at $\epsilon = 1$, while all real surfaces fall in the range $0 \le \epsilon \le 1$. Because emissivity varies with wavelength and the direction of the radiation relative to the radiant surface, the most frequently used value is reported as "total hemispherical emissivity", which has been averaged over all wavelengths and directions.

While no truly ideal radiators exist in nature, several surfaces come very close to blackbody behavior, particularly in selected wavelength bands. Most reported values of ϵ for human skin, for example, are in excess of 0.98; Boehm and Tuft (47) conclude that $\epsilon = 0.993$ is a suitable average ϵ value for all human skin.

The thermal energy emitted by a blackbody is distributed over its wavelength spectrum in the manner shown in Figure 3.18a where the emissive power is shown as a function of wavelength and temperature. With increasing temperature, the curves shift toward the left, putting increasing amounts of energy in the visible and ultraviolet regions. At approximately 700°C, a sufficient percentage of radiant energy lies in the band between approximately 0.6 and 0.7 μ to give the emitting surface a visible dull-red glow.

Fig. 3.18. a, Blackbody emissive power as a function of wavelength and temperature over the range of temperatures employed in infrared radiation therapy; b, Comparison of the spectral distribution of radiant emissive power (E_λ) for real and ideal (blackbody and graybody) surfaces.

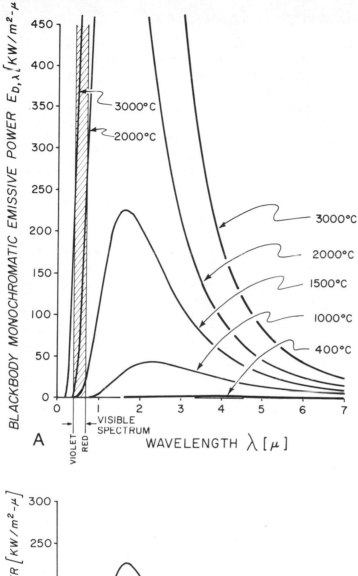

A

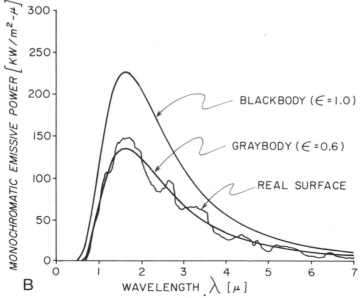

B

Infrared lamps used in physical therapy range in temperature from about 400°C (non-luminous) to approximately 3000°C for tungsten-filament incandescent sources (48). Figure 3.18*b* schematically shows how real surfaces distribute energy over the infrared spectrum in comparison to a blackbody at the same temperature; also shown is the distribution of another theoretically-idealized surface, a *graybody*, which is defined as a radiant surface whose emissivity is constant and independent of wavelength. Treating real radiating surfaces as "gray" greatly simplifies calculation procedures and is often the only way a problem can be solved if sufficient information on the wavelength vs. emissivity relationship is not available. Figure 3.19 shows the spectral variation of emissivity for human skin; note that emissivity is taken to be zero for $\lambda < 1$ μ and unity for $\lambda > 6$ μ. The spectral or "monochromatic" emissivity ϵ_λ should not be confused with ϵ, the total emissivity integrated over all wavelengths (0.993 for skin).

Thus far, only the emission or departure of thermal radiation from a surface has been discussed. The emitting surface is generally also simultaneously irradiated by energy from other sources. Some of this incident energy is absorbed; some is transmitted through the material; and some is reflected. Defining the fraction of incident radiation which is absorbed by a surface as the *absorptivity* α_r, the fraction transmitted as the *transmissivity* τ_r, and the portion reflected as the *reflectivity* ρ_r, it follows from energy conservation considerations that for any surface $\alpha_r + \tau_r + \rho_r = 1$. Since by definition a blackbody absorbs radiation completely, for this idealized surface $\alpha_r = 1$ and $\rho_r = \tau_r = 0$.

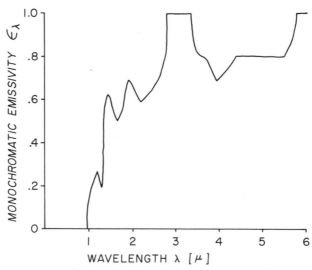

Fig. 3.19. Variation of emissivity with wavelength of radiation for human skin (curve is that of Elam *et al.* as reported in Ref. 47).

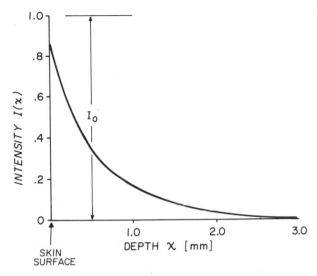

Fig. 3.20. Schematic representation of the absorption of infrared radiation in the skin and subcutaneous layers of excised tissue by 1.2 μ wavelength infrared radiation (from Ref. 50).

The penetration of radiant energy into a medium (*i.e.*, beyond its surface) is expressed mathematically as Beer's law: $I(x) = I_0 e^{-ax}$, where I_0 is the intensity striking the surface of the medium, $I(x)$ is the intensity at a depth x and "a" is an absorption coefficient. Most real solids absorb almost all of the non-reflected incident radiant energy within a depth of between about 1 μ and 2.5 mm from the surface (49) and hence transmit almost none; they are thus considered "opaque" with $\tau_r = 0$. Figure 3.20 shows the Beer's Law absorption of 1.2 μ radiation (the most penetrating infrared wavelength used in therapeutic applications (50)) as it is transmitted into a specimen of excised superficial human tissue. While there is some penetration past the anatomical skin structure, for purposes of thermotherapy, the penetration is considered to be shallow (note that with blood flow, the absorption coefficient a would increase). Consequently, infrared radiation is usually treated as a surface heating modality with $\tau_r = 0$. Thus, as for most real solid surfaces, human skin is characterized by $\alpha_r + \rho_r = 1$.

Up to this point, we have considered a system composed of a single radiant surface. To describe radiant heat "transfer", a second surface is needed, along with some basic definitions. Let two blackbody surfaces of areas A_1 and A_2 be arranged randomly in space such that they "see" each other, as shown in Figure 3.21. To obtain an expression for the net energy exchange between them when they are maintained at different temperatures, the amount of energy which leaves each surface and strikes the other must be determined. Let the fraction of energy leaving surface 1 which

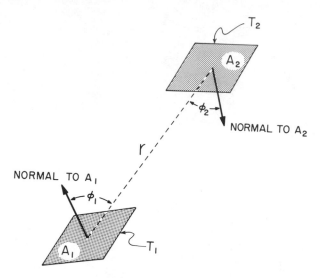

Fig. 3.21. Geometrical relationship of two radiating surfaces in space.

reaches surface 2 be defined as $F_{1\text{-}2}$, the *view factor* from 1 to 2; conversely $F_{2\text{-}1}$ is the fraction of energy leaving surface 2 which reaches surface 1. In terms of their emissive power E_b, the energy leaving surface 1 and arriving at surface 2 is $E_{b_1} A_1 F_{1\text{-}2}$, while that leaving 2 and arriving at 1 is $E_{b_2} A_2 E_{2\text{-}1}$. The net energy exchange, since all energy is absorbed, is

$$q_{1\text{-}2} = E_{b_1} A_1 F_{1\text{-}2} - E_{b_2} A_2 F_{2\text{-}1}$$

In thermal equilibrium, both surfaces are the same temperature and $E_{b_1} = E_{b_2}$, thus, since $q_{1\text{-}2}$ must be zero,

$$A_1 F_{1\text{-}2} = A_2 F_{2\text{-}1}$$

$$(35)$$

which is a property common to all pairs of radiant surfaces and is known as *reciprocity*. From this, the net heat exchange for $T_1 \neq T_2$ is

$$q_{1\text{-}2} = A_1 F_{1\text{-}2}(E_{b_1} - E_{b_2}) = A_2 F_{2\text{-}1}(E_{b_1} - E_{b_2})$$

$$= A_1 F_{1\text{-}2}\sigma(T_1{}^4 - T_2{}^4) = A_2 F_{2\text{-}1}\sigma(T_1{}^4 - T_2{}^4)$$

$$(36)$$

where temperatures are in degrees absolute ($^\circ K$ or $^\circ R$).

If the difference between emissive powers is considered to be analogous to potential difference, the blackbody thermal circuit becomes

$$q_{1\text{-}2} = \frac{E_{b_1} - E_{b_2}}{R_{vf}} = \frac{\Delta E_b}{R_{vf}}$$

$$(37a)$$

where $E_b = \sigma T^4$. The "view factor" (vf) resistance, also termed the "spatial" resistance, is

$$R_{vf} = \frac{1}{A_1 F_{1\text{-}2}} = \frac{1}{A_2 F_{2\text{-}1}} \tag{37b}$$

In detailing the influence of the view factor on $q_{1\text{-}2}$, we must account for two important characteristics of diffuse radiation:[2] First, intensity diminishes in inverse proportion to the square of the distance r between the surfaces. Second, the intensity varies according to the cosine of the angle between a vector normal (perpendicular) to the emitting surface and a vector drawn in the direction of the specified point on the receiving surface (this relationship is known as *Lambert's Cosine Law*). As is demonstrated in basic heat transfer texts, these diffuse radiation properties lead to the following general expression for the view factor between two surfaces 1 and 2 (see Figure 3.21):

$$A_1 F_{1\text{-}2} = A_2 F_{2\text{-}1} = \int_{A_2} \int_{A_1} \frac{\cos \phi_1 \cos \phi_2}{\pi r^2} dA_1 \, dA_2 \tag{38}$$

This integral is evaluated when the specific geometries of surfaces 1 and 2 and their relative orientations are known. As the reader may suspect, this mathematical definition of view factor may be quite complicated for real situations of radiation heat exchange. Some special cases, however, can be dealt with by simple inspection. For example, two parallel planes of infinite extent have view factors $F_{1\text{-}2} = F_{2\text{-}1} = 1$; this because, by definition, all of the emitted energy from each surface strikes the other. Similarly, if one surface ("2") completely encloses another ("1"), the view factor $F_{1\text{-}2} = 1$. The view factors for many different and more difficult geometrical situations have been solved and may be found in standard texts and the heat transfer literature. As an example, Figure 3.22 shows the variation with geometry of the view factor $F_{1\text{-}2}$ between two parallel, concentrically-positioned disks of radii r_1 and r_2 which are separated by a distance L.

Example 9

It is desired to induce cutaneous hyperemia on an area of the back of a patient by heating with a heat lamp designed for large-area irradiation. Assume that the lamp, placed 30 cm above the skin, behaves as a diffusely-radiating 15 cm diameter disk with a uniform effective radiant temperature of 1000°K. Estimate the total net radiant power and the average radiation intensity falling on the patient's back when it has reached an equilibrium

---

[2] "Diffuse" radiation exhibits a scattered quality from an emitting or reflecting surface, as opposed to mirror-like, "specular" reflection.

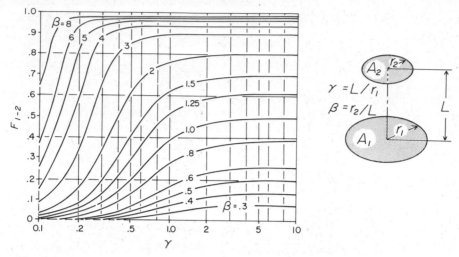

Fig. 3.22. View factor function for two concentric radiating disks in planes parallel to each other separated by a distance L (from Ref. 43, p. 269).

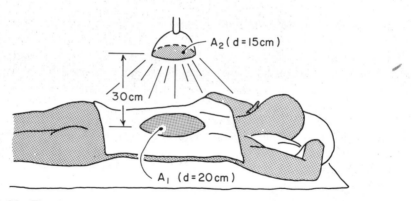

Fig. 3.23. The infrared radiation treatment of a circular region of the back (Example 9).

skin temperature of 45°C. The irradiated area is that exposed by a 20 cm diameter circular hole cut in thick white toweling draped over the prone patient (Figure 3.23).

Solution

Designating the infrared source as surface 2 and the skin as surface 1, we assume that the most efficient orientation of the lamp is employed, which is when the lamp is centered over the exposed skin and the plane of the lamp surface is parallel to the plane of the exposed skin. The net heat exchange is

$$q_{1-2} = A_1 F_{1-2} \sigma (T_1{}^4 - T_2{}^4)$$

where $T_2 = 1000°K$ and $T_1 = 45°C = 318.2°K$. The following parameters define F_{1-2} from Figure 3.22:

$$r_1 = 10 \text{ cm}, \ A_1 = \pi(10^2) = 314.2 \text{ cm}^2$$

$$r_2 = 7.5 \text{ cm}, \ A_2 = \pi(7.5)^2 = 176.7 \text{ cm}^2$$

$$L = 30 \text{ cm}, \ \gamma = 30/10 = 3, \ \beta = 7.5/30 = 0.25$$

and

$$F_{1-2} \approx 0.06$$

Thus

$$q_{1-2} = (0.03142 \text{m}^2)(0.06)\left(5.669 \times 10^{-8} \frac{\text{W}}{\text{m}^2 - °K} \right)$$

$$\cdot [(1000°K)^4 - (318.2°K)^4]$$

$$= 106 \text{ Watts} = 106000 \text{ mW}$$

and the average intensity or flux at the skin is

$$q'' = q/A_1 = \frac{106000}{314.2} = 337 \text{ mW/cm}^2$$

which is within the range required to produce a hyperemic reaction (50). It should be noted that heating lamp reflectors can be designed for varying efficiencies and focusing abilities. The more focused an infrared beam is on a target area of skin, the greater the view factor F_{1-2} will be over that derived from the assumption of diffuse radiation.

A detailed treatment of the analytical methods employed with real (*i.e.*, non-ideal) radiant surfaces is beyond the scope of this introduction. However, these methods can be illustrated by observing the characteristics of surfaces for which the emissivity ϵ and reflectivity ρ are constant (*i.e.*, graybodies). We define the total radiant thermal energy leaving a surface per unit time and unit area as the *radiosity* J (including both emitted and reflected energy). Then, defining the total incident radiation falling per unit time on a unit area as the *irradiation* G, an energy balance yields the radiation surface flux

$$q'' = q/A = J - G \qquad (39)$$

Since radiosity includes both emitted and reflected energy,

$$J = \epsilon E_b + \rho_r G \qquad (40)$$

Eliminating G, the heat transfer q becomes

$$q = \frac{E_b - J}{\left(\dfrac{1 - \epsilon}{\epsilon A}\right)} \tag{41}$$

This provides the basis for a graybody circuit analogy. The numerator, $E_b - J$, can be seen as a potential difference, while $(1 - \epsilon)/\epsilon A$ may be considered to be a resistance related to the surface properties of the radiator. The unknown potential J may be related to the known potential $E_b = \sigma T^4$ by means of this "surface resistance" R_s. The spatial resistance R_{vf} (Equation 37b) between two surfaces is then summed in series with the surface resistances involved to complete the circuit. The circuit analogy for a simple graybody system of two surfaces is shown in Figure 3.24. In this case, the heat exchange "current" between the radiating surface is

$$q_{1\text{-}2} = \frac{E_{b_1} - E_{b_2}}{R_{s_1} + R_{vf} + R_{s_2}}$$

$$= \frac{\sigma(T_1^4 - T_2^4)}{\dfrac{1 - \epsilon_1}{\epsilon_1 A_1} + \dfrac{1}{A_1 F_{1\text{-}2}} + \dfrac{1 - \epsilon_2}{\epsilon_2 A_2}} \tag{42}$$

Radiant heat transfer coefficient: Since it is often desired to determine the radiation and convection heat losses from the body to the ambient environment simultaneously, radiant exchange can be conveniently expressed in a manner analogous to Newton's law of cooling (Equation 17), which requires an effective radiant heat transfer coefficient h_r similar to h_c. The surface heat flux is then

$$q'' = (h_c + h_r)A_s(T_s - T_\infty) \tag{43}$$

This expression is valid only for cases where the radiation and convection surfaces are identical, and where the radiation exchange is from the skin at T_s to a surface (usually an enclosure) which is in thermal equilibrium with the convecting fluid at T_∞. The wall temperatures surrounding a patient, for example, may often be assumed equal to the room air temperature T_∞. Noting that $(T_s^4 - T_\infty^4)$ can be factored into $(T_s^3 + T_s^2 T_\infty + T_s T_\infty^2 + T_\infty^3)(T_s - T_\infty)$ and that the first factor does not vary more than 20 percent over the physiological temperature range, 0 to 50°C, h_r may be assumed

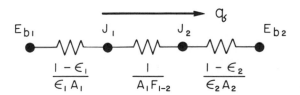

Fig. 3.24. Thermal circuit for two "gray" surfaces which only "see" each other.

approximately constant for applications of relevance to thermotherapy conditions. In general, then, for the extremely simplified situation of heat exchange between the skin and one radiant surface S_1 at T_∞, with a known view factor F_{s-1} between the two, the equation for the radiation heat transfer coefficient becomes

$$h_r = \frac{\sigma(T_s^3 + T_s^2 T_\infty + T_s T_\infty^2 + T_\infty^3)}{A_s\left[\dfrac{1-\epsilon_s}{\epsilon_s A_s} + \dfrac{1}{F_{s-1}A_s} + \dfrac{1-\epsilon_1}{\epsilon_1 A_1}\right]} \qquad (44)$$

UNSTEADY-STATE HEAT TRANSFER

Thus far, we have only dealt with thermal situations which do not change with respect to time. Unsteady-state heat transfer is obviously of significant practical interest for the therapeutic application of heat and cold. Whenever the skin temperature or the skin surface heat flux is changed, or the internal diathermic energy deposition or blood flow conditions are altered, a transient thermal situation ensues. If a steady state is ultimately attained, it may often be viewed as the limiting condition of the transient behavior for large values of time. Perhaps the simplest transient case of interest is that of conduction in a solid, homogeneous sample of superficial tissue at a uniform initial temperature T_i, which has its skin temperature suddenly changed to T_s. If we neglect internal heat production and assume that one-dimensional transfer conditions prevail, Equation 10a yields, for depth x and time t:

$$\frac{\partial^2 T}{\partial x^2} = \frac{1}{\alpha}\frac{\partial T}{\partial t} \qquad (45)$$

If we assume that the region of interest extends only from the skin surface to some arbitrary depth where the tissue temperature does not change from T_i, the temperature response may be described as (5)

$$\frac{T(x, t) - T_s}{T_i - T_s} = \mathrm{erf}\left(\frac{x}{2\sqrt{\alpha t}}\right) \qquad (46)$$

where "erf" designates the Gauss "error function," which varies as shown in Figure 3.25. This is the solution for transient conduction in what is termed a "semi-infinite" solid. Applying Fourier's law (Equation 8b) at the surface ($x = 0$) and noting that $\alpha = \dfrac{k}{\rho c}$, the surface heat flux rate at time t is

$$q''_{x=0} = \frac{\sqrt{k\rho c}\,(T_s - T_i)}{\sqrt{\pi t}} \qquad (47)$$

Example 10

Many modern hot packs are made of a finely woven silicon dioxide matrix with an affinity for water such that every SiO_2 molecule absorbs approxi-

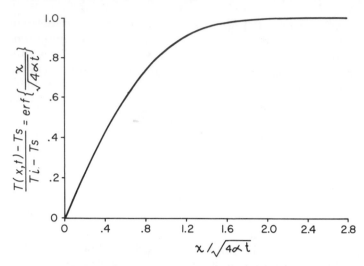

Fig. 3.25. The transient temperature response of one-dimensional passive conduction is described by the so-called "error function" (erf). The boundary condition for which this applies is that of an instantaneous change in surface temperature (see text).

mately 17 molecules of water, when the pouches are soaked in hot water prior to treatment (48). This being the case, the pack behaves as a solid with thermal properties approximating those of water. It is often the practice to apply the packs to the skin at 65 to 90°C using several layers of toweling as insulation. For the case where evaporation from the hot pack is considered to be obstructed, estimate the maximum pack temperature which could be used without toweling which would not burn the patient ($T_s \leq 45°C$), whose skin and subcutaneous tissue may be assumed initially uniform at 30°C.

Solution

Assume that both the hot pack and tissue are semi-infinite solids as shown in Figure 3.26 (this assumption will be checked later). For two semi-infinite solids in contact, with negligible thermal resistance between them, the heat flux out of the surface of the hotter solid must equal that flowing into the cooler body, i.e., $-q''_{hp} = q''_{tissue}$. For heat influx defined as positive heat flow, Equation 47 gives

$$-\left[\frac{\sqrt{k\rho c}(T_s - T_i)}{\sqrt{\pi t}}\right]_{hp} = \left[\frac{\sqrt{k\rho c}(T_s - T_i)}{\sqrt{\pi t}}\right]_{tissue}$$

from which an interesting result is found, this being that the "contact" temperature T_s is independent of time, i.e.,

$$\frac{T_s - T_{tissue,i}}{T_{hp,i} - T_s} = \frac{\sqrt{(k\rho c)_{hp}}}{\sqrt{(k\rho c,)_{tissue}}} \tag{48}$$

The ratio of the changes in temperature at the surface of the tissue versus the hot pack is inversely proportional to the ratio of the square roots of the two $k\rho c$ products. The $k\rho c$ properties (termed *thermal inertias*) for various human tissues and non-biological materials are shown in Table 3.10. As is evident from the tissue values, the presence of blood flow may greatly influence the resulting contact temperature. To provide a conservative estimate for a safe hot pack initial temperature, we will assume poorly perfused subcutaneous tissue composed exclusively of fat ($k\rho c = 4.55 \times 10^{-3}\,W^2 - sec/cm^4\,°C^2$). In this case, for a safe skin temperature of 45°C,

$$\frac{45 - 30}{T_{hp,i} - 45} = \sqrt{\frac{26.7 \times 10^{-3}}{4.55 \times 10^{-3}}} = 2.42$$

from which

$$T_{hp,i} = 51.2°C$$

which is considerably below the temperature of hot packs normally used in conjunction with toweling. If maximal perfusion of the skin is assumed [$k\rho c = 70 \times 10^{-3}\,W^2 - sec/cm^4\,°C^2$], the maximum safe temperature increases to $T_{hp,i} = 69.3°C$!

The general criterion for a semi-infinite solution to apply for a body of

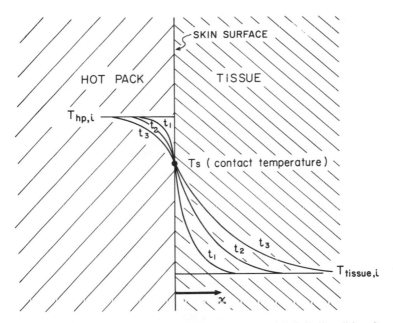

Fig. 3.26. Transient temperature variations in "semi-infinite" solids after being brought into contact with negligible thermal resistance at the contact interface (here representing the tissue and hot pack bodies of Example 10).

TABLE 3.10. *Thermal Inertia (k ρ c) of Various Materials*

Biological Tissues [Watt - sec/cm⁴ - °C²] x 10³		Non-biological Materials [c] [Watt - sec/cm⁴ - °C²] x 10³	
skin (no blood flow)[a]	15.8	water (60°C)	26.7
skin (with blood flow)[a]	15.8 - 70.0	water (0°C)	23.9
forearm skin[b]	22.8	glass (plate)	17.7
average skin[b]	17.5	wood	1.26
finger-tip skin[b]	40.0	steel	1586.
inner forearm skin[b]	24.5	chrome steel	1435.
human fat[a]	4.55	brass	3642.
muscle (excised, moist)[a]	20.0	aluminum	4948.
bone[a]	8.75	copper	13,240.

[a] from ref 14

[b] from ref 19

[c] from ref 4

finite thickness L when subjected to one-dimensional heat transfer is (43)

$$\frac{L}{\sqrt{\alpha t}} \geq 2.0 \qquad (49)$$

Assuming that the fat ($\alpha = 9.62 \times 10^{-4}$ cm²/sec) temperature remains at its initial temperature at a depth of 1 cm ($L = 1$ cm) and beyond, the hot pack application time for which the tissue behaves as a semi-infinite solid is $t \leq L^2/\alpha$, which in this case is 4.3 minutes. This period is long enough so that the cooling losses by convection from both the hot packs and the thigh, and the blood perfusion response, will much more likely limit the validity of the analysis than the assumptions underlying Equation *49*.

Equation *46* may be used to demonstrate the limited depth-penetration produced by surface heating modalities. Assume that surface heating is used on a "semi-infinite" superficial tissue field with negligible fat, *i.e.*, a tissue field of muscle only. As mentioned earlier, the maximum effective conductivity k_{eff} of superficial tissues which can be produced by blood flow augmentation is approximately four times that of the resting conductivity k. This being the case, a reasonable approximation for the maximum thermal diffusivity of muscle is $\alpha = 4 \times (1.62 \times 10^{-3}$ cm²/sec$) = 6.48 \times 10^{-3}$ cm²/sec. For a 20-minute application of surface heating, during which the skin is maintained at the maximum "safe" temperature of 45°C, the initial surface temperature again being 30°C, Equation *46* dictates that the maximum depth which will reach 43°C, the threshold for vigorous therapeutic responses (51), using this elevated value of α, will only be 0.67 cm below the surface! Herein lies the potency of the various diathermy modalities.

Other closed-form analytical solutions of semi-infinite transient conduction problems which are pertinent to thermotherapy may be found in the literature. For example, the transient temperature response of a tissue whose skin is in contact with a convecting fluid may be expressed in terms of the convective coefficient of heat transfer h_c, fluid temperature T_∞, tissue depth x, initial tissue temperature T_i and the thermal properties of the tissue, k and α (4):

$$\frac{T - T_i}{T_\infty - T_i} = 1 - \text{erf } X - e^{\left(\frac{h_c x}{k} + \frac{h_c^2 \alpha t}{k^2}\right)} \cdot \left[1 - \text{erf}\left(x + \frac{h_c \sqrt{\alpha t}}{k}\right)\right] \quad (50)$$

where $X = x/2\sqrt{\alpha t}$ and t is time. This complex solution is presented graphically in standard texts. (4, 40) Similarly, for a sudden exposure of the skin surface to a constant input heat flux q_0'', the temperature at depth x may be expressed as (4)

$$T - T_i = \left(\frac{2q_0''}{k} \sqrt{\frac{\alpha t}{\pi}}\right) \cdot e^{\frac{-x^2}{4\alpha t}} - \frac{q_0'' x}{k} (1 - \text{erf } X) \quad (51)$$

Buettner (52) solves this equation both for non-penetrating and penetrating radiation exposures to the skin. Dussan and Weiner (53) and Buettner (52) solve the problem of transient conduction to superficial tissue through a protective layer, as might be the situation for radiation or hot pack applications employing protective toweling.

The analytical solutions for transient one-dimensional conduction in "finite" solids of regular geometry without internal heat generation are covered thoroughly in the literature (4, 40, 41) and are beyond the scope of this chapter. Of greater interest for our purposes are cases which involve heat generation effects and conduction in more than one direction. Shitzer and Chato (54) apply transient analysis to biological tissue in which heat generation, blood flow heat dissipation effects and changes in the skin surface heat transfer rate are all accounted for. While their assumptions in rectangular and cylindrical tissue segments in one- and two-dimensional heat transfer are very idealized (e.g., uniform, step-like changes in heat generation, blood flow rate and skin heat loss; single component homogeneous tissue with constant properties, etc.), their work serves to illustrate the complexity of the purely analytical process in such transient problems and to provide considerable insight into the transient behavior of perfused biological tissue. In addition, these authors briefly review the previous analytical work in the area of transient heat transfer behavior of tissue.

For more accurate and useful predictions of heat transfer and tissue temperature relevant to the complex contemporary modalities of thermotherapy, the thermal analyst and physiatrist must resort to "numerical" techniques and the digital computer. This is particularly true for modeling irregularly shaped body segments with varying tissue properties and blood flow, and for the complicated energy deposition patterns associated with diathermy. The computer solution approach will be discussed in Chapter 4.

REFERENCES

1. FOURIER, J. B. J. *Théorie Analytique de la Chaleur.* Paris, 1822 (English translation by A. Freeman, Dover publications, Inc., New York, 1955).
2. SEAGRAVE, R. C. *Biomedical Applications of Heat and Mass Transfer.* Iowa State University Press, 1971, p. 66.
3. BROWN, A. C. Energy metabolism. Chapter 4 *In: Physiology and Biophysics.* Vol III. Ruch, T. C. and Patton, H. D. (Eds). W. B. Saunders, Philadelphia, 1973, p. 89.
4. HOLMAN, J. P. *Heat Transfer.* 4th ed, McGraw-Hill Book Co., New York, 1976.
5. MYERS, G. E. *Analytical Methods in Conduction Heat Transfer.* McGraw-Hill, New York, 1971.
6. ZEITER, W. J. Clinical application of the paraffin bath. *Arch. Phys. Ther., 20:* 469–472, 1939.
7. READER, S. R. The effective thermal conductivity of normal and rheumatic tissues in response to cooling. *Clin. Sci., 11:* 1–12, 1952.
8. KELLER, K. H. AND SEILER, L. An analysis of peripheral heat transfer in man. *J. Appl. Physiol., 30:* 779–786, 1971.
9. POPPENDIEK, H. F., RANDALL, R., BREEDEN, J. A., CHAMBERS, J. E. AND MURPHY, J. R. Thermal conductivity measurements and predictions for biological fluids and tissues. *Cryobiology, 3:* 318–327, 1966.
10. CHATO, J. C. Heat transfer in bioengineering. *In: Advanced Heat Transfer.* Chao, B. T. (Ed). University of Illinois Press, 1969, pp. 404–406.
11. GORDON, R. G., ROEMER, R. B. AND HOWATH, S. M. A mathematical model of the human temperature regulatory system—transient cold exposure response. *IEEE Trans. Biomed. Engin., BME-23:* 434–444, 1976.
12. AHUJA, A. S. Acoustical properties of blood: a look at the basic assumptions. *Med. Phys. 1:* 312, 1974.
13. COOPER, T. E. AND TREZEK, G. J. Correlation of thermal properties of some human tissues with water content. *Aerospace Med., 42:* 24–27, 1971.
14. LIPKIN, M. AND HARDY, J. D. Measurement of some thermal properties of human tissues. *J. Appl. Physiol., 7:* 212–217, 1954.
15. COHEN, M. L. Measurement of the thermal properties of human skin. A review. *J. Invest. Dermatol., 69:* 333–338, 1977.
16. NEVINS, R. G. AND DARWISH, M. A. Heat transfer through subcutaneous tissue as heat generating porous material. Chapter 21. *In: Physiological and Behavioral Temperature Regulation.* Hardy, J. D. Gagge, A. P. and Stolwijk, J. A. (Eds). Charles C Thomas Publisher, Springfield, Il, 1970, pp. 281–301.
17. EDWARDS, R. H. T., HILL, D. K. AND JONES, D. A. Heat production and chemical changes during isometric contractions of the human quadriceps muscle. *J. Physiol., 251:* 303–315, 1975.
18. MINARD, D. Body heat content. Chapter 25 *In: Physiological and Behavioral Temperature Regulation.* Hardy, J. D. Gagge, A. P. and Stolwijk, J. A. (Eds). Charles C Thomas Publisher, Springfield, Il, 1970, pp. 345–346.
19. BUETTNER, K. Effects of extreme heat and cold on human skin. II Surface temperature, pain, and heat conductivity in experiments with radiant heat. *J. Appl. Physiol., 3:* 703–713, 1951.

20. VENDRIK, A. J. H. AND VOS, J. J. A method for the measurement of the thermal conductivity of human skin. *J. Appl. Physiol.*, *11:* 211–215, 1957.
21. ROOT, W. S. The flow of blood through bones and joints. *Handbook of Physiology.* Sec 2, Vol II. American Physiological Society, Washington, D.C., 1963, p. 1657.
22. GUY, A. W., LEHMANN, J. F. AND STONEBRIDGE, J. B. Therapeutic applications of electromagnetic power. *Proc. IEEE*, *62:* 60, 1974.
23. NEWBURGH, L. A. *Physiology of Heat Regulation and the Science of Clothing.* Hafner Publishing Co., New York, 1968, p. 120.
24. PERL, W. Heat and matter distribution in body tissues and the determination of tissue blood flow by local clearance methods. *J. Theoret. Biol.*, *2:* 201–235, 1962.
25. DALY, M. J., HENRY, R. E., PATTON, D. D. Measurement of skin perfusion with Xenon-133. *J. Nuclear Med.*, *19:* 709, 1978.
26. STERN, M. D., LAPPE, D. L., BOWEN, P. D., CHIMOSKY, J. E., HOLLOWAY, G. A., KEISER, H. R. AND BOWMAN, R. L. Continuous measurement of tissue blood flow by laser-Doppler spectroscopy. *Am. J. Physiol. 232:* H441–H448, 1977.
27. LEHTOVIRTA, P. AND REKONEN, A. Peripheral blood flow in normal subjects evaluated by plethysmography and Xe[133] clearance at rest and during hyperaemia. *Ann. Clin. Res.*, *6:* 234–240, 1974.
28. LARSEN, O. A., LASSEN, N. A. AND QUAADE, F. Blood flow through human adipose tissue determined with radioactive Xenon. *Acta Physiol. Scand.*, *66:* 337–345, 1966.
29. LASSEN, N. A., LINDBJERG, J. AND MUNCK, O. Measurement of blood flow through skeletal muscle by intramuscular injection of Xenon-133. *Lancet*, *1:* 686–689, 1964.
30. SEKINS, K. M., DUNDORE, D., EMERY, A. F., LEHMANN, J. F., MCGRATH, P. W. AND NELP, W. B. Muscle blood flow changes in response to 915 MHz diathermy with surface cooling as measured by Xe[133] clearance. *Arch. Phys. Med. Rehabil. 61:* 105–113, 1980.
31. SEKINS, K. M., DELATEUR, B. J., DUNDORE, D., EMERY, A. F., ESSELMAN, P., LEHMANN, J. F., AND NELP, W. B. Local muscle blood flow and temperature responses to 915 MHz diathermy as simultaneously measured and numerically predicted. *Arch. Phys. Med. Rehabil.* (submitted 1981).
32. BONNEY, G. L. W., HUGHES, R. A. AND JANUS, O. Blood flow through normal human knee segment. *Clin. Sci. 11:* 169–181, 1952.
33. NIELSEN, S. L. Measurement of blood flow in adipose tissue from washout of Xenon-133 after atraumatic labelling. *Acta Physiol. Scand.*, *84:* 195, 1972.
34. WULFF, W. The energy conservation equation for living tissue. *IEEE Trans. Biomed. Engin.*, *BME-21:* 494–495, 1974.
35. CHEN, M. AND HOLMES, K. R. Microvascular contributions in tissue heat transfer. Presented at the New York Academy of Sciences, Mar 14–16, 1979. To be published in the Annals of the New York Academy of Sciences.
36. CHATO, J. C. Heat transfer to blood vessels. ASME Paper 79-WA/HT-68, 1979.
37. PENNES, H. A. Analysis of tissue and arterial blood temperatures in the resting human forearm. *J. Appl. Physiol.*, *1:* 93–122, 1948.
38. PRIEBE, L. Heat transport and specific blood flow in homogeneously and isotropically perfused tissue. Chapter 20. *In: Physiological and Behavioral Temperature Regulation.* Hardy, J. D. Gagge, A. P. and Stolwijk, J. A. (Eds). Charles C Thomas, Publisher, Springfield, Il, 1970, pp. 272–280.
39. WEINBAUM, S. AND JIJI, L. M. A two phase theory for the influence of circulation on the heat transfer in surface tissue. *In: 1979 Advances in Bioengineering.* ASME, New York, 1979, pp. 179–182.
40. KREITH, F. *Principles of Heat Transfer.* Intext Educational Publishers, New York, 1973.
41. CHAPMAN, A. J. *Heat Transfer.* Macmillan Publishing Co., New York, 1974.
42. TALBOT, L. AND BERGER, S. Fluid mechanical aspects of the human circulation. *Am. Scient.*, *62:* p. 677, 1974.

43. PITTS, D. R. AND SISSOM, E. *Schaum's Outline of Theory and Problems of Heat Transfer.* McGraw-Hill, New York, 1977, p. 77.

44. RAPP, G. M. Convective mass transfer and the coefficient of evaporative heat loss. Chapter 6. *In: Physiological and Behavioral Temperature Regulation.* Hardy, J. D. Gagge, A. P. and Stolwijk, J. A. Charles C Thomas, Publisher, Springfield, Il, 1970, pp. 55–80.

45. MITCHELL, J. W. AND MYERS, G. E. An analytical model of the counter-current heat exchange phenomena. *Biophys. J.,* 8: 897–911, 1968.

46. ROHSENOW, W. M. AND CHOI, H. Y. *Heat, Mass and Momentum Transfer.* Prentice-Hall, Inc., New Jersey, 1961, p. 416.

47. BOEHM, R. F. AND TUFT, D. B. Engineering radiation heat transfer properties of human skin. ASME Paper 71-WA/HT-37, 1971.

48. GRIFFIN, J. E. AND KARSELIS, T. C. *Physical Agents for Physical Therapists.* Charles C Thomas, Publisher, Springfield, Il, 1978, p. 164.

49. SUCEC, J. *Heat Transfer.* Simon and Schuster, New York, 1975, p. 237.

50. STONER, E. K. Luminous and infrared heating. Chapter 9. *In: Therapeutic Heat.* Licht, S. (Ed). Vol II in Physical Medicine Library Series, Elizabeth Licht, New Haven, 1958, p. 236.

51. LEHMANN, J. F., GUY, A. W., STONEBRIDGE, J. B. AND DELATEUR, B. J. Evaluation of a therapeutic direct-contact 915 MHz microwave applicator for effective deep-tissue heating in humans. *IEEE Trans. Microwave Theory Tech., MTT-26:* 556, 1978.

52. BUETTNER, K. Effects of extreme heat and cold on human skin. I. Analysis of temperature changes caused by different kinds of heat application. *J. Appl. Physiol.* 3: 691–702, 1951.

53. DUSSAN, B. I. AND WEINER, R. I. Study of burn hazard in human tissue and its implication on consumer design. ASME Paper 71-WA/HT-39, 1971, pp. 1–7.

54. SHITZER, A. AND CHATO, J. C. Analytical solutions to the problem of transient heat transfer in living tissue. ASME Paper 71-WA/HT-36, 1971, pp. 1–11.

4

Computer Modeling of Thermotherapy[1]

ASHLEY F. EMERY
K. MICHAEL SEKINS

Nomenclature

A_{bl}	Convective surface area exposed to the blood (m^2)
A_{ij}	Surface of a nodal volume through which heat is conducted from node i to node j (m^2)
A_w	Surface area of skin at which evaporation is taking place (m^2)
c	Specific heat capacity of tissue (kJ/kg-°C)
c_{bl}	Specific heat capacity of blood (kJ/kg-°C)
f_b	Blood perfusion rate per unit mass (kg/sec-kg)
F_{12}	Radiation view factor between surfaces 1 and 2
h_s	Heat transfer coefficient at the skin surface (W/m^2-°C)
h_{bl}	Heat transfer coefficient for blood flow (W/m^2-°C)
h_w	Evaporative mass transfer coefficient at the skin surface (kg/m^2-mm Hg)
h_e	Evaporative heat transfer coefficient at the skin surface (W/m^2-mm Hg)
k	Thermal Conductivity of tissue (W/m-°C)
K	Constant coefficient in tissue system energy equation
k_{eff}	Effective thermal conductivity of tissue (W/m-°C)
k_{ij}	Thermal conductivity (W/m-°C) of tissue between nodes i and j
L	Latent heat of water (kJ/kg)
$\dot{m}_{bl}, \dot{m}_{bl_i}$	Mass flow rate of blood, of blood stream i (kg/sec)
$\dot{m}_w$	Mass flow rate of evaporation (kg/sec)
$\dot{M}_D$	Diathermic power absorption (W/kg)
$\dot{M}_o$	Basal metabolic heat generation rate (W/kg)
$\dot{M}_t$	Total energy generated and deposited in a nodal volume (W/kg)

[1] This chapter is in part based on research supported by Research Grant #G008003029 from the National Institute of Handicapped Research, Department of Education, Washington, D.C. 20202.

133

$\dot{M}_{bl}$ Metabolic heat generation in the blood (W/kg)
$\dot{M}_M$ Metabolic heat generation rate in tissue (W/kg)
p Vapor pressure of water (mm Hg)
q'' Heat flux through a surface (W/m²)
q_s'' Heat flux through the skin surface (W/m²)
q_r'' Radiant heat flux (W/m²)
q_e'' Evaporative heat flux (W/m²)
q''' Heat generation rate per unit volume (W/m³)
Q_s Energy flow through a nodal volume surface (W)
Q_{cv} Convective heat flow through a surface (W)
Q_{bs} Heat flow through a boundary surface (W)
Q_{cd} Conductive heat flow through a nodal volume surface (W)
S Diathermic power amplitude (W/kg)
T Temperature (°C)
T_{bl}, T_{bl_i} Blood temperature, of blood stream i (°C)
T_s Skin surface temperature (°C)
T_{fl} Fluid temperature (°C)
t Time (sec.)
U Internal energy (J)
V Volume (m³)
ε Radiative emissivity
ρ Density (kg/m³)
σ Stephan-Boltzmann constant: $5.669 \times 10^{-8} \dfrac{W}{m^2 - °K^4}$
Δl_{ij} Distance between nodal points (m)
ΔT Temperature change in tissue relative to a particular reference temperature
ΔT_{ij} Temperature difference between nodal points i and j (°C)

SUBSCRIPTS

bl Blood
bs Boundary surface
cv Convection
D Diathermy
fl Fluid
i, j Nodal numbers
$m\text{-}f$ Muscle-fat interface
m Muscle
M Metabolism
s Skin, surface
t Total
ti Tissue
w Wetted surface
∞ Denotes ambient conditions

Introduction

In spite of the ever-expanding knowledge of thermophysiology and the significant advances being made in techniques and devices used for diathermy, surface heating and surface cooling modalities, the clinical practice of thermotherapy remains a somewhat quasi-quantitative science. This is due, in part, to the complex interactions of diathermy energy fields with treated tissue, and to the equally involved physiological responses to changing tissue temperatures. It is also a result of the difficulties associated with clinically measuring such principal phenomena as local blood flow and deep tissue temperature during treatment (this problem stemming from both the difficulties of instrumentation and the invasive, traumatic nature of such measurements). A need clearly exists for developing valid thermotherapy models which would provide improved quantitative information for specifying dosimetry, and for predicting the behavior of such clinically significant physiological parameters as blood flow and tissue temperature. Such information would also provide yardsticks by which the consistency and validity of experimental data could be gauged. A promising approach to this need lies in the methods of engineering thermal analysis and the associated "numerical" computer techniques. To logically develop this approach requires that we begin with some basic definitions.

The term "model" is associated with any representation (conceptual or physical) that describes the behavior of a system under study (prototype) in terms of the variables of interest. The intent of "thermal modeling" is to simulate a system in such a way that thermal information (usually temperature and/or heat transfer rates) about the prototype may be obtained. Originally the simulation was done by experimenting with small scale models of the prototype, hence the term modeling. Currently, in the physical sciences and engineering, most modeling of physical phenomena is done through mathematical conceptual models. The sample problems of Chapter 3, for example, were simplified mathematical models of various thermal processes relevant to thermotherapy. For these models the solutions were frequently obtained in exact (*i.e.*, "closed") form. While these particular models were valuable for didactic purposes and for establishing estimates and limits on thermal processes, only a small fraction of practical thermal problems can be modeled in such a way that their behaviors can be expressed in closed form. Models of more useful and complex situations and phenomena are usually constructed by applying the pertinent physical principles to a collection of many discrete small sub-regions (*e.g.*, areas or volumes) which collectively make up the problem domain of concern. This type of analysis, in which a problem domain is "discretized" (*i.e.*, sub-divided into these many sub-volumes or areas), normally results in large sets of interrelated differential equations which theoretically describe, in space and time, the thermal processes over the entire domain of interest. If the methods of classical mathematics were used in seeking simultaneous solutions to these equations, there would be little hope of solving problems of practical interest. Fortunately however, the evolution of "numerical methods"[2] and the advent of the large, high-speed digital computer have rendered tractable a large range of practical thermal problems. Over the past several decades, the validity of the numerical solution to properly defined mathematical thermal models has been demonstrated to the point where numerical thermal modeling is now used routinely to predict the behavior of non-biological thermal systems (3–5). Its use for biological systems, however, has not yet matured to the point of routine application.

There are two typical uses of modeling: The first compares a model's results to situations which are well defined, and whose results are clearly known or which can be accurately estimated by other methods. The second applies modeling techniques to predict the behavior of existing or hypothetical situations or systems. The former is used to prove the accuracy of the model (i.e., its validity), while the latter is used for prediction to eliminate the need either to find information experimentally or to subject tissue to unusual, unexplored, or perhaps dangerous conditions. While modeling usually consists of estimating temperature, the problem can also be considered in reverse, where the temperatures are known, and the investigator attempts to draw conclusions about the system's thermal properties or about its boundary conditions.

This chapter is not intended to teach the reader in great detail how to construct thermotherapy computer models nor how to execute such model simulations. A detailed "how-to" of numerical thermal modeling would require far more space than a single chapter and a comprehensive mathematical background. The purpose of this chapter is rather to familiarize the reader with the basis of thermal modeling, to delineate its strengths and limitations as a research tool in physical medicine, and to present some modeling examples to help illustrate its utility for thermotherapy. Successful modeling requires close cooperation and communication between the physician and the modeling practitioner (the thermal analyst). The accuracy of a simulation depends strongly on the correctness and completeness of the model, and on the applicability of the model and its basic assumptions to the system being modeled. Frequently, a simulation fails because the model is inapplicable or because the prototype is too complicated or too poorly understood to be accurately simulated. It is, in large measure, the responsibility of the analyst to determine if the system and its processes can be modeled and which is the best model (based on medical information,

---

[2] Techniques which involve repetitive calculations of algebraic equations, and thus lend themselves to use on digital computers, are commonly called "numerical techniques." The solution of large sets of simultaneous equations in approximate form is, today, a routine application of numerical analysis (1, 2).

physiological data, and the problem definition supplied by the physician). It is often not known *a priori* if a single model is adequate. Thus, a series of models is sometimes developed to determine the best one or the range of most-probable appropriate models.

While the current state of the modeling art is such that the process is too complex to be quickly and inexpensively used in the clinic for individual patient treatments, continued development and refinement in the research arena will likely lead to sophisticated modeling "packages" (hardware and software) such that the direct use of thermal modeling by the clinician will be commonly employed to aid in the selection of optimal treatment modalities and protocols.

The remainder of this chapter presumes some familiarity with the basic principles of heat transfer. To assist the reader with these fundamentals as they apply to thermal modeling, occasional reference is made to material in Chapter 3.

The Basic Model

THE MESH

Although real thermal systems are three-dimensional, we will treat only anatomical sections which can be approximated with some confidence as being two-dimensional systems for ease and clarity of exposition. Every tissue system will thus be considered to be composed of a cross-section of unit thickness, as shown in Figure 4.1, with all properties and temperatures assumed to be constant across the thickness.

The cross-section will be subdivided into a series of small volumes, as shown in Figures 4.2 and 4.3, each of which is of unit thickness. Figure 4.3 indicates that each volume (*shaded area*) is represented by a point called a node (here node j), and is surrounded by enclosing surfaces (denoted by *dashed lines*). A node is a fictitious point to which we ascribe properties (density, thermal conductivity, etc.) that represent the average values of the volume, henceforth called the "nodal volume." The nodal temperature T_j is the average value of the tissue in the *shaded area* around the point j (Figure 4.3). The *solid lines* of Figure 4.3 which connect the nodes represent heat paths, while the *dashed lines* represent the surfaces which enclose the nodal volume and through which the heat flows. The accuracy and adequacy of any model depends strongly on the size and shape of the nodal volumes. The lines which either demarcate the nodal volumes or connect the nodes are usually termed the "mesh", the size of the elements defines the "mesh size", and the process of establishing these lines and the location of the nodal point is referred to as "meshing." Cross-sections modeled by large, coarsely-defined meshes cannot represent the system as well as more refined meshes which contain a greater number of nodal volumes. On the other hand, the finer the mesh, the greater the number of nodes, and the greater

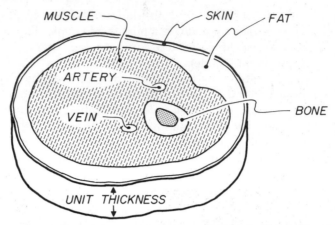

Fig. 4.1. Cross-section of a typical limb tissue section showing the thermally important features.

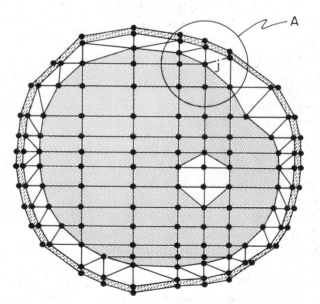

Fig. 4.2. Subdivision of the limb by a nodal mesh into discrete nodal volumes. The region *A* corresponds to the detailed mesh shown in Figure 4.3.

the cost of performing a model simulation. Just how much to refine a mesh is generally difficult to determine and is usually left to the subjective decision of the analyst. Since the accuracy with which the temperatures (evaluated at the nodes) represent the true solution to the mathematical equations depends on the fineness of the mesh, the analyst can repeat calculations with a sequence of meshes of increasing degree of refinement until the results become insensitive to the mesh. The solution is then said to be independent of the mesh and is taken to be the final solution. The thermal analyst usually uses the term "to model"[3] as meaning constructing the mesh and assigning the thermal properties and the thermal conditions to be used on the exterior (*i.e.*, boundary) of the mesh.

THE NODAL VOLUME ENERGY EQUATIONS[4]

All thermal systems are governed by two laws of conservation, the conservation of mass and energy, and by the second law of thermodynamics which dictates the direction in which a thermal process will naturally proceed. These principles relate the temporal and spatial variations of the temperature in a system to its thermal properties and to the initial and boundary conditions which are imposed on the system.

The principle of conservation of energy (the first law of thermodynamics) as applied to any nodal volume of the mesh, in the absence of work and any effects other than thermal effects, states

$$
\begin{bmatrix}
\text{The rate at which internal} \\
\text{energy } (U) \text{ is stored in a} \\
\text{nodal volume over time } \Delta t \\
\left(\dfrac{\Delta U}{\Delta t}\right)
\end{bmatrix}
=
\begin{bmatrix}
\text{the rate at which energy} \\
\text{flows in through the sur-} \\
\text{faces of the nodal volume} \\
(Q_s)
\end{bmatrix}
+
$$

$$
\begin{bmatrix}
\text{the rate at which energy is} \\
\text{generated and deposited} \\
\text{within the volume} \\
(\rho V \dot{M}_t)
\end{bmatrix}
\qquad (1)
$$

Internal Generation of Energy

For our purposes, energy is considered to be generated in a nodal volume of tissue only by metabolism and diathermy. The total rate at which energy is generated and deposited is denoted by $\dot{M}_t$ where

$$
\dot{M}_t = \dot{M}_M + \dot{M}_D \qquad (2)
$$

and the subscripts M and D refer to metabolism and diathermy respectively. The tissue density ρ, although theoretically a function of temperature and position, may usually be treated as independent of temperature for most

---

[3] The reader should be aware that the verb "to model" is often used in more than one sense. To model can refer to the completeness with which the conceptual model represents all of the significant characteristics of the prototype; to the accuracy with which the mathematical equations represent the physical processes; or to the accuracy with which the numerical analysis represents a solution of the mathematical equations.

[4] A good introduction to the various heat transfer modes and the theory underlying them can be found in Chapter 3 and in the References (6, 7). Reference 7 contains a broad background of information relevant to the physiological aspects of temperature regulation and biological heat transfer.

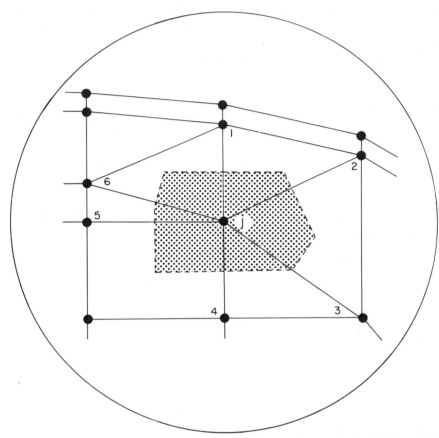

Fig. 4.3. Schematic drawing of a nodal volume, its node (point j) and the neighboring nodal points.

biological systems. In the case where its temperature dependence must be considered, the volume V must change, since the term ρV, representing the mass of the nodal element, will remain constant unless there is a physical addition or subtraction of mass (such as in tissue edema). Although simulations of nonbiological systems often express the heat generation term as Vq''', where q''' is the generation per unit volume, for biological systems, the mass representation is preferred since the chemical generation of heat is directly related to the mass of the reacting tissue. $\dot{M}_M$ is generally a function of temperature, as demonstrated by the simple formulae given in Chapter 3 (Equations $5a$ and $5b$) and by Equation 19 in this chapter.

Energy Storage

The nodal energy storage may be related to a change in nodal temperature ΔT by

$$\text{Energy stored} = \rho c V \cdot \Delta T \qquad (3)$$

where c represents the specific heat capacity of the material, and is normally a function of the local tissue temperature. Using Equation 3, the rate of storage is thus

$$\frac{\Delta U}{\Delta t} = \rho c V \frac{\Delta T}{\Delta t} \tag{4}$$

Surface Heat Flux

The means by which energy enters through the surfaces of the nodal volume must be separated into three distinct parts: internal conduction, internal convection, and energy flowing into the volume through an area which is part of the mesh boundary (the latter obviously applies only to nodal volumes which are part of external or internal boundaries).

INTERNAL CONDUCTION

In numerical methods known as "finite difference" techniques (8), the derivatives which appear in the thermal energy differential equations may be expressed in algebraic, rather than differential form. To briefly illustrate how this is done, let us assume that the true temperature profile between two points in a tissue region, say corresponding to nodes i and j in the mesh, is represented by the solid curve of Figure 4.4. From the law of heat conduction, we know that the magnitude of heat transported by conduction across the interface surface area between the nodal volumes (A_{ij}) must be:

$$Q_{cd} = k A_{ij} \frac{dT}{dx'} \tag{5a}$$

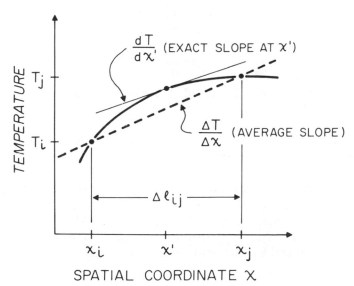

Fig. 4.4. "Central difference" approximation of the derivative dT/dx.

where k = the thermal conductivity of the material in the region between the nodes and

$\dfrac{dT}{dx}$ = the derivative of the temperature with respect to position at the interface position x'.

A frequently used finite difference expression for this derivative involves approximating the temperature profile slope at x', dT/dx, by the average slope between the nodes, that is

$$\left. \frac{dT}{dx} \right|_{x=x'} \approx \frac{(T_j - T_i)}{(x_j - x_i)} = \frac{\Delta T_{ij}}{\Delta l_{ij}} \tag{5b}$$

where

ΔT_{ij} = difference between the temperatures at the respective nodal points i and j and

Δl_{ij} = distance between the two nodal points i and j.

Thus, in this finite numerical form, the rate at which heat is conducted internally (between nodes) may be expressed algebraically, not differentially, as

$$Q_{cd} = k_{ij} A_{ij} \frac{\Delta T_{ij}}{\Delta l_{ij}} \tag{5c}$$

where k_{ij} is the average thermal conductivity of the material between nodes i and j, and A_{ij} is the area of the interfacial surface. For most materials, k is a function of temperature and direction. This is particularly true of biological materials which have a decided orientation of subcomponent materials. Chapter 3 contains a thorough description of typical variations of k for biological tissues. If k_{ij} is independent of direction, the material is said to be isotropic; if it has three distinct values associated with three mutually perpendicular directions, it is termed orthotropic. Equation 5c is an approximation to the differential form, Equation 8b of Chapter 3, and is strictly true only for temperature distributions which are linear in space, and for systems in which the surface area A is constant between the nodes. For nodes which are proximate, however, it is usually a reasonable approximation.

Figure 4.3 illustrates a typical two-dimensional mesh with the areas A_{ij} and distances Δl_{ij} between the nodes. We note that a nodal volume conducts heat only to those nodal volumes which adjoin it, and not to any which are removed from it. For a node j, surrounded by a total of N nodes, the total heat conducted into the nodal volume of j is given by

$$\sum_{i=1}^{N} \frac{k_{ij} A_{ij}}{\Delta l_{ij}} (T_i - T_j) \tag{5d}$$

where the summation ($\sum$) is over all N of the adjacent volumes of nodes i. The subscripts ij indicate that the heat conducted from any node i to node j may be associated with different conductivities, areas and separation distances.

INTERNAL CONVECTION

Internal convection within a biological thermal system is associated with the energy transported into and out of the nodal volume by blood perfusion. We express this in the form

$$Q_{cv} = \dot{m}_{bl}c_{bl}(T_{bl}(\text{in}) - T_{bl}(\text{out})) \qquad (6a)$$

where $\dot{m}_{bl}$ = mass flow rate of the blood through the nodal volume (no accumulation of blood or fluid within a nodal volume is considered)

c_{bl} = specific heat capacity of the blood

$T_{bl}(\text{in})$ = temperature of the incoming blood

$T_{bl}(\text{out})$ = temperature of the outgoing blood

If there is more than one stream of blood, Equation 6a is replaced by

$$Q_{cv} = \sum_{i} \dot{m}_{bl_i}c_{bl}[T_{bl_i}(\text{in}) - T_{bl}(\text{out})] \qquad (6b)$$

where the summation takes place over all i streams. The flow of blood through the volume $\dot{m}_{bl}$ is expressed in terms of a per-unit-mass flow by

$$\dot{m}_{bl} = f_b \rho V \qquad (6c)$$

where f_b is discussed in Chapter 3.

The blood itself is a thermal system which can be represented by an energy balance of the form

$$
\begin{bmatrix}
\text{rate of internal energy} \\
\text{stored in a unit mass of} \\
\text{blood} \\
\dfrac{\Delta U_{bl}}{\Delta t}
\end{bmatrix}
=
\begin{bmatrix}
\text{rate of energy generated in} \\
\text{a unit mass} \\
(\dot{M}_{bl})
\end{bmatrix}
$$

$$(7a)$$

$$
-
\begin{bmatrix}
\text{rate at which energy leaves} \\
\text{the blood and flows into} \\
\text{the surrounding tissue} \\
(Q s_{bl})
\end{bmatrix}
$$

Since we must be able to calculate the rate of energy loss to the tissue from the blood to estimate the temperature of the blood leaving a nodal volume, which depends upon the local tissue temperature (the calculation of which requires a knowledge of the energy gained from the tissue by the blood), we have reached an apparent impasse. Highly complex relationships are available to estimate the energy lost from the blood to the tissue, but normally the following simple relationship is used:

$$Q_{cv} = h_{bl}A_{bl}(T_{bl} - T_{ti}) \qquad (7b)$$

where T_{bl} = local blood temperature

$\quad T_{ti}$ = local tissue temperature

$\quad A_{bl}$ = surface area of the tissue surrounding the blood

$\quad h_{bl}$ = a constant of proportionality, called the heat transfer coefficient.

This relationship is Newton's law of cooling, which is used for any thermal energy transfer between a fluid and a solid surface, whether blood and tissue, air and skin, or water vapor and the lungs (see Equation 17, Chapter 3). The use of Equation 7b is inhibited, however, by the need to know both h_{bl} and A_{bl}. Although for many situations A_{bl} can be estimated (for example, in larger arteries and veins), much of the body's tissue is so interwoven with arterioles, venules, and capillaries, whose size and surface area are constantly changing and complexly distributed, that an accurate estimate of A_{bl} cannot be made. By the same token, the heat transfer coefficient h_{bl} is strongly dependent on the nature of the fluid flow—laminar, turbulent, helical, steady, pulsatile; the nature of the inner vessel surfaces—smooth, rough, regular; the type of vessel fluid flow cross-section—round, oval, irregular, or constant or variable with respect to vessel length; the physical properties of the fluid—viscosity, composition, etc. Thus, h_{bl} must be estimated and can rarely be known exactly. Many of the differences which occur between the results of different simulations of identical problems are due to the use of different assumptions regarding the values and distributions of h_{bl} by different analysts.

Once estimates are made of h_{bl} and A_{bl}, or at least the $h_{bl}A_{bl}$ product, we can evaluate the energy transfer between the tissues in a nodal volume and the blood which perfuses this volume.

The equations which represent energy flow through the mesh boundary Q_{bs} are discussed later in this chapter.

Summary of Equations

From Equation 1, noting that we can express time as well as spatial derivatives in finite difference form, we can sum the energy inputs into the nodal volume of node j.

$$(\rho c V)_j \frac{[T_j(t + \Delta t) - T_j(t)]}{\Delta t}$$

$$= \sum_i k_{ij}A_{ij}\frac{(T_i - T_j)}{\Delta l_{ij}} + \sum_i h_{bl_i}A_{bl_i}(T_{bl_i} - T_j) + (\rho V)_j \dot{M}_j + \sum Q_{bs} \qquad (8a)$$

and for the blood in the nodal volume from Equation 7a we find

$$(\rho c V)_{bl} \frac{[T_{bl}(t + \Delta t) - T_{bl}(t)]}{\Delta t} = (\rho V)_j \dot{M}_{bl_j} - \sum_i h_{bl_i} A_{bl_i} (T_{bl_i} - T_j) \quad (8b)$$

Here the term $\frac{\Delta U}{\Delta t}$ has been replaced by its finite numerical equivalent (Equation 4), and the summation signs are used to account for multiple energy flow paths. The term $\sum Q_{bs}$ refers to the boundary surface energy flow through the portions of the mesh boundary which are associated with the volume of node j.

This development, involving two interdependent energy equations for each nodal volume, one for the tissue and one for the blood, illustrates the conventional engineering modeling approach for a system with internal convection. This classical and rigorous method leads to very complicated analysis. Consequently, most tissue thermal modeling makes use of the simplified approximation introduced by Pennes (9) who suggested, because in most vascular beds the tissue area in contact with the perfusing blood is extremely large, that the term $h_{bl}A_{bl}$ must become effectively infinite. The blood must thus quickly come to complete equilibrium with the local tissue temperature. The result of these assumptions is that Equations 8a and 8b may be replaced by the single equation

$$(\rho c V)_j \frac{[T_j(t + \Delta t) - T_j(t)]}{\Delta t}$$

$$= \sum_i k_{ij} A_{ij} \frac{(T_i - T_j)}{\Delta l_{ij}} + \sum_i \dot{m}_{bl_i} c_{bl} (T_{bl_i}(\text{in}) - T_j) + (\rho V)_j \dot{M}_j + \sum Q_{bs} \quad (9)$$

where Equation 6a has been used with the condition that $T_{bl_i}(\text{out}) = T_j$. This is equivalent to modeling the effect of blood flow as a temperature dependent source (or sink) for internal heat generation (an approach discussed in Chapter 3, see Equation 7a). Of course, this simplification cannot be made if the purpose of modeling is to study the variation and interdependence of blood and tissue temperatures. For most situations of interest to us, such fine discrimination will not be required; we will be satisfied to represent only the average temperature of the perfused tissue.

Initial and Boundary Conditions

What remains is to establish what are known as the "initial" and "boundary" conditions. All thermal systems start from some initial temperature state, and change in accordance with the thermal conditions which are subsequently imposed upon them. Although most analytical thermal studies assume that the system has a uniform and constant initial temperature, this is rarely satisfactory for biological studies (except for the most localized regions) for which the initial temperature distribution, determined by the interaction between blood flow, metabolism and surface heat transfer, is an important part of the problem. Because this initial state is rarely known with sufficient precision, one usually assumes an approximate temperature profile and repeatedly applies Equation 9 until the computed temperature distribution becomes constant with time (i.e., until $T_j(t + \Delta t) \approx T_j(t)$). This steady state distribution (the initial condition) is then taken as the state from which changes occur due to the effects of various boundary and system changes.

The thermal boundary conditions (B.C.'s) are usually divided into five categories:
1. Prescribed temperature
2. Prescribed heat flux
3. Convection
4. Radiation
5. Diffusion and evaporation

PRESCRIBED TEMPERATURE

$$T_s = T_{\text{prescribed}} \qquad (10)$$

This, the simplest of all boundary conditions to model, is the most unlikely condition to be found in thermotherapy. To say that a portion of the tissue surface is maintained at a specified temperature during treatment, while an attractive condition, ignores the reality of how such a state is achieved. Nevertheless, it is a popular concept in thermal modeling because of its mathematical simplicity, and because it usually represents a limiting condition which is easy to visualize. Many experiments in the physiology of thermoregulation are designed to create this kind of boundary condition (e.g., immersion in isothermal baths); successful modeling of such experiments depends on the degree to which this condition is attained.

PRESCRIBED HEAT FLUX

$$q_s'' = q''_{\text{prescribed}} \qquad (11)$$

Just as in the case of a prescribed boundary temperature, this is also an unusual condition. Probably the only case in which it can be accurately used is when one assumes that a known-output heater is completely enclosed by a surface of the system (see Example 3 in Chapter 3). Then, since all of the heat generated must flow through the surface, the heat flux is known (in fact, this is also a simplification which depends upon the thermal capacitance of the heater and whether or not a steady state has truly been achieved).

CONVECTION

A surface is generally maintained at a constant temperature by bathing it with a fluid of constant temperature under constant flow conditions. The heat transferred to the surface is given by Newton's law of cooling as

$$Q_{cv} = h_s A_s (T_{fl} - T_s) \qquad (12)$$

Since heat transfer for a skin surface is limited by the ability of the tissue to accept heat or cold, as h_s is increased with a fixed value of A, the term $T_{fl} - T_s$ must approach zero, *i.e.*, the surface temperature must come to equal the fluid temperature. Thus, it is interesting to note that the limiting cases of $h_s A_s$ becoming either very large or approaching zero correspond to a prescribed surface temperature b.c. or a zero heat flux b.c., respectively. For the numerical modeling of irregularly shaped surfaces (*i.e.*, other than planes, cylinders, spheres, etc.), a purely analytical determination of h_s (its magnitude and distribution) is usually very difficult; thus, most of the time experimental measurements of h_s are made using physical models which are subjected to conditions similar to those of interest. Special techniques are then used to extrapolate the measured values of h_s to those values which are appropriate to the prototype. Unfortunately, such an extrapolation is not always possible or practical; and the analyst must frequently make rather rough assumptions to estimate the proper values of h_s to use for the numerical model. We must also recognize the possibility that sometimes minute differences between the physical model experiment and the proto- type experiment may render such an extrapolation invalid. For example, the loss of heat by a motionless person can be changed by several hundred percent by the existence of a draft in the space surrounding the human body being simulated. For this reason, it is often necessary to make h_s measure- ments on the real human prototypes in the exact prototypical environments desired, rather than rely on physical model experimental results. Because of this rather arduous task, or sometimes because convective surface heat transfer is not an especially important aspect of the problem, analysts may often use rather simple surface shapes and very crude estimates of h_s. For example, an arm is often represented by a simple cylinder or two and the head perhaps by a sphere; then, values of h_s pertinent to these regular shapes, as determined from heat transfer experiments and analysis (*e.g.*, Examples 5 and 6 in Chapter 3), are used, even though air currents around an actual arm and head may be strongly modified by the presence of the rest of the body. Because of the complexity of some situations, the analyst has no accurate way of determining values of h_s; in such a case, he simply chooses values he feels are roughly representative. For example, the con- vective heat loss from the human body in other than standing or supine positions is not well known; and there are basically no accurate models which approximate such postures.

RADIATION

Another of the conventional boundary conditions is the transfer of heat by electromagnetic radiation in the thermal spectrum, for example, from infrared lamps, fireplaces, the sun, electric heaters, or to cold window or wall surfaces. Radiant heat transfer between two surfaces S_1 and S_2 is represented by (see Equations *34* to *36*, Chapter 3)

$$q_r'' = \sigma\epsilon F_{12}(T_{S_1}^4 - T_{S_2}^4) \tag{13}$$

Because of the presence of the fourth power of the absolute surface temperatures, this mode of heat transfer becomes dominant as surface temperatures increase. The factor F_{12} represents the proportional view that each surface has of the other. The analytical determination of this "view factor" is very difficult and time-consuming, so recourse is generally made to experiments. Also, since F_{12} is often strongly affected by small changes in position, it is rarely known with exactness; consequently, appropriate approximations must usually be made. This is particularly true for the human body, for which slight changes in posture or orientation cause substantial changes in the view factor. Although this poses a problem for the analyst, it is important to our physical well-being, since we can avoid many undesirable thermal effects with relatively small changes in position or posture (*e.g.*, a slight change in facial orientation can be used to eliminate sun burning, etc.). The constant of proportionality σ is the Stephan-Boltzmann constant; the emissivity factor ϵ represents the effect of surface radiation properties. For most tissues, ϵ may be taken to be approximately unity (see Chapter 3).

DIFFUSION AND EVAPORATION

The last of the usual boundary conditions is associated with the evaporation of liquid from the tissue surface. As each unit of liquid evaporates, it requires L units of heat (its latent heat) to vaporize it. This heat comes either from the surrounding air or from the tissue surface. For the purposes of physical medicine, the two most common diffusion effects are those associated with the passive diffusion of water vapor through the skin and with the thermoregulatory action of sweating. Regardless of whether moisture arrives at the skin surface passively or actively, once it evaporates from the surface, the laws of diffusion determine its subsequent movement. If it evaporates but remains at the surface, further evaporation is inhibited, requiring any such extra liquid to be removed by dripping or other means; however, since liquid removed in this manner does not evaporate, no heat is required, and thus none is removed from the tissue. Any such non-evaporative excess liquid loss is thus not part of these thermal modeling considerations. That portion which does evaporate diffuses away from the skin in accordance with

$$\dot{m}_w = h_w A_w (p_s - p_\infty) \tag{14a}$$

giving rise to a heat loss of

$$q_e = h_w A_w L (p_s - p_\infty) = h_e A_w (p_s - p_\infty) \tag{14b}$$

where p represents the water vapor pressure, a function of temperature (see Figure 3.17); h_w is the coefficient of mass transfer for water in air, which is affected by all of the same variables which affect the skin surface heat transfer coefficient h; and A_w represents the wetted surface area. Frequently, the analyst makes use of an approximation which states that h_w is proportional to h_s (e.g., Equation 31, Chapter 3). For those conditions in which this approximation is valid, one need not determine h_w, but instead can use h_s together with whatever approximations are felt to be valid in determining h_s. Although these approximations may be imprecise for some situations, this approach has the merit of treating both convective heat loss and surface mass transfer in a mutually consistent fashion.

SUMMARY OF THE ENERGY AND BOUNDARY CONDITION EQUATIONS

For a nodal volume associated with an arbitrary node j, the modeling equations are a) the tissue energy balance:

$$(\rho c V)_j \frac{[T_j(t + \Delta t) - T_j(t)]}{\Delta t}$$

$$= \sum_i k_{ij} A_{ij} \frac{(T_i - T_j)}{\Delta l_{ij}} + (\rho V)_j \dot{M}_j + \sum_i \dot{m}_{bl_i} c_{bl} (T_{bl_i} - T_j) + \sum Q_{bs} \quad (9)$$

and b) the problem domain boundary conditions:

$$T = T_s$$
on A_t (portion of boundary surface area with specified temperatures) $\quad (10)$

$$q'' = q''_{bs}$$
on A_q (portion with specified heat flux) $\quad (11)$

$$q'' = hA_h(T_s - T_\infty)$$
on A_h (portion with convection) $\quad (12)$

$$q'' = \sigma \epsilon F_{12} A_r (T_{S_1}^4 - T_{S_2}^4)$$
on A_r (portion with radiation) $\quad (13)$

$$q'' = h_e A_w L (p_s - p_\infty)$$
on A_w (portion with evaporation) $\quad (14)$

A brief example may further clarify the manner in which relationships of the form of Equations 9 to 14 are used to construct a thermal model. Assume, for instance, we have a simplified tissue system which may be represented by the nine-node mesh of Figure 4.5. To further simplify the discussion, let us focus our attention only on the thermal interactions of a single node, say node 6. Inspection of the figure shows that node 6 communicates thermally with the contiguous volumes of nodes 3, 5, and 9 (both through conduction and, if applicable, blood flow). Being a surface node, the external surface area of the node (A_s) will have a boundary condition

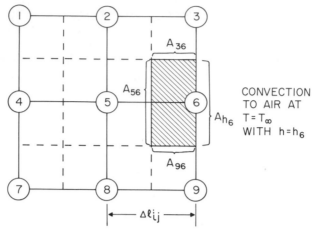

Fig. 4.5. Simplified thermal tissue system made up of a nine-node, rectangular mesh. The energy equations for node 6 typify those for the entire nodal network.

applied to it. Again, for simplicity, we shall assume only a single boundary condition, namely convection with ambient air at a temperature T_∞; thus, $\sum Q_{bs} = h_6 A_{s_6}(T_6 - T_\infty)$. Note that for this tissue system, all nodal volumes except that associated with node number 5 will require a boundary condition.

We can now apply Equation 9 to the node of concern; here $j = 6$ and $i = 3, 5, 9$. Thus

Rate of energy storage $\quad \rho_6 c_6 V_6 \dfrac{[T_6(t + \Delta t) - T_6]}{\Delta t} =$

Conduction $\quad k_{3\text{-}6} A_{3\text{-}6} \dfrac{(T_3 - T_6)}{\Delta l_{36}} + k_{5\text{-}6} A_{5\text{-}6} \dfrac{(T_5 - T_6)}{\Delta l_{56}} + k_{9\text{-}6} A_{9\text{-}6} \dfrac{(T_9 - T_6)}{\Delta l_{96}}$

Blood flow $\quad + \dot{m}_{bl_3} c_{bl}(T_{bl_3} - T_6) + \dot{m}_{bl_5} c_{bl}(T_{bl_5} - T_6) + \dot{m}_{bl_9} c_{bl}(T_{bl_9} - T_6)$

Internal heat generation (metabolism + diathermy) $\quad + \rho_6 V_6 \dot{M}_6$

Convection boundary condition $\quad + h_6 A_{s_6}(T_\infty - T_6)$ $\hfill (15a)$

Inserting the known or assumed values for the various thermal properties, blood flow rates, internal heat generation rate, blood and ambient air temperatures, heat transfer coefficient h_6 and the time interval Δt, after rearrangement, an equation for node 6 results, which is of the form

$$K_0{}^6 T_6(t + \Delta t) = K_3{}^6 T_3 + K_5{}^6 T_5 + K_6{}^6 T_6 + K_9{}^6 T_9 + K_\infty{}^6 T_\infty \quad (15b)$$

where the K's denote constant coefficients made up of the appropriate combinations of the parameters appearing in Equation 15 (the superscripts indicate which nodal equation we are dealing with). Equation 15b can also be expressed in more general form as

$$K_0{}^6 T_6(t + \Delta t) = K_1{}^6 T_1 + K_2{}^6 T_2 + K_3{}^6 T_3 + K_4{}^6 T_4 + K_5{}^6 T_5$$
$$+ K_6{}^6 T_6 + K_7{}^6 T_7 + K_8{}^6 T_8 + K_9{}^6 T_9 + K_\infty{}^6 T_\infty \quad (15c)$$

where, since only nodes 3, 5, and 9 communicate with node 6, $K_1{}^6 = K_2{}^6 = K_4{}^6 = K_7{}^6 = K_8{}^6 = 0$.

Since we are dealing with a total tissue system of nine nodal volumes, the mathematical model is thus composed of a system of nine nodal temperature equations of the form of Equation *15c* (equivalent to Equation *9*), each with its own combination of zero and non-zero constants K. The temperatures T_1, T_2, ... T_9 must be found such that all nine nodal equations are solved simultaneously for a particular value of time t. A series of such solutions for several values of time, progressing from the initial condition at $t_0 = 0$ through $t_1 = 0 + \Delta t$, $t_2 = t_1 + \Delta t$ etc., would constitute a simple transient simulation for this tissue system.

It should be recognized that a variety of mathematical methods can be used to arrive at algebraic equations to approximate the energy differential equations; Equation *9* is only one example, formed by one particular type of "finite difference" approximation. The two most common approaches to forming such approximate solutions are a variety of finite difference methods and the so-called "finite element" method (10, 11). While these various approaches may differ in their mathematical basis and detail, all involve division of the problem's spatial domain into smaller discrete subunits, as we have done in our development, and require the solution of large systems of simultaneous algebraic temperature equations. The reader may regard Equations *9* to *14* as typical of those used to simulate the thermal behavior of tissue. The remainder of this chapter will be devoted to presenting some model solutions based on these equations, to acquaint the reader with some of the solution characteristics and to illustrate many of the advantages which accrue from the use of such simulations.

Thermal Modeling of Limb Tissues under Various Physiological Conditions

Although most tissue sections are complex in substance and shape, we consider in this section the very simple case of the superficial region of a perfectly circular limb cross-section which is subject primarily to metabolic heating (*i.e.*, in the absence of diathermy). The series of simplified models and simulations which follow demonstrate the facility with which we can quantitatively study the energy interactions of a tissue region by these methods. Specifically, we wish to investigate the effects of the following variables on the tissue temperatures:

a) blood perfusion (in the muscle, subcutaneous fat and skin)
b) tissue metabolism

c) fat thickness
d) surface heat transfer coefficient h_s
e) sweating

The calculations are to be based on the conditions listed in Table 4.1, which constitute a reasonable simulation of an idealized cylindrical human thigh. Note that we assume that at some depth, the tissue temperature is equal to the deep core temperature, here 36.5°C.

EFFECTS OF METABOLISM AND SKIN SURFACE HEAT TRANSFER

Based upon an ambient air temperature of $T_\infty = 22°C$ and a surface heat transfer coefficient at 15 W/m² − °C (comprising both free convection and radiation), Figure 4.6 illustrates typical computed steady state temperature profiles for this model for the cases both with and without metabolic heat generation. These temperature computations were made by holding the muscle-core interface temperature constant at 36.5°C (a specified temperature boundary condition). Calculations made by assuming that no heat was transferred from the core to the muscle (a specified heat flux condition) gave virtually the same profiles. Note the small change in the muscle temperature (1.5°C), the substantial temperature drop through the fat layer (3.3°C), the small drop through the skin (0.5°C), and the large temperature difference between the skin surface and the ambient air (9.2°C). The thermal effect of including metabolism in the basal case then is to increase only slightly the overall temperature profile. A comparison of the curves shows that the temperature profile depends primarily on the heat supplied by the blood rather than on that generated through metabolism.

Since steady-state heat loss from the tissue is primarily governed by metabolic heat production and blood perfusion, any changes in geometry or surface conditions cannot be expected to substantially change the overall heat loss. Thus, since the steady-state heat loss is constant and given by Q_{bs}

TABLE 4.1. *Cylindrical Thigh Simulation: Basal Conditions*

Layer	Skin	Fat	Muscle	Core
Thickness	0.2 cm	1.0 cm	4.0 cm	
Outer radius	8.0 cm	7.8 cm	6.8 cm	2.8 cm
k(W/m-v°C)	0.376	0.190	0.642	
$\rho\left(\dfrac{kg}{m^3}\right)$	1000	850	1050	
$c\left(\dfrac{kJ}{kg-°C}\right)$	3.77	2.30	3.75	Temperature maintained at 36.5°C
$\dot{M}\hat{m}\left(\dfrac{kW}{kg}\right)$	1.0	0.38	0.67	
$f_{bl}\left(\dfrac{ml}{min-100g}\right)$	9.8	1.5	2.6	

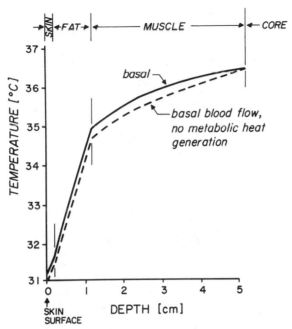

Fig. 4.6. Temperature profiles for an idealized thigh model showing the effect of metabolic heat generation ($h = 15$ $W/m^2 -$ °C, fat thickness = 10 mm).

$= h_s A_s (T_s - T_\infty)$, any changes in h_s will cause corresponding but opposite changes in $(T_s - T_\infty)$. Figure 4.7 shows the temperature profiles to be expected for several different surface heat transfer coefficients ranging from 5 $W/m^2 -$ °C (corresponding to a somewhat insulated skin covering) to 25 $W/m^2 -$ °C (corresponding to a significant draft). Note that the skin temperature is most affected, changing by 5°C, while the superficial muscle temperature, which is insulated by the fat layer, shows markedly less change (1.6°C). The table included in Figure 4.7 indicates the portions of heat loss from the skin surface to the environment which come, respectively, from blood flow, metabolism, and conduction from the core. Even when the most severe temperature gradients exist, conduction from the core supplies only 3 percent of the total heat loss. The blood-supplied heat ranges from 66 percent to 85 percent, and is nearly constant for the higher values of h_s, emphasizing again the dominant role that blood flow plays in maintaining the superficial basal temperature profile. Since most of the limb thermoreceptors are located in the skin, it can be seen that changes in h_s could induce significant thermoregulatory responses: vasodilation and sweating, or vasoconstriction and shivering. Although the range of h_s here is small compared to that found in most non-biological conditions of engineering interest, its physiological effects are likely quite large, thus, indicating the importance of accurately estimating appropriate values of h_s for each condition.

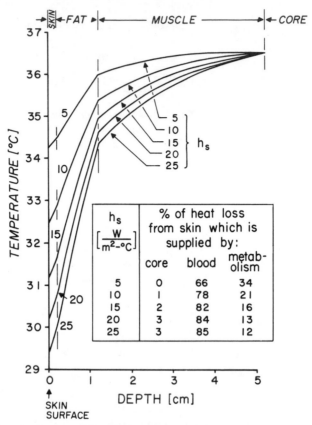

Fig. 4.7. Temperature profiles for the thigh model showing the effects of different surface heat transfer coefficients (fat thickness = 10 mm).

EFFECTS OF SUBCUTANEOUS FAT THICKNESS

The precise effects of varying fat thickness are difficult to estimate because the fat layer is normally not uniform in a human limb, and because local blood perfusion varies (in magnitude and direction) in the fat layer. If, for instance, the blood enters and exits the fat layer in a direction parallel to the longitudinal axis of the limb, the thermal effects are much different than if it flows radially, since in the latter case, the blood temperature upon entry into the fat is conditioned by muscle temperature. Similarly, the exiting (venous) blood in radial flow carries temperatures representative of the fat and skin, and transports this energy directly to the underlying tissue. Since only radial conduction of heat is significant in our two-dimensional model, radial blood flow acts to modify the effective thermal conductivity k_{eff} of the tissue, while axial perfusion corresponds more to a modification in the heat generated within the fat and superficial tissue. The analyses of this

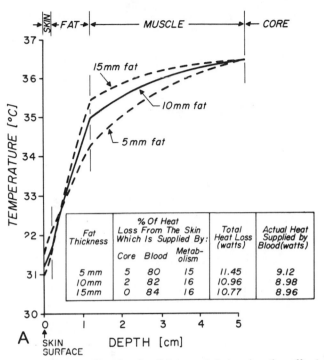

Fig. 4.8a. Temperature profiles for the thigh model showing the effect of different fat thicknesses ($h = 15\ W/m^2 - °C$) plotted versus normalized depth. Temperature profiles for the thigh model showing the effect of different fat thicknesses ($h = 15\ W/m^2 - °C$) plotted versus actual depth.

chapter assume that blood flow can be represented as a variable heat source or sink, as previously mentioned.

Figure 4.8a illustrates the temperature profiles to be found for different fat thicknesses for the basal properties given in Table 4.1, assuming a constant 4.0 cm muscle thickness. (In viewing the figure, note that the fat layers are shown as each having the same constant thickness (*i.e.*, they are scaled); this was done to emphasize the variation in the fat-muscle interface temperature). Note the strong insulating effect of the fat in increasing the interface temperature and in reducing skin temperature as the fat thickness increases. The skin temperature reduction with increasing fat thickness is a consequence of surface heat transfer, expressed as

$$\text{surface heat loss} = Q_{bs} = h_s A_s (T_s - T_\infty) \qquad (16)$$

which, for constant h_s and A_s, requires that T_s diminish as the heat loss diminishes. As indicated by the tabular values in Figure 4.8a, the heat loss is reduced by only 6 percent for a three-fold increase in fat thickness, a three-fold increase in fat thermal resistance—again emphasizing the dominant role of the blood in maintaining the basal temperature distribution,

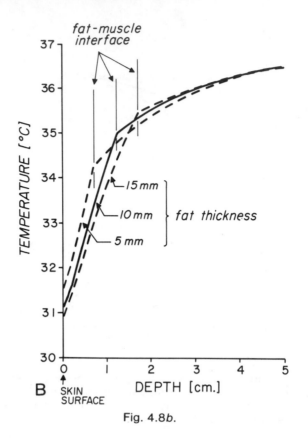

Fig. 4.8b.

and the minor role played by conduction from the core. It is interesting to note that the relative amount of energy supplied by the blood actually increased from 80 to 84 percent, although the absolute amount decreased from 9.12 to 8.96 Watts. This percentage increase came as a consequence of the reduction in the heat conducted outward from the core, which was reduced from 5 to 0 percent.

As a consequence of the reduction in energy supplied by the blood, which you recall may be expressed as

$$Q_{cv} = \dot{m}_{bl} C_{bl} [T_{bl}(\text{in}) - T_{bl}(\text{out})] \tag{6a}$$

the average temperature of the blood departing the subcutaneous fat increases, although not as much as may be suggested by Figure 4.8a, which, because of the scaling in depth, tends to exaggerate the profiles. Figure 4.8b shows temperature profiles plotted against depth from the surface and clearly illustrates that the skin temperature, and therefore the departing skin blood temperature, decreases as the fat thickness increases, while the average muscle, fat, and venous blood temperatures in these regions increase with increasing fat thickness. It might be argued, therefore, that there would be a greater central thermoregulatory drive in a fat person than in one thinner, which would serve to dilate the subcutaneous capillary beds to provide greater cooling of the departing venous blood stream. At the same time, it would appear that the concommitant lower skin temperatures might act to vasoconstrict this capillary region due to the drive from surface thermoreceptors. Experimental data show that thicker layers of subcutaneous fat usually have lower levels of perfusion (see Table 3.5), indicating a shunting of blood away from the fat, and supporting the view that skin thermoreceptor drives normally dominate those of central receptors.

BLOOD FLOW EFFECTS

Figure 4.9 illustrates the effect of altering blood flow to the skin and fat. Several different conditions are shown. The lowest curve is the temperature profile which would exist without heat supplied by either metabolism or blood perfusion, and displays the concave upward shape associated with

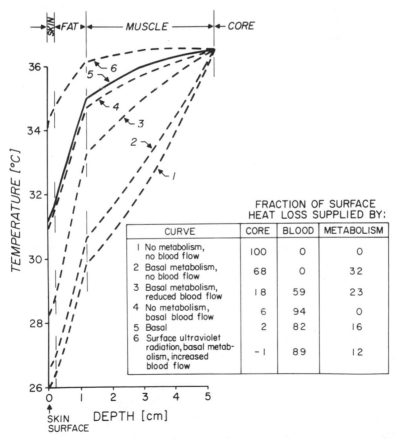

CURVE	FRACTION OF SURFACE HEAT LOSS SUPPLIED BY:		
	CORE	BLOOD	METABOLISM
1 No metabolism, no blood flow	100	0	0
2 Basal metabolism, no blood flow	68	0	32
3 Basal metabolism, reduced blood flow	18	59	23
4 No metabolism, basal blood flow	6	94	0
5 Basal	2	82	16
6 Surface ultraviolet radiation, basal metabolism, increased blood flow	-1	89	12

Fig. 4.9. Temperature profiles for the thigh model showing the effect of metabolism, blood flow and surface heating ($h = 15\ W/m^2 - °C$, fat thickness = 10 mm).

pure radially directed conduction. The next curve illustrates the effect of adding basal metabolism. The table in the figure lists the fraction of surface heat loss supplied by metabolism and blood flow; although approximately 30 percent is generated by metabolism, the temperature elevation is minimal. Note that the third curve models a thigh with significant overall vasoconstriction (perfusion = 1.3, 0.75, and 0 ml/min-100g for muscle, fat, and skin, respectively), while the upper curve represents substantial superficial vasodilation (perfusion = 2.6, 3.0, and 55.0 ml/min-100g, respectively) as found for ultraviolet heating of the skin (12). In the latter case, the increased blood flow to the fat raises its temperature and blocks heat flow from the muscle to the skin. Muscle metabolism, then, increases muscle temperature above the core temperature, thus conducting some heat to the core (the fraction of the heat lost from the skin which is supplied by conduction from the core is the difference between 100 percent and the sum of blood flow and metabolism contributions). This collection of curves graphically demonstrates the role that the three physiological sources of thermal energy—conduction from the core, metabolic generation and heat supplied by the blood—have in establishing the temperature profile in a limb tissue system. The curves and tabular values indicate the result of the interplay between these mechanisms and underscore the role of the arterial supply in maintaining an acceptable temperature distribution.

SWEATING AND METABOLISM-RELATED EFFECTS

In the various simulations presented thus far, the effects of thermoregulatory sweating have not been included. Here we will illustrate the effects of sweating and the increased metabolic heat generation associated with exercise by examining the simulation of an exercising thigh.

When an exercising thigh is simulated, and is treated as independent of the rest of the body, the muscle temperature is found to increase while the skin temperature decreases. The skin temperature decrease occurs because the energy which must be dissipated from the skin is less, even though the heat generated in the muscle has increased due to exercise. This energy reduction is caused by increased muscle blood flow which serves to transport more energy out of the entire tissue section than the exercise has generated, with a concommitant increase in the average exit blood temperature. An increase in this venous temperature would raise the central blood temperature and, through the central nervous system, may elicit a thermoregulatory sweating response, which in turn would tend to further lower the skin temperature. These results, however, are inconsistent with reality. This state of affairs brings us to recognize that since the incoming arterial blood temperature is a major ingredient in determining tissue temperature, even in heavy exercise, it is important to account for any systemic changes in the arterial blood temperature which might occur during its circulation through the body prior to entering the tissue region of interest. Consequently, it is not feasible to accurately simulate a section of limb tissue when it is isolated from the rest of the body because there is no way of properly accounting for systemic temperature changes in the arterial blood and their effects on central thermoregulatory mechanisms.

It is precisely for complicated thermal problems of this type that thermal modeling is particularly advantageous. The analyst can use whole-body thermal models (13–16), and then study the effects of changing the values of selected parameters associated with systemic circulation, sweating or other thermal mechanisms. Let us consider, for example, the case where local muscle blood flow increases in direct proportion to the increase in metabolism during exercise at a rate of 4.42 ml/min/100g for every 100 percent increase in metabolism over the basal rate (as found from experimental measurements (17). As tissue temperatures increase, we may assume that blood flow to the skin also increases according to the model (18)

$$\dot{m}_{bl} = (\dot{m}_{bl})_{basal} + k_{bl}(T_s - T_s^{set}) \qquad (17)$$

where T_s^{set} represents a skin set-point temperature above which vasodilation occurs. Suppose further that the surface is cooled by sweating, where sweat rate is modeled by the simple equation (18)

$$m_{sw} = k_{sw}^{sk}(T_s - T_s^{set}) + K_{sw}^c(T_c - T_c^{set}) \qquad (18)$$

Here, T_s^{set} represents another set-point for the skin (which is generally different than the value for vasodilation); and T_c^{set} represents the set-point for the core. Although these simple equations, 17 and 18, may not be

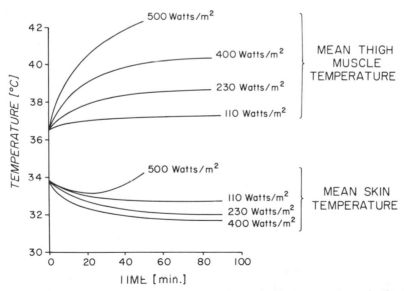

Fig. 4.10. Transient history of mean muscle and skin temperatures in the thigh model for different levels of exercise, showing the effect of whole-body thermoregulation. Exercise is expressed per unit of body surface area.

representative of all conditions, they permit us to observe and systematically study some of the effects of the thermoregulatory system appropriate to our exercise model. In reality, the nature of the sweating response is incompletely defined for all circumstances, and in fact, a number of different investigators have suggested a variety of equations (18–21).

An example of the simulation of a non-isolated thigh, that is, one subject to whole-body thermoregulatory mechanisms, is illustrated in Figure 4.10. This figure shows the use of a selected sweating equation in computing the transient history of thigh temperature, when the body starts at a resting condition and thereafter maintains a constant level of exercise. The onset of sweating is clearly indicated by the relative constancy of the skin temperature (*lower curves*) after a period of reasonably rapid change. The figure also shows the consequence of diffusion-limited sweating (here at 500 Watts/m^2), when the temperature continues to rise and does not achieve a steady-state for the assumed value of h_s. Examination of Equations *12* and *14* shows that a steady-state can be achieved only by changes in the convective coefficients h_s and h_e, *in* T_∞ or in the ambient humidity parameter p_∞, which will increase the heat transferred from the surface and thus, permit a steady-state temperature.

The Simulation of Diathermy

SIMPLE ENERGY DEPOSITION IN PLANAR TISSUES

Consider the simplified plane-wave microwave diathermy deposition pattern shown in Figure 4.11 (only muscle deposition is considered) along with the resulting typical temperature profiles occurring for a constant blood flow and for varying power deposition rates. The discontinuous jump of deposited thermal energy at the fat-muscle boundary, due to the wave reflections from this interface, is clearly apparent. From these conditions, the fat thickness and blood perfusion in the fat are more important than in the previous non-diathermy examples (Figures 4.3, 4.6 to 4.9) since intense energy deposition occurs close to the fat layer. Figure 4.11 illustrates the effects of varying fat thickness and power level on the resulting temperatures. Since low deposition rates ($S = 10$) only increase the temperature slightly above the basal state, it is clear that deposition must be increased substantially to achieve therapeutic temperature levels. When this is done, temperature elevation above the initial temperature roughly parallels the deposition pattern; and deposition becomes effective only near the fat-muscle interface, with the point of maximum temperature moving closer to the fat-muscle interface as the fat thickness increases, in accordance with experimental findings (22).

To develop higher temperatures deeper in the tissue, it seems necessary to either a) increase deposition at deeper areas by increasing overall power, or b) shift the point of maximum deposition. The option to increase power, and therefore, treatment depth, is in fact limited by the high fat-muscle

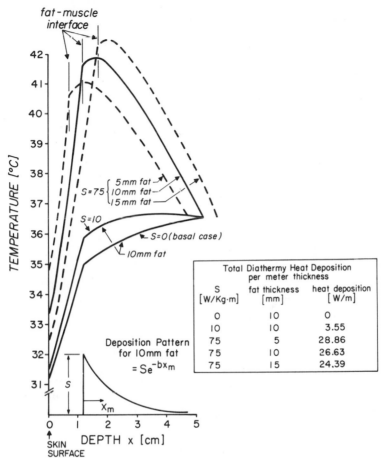

Fig. 4.11. Temperature profiles for the thigh model showing the effects of different diathermy deposition levels and fat thicknesses ($h = 15$ $W/m^2 - °C$). Note that S is the deposited energy intensity at the fat-muscle interface. The solid temperature curves are those for 10 mm fat thickness.

interface temperatures which result, and which are strongly affected by the thickness of the fat layer. Shifting the maximum deposition point, however, can be done either by focusing the electromagnetic waves through the use of multiple microwave sources (23), or by changing the microwave frequency. A third option, shifting the point of peak temperature inward (as opposed to shifting power deposition), can be achieved by surface cooling of the skin and the fat. It is this last method which will be applied in our present diathermy model. Figure 4.12 illustrates the steady-state temperatures produced by a simultaneous application of skin cooling and diathermic heating for constant blood flow. The inward shift of the temperature curve through this "thermal focusing" is easily discernible. The maximum muscle

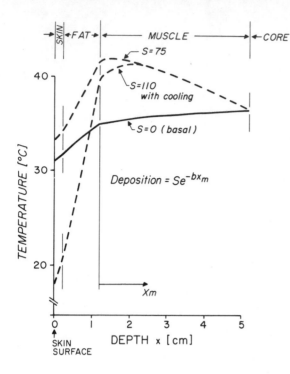

Fig. 4.12. Temperature profiles for the thigh model exposed to diathermy and surface cooling ($h = 15$ W/$m^2 - $ °C, fat thickness = 10 mm, ambient temperature = 5°C).

temperature which can be achieved and its depth are related to the interplay between the diathermic power level, the surface cooling rate and the blood flow rate. This type of thermal model permits the systematic study of this interplay.

DIATHERMY OF THE THIGH

The results shown in Figure 4.12 were qualitative and for an unusually simple situation. Now, the use of thermal modeling will be demonstrated by simulating an actual experimental diathermy treatment of a human thigh. Figure 4.13 presents the mesh, composed of 129 nodes representing a cross-sectional "slice" taken through the proximal portion of the thigh. The anterior (*upper*) surface of the thigh is flattened and the underlying layer of subcutaneous fat narrowed to simulate tissue distortion due to the weight of the 915 MHz direct-contact microwave applicator (24) used in the experiment (Figure 4.14). The treatment protocol to be modeled consisted of 5 minutes of skin pre-cooling with 5°C air (pumped through the applicator and onto the skin surface through a perforated plastic grid), then followed by 20 minutes of diathermic heating at 40 Watts net (absorbed) power, with simultaneous skin cooling.

As indicated in Figure 4.13, depending on its location, an individual nodal volume of the network is assigned the thermophysical properties of either subcutaneous fat, skeletal muscle or bone (typical values are found in Table

FINITE ELEMENT
THERMAL MODEL OF THE HUMAN THIGH

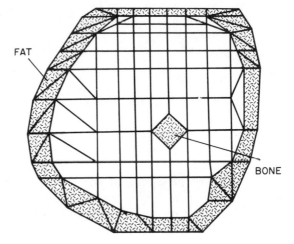

Fig. 4.13. Mesh of the human thigh model.

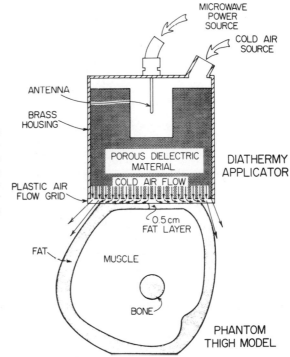

Fig. 4.14. Diagram of the 915 MHz direct-contact microwave applicator on the thigh. Phantom models are used for experimental determination of diathermy power deposition and convective cooling distributions (26).

3.3). In the absence of diathermy, the heat generation and dissipation effects within the tissue are those due only to metabolism and perfusion. Both of these effects are functions of the instantaneous local (nodal) temperature and are assigned on the basis of the mass associated with each respective node. The heat convected by blood flow is represented by Equations 6a and 6b. A unit mass generates heat metabolically according to (see Equation 5b, Chapter 3)

$$\dot{M}_M = \dot{M}_0(1.1)^{\Delta T} \tag{19}$$

where ΔT is the difference between the nodal temperature and its initial basal temperature. The basal nodal temperatures are those derived from the steady state solution to Equations 9 to 14 under basal conditions. The basal metabolic heat output $\dot{M}_0$, of course, varies according to tissue type (see Table 3.4).

The complex geometry of the thigh cross-section and of the square aperture microwave source preclude an accurate theoretical specification of the spatial distribution of the power deposited by the microwave field. Using the materials and methods developed by Guy (25) and described further by Emery et al. (26), the power deposition or "primary heating" pattern in this case was determined through experiments on phantom models as shown in Figure 4.14. The thigh models were constructed in two cross-sectional halves and were irradiated at high power (420 Watts net) for a short period (15 seconds) to minimize the effects of thermal conduction. The microwave power was turned off, the model halves were quickly split apart, and the resulting cross-sectional temperature distribution was immediately "photographed" with a scanning infrared camera (thermograph). The pattern of isotherms thus determined (Figure 4.15) was then converted to diathermic power absorption $\dot{M}_D(W/Kg)$ by assuming no conduction between nodes, i.e.,

$$\dot{M}_D = \rho c V \frac{dT}{dt} \cong \rho c V \frac{\Delta T}{\Delta t} \tag{20}$$

where ΔT was the local temperature rise in the phantom, and Δt the irradiation period (here 15 seconds). The energy deposition was then scaled by the ratio of the power used in the actual human experiment (40 Watts net) to that used in the phantom experiment. Taken over the entire assembly of nodes, Equation 20 thus provided a distribution of heat sources representing the electromagnetic power absorption pattern of the particular applicator, power level, and thigh geometry studied.

As noted previously, temperature profiles are sensitive to the surface heat transfer coefficient. Due to the complex nature of the air flow surrounding the thigh, it was difficult to determine the local variations in h_s analytically. By cooling the phantom thigh at the same air flow rate and temperature conditions as were employed in the human experiments, however, a combined experimental and numerical determination of h_s was possible: after

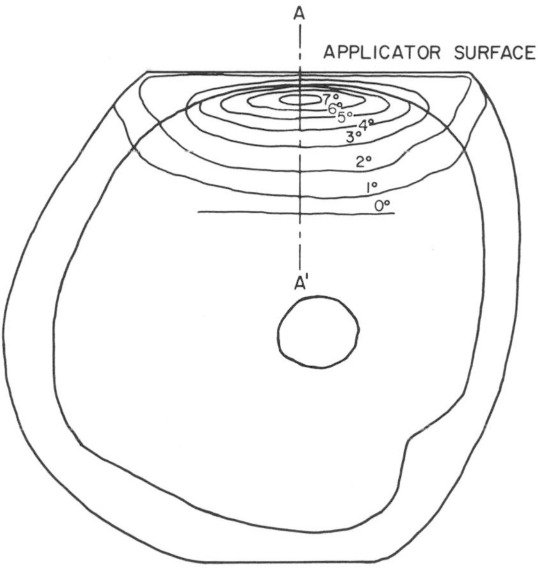

Fig. 4.15. Power deposition pattern (in terms of temperature rise ΔT above initial model equilibrium temperature) as measured by thermography for the 915 MHz heating of the thigh phantom model (26).

the phantom was cooled for the 5-minute pre-cooling period, the model halves were separated and a thermographic measurement of the temperature distribution over the thigh cross-section was made as before. The numerical model was then used to predict the temperature profiles which occurred in the phantom model under the cooling test conditions by a series of simulations in which the values of h_s were systematically varied. The series was continued until the numerical and phantom temperature profiles matched, thereby establishing the h_s distribution, both for the phantom and the human thigh.

Having introduced the thermal contributions of tissue properties, metabolism, electromagnetic energy deposition and the surface cooling convective boundary conditions, we may now proceed to the simulation of the actual thigh diathermy experiment. A series of simulations was made using several different blood flow models. Figure 4.16 shows the numerical temperature profiles predicted along the thigh centerline (corresponding to line A-A' of Figure 4.15) compared with the temperatures measured along the same line by thermistors in the actual thigh of the human subject (26). The blood flow behavior functions which yielded the best agreement between the experiment and computational profiles were a) a gradual, linear onset (in time) of vasoconstriction in the skin and subcutaneous fat, which was complete at the end of the pre-cooling period ($t = 5$ minutes) and b) the muscle blood flow (MBF) algorithm shown in Figure 4.17. This expression for the perfusion of the muscle bed was primarily a function of local temperature elevation ΔT above a core temperature set point ($\Delta T = T - 37°C$). The MBF was held at its basal level (2 ml/min-100g) until a threshold

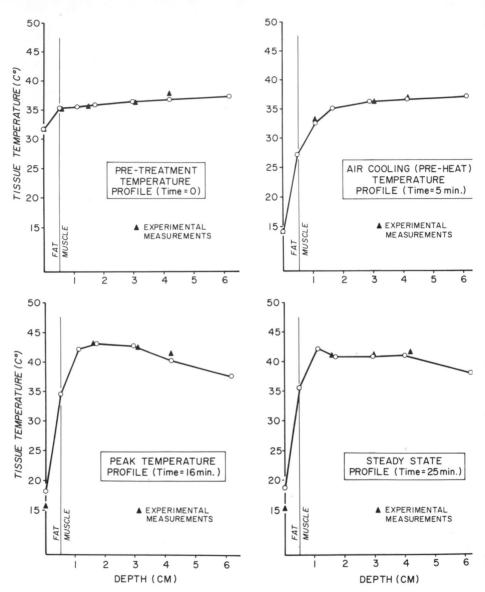

Fig. 4.16. Agreement between numerically predicted temperature profile (*solid line*) and profiles measured experimentally in the human thigh being modeled, for four times during the treatment: a) the basal temperatures existing before treatment (*t* = 0 minutes); b) the profile resulting from 5 minutes of surface pre-cooling (*t* = 5 minutes); c) the maximum temperature profile, occurring at 11 minutes into the heating phase (*t* = 16 minutes); and d) the steady state temperatures existing at the end of the 20 minute heating period (*t* = 25 minutes).

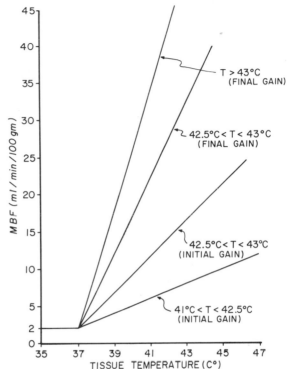

Fig. 4.17. Blood flow response algorithm employed in the numerical thigh model (see text). Based on data reported in Reference 26.

temperature of 41°C was reached, at which point the first (*bottom*) linear function labeled "initial gain" was followed until $T = 42.5°C$. For temperatures above 42.5°C, the next initial gain curve was applied, and then the gain was smoothly increased over 5 minutes time to the "42.5°C $<T<$43°C final gain" curve. For temperatures above 43°C, the (*top*) final gain curve was used. Once the blood flow at any node was represented by a final gain curve, that blood flow rate remained in effect as the tissues cooled for the remainder of the treatment period (to $t = 25$ minutes), since it is common for elevated perfusion to be sustained for several minutes after a temperature stimulus has been removed. The agreement demonstrated in Figure 4.16 shows that the model reasonably simulated the diathermy experiment.

The model points out that the temperatures produced by this protocol in this particular experiment would be only marginally therapeutic, since the tissue region in the thigh cross-section where temperatures exceeded 43°C was small, and this was of short duration. Accordingly, several other hypothetical protocols were simulated. Figure 4.18 shows the predicted temperature field at the time of peak temperatures resulting from a protocol using a pre-cooling period which was extended to 10 minutes and a net microwave

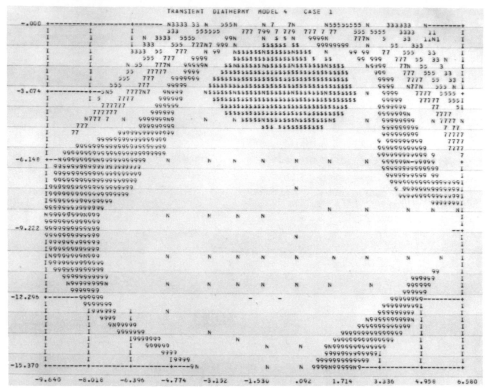

Fig. 4.18. Computer printout of the peak cross-sectional temperature field predicted for a protocol employing 10 minutes of pre-cooling followed by microwave heating at 100 W. (Values of isotherms are: 1 = 2.15°C, 3 = 10.44°C, 5 = 18.73°C, 7 = 28.68°C, 9 = 35.76°C and $ = 44.15°C).

power of 100 Watts. The figure shows a well-defined therapeutic zone in which temperatures are high enough for adequate therapy (>43°C) and yet remain safe (<45°C).

It should be emphasized that the results obtained through the first simulation and their agreement with measured temperatures (as illustrated in Figure 4.16) do *not* justify the blood flow model or any other feature of the simulation in the sense that these features are applicable to all subjects and conditions. They simply represent the results of the analyst's best estimates of the model's parameters, with modifications made to ensure that the calculated results agreed with measured values. Once agreement was reached at a given level of complexity, the model was used to predict further results. In this example, since agreement was good, one may accept the model and the modeling procedure as correct within the limits established for the problem. If the agreement had not been satisfactory, one would then have had to either modify the parameters, keeping in mind that all previous agreements must be maintained, or, if agreement could not be achieved, introduce new mechanisms into the model. Each new mechanism would likely require additional experiments to quantify it; and the lack of such accurate experiments would restrict the use of a model which incorporated these new mechanisms.

Conclusions

Thermal modeling plays two roles in the study of the human thermal system. The first is a predictive role, while the second is investigative. In the predictive mode, we assume that the model has been verified by comparison of computed results with experimental measurements, and that the analyst has made whatever other thermal checks are required to ensure the model's accuracy or validity. Since the boundary conditions are an integral part of the model, this verification may call for comparison with a number of non-biological cases to test the model against standard thermal systems. Once verified, the model may then be used as a predictor. For example, optimal thigh diathermy treatment protocols could be determined by using the model we have developed here to estimate the power levels, pre-cooling times and the necessary treatment times required to reach certain desired temperature levels at specified depths.

In the investigatory mode, the model is normally used to determine the sensitivity of a thermal system to differing parameters or mechanisms. For example, one may wish to determine how strongly the fat thickness affects the peak temperature, what effect the ambient air temperature has, if sweating of the non-cooled portion of the thigh has any meaning, or if the existence of a neighboring artery has any significance. The analyst then modifies the model appropriately and calculates the response. If a postulated mechanism is found to affect the results substantially, then changes in experimental protocol or in the choice of pathologies to be treated can be considered. In this case, one would assume that the basic model had been verified, but it may not be necessary that the new mechanism be precisely modeled. One may wish to consider the new mechanism from several different points of view, and may in fact find that the model's sensitivity is strongly affected by assumptions made about the new feature. For example, an increased subcutaneous fat thickness may alter the temperature profile substantially, but if a fat blood flow model is incorporated the fat thickness may be found to have little effect, suggesting that the blood flow dominates the effects of fat thickness. This would then point to a series of physiological experiments which would be needed to determine if and how much the perfusion of fat does vary. If, on the other hand, different fat blood flow models do not exhibit strong effects, then one can dismiss fat blood flow as an important mechanism under the stated conditions.

Irrespective of the mode in which the numerical thermal model is used, the successful use of modeling in thermotherapeutic applications currently requires a harmonious marriage of the talents of the physician and the experienced thermal analyst. While modeling is conceptually simple, its effective use requires an accurate definition of the system and its properties, and a detailed thermal specification of both the treatment protocol and the ambient conditions. Without these, the model is only an instrument for approximate and qualitative use. The analyst must depend on the physician for precise anatomical and physiological information, but must also be able to understand what facets of the biological system are necessary in specifying a model. Based on this knowledge, he must be able to ask the physician the right questions and not demand detailed information which is of low thermal importance. At the same time, he must be able to assist the medical staff in designing the proper experimental or treatment protocols and to define the necessary conditions from a thermal point of view. Once the team members recognize each other's limitations, the model can be an effective tool in thermotherapy research.

REFERENCES

1. CARNAHAN, B., LUTHER, H. A. AND WILKES, J. O. *Applied Numerical Methods.* John Wiley and Sons, New York, 1969.
2. GERALD, C. F. *Applied Numerical Analysis.* Addison-Wesley, Reading, Massachusetts, 1978.
3. MEYERS, G. E. *Analytical Methods in Conduction Heat Transfer.* McGraw-Hill, New York, 1971.
4. MINKOWYCS, W. J. (ed.). *Numerical Heat Transfer.* Hemisphere Publisher, New York, 1979.
5. PATANKAR, S. V. *Numerical Heat Transfer and Fluid Flow.* McGraw-Hill, New York, 1980.
6. HOLMAN, J. P. *Heat Transfer.* McGraw-Hill, New York, 1976.
7. HARDY, J. D. GAGGE, A. P. AND STOLWIJK, J. A. J. (eds). *Physiological and Behavioral Temperature Regulation.* Charles C Thomas Publisher, Springfield, Il, 1970.
8. FORSYTHE, F. E. AND WASOW, W. R. *Finite Difference Methods for Partial Differential Equations.* John Wiley and Sons, New York, 1960.
9. PENNES, H. A. Analysis of tissue and arterial blood temperatures in the resting human forearm. *J. Appl. Physiol. 1:* 93–122, 1948.
10. HUEBNER, R. H. *The Finite Element Method for Engineers.* John Wiley and Sons, New York, 1975.
11. BATHE K. J. AND WILSON, E. L. *Numerical Methods in Finite Element Analysis.* Prentice-Hall, Inc., Englewood Cliffs, New Jersey, 1976.
12. STERN M. D., LAPPE D. L., BOWEN P. D., CHIMOSKEY J. E., HOLLOWAY, G. A., KEISER J. R., AND BOWMAN, R. L.: Continuous measurement of tissue blood flow by laser-Doppler spectroscopy. *Am. J. Physiol. 232:* H441–H448, 1977.
13. WISSLER, E. H. The use of finite difference techniques in simulating the human thermal system. *In: Physiological and Behavioral Temperature Regulation.* Hardy, J. D., Gagge, A. P., and Stolwijk, J. A. J. (eds). Charles C Thomas, Springfield, Il, 1970, pp. 367–388.
14. STOLWIJK J. A. J.: Mathematical model of thermoregulation. *In: Physiological and Behavioral Temperature Regulation.* Hardy, J. D., Gagge, A. P., and Stolwijk, J. A. J. (eds)., Charles C Thomas, Springfield, Il, 1970, pp. 703–721.
15. FAN L. T., HSU F. T., AND HUANG C. L.: A review on mathematical models of the human thermal system. *Trans. IEEE, BME-18:* 218–234, 1971.

16. HWANG, C. L., AND KONZ, S. A.: Engineering models of the human thermoregulatory system—a review. *Trans. IEEE, BME-24:* 309–325, 1977.
17. GRIMBY, G., HAGGENDAL, E., AND SALTIN B.: Local Xenon 133 clearance from the quadriceps muscle during exercise in man. *J. Appl. Physiol., 22:* 305–310, 1967.
18. EMERY, A. F., SHORT, R. E., GUY, A. W., KRANING K. K., AND LIN, J. C.: The numerical thermal simulation of the human body when absorbing non-ionizing microwave radiation— with emphasis on the effect of different sweat models. *J. Heat Transfer, 98:* 96–118, 1976.
19. NADEL, E. R., BULLARD R. W., AND STOLWIJK, J. A. J.: Importance of skin temperature in the regulation of sweating. *J. Appl. Physiol., 31:* 80–87, 1971.
20. SALTIN, B., GAGGE, A. P., AND STOLWIJK, J. A. J.: Body temperatures and sweating during thermal transients caused by exercise. *J. Appl. Physiol. 28:* 318–327, 1970.
21. STOLWIJK, J. A. J., SALTIN, B., AND GAGGE, A. P.: Physiological factors associated with sweating during exercise. *Aerospace Med., 39:* 1101–1105, 1968.
22. LEHMANN, J. F., GUY, A. W., STONEBRIDGE, J. B., DELATEUR, B. J.: Evaluation of a therapeutic direct-contact 915 MHz microwave applicator for effective deep-tissue heating in humans. *Trans IEEE, Microwave Theory Tech., MTT-26:* 556–563, 1978.
23. HANNEMANN, R. J.: Thermal analysis and design considerations for a dual-beam microwave applictor for hyperthermia research. ASME paper 78–WA-Bio-7. Presented at the 1978 Winter annual meeting, San Francisco, Cal.
24. GUY, A. W., LEHMANN, J. F., STONEBRIDGE, J. B., AND SORENSEN, C. C.: Development of a 915-MHz direct-contact applicator for therapeutic heating of tissues, *IEEE Trans Microwave Theory Tech., MTT-26:* 550–556, 1978.
25. GUY, A. W.: Analysis of electromagnetic fields induced in biological tissues by thermographic studies on equivalent phantom models. *IEEE Trans. Microwave Theory Techn. MTT-19:* 205–214, 1971.
26. EMERY A. F., STONEBRIDGE, J. B., SEKINS, K. M., AND LEHMANN, J. F.: Experimental and numerical studies of the elevated temperatures induced in a human leg by microwave diathermy with surface cooling. *Radio Sci. 14:* 297–304, 1979.

5

Temperature Regulation, Exposure to Heat and Cold, and Effects of Hypothermia

JAMES D. HARDY

Body Temperatures and their Normal Variations

Since the early seventeenth century, when Sanctorius introduced thermometry to medicine, experience has shown that most vital functions of the body are carried out best when the internal body temperature is maintained at a relatively constant level near 37°C. Significant departures from a "normal range" of central core temperature are associated with unusual stresses and illness, and if prolonged, can result in death. Keeping in mind that the body has many temperatures, *e.g.*, higher in the core and lower in the skin and extremities, a range of normal internal body temperatures can be specified. Figure 5.1 shows the range of rectal temperatures usually considered to be physiological, together with some of the factors which affect temperature under particular conditions (1).

In resting man, the temperature is lowest (−0.5°C) in the early morning hours and highest (+0.5°C) in the afternoon. This daily or circadian rhythm of temperature is associated with changes in activity, food intake, and possibly hormonal changes, and is observed even in patients on complete bed rest. The usual range of "normal" indicated in Figure 5.1, roughly 36 to 38°C, allows for this daily rhythm, moderate changes in activity, food, menstrual cycle in women, and age; temperatures out of this range require explanation in terms of unusual activity, disease, or exposure to environmental conditions beyond the thermoregulatory capacity. Some of these conditions may require action by the physician because fever or failure of thermoregulation for any reason may be fatal.

172

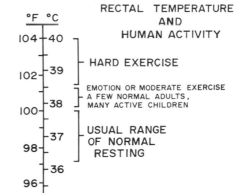

Fig. 5.1. Ranges in rectal temperatures found in normal persons. (Modified from DuBois (1)).

REGULATION OF BODY TEMPERATURE

In view of the vulnerability of body tissues to (extremes of) temperature, it is not surprising that humans have evolved an elaborate mechanism for regulating temperature. As Claude Bernard stated in 1865, "La fixité du milieu intérieur est la condition de la vie libre" (2). For example, the ability to preserve body temperatures near their normal levels enables man to brave the cold depths of outer space or to explore the furnace-hot surface of the moon. To accomplish this regulation, two distinct control systems are employed: behavioral regulation, involving the conscious, voluntary use of all available means; and physiological regulation, employing the involuntary responses of the body that tend to maintain constant temperatures. The relationships between these systems are indicated in Figure 5.2 as they provide for the control of body temperatures in the environmental extremes of terrestrial and near-space environments. By using protective clothing and air conditioning, man can live for extended periods in the coldest or hottest terrestrial climates and make excursions into space. Physiological regulation, in this context, provides fine control of body temperature for the normal resting man, and is the principal means of temperature control during exercise.

HEAT BALANCE IN THE BODY

The overall energy exchange of man may be roughly characterized by the balance diagram shown in Figure 5.3. In the steady state, heat produced in the body is balanced by heat loss to the environment, so that over an extended period the internal body temperature tends to remain near 37°C. The action of the thermoregulator maintains internal temperature near 37°C, since in theory the balance between heat production and heat loss could occur equally well at any body temperature. Thus, chemical energy made available by the combustion of carbohydrates, fats, and proteins in body tissues is converted into heat or external work. The heat is dissipated

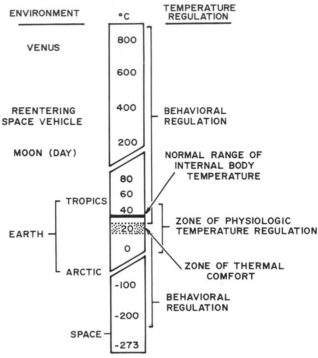

Fig. 5.2. Environmental temperatures on earth and in near space as related to physiological and behavioral regulation of body temperature. (Modified from Hardy (3)).

into the environment by convection, radiation, and the evaporation of water from the skin and respiratory tract. In the unsteady state, the internal body temperature may vary from 35 to 41°C, depending on the circumstances, but when normal conditions prevail, the temperature will return to its resting level near 37°C by thermoregulator action.

BODY HEAT STORAGE

In the resting or sedentary man, changes in body heat content normally take place entirely in the peripheral tissues, as shown in Figure 5.4. With cold exposure, selective vasoconstriction reduces the supply of blood to the skin and peripheral tissues, and diverts blood to the visceral organs. This increase in central blood volume evokes a temporary "cold" diuresis. Under conditions of mild cold exposure, the mean body temperature will decrease, although the rectal temperature may increase or remain near 37°C. The cold, relatively bloodless peripheral tissues provide good insulation to vital internal structures. On exposure of a chilled individual to a warm environment, vasoconstriction may be released so rapidly that warm blood from the core will begin to perfuse the cold tissues and return as cold blood to the

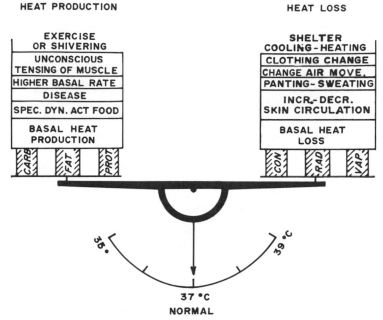

Fig. 5.3. Balance between factors increasing heat production and heat loss. (Modified from DuBois (1)).

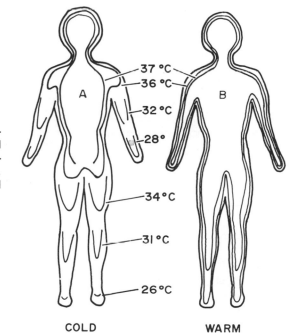

Fig. 5.4. Distribution of internal body temperatures and thermal gradients after exposure to cold (A) and heat (B). (Modified from Aschoff and Wever (4)).

heart. The internal body temperature may then decrease substantially (depending upon the previous cold exposure), causing shivering, nausea, cardiac arrhythmia, or even collapse.

Exposure to heat results in relatively small changes in internal body temperature as long as thermoregulation is effective. Even in an environment of 38 to 40°C (100 to 104°F), the resulting positive body heat storage may cause rectal temperature to increase less than 0.5°C. As shown in Figure 5.4B, under these conditions the isotherms for 36°C and 37°C move out to the extremities. The effector systems for physiological temperature regulation are a) the controls for metabolic heat production, b) the flow of blood from the interior of the body to the skin (vasomotor control), and c) the sweating rate.

METABOLIC RATE

In the quiet, resting man, most heat is produced in the body core—the trunk viscera and brain—even though these constitute only a little over one third of the body mass (see Table 5.1). Thus, heat is supplied to the tissues of the resting man primarily from the central organs; and the escape of this heat from the body is easily controlled by the vasomotor system. During work, the principal site of heat production shifts to the musculature. The actual values for metabolic rates depend on the work being performed and on various physiological factors such as age, sex, and size. They may range from 40 W/m^2 to 800 W/m^2, depending on activity level and condition of physical fitness. On exposure to cold, shivering is stimulated to increase the level of heat production. For short periods, shivering can produce 160–200 W/m^2, but for exposures of several hours, a doubling of the resting metabolism is all that can be expected on the average.

VASOMOTOR CONTROL

Convective heat transfer by the blood stream from deep tissues to the skin is of vital physiological importance, and is under control of the sympathetic nervous system. For each liter of blood at 37°C that flows to the skin and returns to the body core at 36°C, the body loses rapidly 1 kcal or

TABLE 5.1. *Relative masses and rates of metabolic heat production of various body compartments at rest and during exercise.*[a]

	Body mass (percent)	Heat production (percent)	
		Rest	Work
Brain	2	16	1
Trunk viscera	34	56	8
Muscle and skin	56	18	90
Other	8	10	1

[a] Modified from Stolwijk and Hardy (5).

1.16W·h of heat. Thus, when the body is exposed to cold, vigorous vasocon-striction nearly shuts off blood flow to the arms, legs, and skin of the trunk. This action ensures that body heat from the core can be lost only by conduction through muscle and fatty tissues, which are reasonably good insulators. The heat flow cannot be stopped, but can be reduced to between 5 and 9 W/m^2 for each degree of thermal gradient between core and skin (the actual value will depend to some extent on the amount of fat in the body). In the heat, during vigorous exercise, blood flow to the skin can increase this heat flow almost ten-fold, providing an effective channel for heat transfer from the body. Indeed, exercising muscles cannot get rid of their metabolic heat rapidly enough without this increase in convective heat transfer.

Figure 5.5 shows the results of studies in the basal state on heat balance in men and women exposed nude to temperatures of 22 to 36°C. At the bottom are plotted the changes in tissue "conductance." Conductance is the

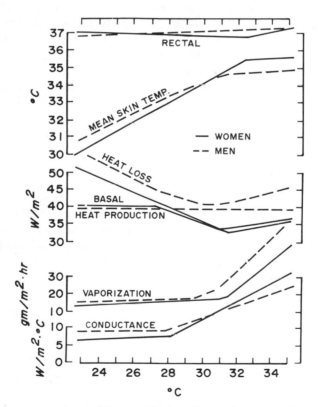

Fig. 5.5. Average values of thermal factors for nude men and women in near steady state at different environmental temperatures. (Modified from Hardy *et al.* (6)).

combined effect of the two heat transfer channels—conduction of heat through muscle and fat layers, and convective heat transfer by the blood. This conductance can be estimated on the assumption that all the body heat is produced in the body core, conducted to the skin, and then transferred to the environment. That is, $H_L = K(T_{re} - \bar{T}_s)$, where H_L is the heat loss (except for a small amount from the respiratory tract), K is the effective conductance, T_{re} is the rectal or core temperature and $\bar{T}_s$ is the mean skin temperature. In the cold (22 to 28°C), the conductance is not greatly affected by ambient temperature, and represents the vasoconstricted state in which cutaneous blood flow is minimal. The layer of subcutaneous fat in women is clearly seen to reduce their conductance below that of men during cold exposure. In the heat (30 to 36°C), the conductance increases progressively, with women having a steeper increase, indicating their greater control of peripheral blood flow.

The rate of "effective" blood flow can be estimated by using the value of conductance in the cold as the condition for "no blood flow", and assuming that any increase above this minimum is due to increased flow of blood from core to skin. As the warm blood leaves the body core via the arteries, it soon flows adjacent to veins carrying cooler venous blood returning from the skin and other peripheral tissues. Heat exchange then begins, returning some of the heat in the arterial stream to the body core. This process is known as "counter-current exchange." Its effect is to reduce convective heat transfer, or to require more blood flow to cause the same heat transfer as would be produced without counter-current exchange. In general, measurement of heat transfer can only give values for the *minimum* blood flow rate which could produce the observed heat flow. The actual blood flow may be, and usually is, greater because accurate data on counter-current heat exchange are not available. For example, the blood flow increase indicated in Figure 5.5 is between three- and four-fold, whereas it has been shown that foot blood flow in the 15 to 44°C range increases almost 80-fold with rising temperature, the major increase occurring above 29°C (7). Also, since skin and muscle blood flow both contribute to conductance changes and are controlled by different mechanisms (8), each part of the body must be considered separately as it contributes to the overall value of thermal conductance (9). Skin blood flow is under control of the central thermoregulatory centers via the sympathetic nervous system, but muscle blood flow is principally determined by the local muscle metabolic rate. Thus, for the working man in hot environments, the two systems act together to increase thermal conductance and to supply muscle metabolic substrates; for resting man, the changes in conductance are entirely due to alterations in skin blood flow.

CONTROL OF SWEATING

When water is converted into vapor at body temperature, 0.7 W·h (0.6 kcal) of heat/gm of water is absorbed in the process. Thus, evaporating water (sweat) from the skin is an efficient way of losing heat, even in an environment hotter than the skin. In this case, the evaporative heat loss must compensate for both the metabolic heat and the heat absorbed by radiation and convection from the hot environment. The body always loses some heat by evaporation from the skin and respiratory tract, even in very cold weather when the problem is to retain body heat. As indicated in Figure 5.5, at ambient temperatures below 30°C evaporation is fairly constant at 12 to 15 gm/m^2·hour, about half of which is due to loss of moisture in breathing, and half to the slow transudation of water through the almost-dry skin. Even though the skin appears dry, moisture continually diffuses through the outer skin layers and evaporates. In a dry environment, this drying effect can be troublesome, causing skin scaling and itching as well as nasal and pharyngeal discomfort. At 30°C, evaporative heat loss amounts to about 25 percent of the total heat loss, which at this neutral temperature equals basal heat production.

Above 30°C, evaporative heat loss increases linearly with temperature, as active sweating is stimulated to compensate for decreased heat loss by radiation and convection. When environmental and skin temperatures are equal, there can be no heat loss by radiation and convection, since the thermal gradient is zero; in this case, usually at an ambient temperature of 35 to 36°C, all of the metabolic heat must be lost through evaporation.

SWEAT GLANDS

The overriding importance of eccrine sweat gland function in preventing dangerous hyperthermia in warm climates is clearly evident. The secretory activity of these glands, which in the average man number something like 2.5 million, is under control of the CNS (central nervous system) via sympathetic innervation. When skin disease—ichthyosis for example—interferes with sweating, exposure to heat, and especially exercise in the heat, may raise the internal body temperature to lethal levels. Such individuals are completely dependent on behavioral temperature regulation in stressfully warm conditions, and must repeatedly dampen clothing with water even during normal sedentary activity.

For the exercising man, sweating is even more important than for the resting or sedentary individual, because the rate of heat production can reach high values during heavy work; and heat must be eliminated rapidly. To provide for this high heat flux, it is first necessary to stimulate the vasomotor system to transfer heat from the muscles and body core to the skin; second, the sweat glands must be activated to eliminate heat from the skin surface. The dependence of both sweating and vasodilation on internal temperature is illustrated in Figure 5.6 for men resting and exercising at 25, 50, and 75 percent of their maximum oxygen uptake at 10, 20, and 30°C (10). During exercise, the internal body temperature must increase even though the environment is cold because it is necessary to activate vasodilation to transfer the heat to the skin. Since the internal temperature

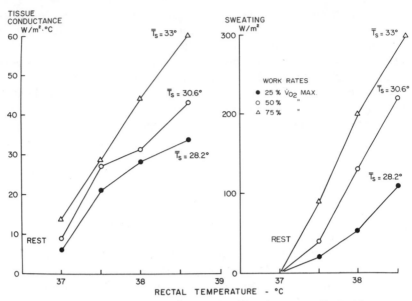

Fig. 5.6. Tissue conductance and sweating heat loss, as affected by mean skin temperature (T_s) and rectal temperature. (Modified from Stolwijk *et al.* (10)).

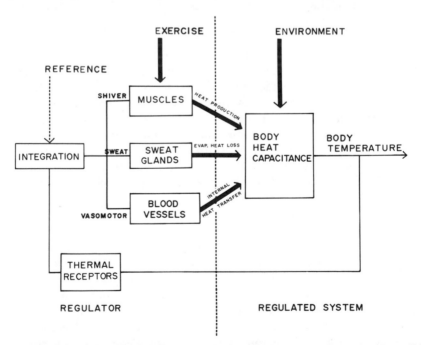

Fig. 5.7. Simplified block diagram of the human thermoregulatory system. (Modified from Stolwijk (11)).

increases in proportion to the work rate (Watts per square meter), regardless of external temperatures (within ranges of possible heat balance), we can assume that the temperature controller action is of the "proportional control" type.

The action of the human thermoregulatory system shown schematically by a flow chart, such as Figure 5.7, which is derived from data from both neurophysiology and thermal physiology. To the *right* in the figure is the "regulated" or "passive" system, which is the body of the person whose temperature is being controlled. Complete characterization of the passive system for temperature regulation involves description of the cardiovascular, respiratory, endocrine, metabolic, and other systems, as well as the heat transfer for the passive system and the detection, transfer, and integration of information concerning body temperatures in the controlling system. In Figure 5.7, the *heavy lines* indicate energy transfer while the *thin lines* represent information transfer. The body produces heat, exchanges thermal energy within itself and exchanges thermal energy with the environment. The temperature receptors in the skin and body core detect the level and rate of change of temperature; and they transmit this information through nerve channels to the hypothalmus in which much of the integration occurs. When deviations are noted, effector signals are generated to modify heat flow in the body by changing the distribution of the circulation, by increasing heat production through shivering, or by altering the rate of heat removal from the skin by sweating.

BEHAVIORAL TEMPERATURE REGULATION

The distinguishing characteristic of behavioral regulation is the participation of directed effort in the control of a variable. Essential elements of such control are sensory detection of the variable, motivation for control, and the employment of energy sources within the body or from the environment to effect control. In the case of temperature regulation, man has available to him many energy sources and means of application (by virtue of his technological and engineering capabilities). Pain and thermal discomfort are sensations with strong motivational components for stimulating conscious behavior. Available data from combined physiological and behavioral studies indicate that the aim of behavioral control is to reduce the sensory and physiological stresses of thermoregulation by providing a comfortable microclimate around the body. Sensations of warmth and cold are felt as either comfortable or uncomfortable, depending on whether they provide decreased or increased physiological strain. For example, to a person who has been exposed to a cold environment, the sensation of warmth from coming indoors to a warm room is pleasant and comfortable, whereas the same warmth sensation would be interpreted as unpleasant if the previous exposure had been to a hot July sun. Diagrammatically, this constellation

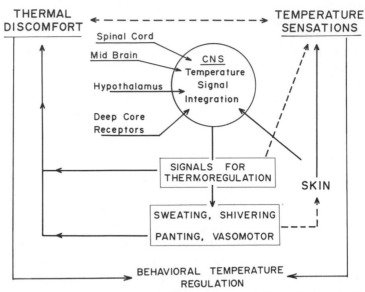

Fig. 5.8. Representation of thermal sensations and discomfort. *Solid lines* refer to major information channels; *dashed lines* refer to interactions.

of sensation and sensory inputs can be represented as shown in Figure 5.8. In this figure, the sensations of warmth, cold, and pain evoked by stimulation of the skin are perceived at the level of consciousness, but neural signals are also transmitted to the temperature-regulating center in the hypothalamus. There, the signals interact with temperature signals from the brain and other body structures to produce the signals which control sweating, shivering, and vasomotor activity, and which at the same time are perceived at the conscious level as thermal discomfort. It has also been shown that the physiological activities of sweating, shivering, and vasomotor action can be felt in the skin. These sensations may contribute to a sense of discomfort and possibly also to thermal sensation, itch, pain, etc.

The close relationship between physiological and behavioral regulation is apparent from Figure 5.8, since the temperature sensing systems and information channels are common to both.

Exposure to Heat (12)

LOCAL EFFECTS

The skin is the body area principally concerned with increases in temperature from environmental exposure. Burns resulting from application of various forms of heat have been studied extensively because of the pain and disfiguration which accompany these serious injuries. Moritz and Henriques

(13) have shown that skin temperatures above 45°C cause tissue damage, depending on the length of time and hyperthermic exposure. It has also been shown that thermal pain is evoked at 45°C if the skin is exposed to intense thermal radiation, and that the intensity of pain increases with skin temperature up to 65 to 70°C. Henriques (14), in his analysis of the relationship of burn production to skin temperature and exposure time, discovered that the probable cause of skin burns was irreversible damage to proteins in the basal layer of skin cells. A similar analysis of skin pain produced by heating indicated that the threshold for pain and the intensity of pain might be due to similar causes. Figure 5.9 illustrates Henriques' analysis for first and third degree burns and the pain intensity associated with burn initiation. Pain intensity is indicated in "dol" units developed from the psychophysical studies of Hardy *et al.* (15); the intensity is indicated only for the first seconds of exposure. As was shown by later studies of skin pain associated with prolonged exposure to hot water, the intensity of pain is quite variable as exposures are lengthened (16).

HYPERTHERMIA

When the body core temperature is raised to a level significantly higher than the mean resting value, a human or animal is said to be hyperthermic. For man, exposure to heat, work, and fever are the three most common

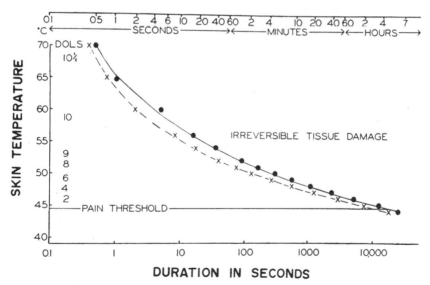

Fig. 5.9. Relationship of skin temperature, duration of elevated skin temperature, and production of tissue damage. Pain intensity corresponding to various skin temperatures is noted for comparison. *Dashed line,* threshold for transient erythema; *solid line*, threshold for "dermal necrosis." (Modified from Moritz and Henriques (13)).

causes of hyperthermia. The general effects of hyperthermia have been classified by Leithead and Lind (17) and by the World Health Organization, and are briefly as follows:

HEAT SYNCOPE

Heat syncope, or heat exhaustion, is caused by temporary circulatory failure due to prolonged standing or postural changes which can result in venous pooling and decreased return of blood to the right heart. Body temperature may be slightly elevated, skin wet and cool. Placing the person in a supine position in the shade results in rapid recovery. The previous state of physical fitness of the subject has a marked effect on susceptibility to heat syncope. Patients with cardiovascular problems receiving special medication for hypertension are prone to heat syncope and should exercise caution when standing in line in crowds, etc.

WATER AND SALT DEPLETION

Dehydration is associated with water loss from the sweat glands, which can amount to more than one liter per hour during work in the heat. Complete replacement of body water is not easy, as repeated tests on marching soldiers have shown (there is a gradual loss of body water during a prolonged march). An associated problem is the loss of body electrolyte due to the salt carried out in the sweat; as much as 0.5–0.75 gm/kg body weight (17) of salt may be lost per day with resulting hemoconcentration. Even if water is supplied, the subject will be prone to giddiness and muscle cramps. Intravenous administration of normal saline may be called for in severe cases. Drinking of water during heat exposure can be useful in preventing dehydration, especially if salt is added.

HEAT STROKE

The most severe and dangerous syndrome associated with heat exposure is the sudden onset of hyperthermia, generalized convulsions and coma, probably due to failure of the thermoregulatory system. Hot and dry skin are typical signs; treatment should be started at the earliest possible moment. Placing the patient in a cold bath 18 to 20°C to immediately lower body temperature, and together with other supportive therapy, may be life-saving.

These "thermal disorders", and the difficulties of diagnosis and classification, were noted by Leithead and Lind (17); the physiological pathology of heat stroke is not well understood. Bridger and Helfand (18) made an epidemiological study of the 1966 heat wave in Missouri and southern Illinois, July 1 to 31, and related the death rates of various age groups to the weather data. Current disease state, if any, reported cause of death, and sex were also noted for the three heat spells—July 1 to 7, July 9 to 15, and the last transient spell that had the highest temperature on July 18. In analyzing their data, the authors used July 1965 as a "normal" period. Figure 5.10 shows the relative effect of the 1966 heat wave on the weekly deaths in St. Louis, and the percentage of deaths of those 65 years and older. In their analysis, the authors noted a 33 percent increase in mortality during the first spell, a 36 percent increase during the second, and a 10 percent increase during the third; the "sliding" averaging method resulted in the curve shown at the top of Figure 5.10.

As expected, of the population at risk, people 65 years of age and over suffered the greatest mortality, which was attributed largely to lesions of the vascular system, lesions of the brain, and other diseases of the circulatory system (excluding heart diseases). Circulatory impairment can lead rapidly to failure of physiological thermoregulation, on which these individuals were entirely dependent. The authors also noted that the heat wave was sudden in onset, that it was the first truly hot spell of the year, and that the effect of such heat exposure on an essentially unacclimatized population might thus be severe.

Acclimatization to heat consists of two parts—the development of additional capacity for cutaneous vasodilation, and the capacity for an earlier

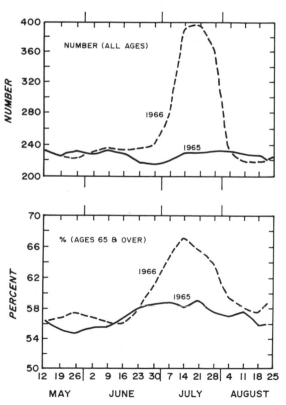

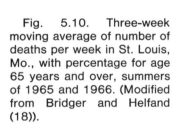

Fig. 5.10. Three-week moving average of number of deaths per week in St. Louis, Mo., with percentage for age 65 years and over, summers of 1965 and 1966. (Modified from Bridger and Helfand (18)).

onset and maintenance of sweating. When these physiological developments are added to acquiring additional physical fitness, the results can be dramatic. Figure 5.11 illustrates the combined effects of developing heat acclimatization and physical fitness in young men who were tested for 12 days during a 4-hour programmed period of work and heat exposure (19). None of the four subjects could complete the test on the first day. Internal body temperature rose rapidly to unacceptable levels; pulse rate was high; and sweat rate declined before reaching required levels. At the end of 12 days, all subjects completed the work period with apparent ease, without undue elevations of body temperatures or pulse rates, and with sweat rates at higher levels. The metabolic rate also decreased, perhaps partly due to increased physical fitness.

The requirement to produce heat acclimatization is repeated exposure to heat which results in both elevation of the internal body temperature (most easily accomplished by exercise) and moderate or profuse sweating. Exposure of 1 to 4 hours for 5 to 7 days is usually sufficient. The failure to develop acclimatization to heat may underly a number of problems encountered by young athletes during the football season, particularly in the northern United States. Heat acclimatization is transient, usually disappearing in 3 to 4 weeks if not maintained by repeated exposures to heat.

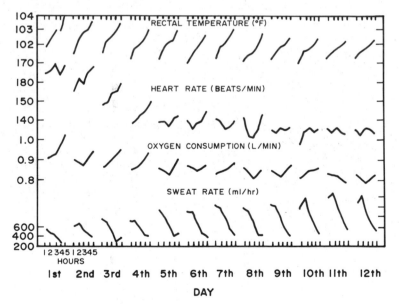

Fig. 5.11. Combined effects of heat acclimatization and physical training on five young men during four-hour heat-work exposure. Dry and wet bulb temperatures were 36 and 34°C, respectively; wind velocity was 40 n/min. (Modified from Strydom *et al.* (19)).

Exposure to Cold (20)

LOCAL EFFECTS

The initial response to rapid local cooling is generally an intense cold sensation and pain. If a hand is put into water at 18°C or lower, aching pain will occur after some seconds, the intensity of pain increasing with lowering temperatures (7). However, the pain will usually subside after a few minutes, possibly because of low temperature nerve block or local adaptation. Vasoconstriction is induced locally, and after some minutes if followed by vasodilation which occurs cyclically (the so-called Lewis reaction). Prolonged exposure to temperature near freezing may cause injuries which appear after some hours: first degree damage or skin reddening, second degree damage with development of edema and separation of the epidermis, or third degree damage consisting of necrosis of the deep tissue (frostbite). The cause of cold injury is not well understood at this time, but seems to be associated with the formation of ice crystals in the tissues, damage to the blood vessels, and dehydration of the intracellular spaces (12). It used to be thought that slow rewarming was the best way to treat frostbite, but experience has shown that necrosis of tissue is reduced by rapid rewarming in hot water 40 to 42°C.

ACCLIMATIZATION AND ADAPTIVE RESPONSES TO COLD

When endotherms (warm-blooded animals) are exposed to environmental temperatures below those in which they can maintain body temperature while in the resting state, significant physiological and behavioral changes generally occur. As classified by the International Union of Physiological Sciences, these changes are:

Acclimatization—physiological changes occuring within the lifetime of the organism which reduce the environmental strain and thus, enhance survival in a stressful natural climate.

Genetic Adaptation—a genetically-fixed condition of a species, or of its evolution, which favors survival in a particular total or natural environment.

There has always been great interest in human acclimatization and genetic adaptation to cold. The Eskimo, Lapplander, Australian aborigine, and the African Kalahari bushman have been studied for genetic adaptive changes; white and negro U.S. soldiers stationed in cold climates such as Alaska have been observed to determine any changes that might be attributed to short-term cold acclimatization. The possibility of acclimatization by a change in metabolic rate was studied as a likely change; and measurements were made of heat loss and heat production in members of a nudist cult in the Russell Sage Calorimeter. Although the young men and women studied were accustomed to sleeping out-of-doors in cold weather nude and without bedding, no changes in metabolic rate from normal standards could be observed. Others could find no alteration in the basal metabolic rate (BMR) of soldiers during a winter at Fort Churchill, Canada, and no change in the BMR in 5 men living for 14 days at 15°C with minimal clothing (7). All evidence available indicates that humans living in the north temperate zone do not undergo a "metabolic" acclimatization to cold such as seen in the rat and other small mammals. However, Scholander *et al.* (21) did note a "slight rise" in the BMR in eight subjects they studied during September and October in the Norwegian mountains. Their subjects were occupied with hiking, hunting, and fishing, and developed a capacity to sleep during the night, even though shivering to maintain a warm skin and normal internal temperature. Unacclimatized subjects did not have this capacity to sleep while shivering. It is perhaps proper to think of these changes, which Scholander terms "cold-hardiness", more as a habituation to cold than acclimatization to cold. LeBlanc (20) used a standard cold exposure to test changes in metabolism in soldiers exposed for four months in the Artic. He reported that at the end of the winter, the increase in heat production caused by a standard cold stress was less than in the fall. From these data, he suggested that acclimatization to cold is associated with a lowering of the body thermostat to more economical levels, a type of response seen in small birds. No changes in basal metabolic rate were seen in members of the Armed Forces in Alaska after some months of duty in the winter season; the Alaskan Eskimo does not have an elevated BMR. The high protein diet of the Eskimo tends to raise his metabolic rate for as long as 14 hours postprandial, but placing the Eskimo on a normal military diet for a week eliminated this effect: there are no adaptive changes in the human to cold which result in increased levels of basal heat production (6). This is confirmed by LeBlanc, although he describes effects resulting from ascorbic acid administration to men on a survival ration (20). Several authors have called attention to the fact that human inhabitants of the very cold regions of the Earth do not expose themselves to cold any more than can be helped. It is likely that the extreme rates of cooling that would occur on exposure to −40°C are such that peripheral tissue damage would occur as a limiting factor before a decrease in internal body temperature became important. Cooling of the extremities was studied in both Eskimos and soldiers. Under a standard cold stress, the hands and feet of the Eskimo were found to maintain significantly higher temperatures than those of U.S. soldiers. This vasomotor adaptation to cold may be of vital importance in preventing frostbite and loss of fingers or toes.

A study of cold adaptation in humans exposed to moderate cold was undertaken by Scholander *et al.* (21) on the Pitjandjara tribe of Australian aborigines and by Wyndham and Morrison (22) on the African bushman of the Kalahari desert. Scholander *et al.* found that the Australian aborigine permitted his skin temperature to drop during the night to levels much below that tolerated by white men, thus considerably reducing heat loss from his body. This enabled the native to sleep throughout the night without elevation of metabolic rate, although white control subjects shivered involuntarily. In fact, the metabolic rate of the natives showed a decrease as body temperature fell. These authors found, however, that both white men and aborigines could sleep comfortably enough outdoors naked on the ground, provided that they slept between the fires used by natives. It was only when they were tested against a standard cold environment that the changes induced by cold adaptation became evident.

Wyndham and Morrison (22) studying environmental effects on the Kalahari bushman, concluded that there was no physiological change in these men due to cold exposure, and that these natives become behaviorally acclimatized to cold rather than adapted to cold. Thus, it is possible that man adapts behaviorally in a different manner to each cold climate, and that there is only a very limited range to his physiological response. Indeed, in the severe cold of the Artic, there is a vasodilatation of the hands, an adaptation which sacrifices some body heat, but which preserves the tissue integrity of the extremities; in the bush of Australia, there is inhibition of shivering with a modest loss of total body heat, which can carry the aborigine over a chilly night until a warm sun the next morning restores body heat; in the windy African high plateau, there is appropriate individual and tribal behavior which involves maintaining minimum shelter to preserve body heat.

Hypothermia

Internal body temperatures markedly lower than those usually encountered in the normal range are termed hypothermic. Rectal temperatures below 35°C in man indicate hypothermia; such temperatures can result from prolonged cold exposure, premortal states (shock), toxic substances (alcohol, narcotics, large amounts of pyrogens, etc.) or from extra-corporeal cooling of the blood for experimental or medical purposes. Hypothermia may thus be of physiological, pathological, or artificial origin; the most careful studies of human hypothermia have been carried out on surgical patients.

Artificial hypothermia was introduced as a technique of modern surgery by Fay and Henry in 1938 (23). These authors were interested in alleviating pain in cancer patients, and in the possibility of reducing the viability of carcinomatous tissues relative to normal tissues by maintaining body temperatures below the normal range. Following carefully-controlled studies in many hospitals throughout the world, this latter hope failed to develop, and so artificial hypothermia was largely abandoned as a clinical tool in this area. About two years later, artificial hypothermia was revived as a surgical procedure by Bigelow et al. (24), who called attention to the marked reduction in oxygen consumption of the brain at low temperatures, and proposed hypothermia as a protection against cerebral hypoxia during intracardiac surgery. The success of this procedure has stimulated physiological and clinical investigation over a wide front. Extensive reports on the subject of artificial hypothermia have been made by Kayser (25), who concludes that hypothermia is useful in certain areas of surgery in which the circulation to the body must be occluded, as for example, during surgery on the heart and brain.

Breaking down the body's defenses against cold is essential to the induction of hypothermia. A combination of three methods are in common use: a) use of drugs in a cool room, b) massive application of cold to the body surface (ice, ice baths) and, c) cooling of blood which is removed from the body and subsequently returned. The first two methods are less rapid and may produce local tissue damage from low temperature. It is generally recognized that patients in the hypothermic state have little or no ability to regulate body temperature, and that this regulation must be provided by the physician. The influence of rate, degree, and duration of cooling has been and continues to be under active study in both man and animals.

The hazards of artificial hypothermia appear to be due primarily to the danger of ventricular fibrillation leading to cardiac arrest. The effects of low temperature on the heart have been studied in dogs, with particular attention given to hypoxia, metabolism and muscular efficiency, conducting system, electrocardiographic changes, and the effects of anti-fibrillatory and other agents on heart action and on blood flow. As the body of a dog is cooled to 28°C, heart rate, coronary blood flow, cardiac output, and blood pressure decrease; and at about 13°C, cardiac activity ceases with only an occasional ventricular contraction (25). The particular values, however, strongly depend on the type and amount of anesthetic agent used. Studies with a heart-lung preparation showed that hypoxia of the myocardium did not contribute to hypothermic arrest, inasmuch as coronary flow was more than adequate at terminal temperatures (19.6°C $\pm$ 0.7°C), and the use of 100 percent oxygen did not further lower this temperature (25). Also, it was found that the hypothermic heart is more efficient, since it is able to perform the same stroke work with less oxygen consumption than the normothermic heart. The increase in efficiency is taken to indicate that low temperature (31.5°C) does not interfere with the aerobic conversion of chemical energy to mechanical energy in heart muscle. Also, the blood remains capable of releasing its oxygen to tissues at low temperatures. The oxygen consumption of the entire animal increases during the initial phases of cooling, due to shivering, but then decreases so that at 17°C oxygen consumption is 15 percent of normal, and the cardiac minute volume is 10 percent of precooling levels. However, the work output of the heart is reduced to 7 to 8 percent of normal, thus, oxygenation is adequate at all temperatures to the point of asystole. However, spontaneous occurrences of fused contractions with apparent summation and incomplete tetanus have been observed in several experiments at low body temperatures. After prolonged periods (14 hours) at low body temperature, the cardiac output and coefficient of oxygen utilization may alter; and after 24 hours, the changes can be profound. Stagnant anoxemia and markedly lowered cardiac output have been observed. Prolonging hypothermia delays the return of the animal to the precooled condition, although following a two-hour period of hypothermia there is generally a prompt return of the cardiac index. Dogs cooled for 12 hours required approximately 12 hours after rewarming to return to normal cardiac output.

The threshold of the heart to electrical stimulation increases as the temperature is lowered. Cooling dogs under pentobarbital and thiopental anesthesia, and dividing animals into a high and a low threshold group, animals with high electrical thresholds could be cooled to the point of asystole at 15 to 18°C, whereas the majority of the low threshold group experienced fibrillation at 19 to 26°C (25). Following ventricular excitability through the cardiac cycle as the dogs were cooled, the ventricular refractory period became greatly prolonged. The increased susceptibility of the hypothermic myocardium to ventricular fibrillation may be due to changes in excitability. Upon rewarming, local electrical activity returned first, followed at higher temperatures by propagated action potentials and contractions; acetylcholine potentiated the development of the action potentials and mechanical tension. Action potentials of excised Purkinje fibers of the heart at low temperature (down to 25°C) have temperature coefficients (Q_{10}) of the membrane of 1.14, and below 25°C, these coefficients are much higher; the duration of the action current is prolonged on cooling. The effect of cooling on the pacemaker was observed in excised rabbit auricles down to 14 to 20°C, at which temperature all electrical and mechanical activity failed. Stimulation of the brain stem reticular system in a paralyzed animal at normal temperature produces cardiac irregularities, and these are potentiated by hypothermia; increased vagal tone cannot account for failure of sinus activity. Cooling of a restricted zone of the myocardium impairs conduction into the cooled zone; and if the cooling is prolonged, there is a reversible depolarization of the area. As the heart is cooled, it becomes progressively more sensitive to calcium; and there may be a relationship of hypothermic death to calcium intoxication of the heart. However, serum potassium rises to high levels in the hypothermic dog; and it seems clear that calcium and potassium changes during hypothermia affect the electrical activity of the cooled heart.

There are marked changes in the electrocardiograms of animals during cooling. These involve changes in PR interval, QPS duration, QT interval, and T wave. Examination of the electrocardiograms, however, cannot be used as a method to predict the fatal outcome in hypothermic dogs. Using a pump oxygenator and cooling the blood in an extracorpeal circuit, it was found that following cooling of the hearts to 1.5°C, with asystole for 35 minutes, there was complete recovery of all the animals (25). As has been pointed out, the method of cooling makes a difference in the effects of cold on the electrical activity of the heart. Cooling dogs by immersion produces electrocardiographic changes which are quantitatively and qualitatively different from those caused by cooling the blood in an external circuit, but cooling (25°C) the blood can result in marked abnormalities in heart rate and in the pathway of depolarization and repolarization. Many others have found that temperatures below 25°C cause difficulty with heart action and result in a linear decrease in pacemaker activity with decrease in temperature.

For surgical purposes, eliminating or reducing ventricular fibrillation of the hypothermic heart is a vital problem. As Thauer points out (26), this danger increases markedly below 25°C and depends to some extent on the anesthetic agent employed. Cardiac arrhythmias and ventricular fibrillation occur less frequently in dogs under thiopental and ether than under pentobarbital. Adrenergic blockage, venesection, and hypotension do not protect against fibrillation. Acetylcholine has been observed to restore the ability of the isolated rabbit auricle to propagate action potentials and to contract and restore the sinus rhythm in the intact heart. If acidosis is allowed to develop during hypothermia, ventricular fibrillation is more marked, but there are reports of complete protection against fibrillation at 23 to 25°C by maintaining a slightly supernormal pH by controlled ventilation.

Blood pressure in the hypothermic animal remains relatively high although the heart rate and cardiac output decrease greatly. An increase in blood viscosity, a possible decrease in blood vessel diameter due to direct action of the cold, and loss of plasma from the blood all contribute to this effect. Thauer and his colleagues (26) note that in the hypothermic dog, the relationship between the heart minute volume and arterial blood pressure does not follow the Poiseuille law as might be expected from conditions noted above. They also note that blood flow depends upon the depth and type of anesthesia—the flow being greater with deep anesthesia.

Respiration is markedly affected by hypothermia; the particular responses observed are determined to a large degree by the type and level of anesthesia. With a light anesthesia, hyperventilation, associated with shivering, occurs as the body temperature is lowered to about 30°C. The result is alkalosis and a rise in the arterial pH. As the body temperature is lowered further, there is a prolonged decrease in pH, apparently the result of CO_2 retention at lower blood temperatures. If the initial anesthesia is sufficiently deep, shivering is minimal or entirely lacking, and alkalosis does not appear, but acidosis develops. In this type of cooling, the animal experiences a reduction in respiratory rate and tidal volume. It has been thought that animals first experience primary respiratory failure, followed by circulatory failure as the cause of hypothermic death. There are, however, reasons to question this point of view. Some investigators have found that severe hypoxia with light or no anesthesia gives better results with some animals in the cooling phase, and results in fewer instances of hind limb damage when CO_2 is used in severe hypothermia.

The acidosis of hypothermia has been studied both *in vitro* and *in vivo*. Blood equilibrated with CO_2-air mixtures between 37°C and 26°C shows a relationship between the log pCO_2 and pH at all temperatures, the ratios of which are constant and not temperature-dependent. However, the addition of red cells increases the ratio while the addition of plasma decreases it. When plasma alone is equilibrated with CO_2 at the two temperatures, the ratio is higher at 26°C than at 37°C, presumably because of the greater solubility of CO_2 at the lower temperature. From this, it would seem that the base binding power of hemoglobin which would occur with temperature offsets the potential acidity of CO_2 due to its greater solubility at the lower temperature. In dogs cooled at 26°C by extra-corporeal cooling of the blood, the transfusion of fresh heparinized blood increases the severity of hypothermic acidosis.

Several investigations lead to the conclusion that hypothermic death is not due to anoxia. This conclusion is based upon the facts that lung ventilation at 20 to 25°C is sufficient to oxygenate the blood, and that blood retains its ability to release sufficient oxygen to maintain the metabolic processes of the tissues at this temperature. Oxygen passes from the alveoli into the blood stream more slowly in hypothermia than at normal temperatures, but the diffusion capacity of the lung for O_2 and CO_2 is adequate to meet the metabolic needs of the tissues. In man, the compliance and resistance of the lung-thorax system has been measured in the hypothermic state; there is no significant difference with body temperatures as low as 29°C. The effects of increased blood CO_2 on the control of respiration during hypothermia has been studied by Cranston *et al.* (27). They measured the blood CO_2 tension in dogs with body temperatures as low as 25°C, and tested the effect of breathing 6 percent CO_2 on the respiratory minute volume at 38°C and 25°C. They found that the percent increase in minute volume was about the same at both temperatures, indicating that the respiratory center had not become insensitive to CO_2 even at low temperatures with an elevated H_2CO_3 level. They suggested that CO_2 may affect the respiratory center largely by virtue of its blood-tension level.

Other changes in blood electrolytes in dogs during hypothermia have been measured. Plasma calcium increases whether or not respiration is controlled to maintain a constant pH; and there is also a rise in the Ca/K ratio. Plasma sodium tends to increase if respiration is spontaneous, and to decrease slightly with controlled hyperventilation. Plasma magnesium does not change significantly. It appears that the electrolyte changes observed may offer an explanation for the onset of spontaneous ventricular fibrillation during hypothermia.

The effect of low temperature on the central nervous system is of particular interest because of its importance in regulating body temperature, and because of practical interest in hypothermia as it relates directly to the protection against anoxia afforded to the CNS by the hypothermic state. However, as has been mentioned, body temperature regulation must be accomplished artificially during hypothermia. Thus, body temperature will tend to rise or fall depending entirely on the degree of physical cooling or warming allowed from the environment. There is a decrease in brain volume of about 4 percent and a decrease in cerebrospinal fluid pressure in proportion to the fall in venous pressure. Experimental reports indicate that hypothermia protects the brain of the dog against cerebral infarction following interruption of the middle cerebral artery. The anesthesia used and the method of lowering brain temperature have a pronounced effect on the outcome. For example, cooling the blood flowing to the brain of rabbits causes death at a higher heart and rectal temperature than cooling the blood returning to the heart. The effects of rapidly cooling the brain could be expected to produce effects of this type because the metabolic requirements of the warmer vital organs may be greater than can be provided by the spontaneous respiration produced by a cooled brain stem.

Low temperature has long been known to block nerve impulse transmission; neuromuscular transmission is blocked at 5°C, and complete cessation of cortical electrical activity occurs at 3°C. Differential blocking actions of cold have been observed in the peripheral nerves of cats. A fibers are blocked before C fibers, and in the A group, progressive cooling blocks δ, γ, β, and α fibers in that order. Also, motor fibers are generally blocked before sensory fibers. However, in the temperature range 20 to 40°C, there is no effect of temperature on acetylcholine (ACH) output from a sympathetic ganglion, but there is a significant reduction in ACH output when the temperature is further lowered to 10°C. Nerve conduction is affected more by temperature than by synaptic transmission in the temperature range 27 to 37°C, although there are reports that synaptic transmission is more sensitive to cold than conduction in the post-ganglionic neuron, which is in turn more sensitive than the effector structure of the sympathetic nervous system.

Brooks and associates (28) have noted a hyperexcitability of the spinal cord as the temperature is lowered. They noted that warming depressed the reflex activity, but that mild cooling (25 to 35°C) produced an augmentation of all responses. Below 20°C, reflexes were depressed and ultimately blocked. They noted a retarding effect of cooling on the development of the excitatory processes at the synapse, but found a greater magnitude and duration of synaptic potentials. During the phase of hyperresponsiveness, the component waves of the electroencephalogram and the electrocorticogram increased in amplitude but not in frequency; and all reflex-produced responses were greatly augmented in amplitude and duration.

Coughing, baroceptor, and chemoreceptor reflexes are active at body temperatures of 26 to 30°C, but to a lesser extent than normal. Carotid sinus reflexes have elevated thresholds and act more slowly at 26°C. Responses to anoxia are feeble, although breathing a 5 percent O_2 in N_2 mixture instead of room air evoked a marked increase of chemoreceptor potentials in animals at 26°C.

The effect of hypothermia on conditioned reflexes has also been studied. Few if any effects on the conditioned reflexes or on the usual habits of dogs, rabbits or rats were observed after recovery from hypothermia (25).

Effects of cooling on kidney function have been reported, although short periods of hypothermia (above 20°C) were found to produce few disorders of urinary or digestive function. Oxygen consumption of the kidney is greatly reduced by hypothermia. Attention has been called to the usefulness of hypothermia in protecting the kidney from anoxia when renal circulation must be occluded during surgery. The concentrations of glucose, phosphorus, amino acids, nitrogen, protein, and creatinine in plasma and urine in hypothermic (20°C) dogs have been studied. Upon cooling there was an increase in urine flow, a decrease in serum amino acid nitrogen and creatinine, and a minimal increase in protein excretion in the urine-plasma ratio for phosphorus; all the filtered glucose appeared in the urine. From this, separate transport mechanisms were postulated for reabsorption of amino acids and phosphorus—the latter being temperature sensitive. The transport mechanism for glucose was completely ineffective at low temperatures.

Tissues removed from hypothermic animals and tissues of animals cooled to hypothermic temperatures have been used to study a variety of effects. Studies of the excised tissues of guinea pigs show that on cooling, oxygen consumption of the brain, liver, and muscle are inhibited in the order given. The effects of up to 12 hours of hypothermia on biliary secretion have been studied by measuring the oxygen uptake in liver slices and liver blood flow. A depression was found in bile volume, which returned only slowly after rewarming. No decrease in liver oxygen consumption was produced by cooling for 6 hours, although there was a depression after cooling for longer periods. This is a most unusual finding, indicating a temperature independence of metabolism in tissues, which probably does not exist in the intact animal. A marked decrease in liver glycogen content was seen, associated with an increase in the non-protein nitrogen fraction of liver composition. Tissues of the heart, lungs, kidneys, pancreas, and adrenals of dogs subjected to hypothermia have been examined for pathologic and histochemical changes. Hypothermia with ether anesthesia for periods of up to 24 hours was not attended by pathological alterations which could be interpreted as resulting from anoxia, although depletion of liver glycogen and adrenal cortical lipid was noted. A decrease of water and solids in the adrenals of hypothermic rats was also noted. Resistance of the kidney to hypothermia was indicated by a lack of alteration in renal lipids, tubular succinic dehydrogenase, cytochrome oxidase, and alkaline phosphatase. Focal pancreatitis was seen in less than 10 percent of the forty experimental animals. The metabolism of ventricular slices has been measured in hypothermic rats cooled to 15°C (25). A tendency toward higher oxygen consumption was observed in slices prepared from cooled rats as compared to normal rats; and there were indications of alternation in membrane permeability and accumulation of reduced intracellular metabolites. A study of the mechanical performance of cooled skeletal muscle of the cat showed that as muscle temperature falls, the rate of development of tension and twitch tension decreases while the duration of the twitch increases.

The influence of body cooling on infection has received modest attention. Dogs cooled at 23°C for as long as 12 hours maintained blood sterility; these animals were able to rid the blood within 6 hours of 99 percent of intravenously-injected pathogens (25). The inability to survive prolonged hypothermia, thus, does not seem to be related to bacteremia; the bacterial defense mechanisms of the hypothermic animal apparently are not depressed. However, Muschenheim *et al.* (29) showed that although hypothermia does not predispose animals (rabbits and guinea pigs) to infection, with thermolabile strains of bacteria, a normally avirulent strain may become highly virulent. These authors also noted that local skin inflammatory reactions were specifically inhibited by hypothermia and by local cooling of sites of inoculation of tuberculin and other test sera. This inhibition of the skin reaction, however, did not affect the general course of infection in the body.

Hibernation of mammals has been a fascinating area of study for physiologists for many years, and although there is occasional confusion between hibernation and hypothermia, the differences in these states have been repeatedly noted (12). As the comparative physiology of the hibernator and non-hibernator becomes better understood, temperature regulation itself will become more clearly understood. However, comparing the physiology of the hibernator to the non-hibernator at present does not lend hope to the idea that the non-hibernator could be placed in a state of deep hibernation.

Of special concern is the possibility that elderly people could spontaneously develop hypothermia, particularly among those living alone with inadequate heat. In the U.S., where homes are usually maintained at relatively high temperatures (70 to 80°F), it is not likely that spontaneous hypothermia is a serious problem at present. However, with increasing difficulties in obtaining adequate heating fuel, circumstances may approach those found in poorer homes in Britain, where the clinical importance of hypothermia in the elderly was first noted. Fox *et al.* (30) made a study of this problem for the Medical Research Council, and concluded that elderly persons living alone under conditions of energy scarcity are at risk of developing hypothermia, and that they show evidence of failure of thermoregulation. There is an additional risk to people who are taking medications which block certain normal functions such as vasomotor control or those which induce general relaxation and sleep.

Summary

Human tissues best perform their physiological functions in the temperature range 35 to 38°C; departure of deep body temperature from this range either in hypothermia (27 to 35°C) or hyperthermia (38 to 41°C) is a severe stress upon the normal function of the body as a whole. At low temperature (27 to 30°C), the conducting system of the heart becomes unstable and ventricular fibrillation results. The extremities and other parts of the body function adequately at lower temperatures down to the freezing level; however, intense pain due to vascular spasm occurs with the pain threshold near 18°C and with increasing intensity of pain as the tissue temperature is lowered.

Hyperthermia above 45°C cannot be sustained indefinitely, and destruction of tissue proteins is so rapid that normal metabolic processes cannot repair the damage thus developed, so that burns occur rapidly at tissue temperatures above 50°C.

The vulnerability of body tissues to temperature requires the careful regulation of all parts of the body; this regulation of deep body temperature at $37 \pm 1°C$ is provided by behavioral and physiological mechanisms. Neurons, sensitive to temperature, are found in all parts of the body and when stimulated, give rise to sensations of warmth and cold and evoke autonomic thermoregulatory activity: vasomotor, shivering, or sweating. Loss of any of these activities is a matter of danger to the individual.

REFERENCES

1. DuBois, E. F. Fever and the regulation of body temperature. *American Lecture Series.* Publ. No. 13, Charles C Thomas, Springfield, Il, 1948.
2. Bernard, C. *Introduction à l'étude de la médicine expérimentale.* Bailliere, Paris, 1865.
3. Hardy, J. D. Thermal comfort and health. *ASHRAE J., 13:* 43–51, 1971.
4. Aschoff, J. and Wever, R. Kern und Schale im Wärmehaushalt des Menschen. *Naturwissenschaften, 20:* 477, 1958.
5. Stolwijk, J. A. J., and Hardy, J. D. Temperature regulation in man—A theoretical study. *Pfluger's Arch., 291:* 129, 1966.
6. Hardy, J. D., Milhorat, A. T., and DuBois, E. F. Basal metabolism and heat loss of young women at temperatures from 22°C to 35°C. *J. Nutr., 21:* 383, 1941.
7. Hardy, J. D. Physiology of temperature regulation. *Physiol. Rev., 41:* 521–606, 1961.
8. Cooper, K. E., Edholm, O. G., Fletcher, J. G., Fox, R. H., and MacPherson, R. K. Vasodilatation in the forearm during indirect heating. *J. Physiol., 125:* 57P, 1954.
9. Stolwijk, J. A. J., and Hardy, J. D. Temperature regulation—A theoretical study. *Pflügers Arch., 291:* 129–162, 1966.
10. Stolwijk, J. A. J., Saltin, B., and Gagge, A. P. Physiological factors associated with sweating during exercise. *Aerosp. Med., 39:* 1101, 1968.
11. Stolwijk, J. A. J. Mathematical model of thermoregulation. *In: Physiological and Behavioral Temperature Regulation.* Hardy, J. D., Gagge, A. P. and Stolwijk, J. A. J. (eds). Charles C Thomas, Springfield, Il, 1970.

12. PRECHT, J., CHRISTOPHERSON, J., HENSEL, H., AND LARCHER, W. (eds). *Temperature and Life*. Springer Verlag, Berlin, New York, 1973.

13. MORITZ, A. R., AND HENRIQUES, F. C. JR. Studies in thermal injury II. The relative importance of time and surface temperature in causation of cutaneous burns. *Am. J. Pathol., 23:* 695, 1947.

14. HENRIQUES, F. C., JR. Studies in thermal injury V. The predictability and the significance of thermally induced rate processes leading to irreversible epidermal injury. *Am. J. Pathol., 23:* 489, 1947.

15. HARDY, J. D., WOLFF, H. G., AND GOODELL, H. *Pain Sensations and Reactions*. William & Wilkins, Baltimore, 1952.

16. HARDY, J. D., STOLWIJK, J. A. J., AND HOFFMAN, D. Pain following step increase in skin temperature. Chapter 21. *In: Skin Senses*. Kenshalo, D. (ed)., Charles C Thomas, Springfield, IL, 1968.

17. LEITHEAD, C. S., AND LIND, A. R. *Heat Stress and Heat Disorders*. F. A. Davis Co., Philadelphia, 1964.

18. BRIDGER, C. A., AND HELFAND, L. A. A mortality from heat during July 1966 in Illinois. *Int. J. Biomet., 12:* 51–70, 1968.

19. STRYDOM, N. B., WYNDHAM, C. H., WILLIAMS, C. G., MORRISON, J. F., BREDELL, G. A. G., BENADE, A. J. S., AND VON RADEM, M. Acclimatization to humid heat and the role of physical conditioning. *J. Appl. Physiol., 21:* 636, 1966.

20. LE BLANC, J. *Man in the Cold*. Charles C Thomas, Springfield, Il, 1975.

21. SCHOLANDER, P. F., HAMMEL, H. T., ANDERSEN, K. L., AND LYNING, Y. Metabolic acclimation to cold in man. *J. Appl. Physiol., 12:* 1, 1958.

22. WYNDHAM, C. H., AND MORRISON, J. F. Adjustment to cold of Bushmen in the Kalahari Desert. *J. Appl. Physiol., 13:* 219, 1958.

23. FAY, T., AND HENRY, G. C. Correlation of body segmental temperature and its relation to the location of carcinomatous metastasis. *Surg. Gynecol. & Obstet., 66:* 512, 1938.

24. BIGELOW, W. G., LINDSAY, W. K., HARRISON, R. C., AND GREENWOOD, W. F. Oxygen transport and utilization in dogs at low body temperature. *Am. J. Physiol., 160:* 125, 1950.

25. KAYSER, CH. Physiological aspects of hypothermia. *Ann. Rev. Physiol., 19:* 83, 1957.

26. THAUER, R. Ergebnisse experimenteller Kreislaufuntersuchen bei Hypothermie. *Thoraxchirurgie, 3:* 521, 1956.

27. CRANSTON, W. I., PEPPER, M. C., AND ROSS, D. N. Carbon dioxide and control of respiration during hypothermia. *J. Physiol., 127:* 380, 1955.

28. BROOKS, C. MC., KOIZUMI, K., AND MALCOLM, J. L. Effects of changes in temperature on reactions of spinal cord. *J. Neurophysiol., 18:* 205, 1955.

29. MUSCHENHEIM, C., DUERSCHNER, D. R., HARDY, J. D., AND STOLL, A. M. Hypothermia in experimental infections III. The effect of hypothermia on resistance to experimental pneumococcus infection. *J. Infect. Dis., 72:* 187, 1943.

30. FOX, R. H., WOODWARD, P. M., SMITH-EXTON, A. N., GREEN, M. F., DONNISON, D. V., AND WICKS, M. H. Body temperatures in the elderly: A national study of physiological, social, and environmental conditions. *Brit. Med. J., 1:* 200–206, 1973.

6

Biophysics of High Frequency Currents and Electromagnetic Radiation[1]

ARTHUR W. GUY

Introduction and Historical Survey

Interest in the use of high frequency (HF) currents for diathermy dates back as far as 1892, when d'Arsonval, a physician-physiologist, observed that currents at 10 kHz or greater produced a sensation of warmth without the painful muscle contractions or fatal consequences which could occur at lower frequencies (81) (see Chapter 1). Although d'Arsonval suggested using HF currents for medical applications other than tissue heating, he set the stage for the use of radio frequency (RF) energy for therapeutic heating of diseased tissue. This type of therapeutic heating became popular because HF currents could penetrate deeply into the tissues to produce heat; it was considered superior to hot packs and infrared radiation for deep tissue heating.

One of the oldest applications of electromagnetic (EM) heating, which only recently has received widespread attention, is the treatment of cancer by hyperthermia. This rapidly developing modality made its debut in the early 1900's when HF currents between 0.5 and 3.0 MHz were used for cautery (Chapter 1). As early as 1909, de Keating-Hart (21) used a combination of heat produced by HF electrical current and ionizing radiation for

[1]This chapter is, in part, based on research supported by Research Grant # G008003029 from the National Institute of Handicapped Research, Department of Education, Washington, D.C. 20202.

the treatment of cancer. These combined modalities have been used in the treatment of cancer in humans and laboratory animals over the past seven decades. Work prior to 1920 was summarized well by Rohdenburg and Prime (101); work between 1920 and 1937 was reviewed by Arons and Sokolov (5). The greatest reported success, to date, has resulted from the treatment of tumors by combined diathermy and X-radiation. Some researchers, however, were able to destroy mouse carcinoma by using diathermy alone (82). By 1928, EM radiation approaching 100 MHz (shortwave diathermy) was being used clinically. Schereschewsky (102) was able to inhibit growth in most cases of transplanted mouse carcinoma, and in some cases to completely eliminate the tumors, by treating them with ultra-shortwaves of three-meter wavelength. For the next decade, there was an average of one scientific paper per year reporting on the subject (5, 26, 30, 43, 45, 55, 96, 97, 100, 103).

It is interesting to note that arguments both in support of and against the thesis of athermal affects developed with the early history of therapeutic application of EM waves. In addition to the claimed frequency specific effects in the shortwave treatment of tumors, Danilewsky and Worobjew (20) demonstrated that contractions in frog nerve muscle preparations increased in amplitude when HF currents were applied along with minimum faradic stimuli. When the HF currents were removed, excitability of the nerve rapidly returned to its original value. With increasing current (0.5–1.0 MHz exposure), a point was reached where a depression in excitability resulted. An increase or decrease of excitability was also obtained by irradiating the sciatic nerve of a warm-blooded animal. Audiat (6) asserted that since the excitability of the nerve muscle preparation diminished under the action of the EM waves, it had to be a "specific" effect, since heat would have an opposite effect. It was also claimed by Delherm and Fischgold (23) that HF currents diminished excitability of the nerve-muscle preparation in a manner similar to that produced by the anodic effect of direct current. Later, it was shown by Weissenberg (120) that interrupted HF current applied to a nerve muscle preparation of a frog showed stimulating effects similar to that obtained by a pulsating DC current. It was postulated that the nerve rectified a small portion of the applied HF current. Pflomm (96) stated that if a frog's heart is placed in a shortwave field, the beat becomes slower and the excursions lessen, with the diastolic beat finally ceasing. But if the field is switched off, the heart gradually resumes its activity. Hill and Taylor (46) on the other hand, replicated the work showing that weak HF fields with wavelengths of 600, 22, and 6 meters would increase the excitability of a nerve-muscle preparation, whereas stronger current produced a depression of excitability. They showed that similar effects would be produced by a hot wire placed near the nerve, and concluded that the action of the HF current on the nerve muscle preparation was thermal. These researchers also demonstrated that the effects observed by Pflomm on the frog's heart due to HF fields were identical to that obtained when the frog's heart was warmed.

Between 1931 and 1941, there were many basic problems in using short-waves for the effective therapeutic heating of tissues. Most of these problems were related to the fact that investigators were not able to quantify the actual power absorbed in tissues during treatment. The results of therapeutic treatment were left entirely to chance; and many quantitatively uncontrolled experiments resulted in contradictory statements in the medical literature. The various shortwave generators produced by different manufacturers had variable outputs. It was implied through advertisements that the heating of deeper tissues would be enhanced with greater power output. Since the heating of tissues seemed to vary considerably with frequency, even with the same apparent output, many researchers jumped to the conclusion that there were selective and specific properties of various wavelengths.

A research team consisting of engineers and physicians (87) measured elevations of temperature *in vivo* in tissues as a function of rates and quantities of energy absorbed instead of the output power of the diathermy applicator or the tissue exposure level. The group instrumented a shortwave diathermy generator such that the energy absorbed by the patient under treatment could be measured to within 5 percent. The power level of absorbed energy was correlated with the rise of temperature in the tissues. The results (Table 6.1) relate the absorbed energy, the temperature rise and the Watts per 1000 cc for 0.1°F temperature rise/minute. This work made use for the first time of volume-normalized rates of energy absorption with

TABLE 6.1. *Relationship of Temperature Rise per Minute to Power Absorption*[a]

	No.	Power absorbed (Watts)	Temperature rise/min.	Watts/1000 cc for 0.1°F temperature rise/min.	Deviation against average (Percent)
Subject I—	1	60	0.275	5.75	−1
Thigh volume	2	72	0.310	6.15	+4.8
approximately	3	74	0.300	6.42	+8
3800 cc	4	85	0.384	5.86	0
	5	86	0.390	5.78	+0.7
	6	100	0.460	5.75	+0.7
	7	137	0.652	5.55	+5.2
Subject II—	8	88	0.440	6.15	+4.8
Thigh volume	9	88	0.440	6.15	+4.8
approximately	10	44	0.260	5.20	−13
3280 cc	11	135	0.720	5.75	−0.7
Average of all tests—				5.86	

[a] From Mittleman *et al.* (87).

units (W/liter) closely related to the W/kg now widely accepted for RF dosimetry. The results of the energy-absorption measurements agreed well with theory. The amount of energy absorption per unit of tissue volume that raised the tissue temperature a certain extent in a given period of time was the same in all of the tests. The group conducted another series of measurements in which the patient was exposed under differing wavelengths and techniques of exposure. The results (Figure 6.1) indicated that the temperature rise per minute was proportional to the energy absorbed by the patient. The absorption necessary to raise the temperature of 1000 cc of tissue volume by 0.1°F per minute computed from the results of Figure 6.1 is recorded in Table 6.2, which is in excellent agreement with the results in Table 6.1. It is important to note that a deviation from linearity was found to take place at the end of a 20-minute exposure period in cases where the absorption rate exceeded 100 Watts (calculated absorption rate = 48 W/liter), and where the subject had been treated for a short time previously (curves with index 2 in Figure 6.1). The work by Mittlemann *et al.* (87) clearly demonstrated that the degree of tissue heating depended solely on energy absorption and not on wavelength for similar ratios of deep to superficial heating. It is also significant to note that these authors found a marked difference in the behavior of the temperature curves for high and low wattage. At power levels less than 100 W (calculated absorption = 33–42 W/liter), temperature in the deep tissue was noted to rise along a straight line until near the termination of the 20-minute exposure period. If the power level exceeded 42 W/liter, the final temperature was lower than the previous temperature, due to an increase in blood circulation which rapidly dissipated the heat.

In the first ten years of the development and use of shortwave diathermy, research consisted of measuring the temperatures of superficial and deep tissues of both animal and human subjects exposed to capacitive and inductive applicators with generator wavelengths varying from 6 to 24 meters. The only dosimetric index at the time was monitoring the power level of each device and relating it to temperature measurements in the tissues. A number of researchers believed as a result of their observations of varying temperature rises and heating in tissues exposed to different wavelengths, that the absorption characteristics were wavelength specific. Others, such as Osborne and Coulter (92), thought that the variations depended more on electrode configuration, spacing, and geometry of the tissue being treated than on frequency. It was also observed by these early researchers that it was difficult to produce therapeutic temperature levels of 42 to 45°C in deep tissues, such as muscle and bone marrow, without adversely affecting the skin and the superficial tissues.

During the late 1930's and early 1940's, there was growing interest in the use of even shorter wavelength EM waves for therapeutic purposes. Williams (121) reported that EM waves with wavelengths of a few centimeters could

TABLE 6.2 *Heating Curves Obtained on Four Different Subjects Using Variable Wattages, Different Techniques, and Various Wavelengths*[a]

Volume (cc)	Curve	Wavelength (meters)	Technique	Power absorption (Watts)	Watts/1000 cc for 0.1°F temperature rise/min	Deviation against average (percent)
3280	a1	6	Air Sp.	35	5.35	−9
3280	a2	6	Air Sp.	63	5.83	0
3100	b1	12	Air Sp.	110	6.25	+6.2
3100	b2	12	Air Sp.	70	6.60	+11.0
2400	c2	12	Pancake Coil	115	5.68	−3.0
3600	d1	8	Db Cuffs	80	5.35	−9.0
Average of all tests—					5.83	

[a] From Mittleman et al. (87).

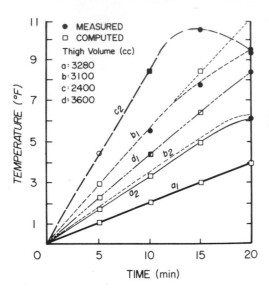

Fig. 6.1. Heating curves for four human subjects exposed to short-wave diathermy, showing that temperature rise is proportional to power absorbed. Several applicators were used at varying power levels. See data in Table 6.2. After Mittlemann *et al.* (87)

be focused; and Southworth (114) pointed out that such radiation could be directed through hollow conducting tubes (waveguides). A proposal to use microwaves for therapeutic purposes originated in Germany when Hollman (50) discussed the possible therapeutic application of 25 cm waves and predicted that the waves could be focused to produce heating of deep tissues without excessive heating of the skin. Similar predictions were made by Hemingway and Stenstrom (44) in the United States. The lack of available hardware at the time prevented clinical application of these concepts; and diathermy treatments continued at frequencies below 100 MHz.

At the end of World War II, when security restrictions were lifted on magnetron sources of microwaves, the first microwave diathermy was developed, operating at a frequency of 3000 MHz. With the new equipment, the first work on therapeutic applications of microwaves began at the Mayo Clinic in 1946 (59, 62). It involved the exposure of laboratory animals to 3000 MHz radiation at 65 W. The temperature distribution in the thigh of experimental dogs was measured with thermocouples before and after exposure to microwaves. In this work (with the thermocouples removed during the period of radiation), it was demonstrated that deep tissues could be heated, resulting in a number of physiological responses, including an increased blood flow to the treated area. But, as with the use of shortwaves, it was noted that the average temperature rise was greater in the skin and subcutaneous fat than in the deeper muscle tissues, although the final temperature in the muscle tissue was higher.

Worden *et al.* (122) found that a monopole antenna with a hemispheric reflector, which was energized by 30 W of 2450 MHz microwave energy, resulted in maximal heating of thighs of dogs after an exposure period of 20 minutes when the antenna was located 2.5 cm from the surface of the thigh. If the period of exposure was extended to 30 minutes, the temperature dropped as a result of a sharp increase in blood flow. This finding is consistent with those found earlier by Mittlemann *et al.* (87). Worden *et al.* (122) also carried out comparative studies on the effects of exposing ischemic tissue and tissue with normal circulation to the same amount of microwave energy over a period of 15 to 20 minutes. They found serious damage resulted in the ischemic area even though the average temperatures recorded were not any higher than those found in tissues with normal circulation.

Siems *et al.* (113) made comparative studies of the effect of shortwave and microwave diathermy on blood flow. Their experiments clearly demonstrated that shortwave and microwave diathermy were equally effective in producing increased blood flow in the extremities of normal dogs. A number of such experiments were carried out, sometimes with conflicting results. Finally, in order to resolve this problem, Richardson *et al.* (98) carried out research on the relationship between deep tissue temperature and blood flow during irradiation of the gastrocnemius muscles of dogs by shortwave diathermy and microwaves. They found that with both modalities, the blood flow in an area depended largely upon the degree of tissue hyperthermia developed. It was necessary to increase the tissue temperatures at 1-cm depth in an extremity of the dog to 42 to 43°C before a consistent increase in blood flow occurred in the femoral artery. The increase in blood flow was sufficient to actually diminish the temperature after reaching a critical temperature. These results are consistent with the findings of Mittlemann *et al.* (87) and have been observed by many researchers since that time.

After 1950 and up until 1965, research on the use of microwaves for diathermy in physical medicine expanded significantly. Clinical and experimental research predominated any quantitative work on dosimetry. Gessler *et al.* (33) appear to be the first group to use RF energy at microwave frequencies in the experimental treatment of cancer. They were able to eradicate spontaneous mammary carcinoma in C3H mice with microwave exposure alone. Five years later, Allen (1) cured Crocker sarcoma 39 in rats with 1500 to 2000 r X-radiation and 12.5 cm microwaves after exposing the animals for 10 to 20 minutes. The microwave exposure produced a temperature of 42°C in the tumors. Crile (19) reported that growth of tumors in dogs and human beings was controlled by microwave diathermy and X-radiation in combination. Crile concluded that prolonged elevation of temperature in certain cancers at levels between 42 and 50°C selectively destroyed the tumors without damaging normal tissues. He believed that it was a secondary inflammatory reaction rather than the primary elevation of temperature that destroyed the tumors. Two years later, Cater *et al.* (12) reported that combined therapy of 2620 r (220 kV X-rays) and subsequent 10-cm microwave irradiation of the tumor (47°C for 8 to 10 minutes) cured some rats with hepatoma 223 transplanted in the leg. The investigators noted that there were no long-term survivors treated by radiation alone or by diathermy alone, and that the tumor size was greater and the mean survival time was significantly shorter than in rats treated by the combined therapies. In the same year, Moressi (88) found that mortality patterns were essentially identical in mouse sarcoma 180 cells exposed to 2450 MHz microwave radiation as those for controls held at the same temperature ranging from 43 to 48°C. He found that cell decay was highly temperature-dependent, as indicated by the "spontaneous" destruction of cellular material. The investigation also showed that in microwave studies concerned with cellular destruction, undetected temperature deviations of no greater than 1°C can lead to erroneous interpretations, and the author pointed out that

> "one may critically question the role of unrecognized temperature discrepancies in many of the previously reported studies in which gross results seemed to indicate the presence of a non-thermal factor. Temperature regulation is thus a major concern in investigations concerned with the effects of high frequency electromagnetic irradiation on biological systems, especially when some form of cellular destruction is involved."(88, p. 250)

Although the use of microwaves for therapeutic heating gained in popularity in the 1950's and early 1960's, interest in the use of shortwaves remained. Birkner and Wachsmann (8) reported regressions and cures in skin carcinoma on patients exposed to shortwaves and X-radiation. Exposures of 82 patients for a period of 2.5 hours to 6-meter shortwaves (tumor temperatures of 42 to 44°C) alone produced regressions but no cures. When the shortwave exposure was combined with X-radiation, however, some cures were observed. Fuchs (31) reported good clinical results when 6-meter shortwave exposures of 10 to 20 minutes were followed by X-radiation exposure. He claimed that the good clinical results were increased radiosensitivity due to hyperemia and acceleration of metabolism as a result of the shortwave exposure.

In addition to the use of combined RF and X-ray therapy, interest developed in the use of microwaves for selectively heating tumors to provide for more effective therapy with injected radioactive materials and chemotherapy. Copeland and Michaelson (18) reported that the heating of Walker carcinoma 256 by selective radiation with 2800 MHz, 260 mW/cm^2 microwaves for 5 minutes induced a substantial increase in the amount of intravenously-injected I^{131} fibrinogen localization in the tumor. They pointed out that this tumor-heating technique could potentially increase tumor radiation therapy dose from I^{131} fibrinogen by 400 percent. Zimmer et al. (123) reported the use of selective electromagnetic heating in tumors in animals in deep hypothermia to enhance the action of chemotherapy. They treated spontaneous mammary tumors in C3H mice and induced mammary tumors in Sprague-Dawley rats. They found that in 20 control mice there were no spontaneous regressions of tumors, and that in 20 mice treated with chemotherapy only, two animals showed regression of tumors with a regression time of 10 days. In the group treated with differential hyperthermia, with a colonic temperature of 4 to 8°C and a treated tumor temperature of 30 to 42°C without chemotherapy, only one tumor regressed with a regression time of 7 days. In the group of 20 mice treated with both differential hyperthermia and chemotherapy, there were 17 tumors that regressed with a regression time of 55 ± 25 days. Similar results were obtained with the rats using 10 animals per group and using S-band instead of X-band microwave heating. In this case, all tumors treated regressed with an average regression time of 22 days.

Overgaard and Overgaard (94) provided an excellent review and reported on very extensive and well conducted experiments with 1200 mice done in their laboratory, where transplanted tumors in the mice were permanently cured without damage to surrounding tissues by treatment with 212 MHz shortwave diathermy. They used a special HF neutral thermocouple embedded in the tumor to provide automatic regulation of the shortwave output. Thus, it was possible to maintain any desired temperature continuously with a variation of about 0.1°C. With carefully controlled elevations in the range of 41.5 to 43.5°C, they were able to work out a quantitative relationship between temperature and exposure time for curing the transplanted tumors. An analysis showed that the treatment induced histological changes in the tumor cells without damaging the stromal and vascular cells in the tumor or in surrounding normal tissue. Immediately after treatment, definite changes were revealed in the mitochondria and lysosomes in the tumor cells. The intensity of these changes was directly related to the elevation of temperature, and became more pronounced within a few hours or days. They noted changes in the nuclei of the tumor cells and the chromosomal and nucleolar chromatin within the first few hours after exposure. They observed severe injury in all tumor cells 24 hours after exposure to a curative dose. Through histological and biochemical observations, they obtained clues that allowed them to assume that the direct effect of the heat was due to an elective activation of the acid hydrolases localized in the lysosomes of the tumor cells. In later work, Overgaard and Overgaard (95) found that the addition of a small dose of local X-radiation produced highly significant intensification of the tumor-deleting effect. They found that successive application of heat and X-radiation doses, both substantially smaller than required in themselves to produce cures, produced large number of total cures. They also noted that intervals of up to 24 hours between applications did not appreciably alter the curative effect.

From the mid-1970's on, interest in using RF fields either alone or in combination with X-radiation increased substantially with a large number of favorable reports on the use of the therapy in frequency symposia proceedings and publications. Among these are the proceedings of the First and Second International Symposia on Cancer therapy by Hyperthermia and Irradiation (99, 116) and a special issue of IEEE Microwave Theory and Techniques Transactions on microwaves and medicine, with accent on the application of electromagnetic energy to cancer treatment (40).

Some examples of more recent shortwave applications are the work of M. von Ardenne (118), Overgaard (93), Kim et al. (57), and LeVeen et al. (61). Continuing success is reported in the use of microwave hyperthermia as an adjunct in the treatment of tumors. Szmigielski et al. (117) reported prolongation of the survival of mice bearing sarcoma 180 tumors when irradiated by 3000 MHz microwaves such that rectal temperatures increased by 3 to 4°C. The inhibitory effect of microwave hyperthermia was enhanced by simultaneous treatment of the mice with interferon and interferon inducers. Mendecki et al. (84) completely eradicated transplanted mammary adenocarcinoma in C3H mice and, in several cases, obtained favorable results in the treatment of basal cell carcinoma, malginant melanoma, and skin metastases of carcinoma of the breast, using both 2450 MHz and 915 MHz microwave radiation. In these studies, the temperatures of the tumors were raised to the hyperthermic range of 42.5 to 43°C. Nelson and Holt (90) and Hornback et al. (51, 52) successfully treated cancers in patients with the ultra-high frequency (UHF) of 433 MHz and ionizing radiation.

Significant research to quantify various biological effects of electromagnetic fields was done by Schwan and associates (105–109) the University of Pennsylvania. Schwan's work on the dielectric properties of biological tissues and absorption by various tissue geometries deserves considerable attention. Schwan demonstrated theoretically that the microwave frequency of 2450 MHz was not a good choice for therapy because of a number of major deficiencies, incluing a) excessive heating in the subcutaneous fat due to standing waves; b) poor penetration into the muscle tissue; and c) poor control and knowledge of energy absorbed by patients due to the large variations in electrical thickness (compared to the wavelength of subcutaneous tissues). He recommended that frequencies be reduced to 900 MHz or less.

Lehmann et al. (70–72, 76) and Guy and Lehmann (34) experimentally verified Schwan's earlier theoretical prediction that 900 MHz or lower frequencies could produce better therapeutic patterns than obtained with 2450 MHz energy. Since 1966, Lehmann et al. (76), deLateur et al. (22), and Guy (35, 36) have developed and clinically tested direct-contact applicators operating at 915 MHz, which have been proven to be therapeutically more effective and safe in terms of leakage radiation than the existing 2450 MHz equipment.

In physical medicine applications, the effects of exposing tissue to electromagnetic fields are believed to be due to simple volume heating. When local elevations of temperature are induced in living tissues, the resulting temperature rise will produce many physiological responses, partly due to direct action on the tissue cells and partly due to thermal action on local nerve receptors. One of the responses is an increase in blood flow due to vasodilatation accompanied by increases in capillary pressure, cellular membrane permeability, and metabolic rate. The latter could result in a further increase in tissue temperature.

Millard (85) measured effects of shortwave irradiation on local blood circulation through the use of radioactive sodium following the method used by Kety (56). He showed that the radioactive sodium remaining at the site of injection decreased along an exponential curve which, when plotted semilogarithmically against time, produced a straight line, the slope of which he called the clearance constant. He found that the skin clearance rate increased approximately 150 percent after exposure, with an average rise in temperature over the injection site of 5.3°C. The muscle clearance rates, on the other hand, were found to increase by 36 percent when the corresponding temperature rise was 5.2°C. In about one-third of the subjects, there was little overall change in the muscle clearance rate and in one-third, there was a decrease followed by an increase.

Harris (42), was able to quantify the effect of shortwave diathermy on the local circulation in normal and rheumatoid knees by using the same method. With the slope K expressed as $K = (0.04343)^{-1} (\log C_1 - \log C_2)(T_2 - T_1)^{-1}$, where C_1 and C_2 are counting rates at times T_1 ad T_2, respectively, he obtained the results shown in Figure 6.2. The results indicate that in normal knees, the increase in circulation averages 100 percent when the knee is

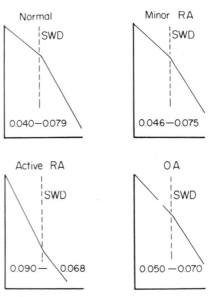

Fig. 6.2. Effect of shortwave diathermy on mean values of sodium clearance from normal, rheumatoid arthritic (minor and major activity) and osteoarthritic knee joints. The slope indicates the value of the coefficient K before and after the onset of shortwave diathermy treatment. After Harris (42).

Normal
SWD
0.040—0.079

Minor RA
SWD
0.046—0.075

Active RA
SWD
0.090— 0.068

OA
SWD
0.050 —0.070

RA – rheumatoid arthritis
OA – osteoarthritis

exposed with shortwave capacitor electrodes, with fields adjusted for maximum skin tolerance to heat. In quiescent rheumtoid knees, the shortwave exposure produced an increase in circulation averaging 60 percent, and in mildly active rheumatoid disease, major increases were not found in four out of five subjects. In active rheumatoid disease, there was a decrease in circulation. Thus, assuming that the rate of sodium clearance is related to the degree of hyperemia, the results indicate it is logical to heat only inactive rheumatoid joints with shortwave diathermy as a local therapy in rheumatoid arthritis.

McNiven and Wyper (83) were able to measure the increase in muscle blood flow in man under treatment by 2450 MHz microwave diathermy, with the power output adjusted to produce maximum comfortable heating. The muscle blood flow was measured using the Xe^{133} clearance technique, where 200 microCuries of inert diffusable radioactive tracer Xe^{133}, dissolved in 0.1 ml of sterile isotonic saline, was injected into the muscle (vastis lateralis). A scintillation counter was use to monitor the count rate of gamma rays/minute from the Xe^{133}. This enabled the rate of clearance of xeon and therefore, the blood flow, to be measured. From a single injection, the muscle blood flow was measured at rest, during application of microwave therapy, and during static exercise. The results are shown in Figure 6.3. Under steady-state conditions, the count rate of Xe^{133}, plotted as a function of time, produces a straight line on semilogarithmic graph paper, as shown in Figure 6.3. From this line, $T_{1/2}$ (the time taken for the count rate to equal

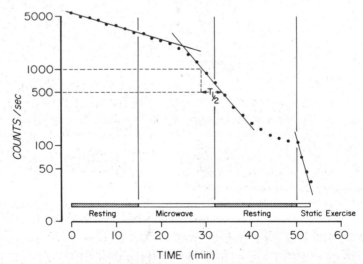

Fig. 6.3. Clearance of xenon-133 from a single intra-muscular injunction. The values of $T_{1/2}$ are 16.7 minutes for the initial resting period, 4.2 minutes at the end of microwave application, and 1.6 minutes during static exercise. The corresponding muscle blood flow values are 2.9, 11.5, and 30.3 ml/100 gm, respectively. After McNiven and Wyper (83).

one-half of the original rate) can be measured. Muscle blood flow F can then be obtained using the equation $F = 48.5 \, (T_{1/2})^{-1}$. If $T_{1/2}$ is in minutes, the units of F will be ml/100 gm/min. The figure indicates that after 8 minutes of microwave exposure, the slope of the clearance curve was observed to increase, corresponding to a rise in the muscle blood flow rate. When this reached a steady-state value, the apparatus was switched off, and it was noted that the flow was maintained at the higher level for about 5 minutes before gradually decreasing. The results of all five subjects (Figure 6.4) show mean values of 2.9 ml/100 gm·min at rest, rising to 11.4 ml/100 gm·min at the end of a microwave application. It was also indicated that blood flow increased to 30.3 ml/100 gm·min during statis exercise. In contrast to the 150 percent increase in blood flow noted by Millard (85) due to shortwave diathermy treatments, the microwave diathermy produced an increase of 400 percent.

Guy *et al.* (38) estimated the increase in blood flow rate in human thighs treated by shortwave diathermy by observing the time dependence of the temperatures measured in the muscle exposed to the shortwave fields. The change in the slope of the temperature curve during shortwave exposure both before and after the blood flow was occluded by a tourniquet provided the quantitative information necessary to predict the increase in blood flow. This method was later used by Lehmann et al. (79) to determine the blood flow in deep muscle exposed to 915 MHz microwave radiation with simultaneous skin surface cooling. Calculated blood flows of 29 ml/100 gm·min

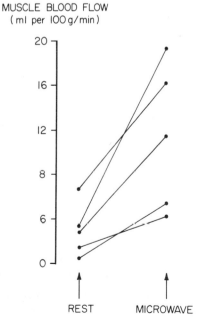

MUSCLE BLOOD FLOW
(ml per 100 g/min)

Fig. 6.4. The values of muscle blood flow during the initial resting period and at the end of microwave therapy in five subjects. After McNiven and Wyper (83).

were obtained when the specific absorption rate in the muscle was 112 W/ kg, producing a maximum temperature between 43 and 45°C. Nearly similar results, calculated maximum blood flows of 32 ml/100 gm/min, were obtained by Sekins *et al.* (111) using the Xe^{133} clearance method in evaluating the same 915 MHz diathermy applicator under the same experimental conditions.

It is believed that these circulatory responses can increase the healing rate in diseased or damaged tissue by increasing the transfer of metabolites across cell membranes, providing for greater concentration of white cells and antibodies, and increasing the transport rate of toxins, engulfed bacteria and debris away from the treated area (104). The heating can promote relaxation in muscles, reduce pain and provide relief of muscle "spasms" (27, 78). Heating can also produce changes in the properties of collagenous tissues, as found in tendon, joint capsule, and scarred synovium. As the collagenous tissue is heated to therapeutic levels, the property of viscous flow becomes predominant, and tension is reduced (77). If a physical therapy program of stretch is used in conjunction with heating, as in patients with hip and shoulder limitations, one can take advantage of the increase in extensibility to produce signficant increases in range of motion (64, 65, 69, 78). Joint stiffness can also be relieved by heating. Backlund and Tiselius (7) have measured the joint stiffness of rheumatoid patients and have shown a decrease in the hysteresis loop after heating the joint.

The temperature of the tissues is the most important factor in determining the extent of the physiological response to heat. Lehmann (78) has shown by animal studies the relation between the percentage of hyperemia (increase in blood volume) and temperature (Figure 6.5). The results indicate that the tissue temperature must be raised above 41°C to produce any

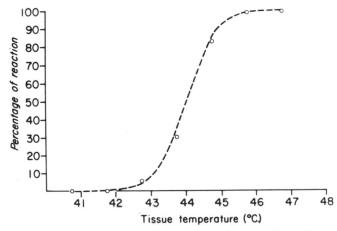

Fig. 6.5. Dependence of hyperemia on tissue temperature. (From *Therapeutic Heat and Cold*, 2nd edition, 1972).

signficant reaction, and a temperature near 45°C is needed for maximal reaction. The overall body metabolic rate will also initially increase with increased temperature ΔT. The factor of increase is approximately $(1.1)^{\Delta T}$ within physiological limits (10) (e.g., with an initial tissue temperature of 34°C, an elevation of temperature to 40°C would produce a 77 percent increase in metabolic rate, assuming that the increase in a specific tissue is comparable to the increase of metabolic rate caused by an increase in the total body temperature. The upper temperature of 45°C probably corresponds closely to the safe upper limit where a further increase could sharply reduce the metabolic rate or stop it altogether (63, 64)). The threshold of thermal pain corresponds to a skin temperature of 45°C, with the pain intensity increasing to a maximum at about 65°C. The threshold for irreversible skin tissue damage is also 45°C, when heat is applied for a sufficiently long period of time (41). For short periods of heat application, the skin can tolerate higher temperatures without damage. For most other tissues, 45°C also appears to be the maximum safe temperature tolerated without damage (58). Certain tissues appear to have a lower tolerance, however. For example, the testicles, which are normally much lower in temperature than other portions of the body, can be affected adversely at temperature equal to the normal 37°C body temperature (53). The lens of the eye is especially vulnerable to radiant-type heating; irreversible damage can occur at elevated temperatures due to the lack of blood circulation and poor tissue repair capabilities (11). Figure 6.5 shows that the therapeutic temperature range is not only narrow, but that it is very close to the damaging temperature level.

Lehmann (78) has also shown that the duration of tissue temperature is important in determining the extent of the biological reaction (Figure 6.6).

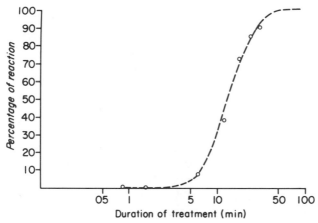

Fig. 6.6. Dependence of hyperemia on duration of treatment. (From *Therapeutic Heat and Cold*, 2nd edition, 1972).

The figure indicates that a minimal effective duration of elevation is 3 to 5 minutes, whereas complete reactions may be obtained with a 30-minute application. It is clear that the rate of temperature rise plays an important role in determining the extent of the biological response, since only the period where an effective temperature level is obtained is therapeutically beneficial. Also, the physiological responses of the nervous system temperature receptors seem to be more pronouned when the rate of temperature elevation is rapid (24, 68).

When surface heat is applied, the skin temperature increases with the accompanying reactions described previously. Although this is beneficial for the treatment of pathological lesions at or near the tissue surface, it is ineffective for treating deeper pathological conditions. The subcutaneous fat acts as a thermal barrier which, combined with the increased surface vasodilatation, prevents the flow of thermal energy into the deeper musculature. No increase in deep tissue blood flow will result; and there may even be vasoconstriction to compensate for the increase in surface blood. Nerve reflexes due to surface heating can produce consensual temperature increases in other parts of the body, e.g., the surface of the opposite extremity, but these are less pronounced than the primary increases (27). Relaxation of the striated skeletal muscles may occur, and muscle spasms may be resolved by the surface heating due to reflex nerve reactions from surface temperature receptors. Thus, in general, surface heating provides only mild physiological and therapeutic reactions; any effects on deeper pathological conditions are reflex in nature.

Effective therapeutic heating of tissues below the skin and subcutaneous fat layer of patients can be accomplished by the use of electromagnetic fields. This requires a choice of frequency, applicator and input power so that the temperature of the deeper tissue can be raised to the maximum level of 44 to 45°C within a 5- to 15-minute period. The time interval to maximum temperature can be controlled by setting the input power level. Just before, or when the temperature reaches this maximum range, vasodilation will produce a marked increase in blood flow. This will limit the rise in temperature in tissues with good vascularity and will produce a decrease in temperature by several degrees. A total exposure period of 20 to 30 minutes is generally required to produce optimum therapeutic benefits.

Methods of Application

Electromagnetic heating of tissues may be accomplished by the four methods shown in Figure 6.7. Figure 6.7a illustrates direct electric heating of muscle tissue by alternating currents, through the use of direct-contact electrodes. The frequency is sufficiently high (greater than 100 kHz) to prevent the excitation of action potentials. Such electrodes have been placed either in direct contact with the tissue surface or interstitially by means of probes as shown in the figure. In general, for frequencies below 27 MHz, volume conduction concepts may be used for quantification of the fields and associated heating patterns. Non-contacting capacitive plates, as illustrated in Figure 6.7b, have generally been used for application of currents at frequencies above 13 MHz. This is one of the types of applicators that has been commonly used for "shortwave" diathermy. Another class of shortwave diathermy applicators (Figure 6.7c) consists of single turn solenoidal or "pancake" magnetic coils that produce alternating magnetic fields. These fields heat tissues by inducing circulating eddy currents. The fourth method of therapeutic heating utilizes radiation fields at UHF or microwave frequencies, as shown in Figure 6.7d.

EM heating mechanisms can best be illustrated by considering the case of a HF current applied to tissue through direct-contact electrodes, as shown in Figure 6.8. Here we consider a slab of tissue of thickness d sandwiched between conducting metal electrodes with surface area A. An alternating current source with RMS voltage V is applied to the electrodes. The resulting RMS current I which will flow through the tissue is given by

$$I = YV \tag{1}$$

where Y is the admittance measured at the metal electrodes. If we assume a uniform electric field and current flow, the admittance may be expressed as

$$Y = j\omega C^* \tag{2}$$

where $\omega = 2\pi f$, f is the frequency of the applied voltage, and C^* represents a complex or "lossy" capacitance:

$$C^* = \epsilon_m{}^* A d^{-1} \tag{3}$$

where $\epsilon_m{}^*$ is the complex permittivity of the tissue given by

$$\epsilon_m{}^* = \epsilon_0 \epsilon_m - j\sigma_m \omega^{-1} \tag{4}$$

$\epsilon_o = 8.85 \times 10^{-12}$ is the permittivity of free space, ϵ_m is the dielectric constant of the tissue, and σ_m is the electrical conductivity of the tissue.

The admittance may also be expressed in the standard form

$$Y = G + jB \tag{5}$$

where G is the conductance and B is the susceptance.

From the previous equations

$$G = \sigma_m A d^{-1} \tag{6}$$

and

$$B = \omega C = \omega \epsilon_o \epsilon_m A d^{-1} \tag{7}$$

where $C = \epsilon_o \epsilon_m A d^{-1}$ is the capacitance for the electrodes, resulting from the real part of the tissue dielectric constant ϵ_m. By Joule's law, the power loss

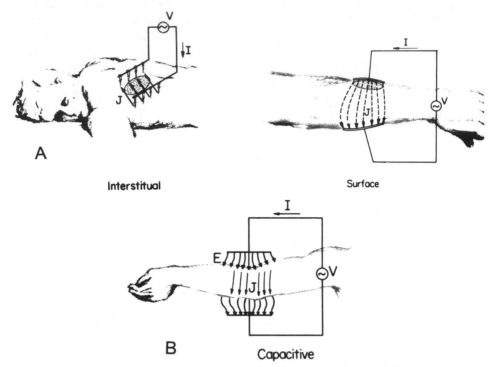

Interstitual

Surface

B

Capacitive

Fig. 6.7 *A* and *B*. Methods of heating tissues by EM fields.

on transfer of electrical energy into heat in the tissue is simply

$$P = GV^2 \tag{8}$$

The tissue-filled capacitor may be represented by the equivalent circuit, shown in Figure 6.8, where the conduction current $I_c = VG$ passing through G is responsible for the tissue heating, and the current $I_d = VB$ flowing through the capacitor C is the displacement current. The current density responsible for the heating is $J = I_c A^{-1}$. Since the electric field strength in the tissue is $E = Vd^{-1}$, we may express the current density as

$$J = \sigma_m E \tag{9}$$

and the power loss in a volume δ^3 of tissue as

$$PA^{-1}d^{-1} = GV^2A^{-1}d^{-1} = \sigma_m E^2$$

$$P = (J\delta^2)(E\delta) = \sigma_m E^2 \delta^3$$

or the power loss per unit volume of tissue as

$$P\delta^{-3} = \sigma_m E^2 \tag{10}$$

The same result may be obtained by considering an elemental cube of

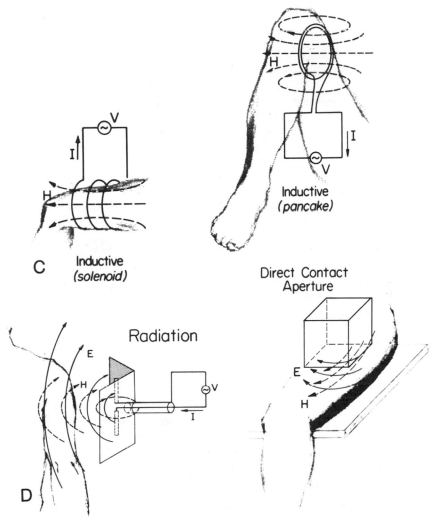

Fig. 6.7 *C* and *D*.

tissue of volume δ^3 within the sample, as shown in Figure 6.8c. The power loss in the cube is simply the product of the current and the impressed voltage, $P = (j\delta^2)(E\delta) = \sigma_m E^2 \delta^3$. The power loss per unit volume is $P\delta^{-3} = \sigma_m E^2$ which is the same as Equation *10*.

The National Council on Radiation Protection and Measurements (NCRP Report No. 67, March 1, 1981) recommends the use of the quantity specific absorption rate (SAR), given in units of watts per kilogram (W/kg) to quantify the rate of energy absorbed per unit mass in tissues exposed to EM fields.

Thus, if we define W as the *SAR*, Equation *10* may be written for any

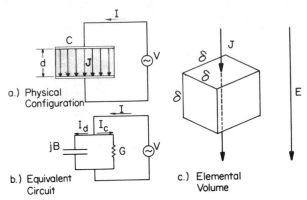

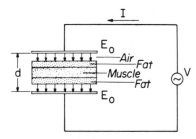

Fig. 6.8. Heating homogeneous tissue with direct-contact, conducting plates.

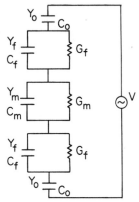

a.) Physical Configuration

Fig. 6.9. Heating multiple layers of tissue with non-contacting capacitor plates.

b.) Equivalent Circuit

tissue with conductivity σ as

$$W = 10^{-3}\rho^{-1}\sigma E^2 \tag{11}$$

where ρ is the density of the tissue in gm/cm^3.

We may consider a more complex geometry of tissue exposed to non-contacting capacitor electrodes as shown in Figure 6.9. In this case, the tissue consists of multiple layers of subcutaneous fat and muscle separated from the metal plates by air gaps. The admittance for this case is

$$Y = [2Y_o^{-1} + 2Y_f^{-1} + Y_m^{-1}]^{-1} \qquad (12)$$

where $Y_{o,f,m}$ are the admittances for the air, fat, and muscle layers, respectively. The total current (displacement and conduction) through the various layers of air and tissue is given by

$$I = YV = Y_o Y_o = Y_f V_f = Y_m V_m \qquad (13)$$

where the V is the applied voltage and $V_{o,f,m}$ are the voltages across the various layers of air and tissue.

From Equations 2 and 3,

$$\epsilon_o E_o = \epsilon_f^* E_f = \epsilon_m^* E_m \qquad (14)$$

where $E_{o,f,m}$ are the electric field strengths in the layers of air and tissue, and $\epsilon_{o,f,m}^*$ are the dielectric constants for these layers. Thus, the electric fields within the tissues will be reduced from that of air, depending on their dielectric constants as follows:

$$E_f = \epsilon_o(\epsilon_f^*)^{-1} E_o \qquad (15)$$

$$E_m = \epsilon_o(\epsilon_m^*)^{-1} E_o \qquad (16)$$

Also, it may be noted that the electric field in each tissue medium is inversely proportional to the dielectric of the medium. This characteristic, which is true for all cases where electric fields or currents are perpendicular to layered tissue boundaries, has important implications in the design and application of shortwave diathermy modalities.

Another important case is the flow of current parallel to tissue boundaries. We may represent this case by placing a muscle-fat tissue between two parallel plate electrodes so that the current flows parallel to the interface between the tissues. The electric fields within the two tissues

$$E_m = E_f = Vd^{-1} \qquad (17)$$

are identical. The current densities are given by

$$J_m = \sigma_m E \qquad (18)$$

and

$$J_f = \sigma_f E \qquad (19)$$

and the SAR in each tissue is

$$W_m = 10^{-3} \rho_m^{-1} \sigma_m E^2 \qquad (20)$$

and

$$W_f = 10^{-3} \rho_f^{-1} \sigma_f E^2 \qquad (21)$$

Thus, for this case, the current density and *SAR* in the layered tissue are directly proportional to the electrical conductivity of the tissue. This has important implications in the design and use of shortwave diathermy modalities.

Although the previous discussion applies to relatively simple plane layer tissue geometries, it introduces some important dosimetric quantities and units that are used for the more complex exposure conditions at frequencies covering both the shortwave and microwave bands. The goal in the use of EM fields for therapeutic heating is to produce electric fields or currents in the region of tissue when the heating is desired, with minimal generation of fields in other regions of tissue. The fields must be maintained at sufficiently high levels to produce an *SAR* that will bring the tissue temperature to the proper level for the desired therapy. In cases where cooling mechanisms such as blood flow are minimal, the required *SAR* will be lower than that needed in other regions where cooling is greater. The *SAR* may be calculated from known field distributions by means of Equation *11*, or it may be measured directly from the rate of temperature rise, which will be discussed later in this chapter.

Electrical Properties of Tissues

In order to understand some of the characteristics of shortwave and microwave interactions with biological material, knowledge of the dielectric properties of biological tissues is necessary. These properties and some important wave parameters which will be discussed later are given in Tables 6.3 and 6.4. The first column lists the properties for frequencies between 1.0 MHz and 10 GHz. The frequencies of 13.65, 27.12, 40.68, 433, 915, 2450, and 5800 MHz are of special interest since they have been allocated for industrial, scientific, and medical (ISM) purposes. The frequencies of 13.65, 27.12, 915, and 2450 MHz are used for diathermy applications in the United States. In Europe, the frequency of 915 MHz is not authorized, but 433 MHz is authorized for ISM purposes. Frequencies below 1 MHz are important for cautery and interstitial heating. The second column in Tables 6.3 and 6.4 lists the corresponding wavelengths in air, and the remaining columns pertain to the wave properties of a tissue group which will be discussed later. Table 6.3 gives data for muscle, skin, or tissues of high water content, while Table 6.4 provides data for fat, bone, and tissues of low water content. Other tissues containing intermediate amounts of water such as brain, lung, bone marrow, etc., will have properties that lie between the tabulated values for the two listed groups. The tables indicate the dielectric properties, the depth of penetration, and the reflection characteristics of various tissues exposed to EM waves as a function of frequency.

The dielectric behaviors of the two groups of biological tissues tabulated in Tables 6.4 and 6.4 have been evaluated thoroughly by Schwan and associates (105–107) and by other researchers including Cook (15–17) and

TABLE 6.3 *Properties of Microwaves in Biological Media*[a]

Muscle, Skin, and Tissues with High Water Content

Frequency (MHz)	Wavelength in air (cm)	Dielectric constant (ε_H)	Conductivity σ_H (S/meter)	Wavelength λ_H (cm)	Depth of penetration (cm)	Reflection coefficient Air-muscle Interface r	Reflection coefficient Air-muscle Interface ϕ	Reflection coefficient Muscle-fat Interface r	Reflection coefficient Muscle-fat Interface ϕ
1	30,000	2,000	0.400	436	91.3	0.982	+170		
10	3,000	160	0.625	110	21.6	0.956	+178		
27.12	1,106	113	0.602	68.1	14.3	0.925	+177	0.652	−11.13
40.68	738	97.3	0.680	51.3	11.2	0.913	+176	0.651	−10.21
100	300	71.7	0.885	27	6.66	0.881	+175	0.650	−7.96
200	150	56.5	1.00	16.6	4.79	0.844	+175	0.612	−8.06
300	100	54	1.15	11.9	3.89	0.825	+175	0.592	−8.14
433	69.3	53	1.18	8.76	3.57	0.803	+175	0.562	−7.06
750	40	52	1.25	5.34	3.18	0.779	+176	0.532	−5.69
915	32.8	51	1.28	4.46	3.04	0.772	+177	0.519	−4.32
1500	20	49	1.56	2.81	2.42	0.761	+177	0.506	−3.66
2450	12.2	47	2.17	1.76	1.70	0.754	+177	0.500	−3.88
3000	10	46	2.27	1.45	1.61	0.751	+178	0.495	−3.20
5000	6	44	4.55	0.89	0.788	0.749	+177	0.502	−4.95
5800	5.17	43.3	4.93	0.775	0.720	0.746	+177	0.502	−4.29
8000	3.75	40	8.33	0.578	0.413	0.744	+176	0.513	−6.65
10,000	3	39.9	10.00	0.464	0.343	0.743	+176	0.518	−5.95

[a] After Johnson and Guy (54).

TABLE 6.4 Properties of Microwaves in Biological Media[a]

Fat, Bone, and Tissues with Low Water Content

Frequency (MHz)	Wavelength in air (cm)	Dielectric constant (ϵ_L)	Conductivity σ_L (mS/m)	Wavelength λ_L (cm)	Depth of penetration (cm)	Air-fat Interface r	Air-fat Interface φ	Fat-muscle Interface r	Fat-muscle Interface φ
1	30,000								
10	3,000								
27.12	1,106	20	10.9 — 43.2	241	159	0.660	+174	0.651	+169
40.68	738	14.6	12.6 — 52.8	187	118	0.617	+173	0.652	+170
100	300	7.45	19.1 — 75.9	106	60.4	0.511	+168	0.650	+172
200	150	5.95	25.8 — 94.2	59.7	39.2	0.458	+168	0.612	+172
300	100	5.7	31.6 — 107	41	32.1	0.438	+169	0.592	+172
433	69.3	5.6	37.9 — 118	28.8	26.2	0.427	+170	0.562	+173
750	40	5.6	49.8 — 138	16.8	23	0.415	+173	0.532	+174
915	32.8	5.6	55.6 — 147	13.7	17.7	0.417	+173	0.519	+176
1500	20	5.6	70.8 — 171	8.41	13.9	0.412	+174	0.506	+176
2450	12.2	5.5	96.4 — 213	5.21	11.2	0.406	+176	0.500	+176
3000	10	5.5	110 — 234	4.25	9.74	0.406	+176	0.495	+177
5000	6	5.5	162 — 309	2.63	6.67	0.393	+176	0.502	+175
5800	5.17	5.05	186 — 338	2.29	5.24	0.388	+176	0.502	+176
8000	3.75	4.7	255 — 431	1.73	4.61	0.371	+176	0.513	+173
10000	3	4.5	324 — 549	1.41	3.39	0.363	+175	0.518	+174

[a] After Johnson and Guy (54).

Cole and Cole (14). The interaction of EM fields with biological tissues is related to these dielectric characteristics. The tissues are composed of cells encapsulated by thin membranes containing an intracellular fluid composed of various salt ions, polar protein molecules, and polar water molecules. The extracellular fluid has similar concentrations of ions and polar molecules, though some of the elements are different.

The action of EM fields on the tissues produces two types of effects that control the dielectric behavior. One is the oscillation of the free charges or ions, while the other is the rotation of dipole molecules at the frequency of the applied electromagnetic fields. The first gives rise to conduction currents with an associated energy loss due to the electrical resistance of the medium; the other affects the displacement current through the medium, with an associated dielectric loss due to viscosity. These effects control the behavior of the complex dielectric constant $\epsilon^*/\epsilon_o = \epsilon' - j\epsilon''$ where $\epsilon'' = \sigma\omega^{-1}\epsilon_o^{-1}$ is called the loss factor of the medium. The effective conductivity σ accounts for both the conduction current and the dielectric losses of the medium. The ratio of conduction to displacement current is called the loss tangent, $\tan \delta = \epsilon''\epsilon'^{-1}$. The complex dielectric constant ϵ^* is dispersive (varies with frequency) due to the various relaxation processes associated with polarization phenomena. This may be illustrated by noting the dielectric properties given in Tables 6.3 and 6.4. The decrease in dielectric constant ϵ_m for tissues of high water content with increasing frequency is due to interfacial polarization across the cell membranes. The cell membranes, with a capacitance of approximately $1\ \mu F \cdot cm^{-2}$, act as insulating layers at low frequencies so that EM-field-induced currents are forced to flow around the membranes through the extracellular medium between the cells. The smaller cross-sectional pathways for the current result in a lower bulk conductivity of the tissues. At sufficiently low frequencies, the charging time constant is small enough to completely charge and discharge the membrane during a single cycle, resulting in a high tissue capacitance and therefore, a high dielectric constant. When the frequency is increased, the capacitive susceptance of the cell increases, resulting in increasing currents in the intracellular medium with a resulting increase in total conductivity of the tissue. The increase in frequency will also prevent the cell walls from becoming totally charged during a complete cycle, resulting in a decrease in ϵ'. At a frequency of approximately 100 MHz, the cell membrane capacitive susceptance becomes sufficiently high that the cells can be assumed to be short-circuited. In the frequency range of 100 MHz to 1 GHz, the ion content of the electrolyte medium has no effect on the dispersion of the dielectric constant so the values of ϵ_m and σ_m are relatively independent of frequency. Schwan (105, 109) has suggested, however, that suspended protein molecules with lower dielectric constants act as "dielectric cavities" in the electrolyte, thereby lowering the dielectric constant of the tissue. He attributes the slight dispersion of ϵ_m to the variation of the effective dielectric constant of

TABLE 6.5. *Temperature Coefficient of Dielectric Constant and Specific Resistance of Body Tissues in Percent per Degree Celsius*[a]

	50 MHz	200 MHz	1000 MHz
a) $100 \dfrac{\Delta\epsilon}{\epsilon}$ °C			
Tissues with high H_2O content	0.5	0.2	−0.4
Fatty tissue		1.3	1.1
0.9 percent NaCl	−0.4	−0.4	−0.4
b) $100 \dfrac{\Delta\rho}{\rho}$ °C			
Tissues with high H_2O content	−2	−1.8	−1.3
Fatty tissue	−(1.7−4.3)	−4.9	−4.2
0.9 percent NaCl	−2.0	−1.7	−1.3

[a] Values at 50 MHz from Osswald, at 200 MHz and 1000 MHz from Schwan and Li. The temperature dependence of resistance is comparable with that of saline solutions for all tissues with high water content. The dependence of the dielectric constant approaches that of saline solutions only at very high frequencies. From Schwan (110).

the protein molecules with frequency. The final decline of ϵ_m and increase of σ_m at frequencies above 1 GHz can be attributed to the polar properties of water molecules which have a relaxation frequency, frequency of maximum σ_m, near 22 GHz.

The dielectric behavior of tissues with low water content is quantitatively similar to tissues with high water content, but the values of the dielectric constant ϵ_f and conductivity σ_f are an order of magnitude lower and are not quantitatively understood as well. This is because the ratio of free to various types of bound water is not known. There is also a large variation in tissues of low water content. Since water has a high dielectric constant and conductivity, its electrical properties will change significantly with small changes in water content.

The values of $\epsilon_{m,f}$ and $\sigma_{m,f}$ also vary with temperature. This variation, which was demonstrated by Schwan (110), is tabulated in Table 6.5.

The dielectric properties of the tissues play an important part in determining the distribution of currents and associated heating patterns resulting from the application of EM fields. They also determine the reflected and transmitted power at interfaces between different tissue media and the amount of total power a given biological specimen will absorb when exposed to EM radiation.

Heating Characteristics

In order to evaluate and understand the therapeutic effectiveness of an applied dose of diathermy energy, one must know the relationship between the rate of absorbed energy or SAR, the tissue cooling mechanisms, and the temperature. The energy equation for the time rate of change of temperature (°C/s) per unit mass of subcutaneous tissue heated with diathermy is

$$\frac{d(\Delta T)}{dt} = \frac{0.239 \times 10^{-3}}{c} [W_a + W_m - W_c - W_b] \qquad (22)$$

where W_a is the SAR given in Equation 11, W_m is the metabolic heating rate, W_c is the power dissipated by thermal conduction, and W_b is the power dissipated by blood flow, all expressed in W/kg; c is the specific heat of the tissue in kcal/kg·°C and $\Delta T = T - T_0$ is the difference between the tissue temperature T and the initial tissue temperature T_0 prior to treatment.

Within the safe therapeutic temperature range, the metabolic heating rate may be expressed as

$$W_m = W_o(1.1)^{\Delta T} \qquad (23)$$

where W_0 is the initial metabolic heating rate (10).

The thermal conduction rate may be expressed as

$$W_c = \frac{k_c}{\rho} \nabla^2 T \qquad (24)$$

where k_c is the thermal conductivity of the tissue in mW/cm·°C and ∇ is the gradient operator.

If it is assumed that blood enters the tissue at arterial temperature T_a and leaves at tissue temperature T, the heat removed by blood flow is

$$W_b = k_2 m c_b \rho_b \, \Delta T' \qquad (25)$$

where $\Delta T' = T - T_a$, c_b is the specific heat of blood, ρ_b is the density of blood in gm/cm³, m is the blood flow rate n ml/100 gm·min, and the constant $k_2 = 0.698$.

Prior to the time the diathermy is applied, it is assumed that a steady-state condition exists where $W_a = T = d(\Delta T)/dt = 0$, requiring

$$W_m - W_c - W_b = 0 \qquad (26)$$

According to the typical values of the physical and thermal properties of tissues given in Table 6.6 (9, 73, 86, 91), the equilibrium values of the terms in Equation 26 under normal conditions are on the order of 1 W/kg for typical resting muscle. When a therapeutic level of EM power, $50 < W_a < 170$ W/kg, is absorbed, ΔT will increase as shown in Figure 6.10 with an initial linear transient period typically lasting about 3 minutes, where by Equation 22:

$$\frac{d(\Delta T)}{dt} \approx \frac{0.239 \times 10^{-3}}{c} W_a \qquad (27)$$

This period is followed by a non-linear transient period usually lasting another 7 to 10 min, where ΔT becomes sufficiently large that blood flow

TABLE 6.6 Thermal and Physical Properties of Human Tissues[a]

Tissue	Subscript	Specific Heat c(kcal/kg·°C)	Density ρ(gm/cm³)	Metabolic rate W_0 (W/kg)	Blood flow rate m(ml/100 gm·min)	Thermal conductivity k_c (mW/cm·°C)
Skeletal muscle (excised)	m		1.07			4.4
Skeletal muscle (living)	m	0.83		0.7	2.7	6.42
Fat	f	0.54	0.937			2.1
Bone (cortical)	bc	0.3	1.79			14.6
Bone (spongy)	bs	0.71	1.25			
Blood	bl	0.93	1.06			5.06
Heart muscle	m			33	84	
Brain (excised)	br			11	54	5.0
Brain (living)	br			20	420	8.05
Kidney	k					
Liver	l			6.7	57.7	
Skin (excised)	s					2.5
Skin (living)	s			1	12.8	4.42
Whole body				1.3	8.6	

[a] From Guy et al. (38).

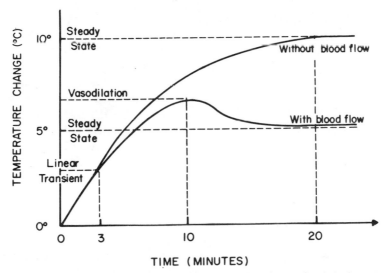

Fig. 6.10. Schematic representation of transient and steady-state temperatures for a typical tissue under diathermy exposure (38).

and thermal conduction become important in dissipating the applied energy (Figure 6.10). In tissues with negligible or insufficient blood flow, the temperature will monotonically approach a steady-state value dictated by the magnitude of W_a as shown on the upper curve, where equilibrium is reached when $W_a = W_c$. For vasculated tissues, however, blood flow plays a significant part in heat dissipation, limiting the slope of the $d(\Delta T)/dt$ curve. In addition, for vasculated tissues, a marked increase in blood flow will occur due to vasodilatation when the temperature passes through the range 42 to 44°C. As a result, the temperature will drop and approach a steady-state value at a somewhat lower level, as shown in the figure, when $W_a = W_c + W_b$. For proper and safe therapeutic action, it is necessary to raise the temperature sufficiently in the deeper vasculated tissue to trigger the vasodilation without exceeding safe levels in the poorly vasculated intervening subcutaneous fat layer. Clinical experience has shown that when normal vasculated tissue is exposed to a diathermy source, pain will be noted by the patient before any tissue damage can occur. In fact, the pain may be used as a guide to indicate that the tissue temperature has reached the required 43 to 45°C for dilatation and associated therapeutic benefits.

The SAR W_a must be sufficiently high so that the therapeutic level of temperature can be maintained over the major portion of the treatment period. If too little power is applied, the period of elevated temperature will be too short for any benefits. If too high a level is applied, the temperature can overshoot the safe level before the vasodilatation can take effect. The pain sensors are a reliable and sensitive means for detecting this temperature range, however, and if the applied power level is set so that only mild pain or discomfort are first experienced by the patient, the vasodilatation will be sufficient to limit or even lower the temperature to a level that is both tolerable and therapeutically effective. If the effective temperature is reached at the surface, it is felt as a mild burning sensation. On the other hand, if it is reached in the deeper tissues, it is felt as a dull aching type of pain. Hardy (41) has shown that the intensity of absorbed non-penetrating radiation at the threshold of pain in the skin is 0.045 gm cal/s$\cdot$cm^2, or 188 mW/cm^2. Various methods of achieving therapeutic levels of tissue heating by EM fields were briefly reviewed at the beginning of this chapter. The two major methods of EM heating, shortwave and microwave diathermy, are discussed in the following sections.

Shortwave Applicators

The earliest diathermy equipment consisted of HF generator, from which currents were applied directly to the tissues by contacting electrodes. As a result of uneven or poor contact, one of the greatest hazards was the production of burns, localized at the electrode-tissue interface. As the operating frequency of diathermy equipment increased, the electrodes were redesigned so that they did not have to make direct contact with the tissues, since displacement currents between the electrode plates and the anatomical surfaces were sufficient to couple energy to the tissue. Although capacitor electrode arrangements such as those shown in Figure 6.11 are still used to

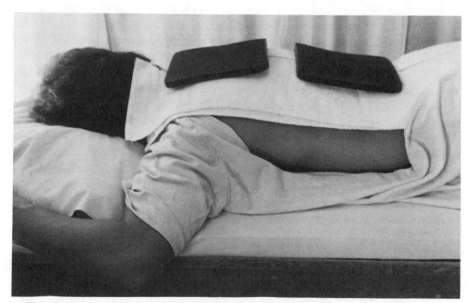

Fig. 6.11. Shortwave diathermy application with capacitor pads to back, with spacing between skin and electrodes provided by layers of terry cloth (38).

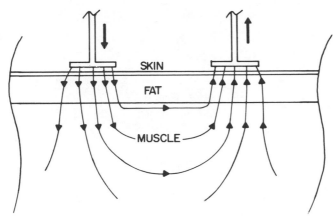

Fig. 6.12. Cross-sectional sketch showing fields in layered tissue exposed to shortwave diathermy capacitor-type electrodes.

treat patients with present day 13.65 and 27.33 MHz diathermy equipment, there are some fundamental problems. Figure 6.12 illustrates how induced conduction currents in the tissue produce much greater power absorption in the subcutaneous fat than in the skin and muscle tissue, and how the divergence of the current tends to concentrate the power absorption in the superficial tissue adjacent to the electrodes. For example, if we neglect the spreading of the fields and note that the electric fields are predominantly normal to the tissue interfaces, the relationship between the fields in the air E_0 and those in the subcutaneous fat E_f and muscle E_m are given in Equation 14.

Evaluation of the SAR W_f and W_m in the fat and muscle, using the physical parameters from Table 6.3 and 6.4 gives

$$W_f = \frac{\sigma_f}{\rho_f} \frac{\epsilon_0^2 E_0^2}{|\epsilon_f^*|^2} \times 10^{-3} = 3.50 \times 10^{-8} E_0^2 \tag{28}$$

$$W_m = \frac{\sigma_m}{\rho_m} \frac{\epsilon_0^2 E_0^2}{|\epsilon_m^*|^2} \times 10^{-3} = 3.68 \times 10^{-9} E_0^2 \tag{29}$$

The results show an order-of-magnitude greater heating in subcutaneous fat than in muscle or skin. Additional selective heating occurs in the fat due to spreading of the fields as a function of distance from the electrodes. This, along with the lower specific heat and density in fat as indicated in Table 6.6, result in a rate of heating more than 17 times greater in fat than in muscle. In addition, the blood cooling rate is significantly less in fat, so the final steady-state temperature would be considerably higher than in muscle.

Other types of shortwave diathermy applicators are induction coil arrangements (Figures 6.13 and 6.14) which induce circular eddy currents in the tissues by magnetic induction. Figure 6.13 shows a large coil of insulated

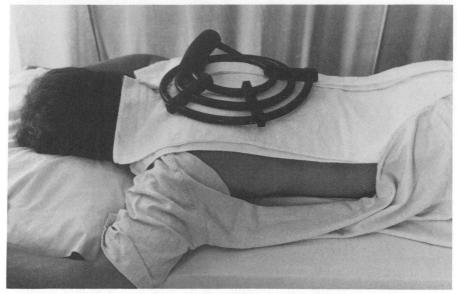

Fig. 6.13. Shortwave diathermy application to back with induction coil ('pancake' coil). Spacing between coil and skin provided by layers of terry cloth (38).

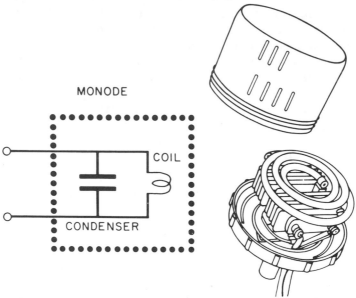

Fig. 6.14. Compact-type induction coil with wiring arrangement (courtesy of Siemens-Reiniger Werke AG).

cable separated from the patient by toweling. The applicator shown in Figure 6.14, called a "monode" by the manufacturer, is a more compact coil and capacitor combination that may be spaced at various distances from the patient by an adjustable supporting arm (not shown). A cross-sectional

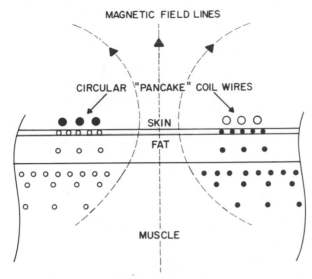

Fig. 6.15. Cross-sectional sketch showing magnetically induced current in tissue exposed to shortwave diathermy pancake coil. *Dark dots* indicate current density vectors directed out of the paper; *open circles* indicate vectors directed into the paper.

view of the induced currents (Figure 6.15) illustrates the superiority of the inductive applicator over the electrode type. For this case, the induced electric fields are parallel to the tissue interfaces, and therefore are not greatly modified by the tissue boundaries, as illustrated by Equations *20* and *21*. Ideally, according to the equations, the current density and heating will be higher in the muscle tissue where the conductivity is maximum, as shown schematically in Figure 6.15.

Under certain conditions where the diameter and spacing of the coil turns are excessive, or when the coil is placed too close to the tissue, more energy may be coupled to the subcutaneous fat than to the deeper vasculated tissues. This is caused by the sharp increase in magnetic field strength near the coils and the high electric field between the coil turns. This latter coupling is illustrated in Figure 6.16.

A typical circuit for shortwave diathermy equipment is shown in simplified schematic form in Figure 6.17. The tank circuit of a high-power, HF generator tuned near 27.12 MHz is coupled to a second parallel resonant circuit with variable tuning. Depending on the method of application, the circuit may be coupled to a pair of capacitor electrodes, an inductive coil, or an inductive coil and capacitor combination, as shown in Figures 6.11, 6.13, and 6.14. Under different clinical conditions, the capacitance between the electrodes and the patient will vary, requiring adjustments in generator tuning. This is generally done automatically, for example, in the manner shown in Figure 6.17. A motor M is used to continually rotate the tuning

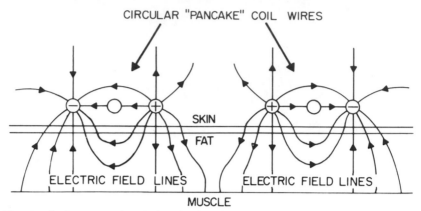

Fig. 6.16. Cross-sectional sketch showing induced fields in tissue due to inter-coil potentials of shortwave diathermy pancake coil (38).

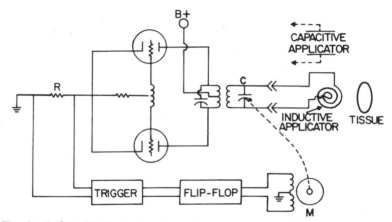

Fig. 6.17. Simplified circuit schematic of shortwave diathermy generator.

capacitor C. As the circuit is tuned through resonance, the change in the plate current sensed by the voltage across resistor R triggers a flip-flop circuit to reverse the direction of rotation of the tuning motor so that the capacitor is again driven through resonance. The hunting action of the tuning capacitor across resonance insures that the circuit stays tuned under varying clinical conditions. A variable-output power control is usually provided, while a timer controls the exposure time of the patient. It is almost impossible, however, for the physician to determine the amount of energy a patient is absorbing from various applicators for different spacings and various power settings.

A great deal of insight and some quantitative information concerning absorbed energy can be gained through a simple theoretical analysis of the coupling characteristics of the applicator to the patient. Since inductive

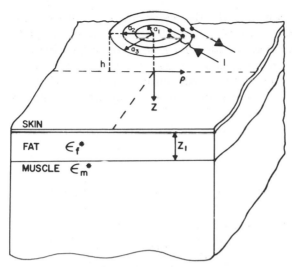

Fig. 6.18. Geometry and coordinates for a skin-fat muscle tissue geometry exposed to a flat pancake diathermy induction coil.

coupling appears most effective, we will examine the case of a planar skin-fat-muscle tissue geometry exposed to a flat pancake coil with coordinates and parameters as defined in Figure 6.18. Since the size of the coil is small compared to the 11-meter wavelength, the mathematics can be greatly simplified by approximating the actual spiral coil with perfect concentric loops connected in series and by assuming quasi-stationary field conditions. The well-known vector potential and magnetic field expressions for a single closed loop (119) may be used to express the vector potential A and magnetic field component H_z of the coil:

$$A_\phi = \frac{\mu I}{\pi (\rho)^{1/2}} \sum_{i=1}^{n} \frac{(a_i)^{1/2}}{k_i} \left[(1 - \frac{1}{2} k_i^2) K(k_i) - E(k_i) \right] \qquad (30)$$

$$H_z = \frac{I}{4\pi(\rho)^{1/2}} \sum_{i=1}^{n} \frac{k_i}{(a_i)^{1/2}} \left[K(k_i) + \frac{a_i^2 - \rho^2 - (z+h)^2}{(a_i - \rho)^2 + (z+h)^2} E(k_i) \right] \qquad (31)$$

where

$$k_i^2 = \frac{4\rho a_i}{(\rho + a_i)^2 + (z+h)^2} \qquad (32)$$

and where $K(k_i)$ and $E(k_i)$ are elliptical integrals of the first and second kind, a_i is the radius of the ith loop, n is the number of loops, I is the loop current, μ is the permeability of free space, and ρ and z are the cylindrical coordinates of the point of observation. The magnetically induced electric field component E may be expressed as $E = j\omega A$, which at shortwave diathermy frequencies can be assumed to penetrate tissues without significant perturbation since the tissues are nearly transparent to the near-field inductive components of the coil. There will also be significant radial and axial components of electric field $\bar{E} = -\nabla\phi$ originating from the potential, due to inter-turn voltages in the coil. Since the fields are maximum in the radial direction between the concentric turns, we will make the first order approximation that each turn i is at a constant potential V_i, but that the voltage between turns i and $i - 1$ is

$$V_i - V_{i-1} = 2\pi f L_i I \tag{33}$$

where

$$L_i = \mu \sum_{i=1}^{n} (a_i + a_j - a_0)\left(1 - \frac{k_{ij}}{2}\right)[K(k_{ij}) - E(k_{ij})] \tag{34}$$

is the inductance of the ith turn

$$k_{ij}^2 = \frac{4a_i(a_j - a_0)}{(a_i + a_j - a_0)^2} \tag{35}$$

and a_0 is the radius of the coil conductor.

The potential of the nth turn V_n is assumed to be

$$V_n = V/2 \tag{36}$$

where

$$V = 2\pi f l \sum_{i=1}^{n} L_i \tag{37}$$

and the inductance of the coil is

$$L = \sum_{i=1}^{n} L_i \tag{38}$$

A rigorous solution of the potential field ϕ in the tissues would require proper accounting for the images of the coil due to tissue interfaces. Since both the fat and the muscle have high dielectric constants, however, the potential distributions above the tissues may be approximated by considering a single perfect image along with the actual coil (119), giving

$$\phi = \sum_{n=1}^{n} A_i \left\{ \frac{K(k_i +)}{[(\rho + a_i)^2 + (z + h)^2]^{1/2}} - \frac{K(k_i -)}{[(\rho + a_i)^2 + (z - h)^2]^{1/2}} \right\} \tag{39}$$

where

$$k_i^2 + = \frac{4\rho a_i}{(\rho + a_i)^2 + (z + h)^2} \tag{40}$$

$$k_i^2 - = \frac{4\rho a_i}{(\rho + a_i)^2 + (z - h)^2} \tag{41}$$

and the values of A_i are found by evaluating the set of simultaneous equations obtained when 39 is evaluated at $z - h$ and $\rho = a_i, a_2, \ldots, a_n$ for the known voltages $V_1, V_2, \ldots, V_n$.

The field normal to the surface of the tissue may be evaluated from the gradient of the potential distribution at $z = 0$. Then, since it was shown previously that the major heating due to a field perpendicular to the tissue interface occurs in the subcutaneous fat, we obtain

$$E_z = \frac{1}{|\epsilon_{f^*}|} \sum_{i=1}^{n} A_i \left\{ \frac{2h}{[(\rho + a_i)^2 + h^2]^{3/2}} \left[K(k_i) - \frac{4\rho a_i}{(\rho - a_i)^2 + h^2} B(k_i) \right] \right\} \quad (42)$$

in the fat where

$$B(k_i) = \frac{E(k_i)}{k_i^2} - \frac{1 - k_i^2}{k_i^2} K(k_i) \quad (43)$$

and k_i is simply k_i^+ evaluated at $z = 0$.

If we ignore the field spreading and other quasi-static field components because of the close proximity of the fat-muscle interface, we may obtain an estimate of the absorbed power in the fat

$$W_a = \frac{\sigma_f}{\rho_f} [E_z^2 + E_\phi^2] \times 10^{-3} \quad (44)$$

due to both the induction field (E_ϕ) and the significant component (E_z) of the quasi-static field.

When evaluating Equation 44, one should keep in mind that the most desirable heating or absorption patterns for therapeutic purposes correspond to minimum relative heating in the fat with maximum relative heating and depth of penetration into the muscle. Figure 6.19 illustrates the calculated results for tissues exposed to a flat coil with the same wire thickness and radii of turns as the commercial applicator (Figure 6.14). Three concentric loops provide the closest approximation for this case. With such few turns, it is more convenient to assume that the total applied voltage calculated from the coil current and inductance was distributed equally among the center, inner, and outer loops. A coil current of 1 A, a fat thickness of $z_1 = 2$ cm, and a spacing of 3 cm between the applicator coil and the surface of the fat are assumed. The results show that the coil induces a toroidal heating pattern with a maximum SAR of 0.665 W/kg in the muscle at a radial distance $\rho = 5.5$ cm from the coil axis with a penetration depth (depth where heating drops by a factor of e^{-2} from the maximum) into the muscle of about 4 cm. The maximum heating in the fat which occurs on axis is approximately one-third of that in the muscle. A second, lower peak occurs in the fat at $\rho = 5.8$ cm. While the former is due to coupling from the electric

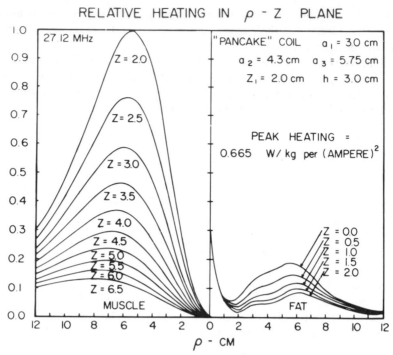

Fig. 6.19. Calculated SAR in plane geometry and muscle tissue layers exposed to shortwave diathermy induction coil (38).

field between the loops, the latter is due to the electric field induced by magnetic coupling. The value of heating for other values of coil current may be obtained by multiplying the results given in the figure by the square of the coil current. The value of coil current varies according to the generator power output setting, the spacing between the coil and the patient, and the geometry of the exposed tissue. Typical values for the five power settings available from the generator (Siemens Ultratherm 608) which powered the applicators chosen are listed in Table 6.7. These were determined by comparing magnetic fields measured with a small shielded loop along the axis of the applicator and calculating the equivalent current from Equation 31 for a theoretical coil which would produce the same field. It is convenient to reduce Equation 31 to

$$H_z = \frac{I}{2} \sum_{i=1}^{n} \frac{a_i^2}{(a_i^2 + z^2)^{3/2}} \tag{45}$$

for this case. Figure 6.20 illustrates the heating patterns calculated for coils spaced 1.5 cm from the tissues surface for a 1-cm thick fat layer. The peak heating for this case is greater by more than a factor of four, the relative fat

TABLE 6.7. *Measured Magnetic Fields (Surface of Exposed Subject) and Calculated Equivalent Induction Coil Current as a Function of Power Setting for Siemens Ultratherm 608 Shortwave Diathermy Equipment*[a]

Power setting	Coil to subject spacing (cm)	Unloaded coil		Exposing human thigh	
		1 (A)	H_z (A/m)	I (A)	H_z (A/m)
1	5.0	3.40	31.5		
2	5.0	5.15	47.5		
3	3.0	7.12	128	5.44	97.8
	5.0	7.12	65.7		
4	5.0	8.85	81.7		
5	1.5	9.87	291	7.39	218
	2.0	9.87	278		
	3.0	9.87	182	7.54	139
	3.5	9.87	152	8.22	127
	4.0	9.87	126		
	5.0	9.87	91.0		

[a] Coil inductance: 0.8 μH (measured), 0.83 μH (theory). From Guy *et al.* (38).

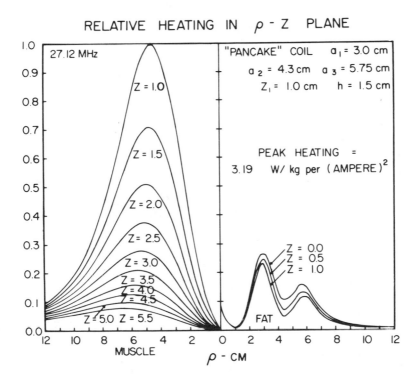

Fig. 6.20. Calculated SAR in plane geometry fat and muscle tissue layers exposed to shortwave diathermy induction coil (38).

heating is increased slightly, the depth of penetration is decreased to approximately 3 cm, and the radius for maximum absorption in the muscle is decreased by 1 cm. Lehmann *et al.* (74) exposed large specimens of thighs from freshly slaughtered pigs to experimentally determine the heating patterns of the commercial applicator, with the results shown in Figure 6.21. The specimens were large compared to the applicator, and contained 2 cm of subcutaneous fat. The applicator coils were placed 3 cm from the specimen, and power (position 3 setting) was applied for 5 minutes. The shapes of the measured temperature curves in the muscle correspond closely to the relative heating predicted theoretically. The absolute values cannot be compared, however, since the actual current was unknown, and exposure time was too long during the experiment for the linear transient relationship to hold. The results of a later experiment conducted by Lehmann *et al.* (75) on live human tissue are shown in Figure 6.22, where the temperature in the exposed tissue in the region of maximum absorption was measured as a function of time. It should be noted, however, that the temperatures were measured with implanted thermistors during the period of exposure. Miniature thermistors were used, with small-diameter high-resistance leads

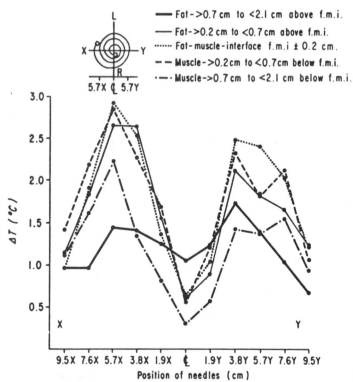

Fig. 6.21. Recording of temperature increase produced by the shortwave inductive applicator applied to pig thigh with $z_1 = 2$ and $h = 3$ (74).

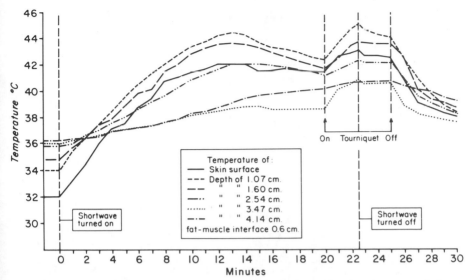

Fig. 6.22. Recording of temperature increase produced by the shortwave inductive applicator applied to human thigh with $z_1 = 0.6$ and $h = 3.5$ (79).

TABLE 6.8. *Comparison of Measurerd and Theoretical Shortwave Power Absorption and Calculated Blood Flow Rate in Human Thigh Muscle[a]*

Distance (cm) z	1.07	1.60	2.54	3.47	4.14
Calculated W_a	61	42.5	21.9	14.9	11
Measured W_a	70	50	24	10	6
Blood flow heat dissipation W_b	81	81	25.4		
Estimated blood flow rate m	13.7	13.7	4.3		

[a] $z_1 = 0.6$ cm, $h = 3.5$ cm, and $I = 8.22$ A. From Guy *et al.* (38).

placed perpendicular to the circulating eddy currents. Although recent studies (54, 60) have shown that serious artifacts can result from the use of metallic probes in the presence of EM fields, the absence of any appreciable artifact was verified by comparing temperatures measured in the field by thermistors with those measured by alcohol thermometers. Extreme care was exercised to maintain artifact-free measurements (74). Maximum power available from the shortwave equipment (position 5, $I = 8.22$ A) and a spacing between coil and tissue of 3.5 cm were used. This also corresponded to a tolerable dose where only mild pain was experienced by the patient after 12 minutes of exposure. The initial transient rise for each temperature curve was used to obtain the SAR from Equation *11* at each point of measurement and was compared with the theoretical calculations, with the results shown in Table 6.8. The skin absorption is not compared with theoretical calculations since the temperature is much more dependent on uncontrollable surface conditions. The complete theoretical curves are shown in Figure 6.23. After a 20-minute exposure to the shortwave appli-

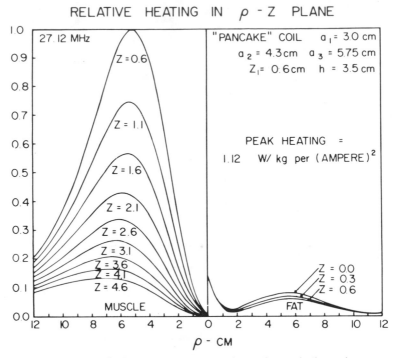

Fig. 6.23. Calculated SAR in plane geometry fat and muscle tissue layers exposed to a shortwave diathermy induction coil (38).

cator, a tourniquet was inflated to obstruct arterial blood flow. After 2.5 minutes, the power was turned off and the blood flow was later restored. The curve for the temperature approximately 0.5 cm below the fat-muscle interface indicates a maximum initial linear increase of nearly 1.1°C/min. This corresponds to a calculated absorbed power of $W_a = 70$ W/kg. After about 12 minutes, when the tissue temperature reached 44°C, corresponding to the point of impending discomfort by the patient, there was a marked change in $d(\Delta T)/dt$ to a negative 0.3°C/min, or an estimated 17 W/kg more heat dissipation needed to maintain a steady-state condition. This necessarily implies by Equation 22 that the blood cooling rate W_b has increased substantially due to an increase in the blood flow rate m. When the arterial blood flow was occluded, $d(\Delta T)/dt$ again changed sharply and became a positive 1.1°C/min, indicating the 70 W/kg of absorbed shortwave power. The results imply that a total heat dissipation of 87 W/kg was provided by blood cooling. If one assumes that arterial blood arrives at the tissue site at core temperature (approximately 6.0°C below local tissue temperature), we may estimate a flow rate by equation 25 of approximately 18.23 ml per 100 gm·min, which is substantially greater than the initial value estimated from Table 6.6. The increase in temperature after occlusion at a depth of 3.47 cm is believed to be due to a transient displacement of heated blood to that particular site by the occlusion process. According to the results, there is sufficient blood cooling reserve under the particular conditions to maintain a constant tissue temperature below 44°C, even with an increase of 10 to 20 percent in applied power. The slow rate of cooling after the applied power is removed indicates the much stronger role of blood flow cooling over that of conduction.

One of the recommended methods of using the inductive shortwave applicator is to place the cover (1.5 cm from coils) directly against the patient with an intervening 0.3-cm-thick terry cloth spacer. The theoretical heating patterns for a case similar to this are given in Figure 6.20; and the measured temperature changes in the human thigh exposed at the same power setting (position 5, $I = 7.39\ A$) with a 1-cm fat thickness are shown in Figure 6.24. The theoretical curves for the $h = 1.5$ cm case can be used for comparison with $h = 1.8$ cm measurements, provided that 0.3 cm is added to the desired value of z. These results clearly show (Table 6.9) the

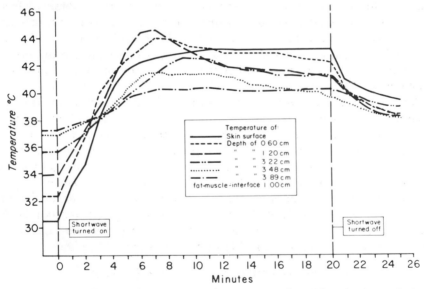

Fig. 6.24. Recording of temperature increase produced by shortwave inductive applicator applied to human thigh with $z_1 = 1.0$ and h = 1.8 (79).

TABLE 6.9. *Comparison of Measured and Theoretical Shortwave Power Absorption in Human Thigh Tissue*[a]

	Fat		Muscle		
Distance (cm) z	0.6	1.2	3.22	3.48	3.89
Calculated W_a (W/kg)	32.6	126	35	27.2	23.5
Measured W_a (W/kg)	99	102	44	26	20

[a] $z_1 = 1.0$ cm, h = 1.8 cm, and I = 7.54 A. From Guy *et al.* (38).

increased absorbed power due to the closer proximity of the coil to the tissue. The results again indicate a triggering of blood flow when the muscle temperature rises above 44°C, which is followed by a $d(\Delta T)/dt = 0.6°C/$ min at a depth of 1.2 cm. In this case, however, the transition took place after only 6 minutes of exposure, coincident with pain, when the temperature exceeded the threshold level. For this reason, the application had to be terminated prematurely with approximately half the subjects tested under these conditions. From the energy balance Equations 22 and from 25, the blood cooling rate was estimated to be 131 W/kg, which would require a flow rate of 27.4 ml/100 gm. min or more. We may note in the first case with the $h = 3$ cm spacing, the deeper muscle tissue reached a higher temperature than the skin surface; whereas, in this latter case, the reverse was true. It appears that the insulating characteristics of terry cloth may have been responsible for preventing skin cooling. The higher heating in subcutaneous fat measured than theoretically predicted can be due to a) errors in measurement resulting from a high thermal gradient near the fat-muscle interface, b) a higher electrical conductivity in living fat than obtained from measurements on dead tissue upon which the theory is based, or c) inaccuracies due to the approximations used in the theoretical equations. We may conclude from the previous study that a) inductive shortwave diathermy applicators are effective in elevating the temperature of deep tissue while maintaining cooler surface tissues; b) the shortwave technique is capable of producing 70 to 100 W/kg of power absorption in the musculature, thereby triggering vigorous blood flow; and c) the blood flow is more than adequate to maintain safe steady-state temperatures within the therapeutic range at or below the pain tolerance level. One of the major disadvantages of the inductive shortwave applicator is the non-uniformity of the toroidal heating pattern, which is awkward to use for treating a small area of tissue. The use of a magnetic loop applicator has gained in popularity, however, in treating deep cancers in the trunk of the body. When such a loop surrounds the trunk, the SAR and induced current at the periphery of the high water content tissues are maximum, and are zero at the axis of the body.

Microwave Applicators and SAR Patterns

When microwave diathermy was first introduced in 1946, there was great hope that it would provide significantly improved heating patterns over those of shortwave diathermy. The shorter wavelength provided the capabilities to direct and focus the power and to couple it to the patient by direct radiation from a small, compact applicator. This was originally believed to be a distinct improvement over the quasi-static and induction field coupling provided by cumbersome capacitor and coil-type applicators. The cross-sectional area of the directed power could be made smaller and used to provide much more flexibility in controlling the size of the area treated.

PLANER TISSUE MODELS EXPOSED TO RADIATION FIELDS

Microwave diathermy had been used for a considerable number of years before any quantitative evaluation was made of the modality. The initial engineering work was done by Schwan (105, 106, 110), who measured the dielectric properties of human tissues over a wide frequency range (from audio through microwave frequencies) from which much of the data in Tables 6.3 and 6.4 were derived. Using these results, Schwan theoretically demonstrated the dependence of relative heating in the tissue on the thickness of the skin, on the thickness of the subcutaneous fat, and on the frequency of a plane wave normally incident at the surface. This can be illustrated by evaluating the expression for absorbed power in each tissue layer of a combination of parallel flat layers exposed to plane waves at normal incidence.

Plane wave propagation characteristics in plane layered biological tissues show how radiation is absorbed when the radius of curvature of the tissue surface is large compared to a wavelength. The propagation constant $k_{m,f}$ for power transmission through biological tissues can be written in terms of the complex dielectric permittivities $\epsilon^*_{m,f}$ and the free space propagation constant k_0 in the standard form

$$k_{m,f} = k_0(\epsilon^*_{m,f}\epsilon_0^{-1})^{1/2} = \beta_{m,f} - j\alpha_{m,f} \qquad (46)$$

where the wavelengths $\lambda_{m,f} = 2\pi\beta^{-1}_{m,f}$ are significantly reduced in the tissues due to the high dielectric permittivities. Tables 6.3 and 6.4 indicate that the factors of reduction are quite large, between 6.5 and 8.5, for tissues of high water content, and between 2 and 2.5 for tissues with low water content. In addition to the large reduction in wavelength, there will be a large absorption of energy in the tissue which will result in heating of the tissue. One may note from the conductivities listed in Tables 6.3 and 6.4 that absorption in tissue of higher water content may be as high as 60 times greater than in that of low water content for the same electric fields. The absorption of microwave power will result in a progressive reduction of wave power density as the waves penetrate into the tissues. We can quantify this by defining a depth of penetration or a distance the propagating wave will travel before the power density decreases by a factor of e^{-2}. We can see from Tables 6.3 and 6.4 that the depth of penetration for tissues of low water content is as much as 10 times greater than that for tissues of high water content.

Since each tissue in a complex biological system such as man has different complex permittivity, there will in general be reflections of energy between the various tissue interfaces during exposure to microwaves. The complex reflection coefficient due to a wave transmitted from a medium of complex permittivity ϵ_1^* to a medium of complex permittivity ϵ_2^* and thickness greater than a depth of penetration is given by

$$\rho = re^{j\phi} = \frac{\sqrt{\epsilon_1^*} - \sqrt{\epsilon_2^*}}{\sqrt{\epsilon_1^*} + \sqrt{\epsilon_2^*}} \qquad (47)$$

The values r and ϕ for various interfaces are listed in Tables 6.3 and 6.4. Note the large reflection coefficient for an air-muscle or a fat-muscle interface. When a wave in a tissue of low water content is incident on an interface with a tissue of high water content of sufficient thickness (greater than the depth of penetration), the reflected wave is nearly 180° out of phase with the incident wave, thereby producing a standing wave with an intensity minimum near the interface. If the wave is propagating in a tissue of high water content and is incident on a tissue of low water content, the amplitude of the reflected component is in phase with the incident wave, thereby producing a standing wave with an intensity maximum near the interface. If there are several layers of different tissue media with thicknesses less than the depth of penetration for ech medium, the reflected energy and standing wave pattern are influenced by the thickness of each layer and the various wave impedances in the tissue. These effects may be obtained from the standard transmission line equations. The distribution of electric field strength E in a given layer is

$$E = E_0[e^{-jkz} + \rho e^{jkz}] \qquad (48)$$

where E_0 is the peak magnitude of the field and ρ is the reflection coefficient.

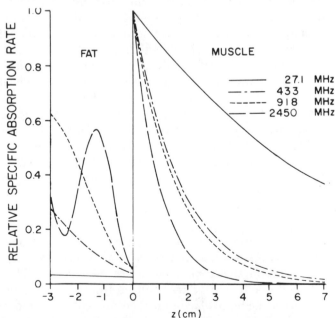

Fig. 6.25. Relative SAR patterns in plane geometry fat and muscle layers exposed to a plane wave source (54).

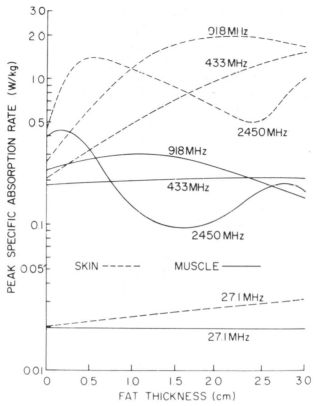

Fig. 6.26. Peak SAR in plane skin and muscle layers as a function of fat thickness (skin thickness = 2 mm) (54).

From Equation *11*, the equation for the SAR in the tissue layer, we obtain

$$P = 10^{-3} \frac{\sigma E_0^2}{2\rho} [e^{-2az} + r^2 e^{2az} + 2r \cos(2\beta z + \phi)] \qquad (49)$$

Schwan (105, 110) has made extensive calculations of these absorption distributions in various tissues. Typical distributions are shown in Figures 6.25 and 6.26 for a wave transmitted through skin, subcutaneous fat and muscle.

The results show typical SAR characteristics from plane wave irradiation of tissue for various diathermy frequencies (433 M Hz authorized only for European use). Figure 6.25 illustrates the results for a wave transmitted through a subcutaneous fat medium into a muscle medium. The absorption is normalized to unity in the muscle at the fat-muscle interface. The relative absorption curves in the fat will remain the same for smaller fat thicknesses (*e.g.*, the portion of the curves between −2 and 0 would correspond to a 2-cm thick fat layer). Figure 6.26 illustrates the SAR in the muscle interface and in a 2-mm thick skin layer as a function of fat thickness for an incident power intensity of 1 mW/cm^2. The values may be used to determine the SAR at other locations in the muscle and fat by relating them to the curves in Figure 6.25. The peak absorbed power density is always maximum in the skin layer for this type of tissue model. The curves illustrate the major deficiencies of 2450 MHz diathermy as originally demonstrated by Schwan: a) absorption is so great in the muscle layer that the depth of penetration is only 1.7 cm; b) the severe discontinuity at the fat-muscle interface produces a large standing wave resulting in a "hot spot" in the fat layer one-quarter wavelength from the muscle surface; and c) the absorbed power density in the deep tissues varies considerably with fat thickness, making it difficult to predict the proper therapeutic level for different patients having a wide variation of fat thicknesses. The curves indicate, however, that these undesirable conditions may be partially eliminated by using lower frequencies, since the depth of penetration increases, and the fat and skin thickness become proportionally smaller compared to a wavelength. The commercially available 2450 MHz diathermy equipment consists of a 0 to 100 W magnetron generator with a variable-power control calibrated in percentage of total power. Various types of standardized dipole and monopole applicators used with this generator are illustrated in Figure 6.27. The radiation power density of the most widely used C director is shown in Figure 6.28 as a function of the distance from the applicator and percentage of power output from the generator. The relationship between percent power and actual power delivered to the antenna is shown in Figure 6.29. It should be noted that the measurements are of "indicated" power density based on the square of the electric field perpendicular to the direction of propagation along the line of maximum intensity (from T-feed section of dipole). The measure-

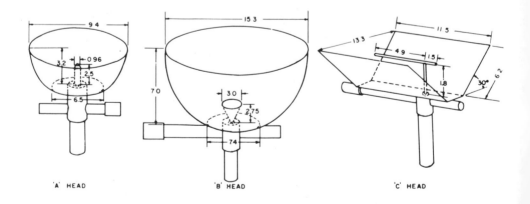

ALL DIMENSIONS IN CENTIMETERS

Fig. 6.27. Applicators used with 2450 MHz diathermy apparatus (38).

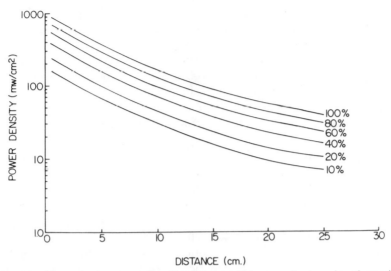

Fig. 6.28. Measured power density versus distance along axis of maximum intensity for Burdick 2450 MHz C director. (Measurements made with Narda microline electromagnetic radiation monitor Model 8100 with distance measured from dielectric cover 1.3 cm from dipole) (38).

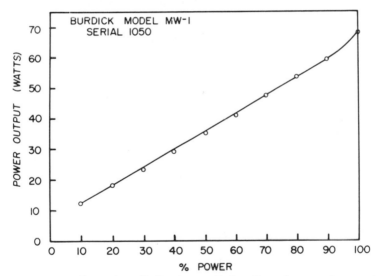

Fig. 6.29. Power delivered to C director as a function of percentage output for Burdick 2450 MHz diathermy apparatus (38).

ments were made with distance measured from the protective plastic dipole cover (1.3 cm from dipole). The characteristics of the power density survey meter are such that neither field components in the direction of propagation nor wave impedances different than 120 ohms are accounted for. Using a meter developed by the National Bureau of Standards (EDM-1C), one can measure the total field in terms of stored energy and compare it to the field oriented in the direction transverse to propagation, as shown in Figure 6.30. The results show that the error of neglecting the fields parallel to the direction of propagation can be appreciable for the normal spacing of 5 cm or more used in the clinic. Thus, the plane wave analysis will not be completely valid for predicting the absorbed power when the applicator is so close to the tissue, since the field and field impedance conditions are considerably different.

A problem of interest in diathermy is determining how effective microwaves are in heating a layer of bone beneath layers of subcutaneous fat and muscle. Figure 6.31 illustrates heating patterns for this case, using diathermy frequencies of 2450 MHz and 918 MHz for a 2-cm thick bone. The results clearly show that absorption in bone is very poor due to both severe reflection and low electrical conductivity. Since a standing wave peak at 918 MHz occurs in the muscle near the bone surface, we would expect significant bone heating due to thermal conduction from the muscle.

NON-PLANER TISSUE MODELS EXPOSED TO RADIATION FIELDS

Spherical tissue layers exposed to plane waves: Both outside and inside body geometries also influence the amount of microwave absorption in the

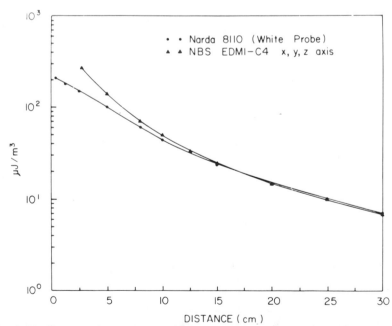

Fig. 6.30. Electric field energy density versus distance along axis of maximum intensity for Burdick 2450 MHz C director. (Measurement made with NBS electric energy density Meter 1-C4 and Narda 8100 electromagnetic radiation monitor with distance measured from dielectric cover 1.2 cm from dipole) (38).

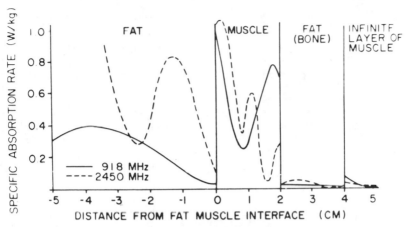

Fig. 6.31. Relative SAR patterns in plane fat, muscle, and bone layers exposed to a plane wave source (54).

human body. If the entire body, or a body member such as the head or arm, is exposed to a microwave beam of large diameter, the amounts of energy absorbed by the tissues are functions of not only the tissue layer thicknesses and cross-sectional area exposed, but also the size of the body or member compared to a free space wavelength and the body surface curvatures. We can illustrate the effects of body size and curvature on absorption characteristics by considering a spherically shaped body composed of tissue with a high water content.

Spherical Models

The electric fields induced in a sphere or spherical layer (shell) of tissue by an incident plane wave field can be calculated from the general vector spherical wave solutions of the wave equation

$$E = E_o e^{j\omega t} \sum_{n=0}^{\infty} (j)^n \frac{2n + 1}{n(n + 1)} (a_n m_{o1n} - jb_n n_{o1n}) \qquad (50)$$

where both the functions m_{o1n} and n_{o1n} are defined and the coefficients a_n and b_n are obtained as described by Stratton (115, pp. 653–567). The equations may be evaluated on a digital computer as described by Anne *et al.* (2–4), and Shapiro *et al.* (112). Figure 6.32 illustrates the relative absorbed power density patterns (called relative heating) for a simplified homogeneous spherical model of a cat or monkey-sized brain and a human-sized brain exposed to a 1 mW/cm² plane wave source. The origin of the rectangular coordinate system used in the figures is located at the center of the sphere, with wave propagation along the z axis, and the E field polarized along the x axis. The maximum absorption (at the peak of the most severe standing wave) and the average absorption along the x, y and z axes are illustrated on each plot. The dielectric properties for brain tissue were based

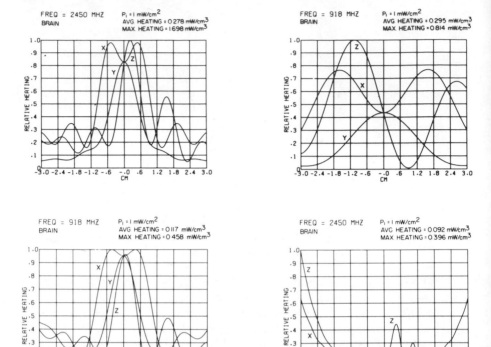

Fig. 6.32. Theoretical SAR patterns along the *x*, *y*, and *z* axis of spherical models of brain tissue exposed to a plane wave source. (Incident power density 1 mW/cm², propagation along the *z* axis, and electrical field polarized along the *x* axis with origin at center of sphere) (54).

on values reported by Schwan (110) ($\epsilon = 35$ and 30.9, and $\sigma = 0.7$ and 1.1 S/m for 918 and 2450 MHz, respectively). The figures clearly illustrate the intense fields and associated absorbed power density directly in the center of the model human head and 1.2 cm off center in the model animal head for 918-MHz exposure. One may note that the maximum absorption in the model animal head is larger by a factor of two than in the model human head. With 2450 MHz exposure, on the other hand, there is maximum absorption in the anterior (front) portion of the simulated human head, while there is maximum absorption in the center portion of the simulated animal head. The model animal head receives a maximum absorption four times that of the human model head. In comparing the plots with Figures 6.25 and 6.26, it is clear that the SAR for exposed body sizes or radii of curvature that are small compared to a wavelength is considerably different than that for larger bodies or plane tissue layers. It is significant to note that for a human brain exposed to 918 MHz EM radiation, the absorption at a depth of 2.3 times the depth of penetration (depth of penetration = 3.2 cm) is twice the absorption at the surface. This corresponds to a factor greater than 200 times that expected based on the plane tissue model. At 2450 MHz, the absorbed power density at a depth approximately equal to 4.7 times the depth of penetration is 0.43 times that at the surface, corresponding to a factor greater than 5000 times that expected from the plane tissue model. The regions of intense absorbed power density are due to a combination of the high refractive index and the radius of curvature of the model, which produces a strong focusing of power toward the interior of the sphere which more than compensates for transmission losses through the tissue. These results are significant in view of the many reported CNS effects at frequencies near 1 GHz. Figure 6.33 illustrates the calculated peak absorbed power density per unit volume and the average total absorbed power density per unit area for various sized spheres of brain tissue as a function of frequency. An incident power of 1 mW/cm^2 is assumed. Note

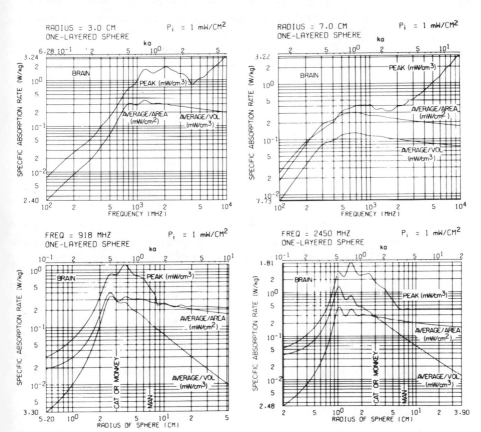

Fig. 6.33. SAR characteristics for spherical models of brain tissue exposed to 1 mW/cm^2 plane wave source (54).

the wide variation in absorbed power characteristics with different sphere sizes and frequencies of exposure. The graphs at the top of the figure indicate that there are sharp rises in peak absorption with increasing frequency, followed by several "peaks" in the absorption curves. These peaks are related to the occurrence of hot spots or maxima in the internal absorption or heating patterns similar to those indicated in Figure 6.32. As the frequency is further increased beyond the values where the peaks in absorption occur, the hot spots disappear, and maximum absorption occurs at the exposed surface of the spheres. This is due to the decreasing depth of penetration with frequency. At frequencies beyond this point, the peak absorption at the surface increases with frequency, since the constant incident power is absorbed in a decreasingly smaller volume. The peak internal heating for the spherical model of the human head is maximum in the UHF frequency range centered near 915 MHz. This, again, is significant in terms of the large number of reported CNS effects for human exposure in the UHF frequency range. The phenomenon of hearing radar pulses is also reported in this frequency range (28, 29). The graph indicates a further increase in peak absorption at frequencies above the UHF range, but this is due to decreasing depth of penetration resulting in increased surface absorption. The curves at the bottom of Figure 6.33 also show some interesting phenomena. They indicate that peak absorption can vary over an order of magnitude, depending on brain size. The curves clearly indicate some important points to consider when one relates research results for different size animals, or human exposed to RF radiation.

Similar calculations have been made for muscle spheres to obtain clues to internal heating effects due to whole body radiation. The results are very similar to the curves for brain tissue given in Figure 6.33. Peak SAR inside the body is important since it is related to the location where localized heating may occur as a function of frequency and body size. The average SAR is important because it is related to the time it takes for an exposed subject's thermoregulatory system to become overloaded, or to the time that a steady-state thermal condition is reached. There is more than an order-of-magnitude variation in this value between a spherical tissue with the same mass as man and that with the same mass as a small animal such as a mouse or rat. The curves showing average power per unit area are important since they are related to the steady-state power an exposed body can absorb without overload of the thermoregulatory system. Although the spheres are only rough approximations of actual biological bodies, they allow estimations of how applied power for producing various effects can be extrapolated from one body size to another as a function of frequency.

Cylindrical Models

Cylindrical tissue layers exposed to plane waves: SAR patterns may also be calculated for other simple tissue geometries representing portions of the anatomy. We can roughly approximate human limbs by concentric cylindrical layers of bone, muscle, fat, and skin, and express the fields in each layer by an infinite series of Bessel functions of the first and second kind as discussed by Stratton (115, pp. 349–374). For example, the electric field parallel to the z axis of the cylinder is expressed as

$$E_z = \sum_{n=0}^{\infty} [A_n J_n(kr) + B_n Y_n(kr)]e^{jn\theta} \qquad (51)$$

where k is the propagation constant in the medium, and the coefficients A_n and B_n are obtained by expanding the plane wave source expression into a series of Bessel functions and applying boundary conditions. Similar equations may be written for the wave polarized with the magnetic field paralled to the z axis. Ho (47) has evaluated the equations and has determined the fields and SAR for cylinders corresponding to human arms and legs exposed to plane waves. The results show the same increases in muscle-to-fat SAR ratio as observed for planar models exposed to lower frequencies. The results also show a greater depth of energy penetration into the muscle due to the curvature of the tissues. Recently, there have been considerable advances in our knowledge of how EM energy is absorbed in the bodies of humans and laboratory animals which are exposed to plane waves. This has been accomplished by mathematical analyses on various models of shapes more sophisticated than simple spheres or cylinders. These include prolate spheroids, arbitrary shaped ellipsoids and models closely approximating the

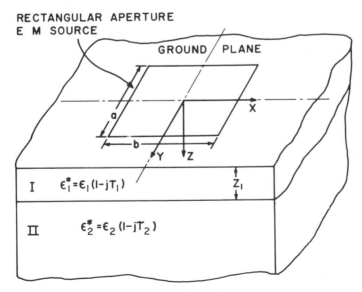

APERTURE SOURCE & TISSUE GEOMETRY
Fig. 6.34. Aperture source and tissue geometry (35).

shapes of humans including the head, the trunk, and limbs (13, 25, 32, 40, 99, 116).

TISSUES EXPOSED TO DIRECT-CONTACT EM SOURCES

Tissues exposed to near-zone fields: If other than a plane wave source is used to expose biological tissues, the absorbed power density patterns are highly dependent on source size and distribution. Many applications of microwave power in medicine and many studies on the biological effects of microwave power require an understanding of the absorbed power patterns in tissues exposed to aperture and waveguide sources. Guy (35) has analyzed the case where a bilayered fat and muscle tissue model is exposed to a direct-contact aperture source of width a and height b as shown in Figure 6.34. A fat tissue layer of thickness z_1 and dielectric permittivity ϵ_f^* in contact with a semi-infinite muscle tissue layer with a dielectric permittivity ϵ_m^* is assumed. The electric fields $E_{f,m}$ in the fat and muscle tissue may be expressed as Fourier integrals

$$E_{f,m}(x, y, z) = \frac{1}{(2\pi)^2} \int_{-\infty}^{\infty} \int_{-\infty}^{\infty} T_{f,m}(u, v, z)e^{j(ux+vy)} \, du dv \qquad (52)$$

where $T_{f,m}$ are the Fourier transforms of the electric fields at the fat and

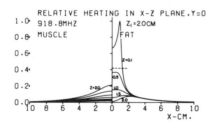

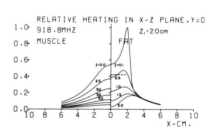

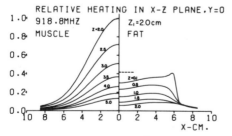

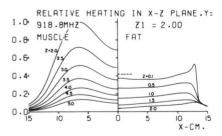

Fig. 6.35. Relative SAR patterns in plane layers of fat and muscle exposed to TE$_{10}$ mode waveguide aperture source with a = 12, f = 918.8 MHz and z_1 = 2 cm for various aperture heights. For (a)–(d), the values of b are 2, 4, 12, and 26 cm, respectively (54).

muscle boundaries, derived from the boundary conditions at $z = 0$ and $z = z_1$ in terms of the Fourier transform of the aperture

$$T_a(u, v) = \int_{-\infty}^{\infty} \int_{-\infty}^{\infty} E_f a_z X(x, y, 0) e^{-j(ux+vy)} \, dxdy \qquad (53)$$

The aperture field is denoted as $E_f(x, y, 0)$, and a_z is a unit vector along the z axis. The expressions may be evaluated numerically and the absorption patterns plotted by means of a digital computer. As an example, we may consider a waveguide aperture source and evaluate it as a diathermy applicator for use at 918 MHz. Figure 6.35 illustrates the relative SAR levels in the $x - z$ plane for $a = 12$ cm and $b = 2, 4, 12,$ and 26 cm. The SAR at the fat surface for a plane wave exposure is denoted by the dashed line in the figures. With small aperture heights, the applicator produces considerable superficial heating, in excess of that produced by plane wave exposure, but with limited heating in the underlying musculature. As the aperture height is increased, the relative heating in the musculature increases greatly, compared to the superficial heating.

The SAR patterns in multilayered cylindrical tissues exposed to an aperture source can also be determined by using a summation of three-dimensional cylindrical waves, expressing the aperture field as a two-dimen-

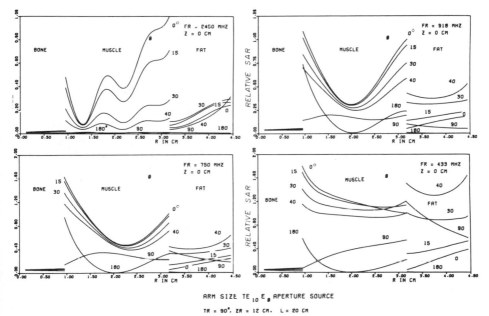

ARM SIZE TE$_{10}$ E$_\phi$ APERTURE SOURCE

TR = 90°. ZR = 12 CM. L = 20 CM

Fig. 6.36. Heating patterns in a cylindrical model of the human arm with a direct-contact cylindrical aperture source (54).

sional Fourier series and matching the boundary conditions. Ho *et al.* (48, 49) have calculated the SAR patterns for a number of different aperture and cylinder sizes. Typical results are shown in Figure 6.36 for a human-arm-sized cylinder exposed to a surface aperture source 12 cm long in the direction of the axis. The patterns are plotted as a function of the radial distance from the center of the cylinder, for various circumferential angles ϕ from the center of the aperture. The patterns are normalized to the values at $\phi = 0°$ at the fat-muscle interface. The differences illustrated between the patterns in cylindrical tissues and plane layered tissues demonstrates the importance of tissue curvature when assessing the effectiveness and safety of devices designed for the medical application of microwave energy.

All of the theoretical results discussed in this section strongly point to the ineffectiveness of 2450 MHz for diathermy, as pointed out in earlier reports by Schwan (105, 106), Lehmann *et al.*, (70–72, 78), and Guy (34–36). Although the lower frequencies of 915 MHz authorized in the United States or 433 MHz authorized in Europe appear to be better choices; the theoretical data show that 750 MHz would be the best choice. By their nature, the frequencies that provide the best therapeutic heating would also be frequencies that could be most hazardous to man in an uncontrolled exposure situation.

Measurement of SAR by Thermography

Guy (36, 37) and Johnson and Guy (54) have described a method for rapid evaluation of SAR in tissues of arbitrary shape and characteristics when they are exposed to various sources, including plane wave, aperture, slot and dipole sources. The method, valid for both far- and near-zone fields, involves the use of a thermograph camera for recording temperature distributions produced in phantom models of the tissue structures. The absorbed power or magnitude of the electric field may then be obtained anywhere on the model as a function of the square root of the magnitude of the calculated heating pattern. The phantoms are composed of materials with dielectric and geometric properties identical to the tissue structures they represent. Phantom materials have been developed which simulate human fat, muscle, brain, and bone. These materials have complex dielectric properties that closely resemble the properties of human tissues reported by Schwan (108). The modeling material for fat may also be used for bone, and the synthetic muscle material can also be used to simulate other tissues with high water content. A simulated tissue structure composed of these modeling materials will have the same internal field distribution and relative heating pattern in the presence of an EM source as the actual tissue structure. Phantom models of various tissue geometries can be fabricated as shown in Figure 6.37. They include circular cylindrical structures consisting of synthetic fat, muscle, and bone, and spheres of synthetic brain to simulate various parts of the anatomy. The models are designed to separate along planes perpendicular to the tissue interfaces so that the cross-sectional relative heating patterns can be measured with a thermograph. A thin (0.00254-cm thick) polyethylene film is placed over the precut surface on each half of the model to prevent evaporation from the wet synthetic tissue. The model is exposed to the same source that will be used to expose actual tissue. The power used on the model will be considerably greater, however, in order to heat it in the shortest possible time. After a short exposure, the model is quickly disassembled and the temperature pattern over the surface of separation is observed and recorded by means of a thermograph. The exposure is applied over a 5- to 60-second time interval, depending on the source. After a 3- to 5-second delay for separating the two halves of the model, the recording is done within a 5-second time interval or less. Since the thermal conductivity of the model is low, the difference in measured temperature distribution

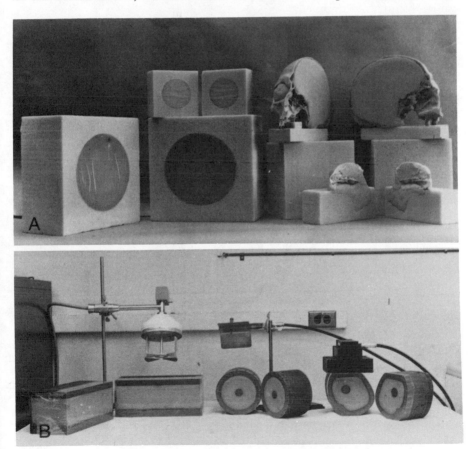

Fig. 6.37. Phantom tissue models (54).

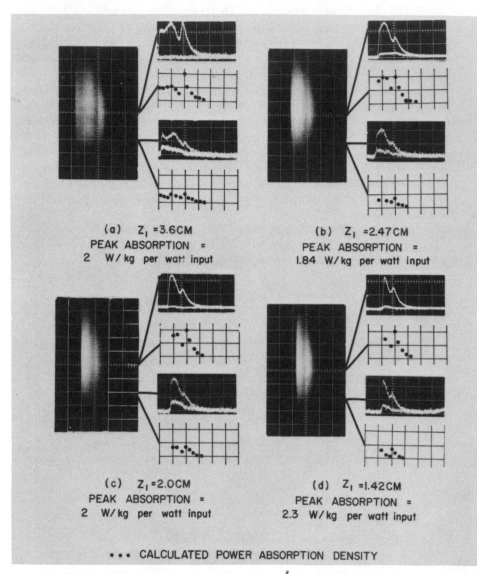

(a) Z_1 =3.6CM
PEAK ABSORPTION =
2 W/kg per watt input

(b) Z_1 =2.47CM
PEAK ABSORPTION =
1.84 W/kg per watt input

(c) Z_1 =2.0CM
PEAK ABSORPTION =
2 W/kg per watt input

(d) Z_1 =1.42CM
PEAK ABSORPTION =
2.3 W/kg per watt input

• • • CALCULATED POWER ABSORPTION DENSITY

Fig. 6.38. Thermograms and relative SAR patterns in rectangular tissue model exposed to 2450 MHz C director. (Vertical scale B scans, 2.5°C/div for midline z_1 = 2.47, 2.00, and 1.42 cm; input power, 1000 W for 10 seconds; spacing, 5 cm). (a) z_1 = 3.6 cm. Peak absorption = 2 W/kg per watt input. (b) z_1 = 2.47 cm. Peak absorption = 1.84 W/kg per watt input. (c) z_1 = 2.0 cm. Peak absorption = 2 W/kg per watt input. (d) z_1 = 1.42 cm. Peak absorption = 2.3 W/kg per watt input. • • • • •, calculated SAR (38).

before and after heating will closely approximate the heating distribution over the flat surface, except in regions of high temperature gradient where errors may occur due to appreciable diffusion of heat. The thermograph technique described for use with phantom models can also be used on test animals.

Figure 6.38 illustrates the absorption patterns measured in this manner for plane fat-muscle tissue layers exposed to the diathermy C director for different fat thicknesses. The spacing between the applicator (plastic cover) and tissue surface was set to the clinically recommended value of 5 cm. The phantom models used for these studies were assembled by first constructing a 30-cm x 30-cm x 14-cm box with ¼ in thick *Plexiglas* sides, top and bottom surfaces consisting of solid synthetic fat of uniform thickness. The box was then separated into two 30-cm by 15-cm by 14-cm halves, each filled with synthetic muscle. The exposed cut surfaces were covered with a 0.00254-cm thick polyethylene film to prevent loss of moisture. The models were constructed with fat thicknesses of 1.42, 2.00, 2.47, and 3.6 cm, and muscle thicknesses greater than 10 cm. The experimental data were taken by first exposing the center of the assembled model to the applicator so that the polarization of the electric field was parallel to the plane of separation of the model. The applicator was then energized with sufficient power over a duration of 5 to 60 seconds, so that the internal temperature rise of the model was sufficient to obtain a thermographic photograph of the plane of separation. The thermograph camera was set to obtain a C scan, displaying a two-dimensional picture of the entire area heated (intensity proportional to temperature) as shown by the large photographs in Figure 6.38. The scale on the oscilloscope indicator was set so that one large division is equal to 2 cm. The horizontal midline with the small subdivisions on the photographs corresponds to a line through the geometric center of the applicator and perpendicular to the flat interface of the phantom tissues. The vertical midline with the small subdivisions corresponds to the fat-muscle interface. After each C scan photo was taken, the model was allowed to cool, and the ambient temperature was first recorded by photographing the B scans along the horizontal midline and also along a parallel line 4 cm below the midline of the model. The B scans consisted of one-dimensional scans with the same horizontal scale as the C scans and a vertical deflection proportional to temperature (scale is given under each figure). The model was then reassembled, exposed to the EM source, again disassembled, and B scans were repeated and photographically superimposed on the previously taken B scans. The photographs of the composite B scans and their relation to the C scans are shown at the right of the large photographs in Figure 6.38. If the difference in specific heat and density of the synthetic fat and muscle are taken into account by Equation 27, the temperature difference ΔT between the superimposed B scan deflections is approximately proportional to the SAR distribution over the region scanned. The accuracy of the estimated

SAR pattern along the midline can be further improved by correcting the error due to heat flow across the interface between the high-temperature muscle and the low-temperature fat observed on all of the thermographs. This can be done in a manner previously described (36) by noting that the SAR discontinuity at the fat-muscle interface must be proportional to the ratio of electrical conductivities of the two media. The corrected curve is shown by the dotted lines in the figure. The peak SAR per mW/cm^2 of incident power density normally measured 5 cm from the applicator is shown under each group. The values are substantially greater than that predicted for a plane wave with the same power density as obtained from the graphs in Figures 6.25 and 6.26, using the applicator properties from Figures 6.28 and 6.29. This shows that the power density measurements of the near-zone fields of the C director cannot be compared to the same level measured for a plane wave source, due to multiple reflections between the applicator and the tissue and to different impedance conditions. This apparently accounts for the reduced sensitivity of the SAR to fat thickness from that of the plane wave source. The experimental data do indicate, however, the problem of excessive heating in the fat due to standing waves, and the relatively small depth of penetration into the muscle. Though the results show that the applicator is capable of producing absorption in excess of 130 W/kg at the surface of the muscle, the superficial heating is excessive, and it has been clinically demonstrated that the tolerance level is dictated by surface heating rather than by deep heating. There are no data in the literature on the SAR in actual human tissues exposed to the C director at the 5-cm spacing. Measurements have been done, however, by Lehmann *et al.* (72) for a fat thickness of 0.8 cm and an applicator spacing of 2 cm from the tissue with the results shown in Figure 6.39. For this case, the applied power was adjusted to the point where discomfort or mild pain was felt temporarily at the surface of the skin. For this case, an input power of 17 W (approximately a 17 percent output setting on the machine) or a measured incident power level of 160 mW/cm^2 was used. Table 6.10 gives the calculated SAR with depth as compared to that which would be produced by a plane wave with identical incident power density.

The deeper SAR levels are somewhat lower than that obtained for the shortwave inductive applicator. With all aspects considered, the heating characteristics of shortwave diathermy discussed in the previous section appear to be superior in terms of therapeutic value to those of the 2450 MHz modality.

Direct-Contact Microwave Applicators

The plane wave SAR characteristics shown in figures 6.25 and 6.26 clearly indicate the superiority of frequencies lower than 2450 MHz in terms of desirable therapeutic heating characteristics. Plane wave or radiating-type sources at these lower frequencies become impractical to use, however, since

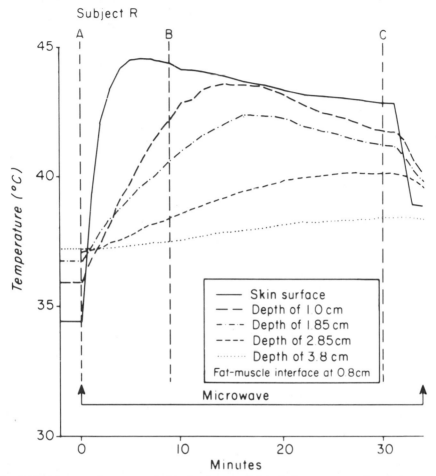

Fig. 6.39. Temperature recorded in the human thigh during exposure to microwaves at 2456 MHz applied with *C* director (72).

the energy is impossible to focus into a beam with reasonable size applicators, and the near-zone fields of the applicators extend to greater distances. Under these conditions, a pure radiation or far-zone field can be maintained only by placing the applicator at distances where large areas of the body would be exposed and excessive power levels would be required. Thus, in order to obtain selective heating with reasonable input power levels (50 to 100 W), one must necessarily expose the tissues to the near-zone fields of the source. The induced fields in the tissue are then highly dependent on the source field distribution and frequency, and may be considerably different from those produced by plane-wave or radiation fields. The aperture source provides a reasonable model for studying the effect of source distribution, size, and frequency on the induced fields in the tissues. With such a

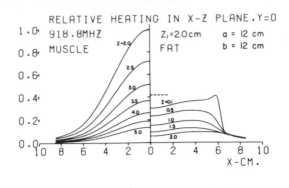

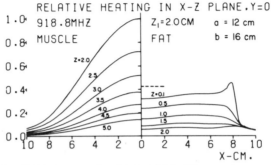

Fig. 6.40. Relative SAR patterns for 91 8.8 MHz TE_{10} mode aperture source (35).

source, the size and distribution of the induced fields may be controlled, resulting in improved diathermy applicators and a more effective SAR distribution.

APPLICATOR DESIGN

The analysis of the aperture source shown in Figure 6.34 and discussed previously provides a method for determining the optimum frequency for therapeutic heating with a clinically sized applicator. Figure 6.40 illustrates the calculated SAR or relative heating patterns for a 12-cm × 16-cm aperture and for a 12-cm × 12-cm aperture with a TE_{10} mode waveguide electric field aperture distribution. The penetration depth of energy into the muscle from such a finite-sized applicator was predicted theoretically to be identical to that of a plane wave. Studies have indicated that a 12- × 12- to 16-cm rectangular aperture with a TE_{10} waveguide mode source distribution should produce the maximum muscle-to-fat heating ratio with the minimum size source at 915 MHz.

A cavity applicator was designed by Guy (39) with special provisions for eliminating the excitation of higher modes. This was accomplished by eliminating the abrupt transitions from the smaller feed guide to the large aperture which contacts the tissue to be treated. Theoretical studies showed

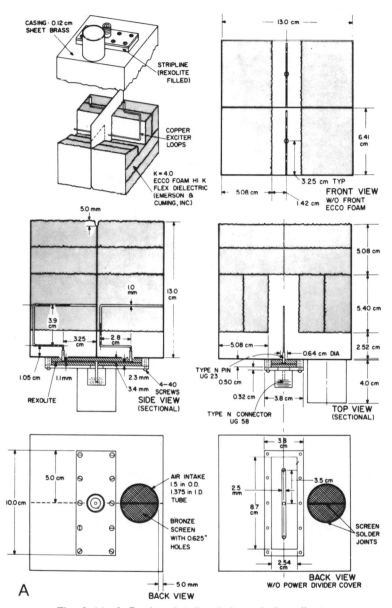

Fig. 6.41. *A*, Design details of air-cooled applicator.

that the heating pattern was nearly optimal for an aperture of 13 cm × 13 cm fed by two separate waveguides formed by a metal bifurcation placed at the center of a square cavity. Based on the improvement of deep heating with surface cooling demonstrated by de Lateur *et al.* (22), a forced-air

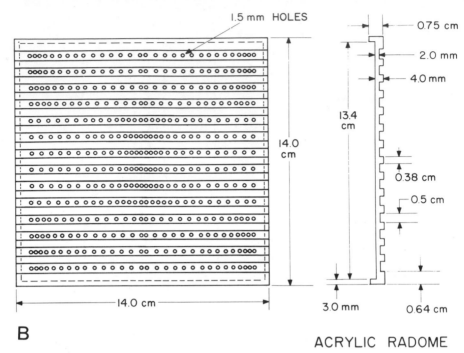

B

ACRYLIC RADOME

Fig. 6.41. *B*, Radome for air-cooled applicator (39).

cooling system was designed as an integral part of the applicator. Details of the application are shown in Figures 6.41 and 6.42. The first figure shows a three-dimensional view of the applicator with its walls removed, as well as other details. The combined waveguides 6.5 cm × 13.0 cm form the 13-cm square aperture source for producing a TE_{10} mode field distribution. Power fed to a coaxial connector is divided by a stripline power splitter for distribution to the independent waveguides by excitation loops. A lightweight Emerson and Cuming, Inc., Ecco dielectric foam with dielectric constant of 4 is used to load the applicator to allow 915 MHz wave propagation in the small sized waveguide feed system. The foam is also porous, which allows cooling air to be blown through the applicator and onto the surface of tissue being treated. At the time of fabrication of the applicator, the size and shape of the loops are adjusted to provide minimum reflection at the coaxial feed section when the applicator is in direct contact with the human thigh.

A metal screened airflow aperture is built into the back of the applicator so that forced air can be directed through the porous dielectric material. An acrylic radome shown in Figure 6.41*b* is placed at the aperture of the applicator to eliminate the hot spots in the tissue by preventing the metal walls of the applicator from contacting the tissue. A system of holes and

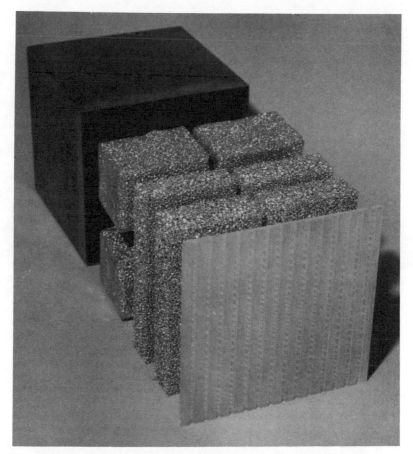

Fig. 6.42. Photograph of 915 MHz air-cooled applicator (39).

ridges was built into the radome to allow for the efficient flow of cooling air over the surface of the treated tissue.

Figure 6.43 shows the applicator as connected for testing in the clinic. Cooling air, from a small portable air conditioning unit attached to the applicator by a flexible hose, may be provided at a wide range of temperatures and flow rates.

Figure 6.44 shows a set of thermograms illustrating the SAR patterns in a muscle phantom model exposed to the applicator. The results show that the maximum absorption in the muscle is 3.27 W/kg per watt input to the applicator. Thus, an input power of approximately 50 W will produce an SAR of approximately 164 W/kg in the tissue, more than adequate for typical clinical applications. Taking density and specific heat into account, the maximum heating in the fat was approximately 40 percent of that in the

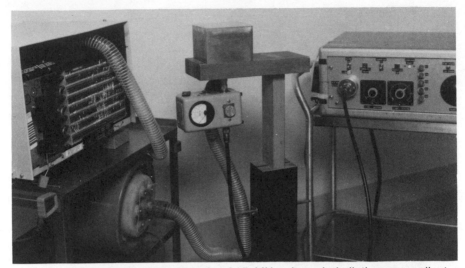

Fig. 6.43. Photograph illustrating the 915 MHz air-cooled diathermy applicator connected to microwave sources for clinical testing (39).

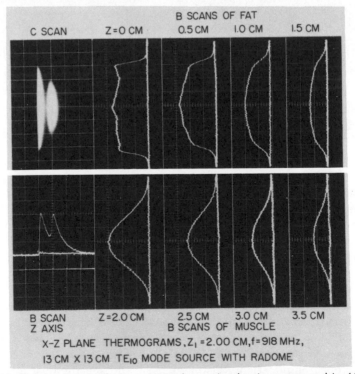

Fig. 6.44. Thermograms of plane fat and muscle phantom exposed to 13-cm × 13-cm aperture source. Maximum absorption in muscle is 3.27 W/kg per watt input. x-z plane thermograms. $z_1 = 2.0$ cm, $f = 918$ MHz. TE_{10} mode source with radome (22).

muscle. The maximum SAR per unit of incident power density was greater than that for a plane wave applicator. This was expected since the applicator was designed to couple all of the applied energy to the tissue, whereas, with a plane wave source, a considerable amount of energy is reflected from the surface. The penetration and minimal fat heating characteristics in phantom models compare favorably with those of shortwave diathermy, with the additional advantage that the heating pattern is reasonably uniform, in contrast with the undesirable toroidal pattern of shortwave diathermy.

CLINICAL TESTS

The 915 MHz UHF applicator was tested under clinical conditions by Lehmann *et al.* (79) by exposing the thighs of human volunteers. The experiments were conducted both with skin surface cooling and without cooling, with the latter providing the best therapeutic heating of deep tissue. In a typical experiment after 5 minutes of cooling, 40 W of 915 MHz power was applied for 20 minutes to the 13-cm × 13-cm aperture applicator. This corresponded to a maximum power density of 473 mW/cm^2 at the center of the applicator. Figure 6.45 shows the results of a typical experiment for a subject with 1 cm of subcutaneous fat. The initial 5 minutes of cooling lowered the skin temperature below 15°C and, to a lesser degree, the fat

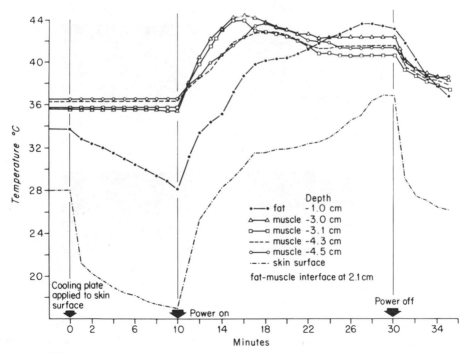

Fig. 6.45. Temperatures in a human thigh at various depths of tissue resulting from treatment with 915 MHz direct-contact aperture source with surface cooling (38).

TABLE 6.10. *Calculated Values of Absorbed Power in Human Muscle*[a]

SAR in W/kg in musculature (1–2 cm)	
RUN	SAR
1	121.60
2	78.17
3	118.70
4	75.27
5	167.93

[a] Incident radiation 555.55 mW/cm² maximum power density. From Lehmann *et al.* (79).

TABLE 6.11. *Calculated Values for Blood Flow in Human Muscle*[a]

Run Number	Blood flow rate ml/100 gm/min
1	28.90
2	28.91
3	25.00
4	23.64
5	29.69

[a] From Lehmann *et al.* (79).

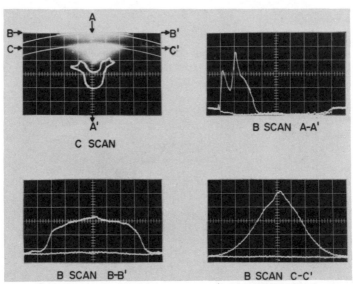

Fig. 6.46. Thermogram recording of phantom back exposed to 2450 MHz C director. (Peak SAR 2.39 W/kg per watt input at surface of muscle, scale 1 div = 2 cm) (54).

temperature to 27°C. The muscle tissue was unaffected. When power was applied, the usual linear transient was observed, from which an absorbed power density of 87 W/kg was calculated for a 1.4 cm depth in the muscle and 54 W/kg was calculated for a 2.1 cm depth in the muscle. A power

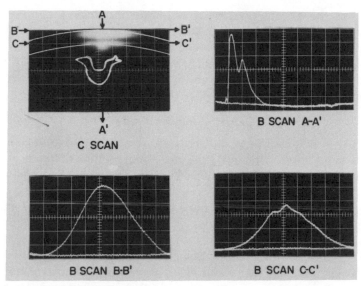

Fig. 6.47. Thermogram recordings of phantom back exposed to 918 MHz 13-cm × 13-cm aperture source with 1 W input. (Peak SAR 3.94 W/kg per watt input at surface of muscle, scale 1 div = 2 cm) (54).

density of 56 W/kg was calculated for the center of the fat layer. During the 20-minute heating period, the muscle temperature versus time curves followed the characteristic trend illustrated in Figure 6.10. The maximum temperature reached 45°C after a typical period of 6.5 minutes after exposure at a location 0.5 to 0.6 cm below the fat-muscle interface. At this time, an increase in blood cooling occurred, resulting in a decrease in tissue temperature. It may be noted, however, that all sites monitored in the muscle attained temperatures in the therapeutic range above 40°C. The temperature curves in muscle are more uniform when cooling is used because of the cooling produced by blood flow.

The SAR was calculated for five subjects who participated in the experiment. These data, calculated from the initial rate of temperature rise, are shown in Table 6.10. The power levels were calculated at one of the thermistor locations 1 to 2 cm from the fat-muscle interface in the musculature. The total power input to the applicator was 40 W, thus, the averaged specific absorption rate (SAR) was 2.81 W/kg per watt input.

In a similar manner, it is possible to estimate the flow rate of blood in the musculature by Equation 25 from the maximum slope of temperature decline after power was removed. The results are shown in Table 6.11.

If it is therapeutically desirable to override this blood-flow cooling effect to maintain maximum temperatures in the tissue, the output of the applicator could be increased during treatment.

Lehmann's (76) experiments carried out on human volunteers demonstrated that the 13-cm square direct-contact microwave applicator with randome and cooling selectively heats musculature, and that the temperature can be brought to a level between 43 and 45°C at 1 to 2 cm in muscle. By increasing power levels sufficiently after blood flow has cooled the tissue, it would be feasible to increase the temperatures back to 43 to 45°C and hold them at these levels for longer periods of treatment.

Safety Considerations

The finite-sized direct-contact apertures are not only advantageous to use for the reasons described, but also allow more efficient application and better control of the energy imparted to the tissues, thereby eliminating unwanted high-level and possibly unsafe side radiation originating from the radiating-type applicators. It should be pointed out that existing commercial diathermy applicators are not high-gain antennas and have broad radiation patterns. The therapeutic effectiveness and leakage radiation of both the 2450 MHz C director and the 915 direct-contact applicator were determined by Guy *et al.* (38) and Lehmann *et al.* (80), while phantom models and actual human tissues were exposed with each applicator in an anechoic chamber. Figures 6.46 and 6.47 illustrate the thermographic recordings of the absorbed power distribution in a phantom back model consisting of synthetic muscle tissue containing synthetic vertebrae and covered with 2 cm of synthetic subcutaneous fat, exposed to the 2450 MHz C director and the 13 cm × 13 cm 915 MHz direct-contact applicator. Figures 6.48 and 6.49 illustrate the power density in the vicinity of the applicator and the models for the two frequencies, as measured with a Narda Model 1800 radiation monitor in the plane parallel to the plane of electric field polarization and

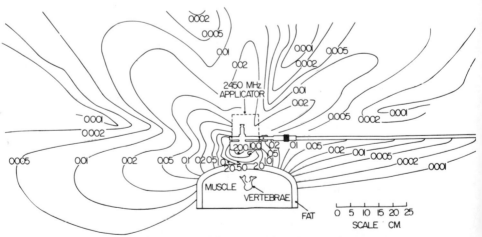

Fig. 6.48. Leakage radiation (mW/cm²) from phantom model of human back exposed to 2450 MHz C director (1 W input) (54).

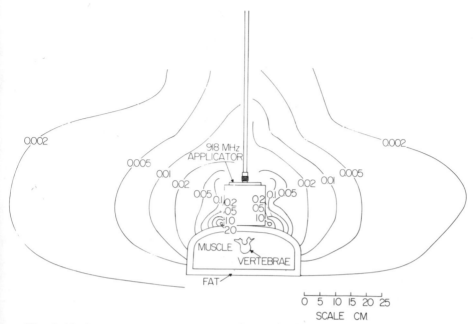

Fig. 6.49. Leakage radiation (mW/cm²) from phantom model of human back exposed to 918 MHz 13-cm × 13-cm square aperture TE₁₀ mode source (1 W input) (54).

perpendicular to the surface of the model. All values for internal SAR and external power density are normalized for 1 W input to the applicator.

The data indicate that an input of 100 W to the 2450 MHz C director would produce a maximum of 239 W/kg absorption at the surface of the muscle and 187 W/kg at the surface of the fat, while at the same time producing a maximum radiation level of 10 mW/cm² at a distance of 25 cm from the end of the applicator at an angle of 45° from the surface of the model. On the other hand, an input of 61 W to the 915 MHz direct-contact aperture source would produce the same maximum 239 W/kg power absorption at the surface of the muscle, but the maximum absorption in the fat would be reduced to 77 W/kg and the outside radiation level would be below 10 mW/cm² at a distance greater than 8 cm from the edge of the applicator. The superiority of the aperture source over the C director, both in terms of therapeutic effectiveness and radiation safety, is apparent.

REFERENCES

1. ALLEN, F. M. Biological modification of effects of roentgen rays. II. High temperature and related factors. *Am. J. Roentgenol.*, 73: 836–848, 1955.
2. ANNE, A. Relative microwave absorption cross sections of biological significance. *In: Biological Effects of Microwave Radiation.* Vol. 1. Plenum Press, New York, 1960.
3. ANNE, A., SATIO, M., SALATI, O. M., AND SCHWAN, H. P. Penetration and thermal

dissipation of microwaves in tissues. Univ. of Pennsylvania, Philadelphia, Pa., Tech. Rep. RADC-TDR-62-244. Cont. AF 3-(602)-2344, ASTIA Doc., 1962.

4. ANNE, A. Scattering and absorption of microwaves by dissipative dielectric objects: The biological significance and hazard to mankind. Ph.D. dissertation, Univ. of Pennsylvania, Philadelphia, Pa., 106 p., Cont. NONR 551505, ASTIA Doc. 408997, 1963.

5. ARONS, I., AND SOKOLOFF, B. Combined roentgenotherapy and ultra-short wave. *Am. J. Surg., 36:* 533-543, 1937.

6. AUDIAT, J. Action des ondes hertziennes sur l'excitabilite electrique des nerfs. (Ondes amorties, entretenues, courtes). *Rev. d'actionol., 8:* 227, 1932.

7. BACKLUND, L., AND TISELIUS, P. Objective measurements of joint stiffness in rheumatoid arthritis. *Acta Rheumatol. Scand., 13:* 275-288, 1967.

8. BIRKNER, R., AND WACHSMANN, F. Uber die Kombination von Rontgenstrahlen und Kurzwellen. *Strahlentherapie, 79:* 93, 1949.

9. BLUESTEIN, M., HARVEY, R. J., AND ROBINSON, T. C. Heat-transfer studies of blood-cooled heat exchangers. *In: Thermal Problems in Biotechnology.* ASME, New York, 1968, pp. 46-81.

10. BROWN, A. C., AND BRENGELMANN, G. Energy metabolism. *In: Physiology and Biophysics.* Ruch and Patton, (Eds). W.B. Saunders, Philadelphia, 1965, pp. 1030-1049.

11. CARPENTER, R. L., AND VAN UMMERSEN, C. A. The action of microwave radiation on the eye. *J. Microwave Power, 3:* 3, 1968.

12. CATER, D. B., SILVER, I. A., AND WATKINSON, D. A. Combined therapy with 220 Kv roentgen and 10 cm microwave heating in rat hepatoma. *Acta Radiol., 2:* 321-336, 1964.

13. CHEN, K. M., AND GURU, B. S. Induced EM fields inside human bodies irradiated by EM waves of up to 500 MHz. *J. Microwave Power, 12:* 173-183, 1977.

14. COLE, K., AND COLE, R. Dispersion and absorption in dielectrics. *J. Chem. Phys., 9:* 34, 1941.

15. COOK, H. The dielectric behavior of some types of human tissues at microwave frequencies. *Br. J. Appl. Phys., 2:* 295, 1951.

16. COOK, H. Dielectric behavior of human blood at microwave frequencies. *Nature, 168:* 247, 1951.

17. COOK, H. A comparison of the dielectric behavior of pure water and human blood at microwave frequencies. *Br. J. Appl. Phys., 3:* 249, 1952.

18. COPELAND, E. S., AND MICHAELSON, S. M. Effect of selective tumor heating on the localization of ^{131}I fibrinogen in the Walker carcinoma 256. II. Heating with microwaves. *Acta Radiol., 9:* 323-336, 1970.

19. CRILE, G., JR. Selective destruction of cancers after exposure to heat. *Ann. Surg., 156:* 404-407, 1962.

20. DANILEWSKY, B., AND WOROBJEW, A. Uber die Fernwirkung elektrischer Hochfrequenzstrome auf die Nerven. *Arch. F. D. Physiol., 236:* 443, 1935.

21. DE KEATING-HART, W. La fulguration et ses resultats dans le traitment du cancer, d'ares une statistique personnelle de 247 cas. Maloine, Paris, 1909.

22. DE LATEUR, B. J., LEHMANN, J. F., STONEBRIDGE, J. B., WARREN, C. G., AND GUY, A. W. Muscle heating in human subjects with 915 MHz microwave contact applicator. *Arch. Phys. Med., 51:* 147-151, 1970.

23. DELHERM, L., AND FISCHGOLD, H. Le courant de d'Arsonval diminuent l'excitabilite neuromusculaire. *Compt. rend. Acad. Sci., 199:* 1688, 1934.

24. DODT, E., AND ZOTTERMAN, Y. Mode of action of warm receptors. *Acta Physiol. Scand., 26:* 345-357, 1952.

25. DURNEY, C. H., JOHNSON, C. C., BARBER, P. W., MASSOUDE, H., ISKANDER, M. E., LORDS, J. L., RYSER, D. K., ALLEN, S. F., AND MITCHELL, J. C. Radiofrequency Radiation Dosimetry Handbook. Second edition. Report no. SAM-TR-78-22, prepared by the Univ. of Utah for USAF School of Aerospace Med., Brooks AFB, TX, 1978.

26. EIDINOW, A. Action of ultra-short waves on tumours. *Br. Med. J., 2:* 332, 1934.

27. FISCHER, E., AND SOLOMON, S. Physiological responses to heat and cold. *In: Therapeutic Heat and Cold.* Licht, S. (Ed). Licht, New Haven, CN. Sec. 4. pp. 126–169, 1965.
28. FREY, A. H. Auditory system response to RF energy. *Aerospace Med., 32:* 1140–1142, 1961.
29. FREY, A. H. Human auditory system response to modulated electromagnetic energy. *J. Appl. Physiol., 17:* 689–692, 1962.
30. FUCHS, G. Uber die Sensibilisierung rontgenrefractarer Neoplasmen durch Kurzwellen. *Strahlentherapie, 55:* 473–480, 1936.
31. FUCHS, G. Zur Sensibilisierung maligner Tumoren durch Ultrakurzwellen. *Strahlentherapie, 88:* 647–653, 1952.
32. GANDHI, O. P., HUNT, E. L., AND D'ANDREA, J. A. Electromagnetic power deposition in man and animals with and without ground and reflector effects. *Radio Sci., 12:* 39–48, 1977.
33. GESSLER, A. E., McCARTY, K. S., AND PARKINSON, M. C. Eradication of spontaneous mouse tumours by high frequency radiation. *Exp. Med. Surg., 8:* 143, 1950.
34. GUY, A. W., AND LEHMANN, J. F. On the determination of an optimum microwave diathermy frequency for a direct contact applicator. *IEEE Trans., BME-13:* 76–87, 1966.
35. GUY, A. W. Electromagnetic fields and relative heating patterns due to a rectangular aperture source in direct contact with bilayered biological tissue. *IEEE Trans., MTT-19:* 214–223, 1971.
36. GUY, A. W. Analyses of electromagnetic fields induced in biological tissues by thermographic studies on equivalent phantom models. *IEEE Trans., MTT-19:* 205–214, 1971.
37. GUY, A. W. Quantitation of induced electromatnetic field patterns in tissue and associated biological effects. *Biologic Effects and Health Hazards of Microwave Radiation, Proc. Int. Symp.,* (Warsaw, Poland, Oct., 1973). Warsaw, Poland: Polish Medical, pp. 203–216, 1974.
38. GUY, A. W., LEHMANN, J. F., AND STONEBRIDGE, J. B. Therapeutic applications of electromagnetic power. *Proc. IEEE, 62:* 55–75, 1974.
39. GUY, A. W., LEHMANN, J. F., STONEBRIDGE, J. B., AND SORENSEN, C. C. Development of a 915 MHz direct contact applicator for therapeutic heating of tissues. *IEEE Trans., MTT-26:* 550–556, 1978.
40. GUY, A. W. (Ed). Special Issue on Microwaves in Medicine, with Accent on the Application of Electromagnetics to Cancer Treatment. *IEEE Trans., MTT-26:* No. 8, 1978.
41. HARDY, J. D. Thermal radiation, pain and injury. *In: Therapeutic Heat and Cold.* Licht, S. (Ed). Licht, New Haven, Cn., Sec. 5, pp. 170–195, 1965.
42. HARRIS, R. The effect of various forms of physical therapy on radio sodium clearance from the normal and arthritic knee joint. *Ann. Phys. Med., 7:* 1–10, 1963.
43. HASCHE, E., AND COLLIER, W. A. Uber die Beeinflussung bosartiger Geschwulste durch Ultrakurzwellen. *Strahlentherapie, 51:* 309–311, 1934.
44. HEMINGWAY, A., AND STENSTROM, K. W. Physical characteristics of short-wave diathermy. *In: Handbook of Physical Therapy.* Amer. Med. Assoc. Press, Chicago, IL, pp. 214–229, 1939.
45. HILL, L. Actions of ultra short waves on tumours. *Br. Med. J., 2:* 370–371, 1934.
46. HILL, L., AND TAYLOR, H. J. Effect of high-frequency field on some physiologic preparations. *Lancet, 1:* 311, 1936.
47. HO, H. S. Energy absorption patterns in circular triple-layered tissue cylinders exposed to plane wave sources [Calculated for sources of 433, 750, 918, and 2450 MHz]. *Health Phys., 31:* 97–108, 1976.
48. HO, H. S., SIGELMANN, R. A., GUY, A. W., AND LEHMANN, J. F. Electromagnetic heating of simulated human limbs by aperture sources. *In: Proc. 23rd Ann. Conf. on Eng. in Med. and Biol.* Washington, D.C., 1970, p. 159.
49. HO, H. S., GUY, A. W., SIGELMANN, R. A., AND LEHMANN, J. F. Microwave heating of simulated human limbs by aperture sources. *IEEE Trans. Microwave Theory Tech.,*

MTT-19: 224–231, 1971.

50. HOLLMAN, H. E. Das problem der behandlung biologisher korper in ultrakurzwellen-strahlungsfel. *In: Ultrakurz-wellen in Ihren Medizinishe-biologischen Anwendundungen.* Sec. 4, Thiem, Leipzig, Germany, pp. 232–249, 1938.

51. HORNBACK, N. B., SHUPE, R. E., SHIDNIA, H., JOE, B. T., SAYOC, E., AND MARSHALL, C. Preliminary clinical results of combined 433 megahertz microwave therapy and radiation therapy on patients with advanced cancer. *Cancer 40:* 2854–2863, 1977.

52. HORNBACK, N. B., SHUPE, R., SHIDNIA, H., JOE, B. T., SAYOC, E., GEORGE, R., AND MARSHALL, C. Radiation and microwave therapy in the treatment of advanced cancer. *Radiology, 130:* 459–464, 1979.

53. IMIG, C. J., THOMSON, J. D., AND HINES, H. M. Testicular degeneration as a result of microwave irradiation. *Proc. Soc. Exp. Biol. Med., 69:* 382–386, 1948.

54. JOHNSON, C. C., AND GUY, A. W. Nonionizing electromagnetic wave effects in biological materials and systems. *Proc. IEEE,* Vol. 60, 1972.

55. JOHNSON, H. J. The action of short radio waves on tissues. III. A comparison of the thermal sensitivities of transplantable tumours *in vivo* and *in vitro. Am. J. Cancer, 38:* 533–550, 1940.

56. KETY, S. S. Measurement of regional circulation by the local clearance of radioactive sodium. *Am. Heart J., 38:* 321, 1949.

57. KIM, J. H., HAHN, E. W., AND TOKITA, N. Combination hyperthermia and radiation therapy for cutaneous malignant melanoma. *Cancer, 41:* 2143–2148, 1978.

58. KOTTKE, F. J. Heat in pelvic diseases. *In: Therapeutic Heat and Cold.* Licht, S. (Ed). Licht, New Haven, Cn. Sec. 18, pp. 474–490, 1965.

59. KRUSEN, F. H., HERRICK, J. F., LEDEN, U., AND WAKIM, K. G. Microkymatotherapy: Preliminary report of experimental studies of the heating effect of microwaves (radar) in living tissues. *Proc. Staff Meeting Mayo Clin., 22:* 209–224, 1947.

60. LARSEN, L. E., MOORE, R. A., ACEVEDO, J. An R.F. decoupled electrode for measurement of brain temperatures during microwave exposure. In: *1973 IEEE G-MTT Int. Microwave Symp.* Univ. of Colorado, Boulder, June 1973, pp. 262–263.

61. LeVEEN, H. H., WAPNICK, S., PICCONE, V., FALK, G., AND AHMED, N. Tumor eradication by radiofrequency therapy: response in 21 patients. *J.A.M.A., 235:* 2198–2200, 1976.

62. LEDEN, U. M., HERRICK, J. F., WAKIM, K. G., AND KRUSEN, F. H. Preliminary studies on the heating and circulating effects of microwaves (radar). *Br. J. Phys. Med., 10:* 177–184, 1947.

63. LEHMANN, J. F., AND VORSCHUTY, R. Die wirkung von ultraschallwellen auf die gewe-beatmung als beitrag zum therapeutischen wirkungsmechanismus. *Strahlentherapie, 82:* 287–292, 1950.

64. LEHMANN, J. F., AND HOHLFELD, R. Der gewebestoffwechsel nach ultraschall und warmeeinwirkung. *Strahlentherapie, 87:* 544–549, 1952.

65. LEHMANN, J. F., ERICKSON, D. J., MARTIN, G. M., AND KRUSEN, F. H. Comparison of ultrasonic and microwave diathermy in the physical treatment of periarthritis of the shoulder. *Arch. Phys. Med., 35:* 627–634, 1954.

66. LEHMANN, J. F., GUY, A. W., DeLATEUR, B. J., STONEBRIDGE, J. B., AND WARREN, C. G. Heating patterns produced by shortwave diathermy using helical induction coil applicators. *Arch. Phys. Med., 49:* 193–198, 1968.

67. LEHMANN, J. F., ERICKSON, D. J., MARTIN, G. M., AND KRUSEN, F. H. The present value of ultrasonic diathermy. *J.A.M.A., 147:* 996–999, 1955.

68. LEHMANN, J. F., BRUNNER, G. D., AND STOW, R. W. Pain thresholds measurements after therapeutic application of ultrasonic microwave and infrared. *Arch. Phys. Med., 39:* 560–565, 1958.

69. LEHMANN, J. F., FORDYCE, W. E., RATHBUN, L. A., LARSON, R. E., AND WOOD, D. H. Clinical evaluation of a new approach in the treatment of contracture associated with hip fractures after internal fixation. *Arch. Phys. Med., 42:* 95–100, 1961.

70. LEHMANN, J. F., GUY, A. W., JOHNSON, V. C., BRUNNER, G. D., AND BELL, J. W. Comparison of relative heating patterns produced in tissues by exposure to microwave energy at frequencies of 2450 and 900 megacycles. *Arch. Phys. Med.*, *43:* 69–76, 1962.

71. LEHMANN, J. F., McMILLAN, J. A., BRUNNER, G. D., AND GUY, A. W. A comparative evaluation of temperature distributions produced by microwaves at 2456 and 900 megacycles in geometrically complex specimens. *Arch. Phys. Med.*, *43:* 502–507, 1962.

72. LEHMANN, J. F., et al. Comparison of deep heating by microwaves at frequencies 2456 and 900 megacycles. *Arch. Phys. Med.*, *46:* 307–314, 1965.

73. LEHMANN, J. F. Ultrasound therapy. *In: Therapeutic Heat and Cold.* Licht, S. (Ed). New Haven, Cn., Licht, Sec. 13, pp. 321–386, 1965.

74. LEHMANN, J. F., GUY, A. W., DELATEUR, B. J., STONEBRIDGE, J. B., AND WARREN, C. G. Heating patterns produced by shortwave diathermy using helical induction coil applicators. *Arch. Phys. Med.*, *49:* 193–198, 1968.

75. LEHMANN, J. F., DELATEUR, B. J., AND STONEBRIDGE, J. B. Selective muscle heating by shortwave diathermy with a helical coil. *Arch. Phys. Med.*, *50:* 117–132, 1969.

76. LEHMANN, J. F., GUY, A. W., WARREN, C. G., DELATEUR, B. J., AND STONEBRIDGE, J. B. Evaluation of a microwave contact applicator. *Arch. Phys. Med.*, *51:* 143–147, 1970.

77. LEHMANN, J. F., MASOCK, A. J., WARREN, C. G., AND KOBLANSKI, J. N. Effects of therapeutic temperatures on tendon extensibility. *Arch. Phys. Med.*, *51:* 481–487, 1970.

78. LEHMANN, J. F. Diathermy. *In: Handbook of Physical Medicine and Rehabilitation.* Krusen, Kottke, Elwood, (Eds). W.B. Saunders, Philadelphia, Sec. 11, pp. 273–345, 1971.

79. LEHMANN, J. F., GUY, A. W., STONEBRIDGE, J. B., AND DELATEUR, B. J. Evaluation of a therapeutic direct-contact 915-MHz microwave applicator for effective deep-tissue heating in humans. *IEEE Trans.*, *MTT-26:* 556–563, 1978.

80. LEHMANN, J. F., STONEBRIDGE, J. B., AND GUY, A. W. A comparison of patterns of stray radiation from therapeutic microwave applicators measured near tissue-substitute models and human subjects. *Radio Sco.*, *14:* 271–283, 1979.

81. LICHT, S. History of therapeutic heat. *In: Therapeutic Heat and Cold.* Licht, S. (Ed). Licht, New Haven, Cn. Sec. 6, pp. 196–231, 1965.

82. LIEBESNY, P. Experimentelle Untersuchungen Uber Diathermie. *Wien. klin. Wchnschr.*, *34:* 117, 1921.

83. McNIVEN, D. R., AND WYPER, D. J. Microwave therapy and muscle blood flow in man. *J. Microwave Power*, *11:* 168–170, 1976.

84. MENDECKI, J., FRIEDENTHAL, E., BOTSTEIN, C., STERZER, F., PAGLIONE, R., NOWO-GRODZKI, M., AND BECK, E. Microwave-induced hyperthermia in cancer treatment: apparatus and preliminary results. *Int. J. Radiat. Oncol. Biol. Phys.*, *4:* 1095–1103, 1978.

85. MILLARD, J. B. Effect of high-frequency currents and infra-red rays on the circulation of the lower limb in man. *Ann. Phys. Med.*, *6:* 45–66, 1961.

86. MINARD, D. Body heat content. *In: Physiological and Behavioral Temperature Regulation.* Hardy, J., Gagge, A., and Stolwijh, J. (Eds). Springfield, Il. Sec. 25, pp. 345–357, 1970. Charles C Thomas, *Medical Physiology*, P. Bard, (Ed). 11th edition. C.V. Mosby, St. Louis, Mo. 1961, p. 240.

87. MITTLEMANN, E., OSBORNE, S. L., AND COULTER, J. S. Short wave diathermy power absorption and deep tissue temperature. *Arch. Phys. Ther.*, *22:* 133–139, 1941.

88. MORESSI, W. J. Mortality patterns of mouse sarcoma 180 cells resulting from direct heating and chronic microwave irradiation. *Exp. Cell Res.*, *33:* 240–253, 1964.

89. MORTIMER, B., AND OSBORNE, S. L. Short wave diathermy—some biologic considerations. *J.A.M.A.*, *104:* 1413, 1935.

90. NELSON, A. J. M., AND HOLT, J. A. G. Combined microwave therapy. *Med. J. Austral.*, *2:* 88–90, 1978.

91. NEVINS, R. G., AND DARWISH, M. A. Heat transfer through subcutaneous tissue as heat generating porous material. *In: Physiological and Behavioral Temperature Regulation.* Hardy, J., Gagge, A., and Stolwijh, J. (Eds). Charles C Thomas, Springfield, Il.: Sec. 21,

pp. 281–301, 1970.

92. OSBORNE, S. L., AND COULTER, J. S. Thermal effects of shortwave diathermy on bone and muscle. *Arch. Phys. Ther.*, *38:* 281–284, 1938.

93. OVERGAARD, J. Biological effect of 27.12-MHz short-wave diathermic heating in experimental tumors. *IEEE Trans. MTT-26:* 523–529, 1978.

94. OVERGAARD, K., AND OVERGAARD, J. Investigations on the possibility of a thermic tumour therapy. I. Short-wave treatment of a transplanted isologous mouse mammary carcinoma. *Europ. J. Cancer, 8:* 65–78, 1972.

95. OVERGAARD, K., AND OVERGAARD, J. Investigations on the possibility of a thermic tumour therapy. II. Action of combined heat-roentgen treatment on a transplanted mouse mammary carcinoma. *Europ. J. Cancer, 8:* 573–575, 1972.

96. PFLOMM, E. Experimentelle u. klinische Untersuchungen Uber die Wirkung Ultrakurzer elektrischen Wellen. *Arch. Klin. Chir., 166:* 251, 1931.

97. REITER, T. Researches sur les ondes ultra-courtes. *Ann. d'Inst. Actinol., 7:* 195–198, 1932.

98. RICHARDSON, A. W., IMIG, C. J., FEUCHT, B. L., AND HINES, H. M. The relationship between deep tissue temperature and blood flow during electromagnetic radiation. *Arch. Phys. Med., 50:* 19–25, 1950.

99. ROBINSON, J. E., AND WIZENBERG, M. J. (Co-Chairmen) International Symposium on Cancer Therapy by Hyperthermia and Radiation, 1975.

100. ROFFO, A. E., JR. Relation entre les ondes electriques et la multiplication cellulaire dans les cultures de tissues *in vitro. Arch d'electric Med, 42:* 466–475, 1934.

101. ROHDENBURG, G. L., AND PRIME, F. The effect of combined radiation and heat on neoplasms. *Arch. Surg., 2:* 116–129, 1921.

102. SCHERESCHEWSKY, J. W. The action of very high frequency upon a transplanted mouth sarcoma. *Public Health Rep., 43:* 937, 1928.

103. SCHLIEPHAKE, E. *Short Wave Therapy* The Actinic Press, London, p. 181, 1935.

104. SCHLIEPHAKE, E. General principles of thermotherapy. *In:* Therapeutic Heat. Licht, S. (Ed). Licht, New Haven, Cn. Sec. 4, pp. 126–169, 1958.

105. SCHWAN, H. P., AND PIERSAL, G. M. The absorption of electromagnetic energy in body tissues, Part I. *Am. J. Phys. Med., 33:* 371–404, 1954.

106. SCHWAN, H. P., AND PIERSAL, G. M. The absorption of electromagnetic energy in body tissues, Part II. *Am. J. Phys. Med., 34:* 425–448, 1955.

107. SCHWAN, H. P. Electrical properties of tissues and cells. *Adv. Biol. Med. Phys., 5:* 147–209, 1957.

108. SCHWAN, H. P. Survey of microwave absorption characteristics of body tissues. *In: Proc. Second Tri-Service Conf. Biol. Effects of Microwave Energy.* pp. 126–145, 1958.

109. SCHWAN, H. P. Alternating current spectroscopy of biological substances. *Proc. IRE, 47:* 1841–1855, 1959.

110. SCHWAN, H. P. Biophysics of diathermy. *In: Therapeutic Heat and Cold.* Licht, S. (Ed). Licht, New Haven, Cn. Sec. 3, pp. 63–125, 1965.

111. SEKINS, K. M., DUNDORE, D., EMERY, A. F., LEHMANN, J. F., McGRATH, P. W., AND NELP, W. B. Muscle blood flow changes in response to 915 MHz diathermy with surface cooling as measured by Xe^{133} clearance. *Arch. Phys. Med. Rehabil. 61:* 105–113, 1980.

112. SHAPIRO, A. R., LUTOMIRSKI, R. F., AND YURA, H. T. Induced fields and heating within a cranial structure irradiated by an electromagnetic plane wave. *IEEE Trans. Microwave Theory Tech* (special Issue on Biological Effects of Microwaves), *MTT-19:* 187–196, 1971.

113. SIEMS, L. L., KOSMAN, A. J., AND OSBORNE, S. L. A comparative study of short waves and microwave diathermy on blood flow. *Arch. Phys. Med, 29:* 759, 1948.

114. SOUTHWORTH, G. C. New experimental methods applicable to ultra short waves. *J. Appl. Phys., 8:* 660, 1937.

115. STRATTON, J. A. *Electromagnetic Theory.* McGraw-Hill, New York, 1941.

116. STREFFER, C. S. (Ed). Cancer therapy by hyperthermia and radiation. Proc. 2nd International Symposium. Urban & Schwarzenberg, Baltimore, Munich, 1978.

117. SZMIGIELSKI, S., BIELEC, M., JANIAK, M., KOBUS, M., LCUZAK, M., AND DECLERCQ, E. Inhibition of tumor growth in mice by microwave hyperthermia, polyriboinosinic-polyribocytidylic, and mouse interferon. *IEEE Trans.*, *MTT-26:* 520–522, 1978.

118. VON ARDENNE, M. On a new physical principle for selective local hyperthermia of tumor tissues. *In: Cancer Therapy by Hyperthermia and Radiation.* Streffer, C. et al. (Eds.), Urban & Schwarzenberg, Munich, pp. 96–104, 1978.

119. WEBER, E. *Electromagnetic Fields.* John Wiley & Sons, New York, pp. 140–144, 1950.

120. WEISSENBERG, E. Soc. Francaise d'Electrotherapie et de Radiologie *10:* 535, 1935.

121. WILLIAMS, N. H. Production and absorption of electromagnetic waves from 3 cm to 6 mm in length. *J. Appl. Phys., 8:* 655, 1937.

122. WORDEN, R. W., HERRICK, J. F., WAKIM, K. G., AND KRUSEN, F. H. The heating effects of microwaves with and without eschemia. *Arch. Phys. Med., 29:* 751, 1948.

123. ZIMMER, R. P., ECKER, H. A., AND POPOVIC, V. P. Selective electromagnetic heating of tumors in animals in deep hypothermia. *IEEE Trans., MTT-19:* 232–238, 1971.

7

Bioeffects of High Frequency Currents and Electromagnetic Radiation[1]

SOL M. MICHAELSON

Introduction

A complete review of the literature on the biological effects of exposure to microwave/radiofrequency (MW/RF) energies is beyond the scope of this chapter. The reader is referred to monographs and reviews by Petrov (266), Michaelson (226–231), Marha *et al.* (216), Presman (273), Schwan and Piersol (302, 303), Gordon (128), Cleary (71), and Baranski and Czerski (28).

Certain organs and organ systems are reported to be affected by MW/RF exposure in terms of functional disturbance, structural alterations, or both. Some reactions to MW/RF exposure may lead to measurable biological effects which remain within the range of normal (physiological) compensation, thus an effect is not necessarily a hazard. Some reactions, on the other hand, may lead to potential or actual health hazards.

Most of the biological reactions elicited by microwave exposure can be attributed to thermal energy conversion, almost exclusively as enthalpic energy (heating) phenomena. This, however, does not provide a predictive model of the biological consequences of non-uniform absorption of energy in animals and humans. The non-uniform, largely unpredictable distribution of energy absorption may give rise to temperature increases and rates of heating that can result in unique biological effects. The non-uniform characteristics of microwave absorption, with differing rates of temperature rise

[1] This chapter is based on work performed under Contract No. DE-AC02–76EV03490 with the U.S. Department of Energy at the University of Rochester Department of Radiation Biology and Biophysics and has been assigned Report No. UR-3490–1948.

in different tissues, results in heating patterns which cannot be replicated with radiant, convected or conducted heat. Furthermore, induced temperature gradients in deep body organs may act as a stimulus to alter normal function both in the heated organ and in other organs of the system. Thus, indirect effects can be mediated in organs far removed from the site of the primary interaction. It should also be pointed out that temperature rises from diverse etiologies may induce chromosomal alterations, mutagenesis, virus activation and inactivation, as well as behavioral and immunological reactions.

Extensive investigations into microwave bioeffects during the last quarter century have shown that for frequencies between 200 and 24,500 MHz, exposure to a power density of 100 mW/cm^2 for several minutes or hours can result in pathophysiological manifestations of a thermal nature in laboratory animals. Such effects may or may not be characterized by a measureable temperature rise, which is a function of thermal regulatory processes and active adaptation of the animal. The end result is either reversible or irreversible change, depending on the irradiation conditions and the physiological state of the animal. At lower power densities, evidence of pathological changes or physiological alteration is non-existent or equivocal. A great deal of discussion, nevertheless, has taken place on the relative importance of thermal or nonthermal effects of radiofrequency (RF) and microwave radiation.

The results of some *in vitro* studies have been considered to be evidence of non-thermal effects of RF radiation. Although some investigators and reviewers question the interpretation of these so-called non-thermal effects (224, 228, 243, 295), several support *non-thermal* interactions between tissues and electric and magnetic fields (129, 174, 216, 266, 273).

Temperature increase during exposure to microwaves depends on a) the specific area of the body exposed and the efficiency of heat elimination; b) the intensity or field strength; c) the duration of exposure; d) the specific frequency or wavelength. These variables determine the percentage of radiant energy absorbed by various tissues of the body (302, 303).

In partial body exposure under normal conditions, the body acts as a cooling reservoir, which stabilizes the temperature of the irradiated part. The stabilization is due to an equilibrium established between the energy absorbed by the irradiated part and the heat carried away from it. This heat transport is due to increased blood flow to cooler parts of the body, maintained at normal temperature by heat-regulation mechanisms. If the amount of absorbed energy exceeds the heat energy that can be handled by the mechanisms of temperature regulation, the excess energy will cause continuous temperature rise. Hyperthermia and, under some circumstances, local tissue destruction can result (302, 303).

Elucidation of the biological effects of microwave exposure requires a careful review and critical analysis of the available literature. This entails differentiating established effects and mechanisms from speculative and unsubstantiated reports. Although most of the experimental data support the concept that the effects of microwave exposure are primarily, if not only, a response to heating or altered thermal gradients in the body, there are large areas of confusion, uncertainty, and misinformation.

Rate of Energy Absorption in Living Systems

Irradiation of biological systems with MW/RF energy leads to temperature elevation when the rate of energy absorption exceeds the rate of energy dissipation. Whether the resultant temperature elevation is diffuse or is confined to specific anatomical sites depends on a) the electromagnetic field characteristics and distributions within the body, and b) the passive and active thermoregulatory mechanisms available to the particular biological entity.

The passive thermoregulatory mechanisms available consist of heat radiation, conduction, convection and evaporative cooling. In fur-bearing animals and clothed humans, heat loss by radiation and evaporative cooling is poor. The efficiency of heat convection between a body and its immediate environment is a function of environmental conditions.

Active thermoregulatory mechanisms make use of passive heat transfer mechanisms by employing internal circulating fluids (such as blood) to transfer heat from internal regions to external regions where passive heat radiation and convection are more effective. In some fur-bearing animals, an efficient mechanism is the movement of internally-warmed blood to the lungs; heat in the lungs is transferred to the inspired air by convection and is then expired into the environment. Another mechanism (especially in man) is cutaneous vasodilation, resulting in the transfer of internal heat to the skin, where it can be radiated and convected into the surrounding environment. Sweating from the skin of humans and the paws and snout of fur-bearing animals provides a means of heat transfer; evaporation of the fluid permits rapid heat loss to the environment.

While respiratory and cutaneous heat transfer is well-documented (55), no information is available on any alteration of vascular perfusion patterns of internal organs in response to local temperature changes. As a result, the possibility of local internal "hot spots" exists if

a) the rate of energy absorption is relatively high compared to the vascular heat transfer capacity of the local region (*i.e.*, lens of the eye, necrotic center of tumor, etc.), and

b) the rate of energy absorption is relatively uniform throughout the region, but the vascular perfusion patterns are such that confluence or pooling occurs (*i.e.*, venous system in the splanchnic region and above the spinal cord).

Principles of Biological Experiments and Interpretation

In order to extrapolate observations in animals to predict results that might occur during human exposure, some method of scaling must be employed. The best method available at present, albeit fraught with over-simplifications, is frequency scaling. This approach assumes the use of shorter wavelengths (higher frequencies) for smaller animals and longer wavelengths (lower frequencies) for larger animals. Approximating the bodies of all animals and man as prolate spheroids, an attempt has been made to ascertain what (lower) frequency must be used with the larger animal if the total absorbed dose rate (at the same plane wave exposure field intensity) is to be the same as that obtained at a higher frequency for a smaller animal (105).

Even by using approaches where absorbed energy patterns in test animals closely approximate patterns that may exist in humans under certain exposure conditions, the intrinsic physical and physiological dissimilarities between species further confound the problem of extrapolating between animals and humans. In addition to the obvious external geometric differences, the differences in internal vascular anatomy and mechanisms of heat dissipation in fur-bearing animals compared to man, must be taken into consideration.

Experimental animal models are used extensively to study physical factors in the environment to assure human health and safety. The best we can do experimentally is to create an arbitrary set of conditions which we consider to be as relevant as possible for the purpose of the study. Many factors such as methods of animal care, the role of seasonal and circadian rhythms, temperature, humidity, etc., as well as psychosocial interactions, must be considered in experimental design and analysis of results. Reliability of laboratory studies depends on the following:

   a) Selection of the animal model, with consideration of its cognitive limits.
   b) Application of methods for investigation of biological processes in animals.
   c) Extrapolation of data from animals to man.

Direct extrapolation from animal experiments to man cannot always be performed a priori. This is due not only to the physiological differences but also to differences in physical dimensions and shape.

Meticulous care must be used in defining the experimental conditions. One of the general problems in studying biological effects is the selection of the most appropriate animal species for extrapolation to man. Animals are quite often selected on the basis of convenience, economy, or familiarity, and without regard to their suitability for the problem under study. Results obtained in small laboratory animals should not be extrapolated to larger animals or man without consideration of size distributions as well as metabolic and physiological differences.

Proper investigation of the biological effects of electromagnetic fields requires an understanding and appreciation of biophysical principles and "comparative medicine." Such studies require interspecies "scaling", the selection of biomedical parameters which consider basic physiological functions, identification of specific and non-specific reactions, and differentation of adaptational or compensatory changes from pathological manifestations. In comparing results of experiments performed in the same or different laboratories, standardization of conditions is mandatory.

The investigator has to determine whether an observed difference can be attributed to the causal factor in question, or whether it might simply have occurred spontaneously. In cases in which no difference is observed, the question is whether any conclusion at all is warranted, and if so, what confidence should be placed in it. For guidance, the investigator often turns to statistical analysis. He or she must appreciate, however, that statistics cannot decide what is true and what is not. Statistical analysis should be considered only as an adjunct to, and an integral part of, experiment and observation. But as with any tool, its usefulness will be enhanced only if its inherent limitations are properly recognized.

The following parameters should be specified when reporting biological effects of MW/RF exposures:

1. Energy Source:
   a. Frequency
   b. Modulation (*e.g.*, pulse frequency, duration, peak power)
   c. Polarization
   d. Incident power density
   e. Energy distribution
   f. Number and schedule of exposures
   g. Duration of exposure
2. Dosimetry:
   a. Field probes
   b. Thermometry
   c. Methods and standards used for calibrating measurement devices
   d. Specific absorption rate
3. Exposure Apparatus:
   a. Source, method of propagation
   b. Animal chamber: materials, dimensions
   c. Exposure chamber: materials, dimensions
   d. Number of animals per chamber
   e. Spatial relations among components
4. Environmental Variables:
   a. Temperature
   b. Humidity

c. Air flow
d. Ambient lighting conditions
e. Ambient noise
f. Time of day
5. Subject Variables:
  a. Species, sex, age, weight, and other attributes
  b. Maintenance conditions
  c. Interventions, such as drugs, electrodes, etc.
  d. Number of subjects

Physical and Physiological Scaling

Much of the research on biological effects of MW/RF has been done with small rodents having coefficients of heat absorption, field concentration effects, body surface areas, and thermal regulatory mechanisms significantly different from man. Adverse reaction in animals does not prove adverse effect in man; and lack of reaction in animals does not prove that man will not be affected. Even closely related species can differ widely in their responses. The literature is replete with "anomalous" reactions. Thus, results of exposure of common laboratory animals cannot be readily extrapolated to man unless some form of "scaling" among different animals species, and from animal to man, can be used in an accurate way to obtain a quantitatively valid extrapolation from the actual data observed.

Proper dosimetry in experimental procedures and realistic scaling factors for extrapolation of data from small laboratory animals to man are clearly necessary. Detailed discussions that serve as bases for scaling are available from several authors (123, 146, 217).

Durney *et al.* (105) have made calculations of the Specific Absorbed Rate (SAR) as a function of frequency for different sizes of laboratory animals and for man. This concept is useful to allow limited extrapolation from one species to another, but it should be used cautiously because of its limitations. Except for spherical models, the bodies studied have uniform properties. Because of the very different properties of bone and muscle, for instance, energy distribution may be much more uneven in animals than the models predict.

Cellular-Chromosome-Genetic Effects

Some investigators have reported chromosomal changes in various plant and animal cells in tissue culture (64, 150, 166, 364). *In vivo* treatment of Chinese hamster bone marrow and testis cells at 30 to 35 MHz for 1 to 9 days induced significant increases of abnormal cells (239). Other investigators have reported no changes (158). Reported chromosomal changes include structural aberrations (64, 364), polyploidy (363), and stickiness (64). Exposures ranged from 7 mW/cm^2 to more than 200 mW/cm^2. In a study of meiotic cells removed from exposed male mice (213), translocations were observed at meiosis I after 0.1 and 0.5 mW/cm^2.

Some investigators have reported chromosome changes in various plant and animal cells, and in tissue cultures (150, 166). These studies have been criticized by others who asserted that the systems were subjected to thermal stress. The chosen parameters of the applied field caused biologically significant field-induced force effects in *in vitro* experiments; many of these experiments have not yet been replicated independently (219, 299). Generally, in studies of the response of cells in culture, undetected temperature deviations between irradiated and control systems of no more than one degree can lead to erroneous interpretations. When investigating the effects of microwave and radiofrequency energies on biological systems, especially when some form of cellular response is involved, temperature control must be a major consideration.

Inferences of apparent genetic effects as a result of chromosome studies should be viewed with circumspection, since chromosome scoring techniques are tedious and require considerable skill (297). Such studies are very complex, and conclusions made from only fragmentary data should be suspect. In general, results such as chromosome stickiness are interesting but unresolved phenomena. Stickiness has been attributed to a spatial dissociation and reorganization of the nucleoproteins, and appears to be reversible.

Although studies of chromosome aberrations are potential early indicators of microwave-induced biological changes, such effects in tissue culture may reflect total response of a specific tissue, but not to genetic injury to the germinal epithelium where it is especially important. Chromosome aberrations may also be referable to somatic mutations, which has no relevance for transmissible genetic mutations.

There are several sources of error in estimating chromosome aberration frequencies and in using these estimates to evaluate microwave exposure. When cells are cultured *in vitro*, aberration frequencies may vary with post-exposure time in culture. There are also many variables in the tissue culture techniques used in various laboratories, which must be considered when comparing and evaluating results. The possible influence of other agents such as viruses, heat, chemicals, etc. which are known to produce chromosome anomalies, should not be ignored. It is possible to measure changes in cells when they are not a part of an integrated living system; it is not always correct, however, to extrapolate these findings to the intact organism, where the cell may be in a different relationship to other cells with differing sensitivities or protective capacities.

There have been some questions concerning the exact magnitude of the fields and temperatures within the receptacles containing cell cultures, blood samples, and solutions during exposure. Often the samples are placed in fields of known strength and power density, but due to the complex shapes of the vessels holding the samples, the actual fields acting on the cells or organisms are unknown. Also, it is difficult in some cases to determine whether the effects are specifically due to the fields or are simply due to a temperature rise. Attempts to measure the temperature of fields within the sample by conventional methods can produce perturbations that can significantly modify the results of the experiment (141).

Effects on mitochondria isolated from exposed animals have been reported (103), but there was no effect on rat liver mitochondria exposed *in vitro* to 2.4 GHz, 1 to 4 W/kg microwaves (111) or 1 to 12 GHz, at a maximum of 2 mW/cm^2 (327). No effect of microwave exposure has been found on a number of enzymes and proteins irradiated *in vitro* (11, 43, 51, 356). Albert *et al.* (9) exposed Chinese hamsters at 2450 MHz, 50 mW/cm^2, for 0.5 to 4.5 hours over a period of 1 to 21 days and found no change in liver ATP.

Miro *et al.* (249) exposed Swiss albino mice to pulsed 3105 MHz at 20 mW/cm^2 average power density (40 W/cm^2 peak) for 145 hours. Stimulation of splenic lymphopoiesis and increased ^{35}S methionine incorporation in spleen, thymus, and liver were found. The authors interpret these results as a sign of stimulation of cells belonging to the reticulo-endothelial system.

Both inhibitory and stimulatory effects on the expression of genetically regulated enzyme synthesis and on bacterial and mammalian cell growth were reported by Webb (357) at 59 to 143 GHz, 10 to 50 mW/cm^2; a frequency-dependent periodicity of the effects was described. Hill *et al.* (154) found no effect on growth of *Echerichia coli* exposed to 10 to 70 mW/cm^2 at 65 to 75 GHz. Other reports show interference with genetically controlled synthesis in bacteria (317, 366). Blackman *et al.* (52) reported no effect on bacterial growth at 68, 69, 70, 71, 72, 73, or 74 GHz at an incident power density estimated to be 0.3 mW/cm^2, or at 1.70 or 2.45 GHz between 0.005 and 50 mW/cm^2 (0.008 to 75 mW/g), nor was there any effect on mutagenesis in bacteria exposed to 2.45 GHz (10 and 50 mW/cm^2, 15 and 70 W/kg) or to 1.70 GHz (88 V/m; 3 W/kg) (54).

Baranski *et al.* (25, 29) were not able to attribute mutagenic effects or metabolic changes in Physarum polycephalum or Aspergillus nidulans to specific effects of 10 mW/cm^2, 2450 MHz continuous wave (CW) or pulsed microwaves. Correlli *et al.* (79) also reported no mutagenesis after exposure to 2.6 to 4.0 GHz at 20 W/kg. They investigated the effects of RF on colony-forming ability (CFA) and molecular structure (determined by infrared spectroscopy) of *E. coli B* bacterial cells in aqueous suspension. Cells were exposed for 10 hours at SAR's of 20 W/kg (equivalent to 50 mW/cm^2). No RF-induced effects on either CFA or molecular structure were observed.

The mutagenic potential of microwave energy has been evaluated by various techniques, including the dominant lethal test in mammalian systems (Varma and Traboulay, 1976; (48), genetic transmission in Drosophila (250, 265), and point mutations in bacterial assays (54), with inconsistent results.

Varma and co-workers (351) reported increased mutagenesis, using the dominant lethal test with male mice exposed to 10 and 50 mW/cm^2 1.7 GHz CW for 90 and 30 minutes, respectively. Mice exposed to 2.45 GHz CW at 100 mW/cm^2 for 10 minutes and at 50 mW/cm^2 three times, 10 minutes each within one day, also showed increased mutagenesis. Mice subjected to four exposures of 50 mW/cm^2, 10 minutes each over a period of two weeks, showed no increase of dominant lethality above control levels.

Berman and Carter (48) exposed male rats daily to 425 MHz CW (day 12 of gestation to 90 days of age, 10 mW/cm^2, 4 hours/day) or 2,450 MHz CW at 5, 10, or 28 mW/cm^2 from day 6 of gestation to 90 days of age, 4 or 5 hours/day. No significant evidence of germ cell mutagenesis or alteration in reproductive efficiency was detected. Although Mickey (238) reported increased mutagenesis in Drosophila exposed in a 20 MHz field, no effects on mutagenesis were observed by Pay et al. (265) using 2450 MHz, or by Mittler (250) with 3 MHz and 150 MHz RF energy.

There is no satisfactory evidence of microwave-induced genetic effects at low to modest power densities (28). It is known that the rate of induction of mutations increases with increasing temperature. It is possible, therefore, that artifacts or thermal stress could be factors in some of the reported studies.

Recent experimental studies on primitive organisms (25, 29, 54) and on rodents (185, 351, 352), have confirmed earlier findings that microwave exposure at power densities below 10 mW/cm^2 are not mutagenic in these organisms.

Changes of cell membrane permeability have also been attributed to RF energy (33). Other studies (197) have failed to find effects which are different from those resulting from RF heating. Janiak and Szmigielski (167) likewise reported no significant differences in the sequence and time-course of cell membrane injury between cells treated in a water bath and those heated with 2,450 MHz microwaves.

Overt thermal effects due to radiofrequency and microwave energy absorption have been demonstrated and documented. The reports of effects which appear to depend on specific frequencies and amplitudes or "windows" (2) would imply biological responses that may not always be due to a rise in temperature. Prohofsky (276) has suggested that low-lying longitudinal vibrational modes of DNA molecules could be induced or enhanced by electromagnetic fields at microwave frequencies of 3 GHz or higher. Such induced modes could theoretically produce conformational changes in the DNA molecule and could result in biologically significant functional alterations. Fröhlich (117) has similarly suggested microwave interactions with macromolecular biologically active complexes. Illinger (161, 162) has treated the problem of molecular interaction from a quantum mechanical approach. He suggests the possibility of field-induced quasi-resonant transitions occurring at frequencies higher than 10 GHz from the excitation of coherent vibrational modes. Although some experiments seem to provide results that support such a theory, it has been pointed out that great care must be exercised in differentiating between actual biological interactions and cyclic and multiple resonances in cavity, waveguide and other exposure systems which have the capability of creating multiple reflections (153).

The principal technical problems in studying RF-induced effects on cells is that the studies are often conducted using conventional apparatus designed for cell studies—flasks, dishes, holders, agitators, water baths, incubators, etc. Various elements of this apparatus may distort RF fields in such a way that the SAR of energy in the cell cultures may be considerably higher or lower than field measurements would indicate. Some progress has been made in designing cell culture apparatus that will provide accurate, calibrated exposure to RF fields, but results of much of the earlier work on cell and tissue cultures must be questioned with regard to the actual absorbed RF energy in the cell culture media (141, 225, 230).

The present knowledge of biophysical mechanisms underlying cell membrane function, and functional and structural properties of subcellular components is limited. Interpretation of studies of such phenomena and their biological significance, therefore, requires considerable circumspection. The anomalous behavior of the "bound water" of membranes as reported by Grant (134) may help in providing explanations for such effects.

Growth and Development

There are a few reports which suggest that particular combinations of exposure frequency, duration, and power density produce effects on embryonic development and post-natal growth. Alterations in development have been reported in insects (61), chick embryos (349, 350), and rodents (45, 46, 286, 287, 290).

Olsen (258) has provided a thermal basis for explanation of the microwave-induced teratogenic effects in the meal worm *Tenebrio molitor* reported by Carpenter and Livstone (61), Lindauer *et al.* (196), and Liu *et al.* (198), Olsen (257) and Pickard and Olsen (270) noted the threshold of teratogenesis in *Tenebrio* to be associated with a rise of pupal temperature in excess of 10°C.

Van Ummersen (349, 350) reported inhibition of growth and development of chick embryos exposed to 2,450 MHz (CW) 400 to 20 mW/cm^2, 4.5 minutes to 5 hours (ΔT up to 19°C). Since all embryos in which effects were produced experienced a significant temperature increase, the observed deleterious effects were no doubt due to heating.

Quail embryos exposed to 30 mW/cm^2, 2,450 MHz (CW) for 4 hours on each of the first 5 days of incubation, did not develop gross deformities or changes in hatchability that could be correlated with exposure (221). Microwave-induced temperature within the eggs varied from 34 to 37°C, which is the normal incubation temperature.

In another study, Japanese Quail embryos were exposed during the first

12 days of development to 2.45 GHz microwaves at an incident power density of 5 mW/cm^2 and specific absorption rate of 4.03 mW/g. No gross deformities were observed in the exposed quail when examined and sacrificed at 24 to 36 hours after hatch. No significant changes in the total body weight or weight of the heart, liver, gizzard, adrenals, and pancreas were found in the treated birds. Hematological parameters were also measured in the study. The results showed a statistically significant increase in hemoglobin and a statistically significant decrease in monocytes in birds exposed to microwaves. No statistically significant changes in hematocrit, red blood cells, total white blood cells, lymphocytes, heterophils, basophils, or eosinophils were detected (220).

Rugh et al. (286, 287) reported abnormalities in mouse fetuses exposed in an environmentally controlled waveguide at days 7 to 13 of gestation to absorbed 2,450 MHz (CW) microwaves in the range of 12.6 to 33.5 J/Kg, equivalent to 123 mW/cm^2 incident power. Hemorrhages, resorptions, exencephaly, stunting, and fetal death were observed. Differential effects at different gestations days suggest thermal sensitivity of embryos. In a further study, Rugh and McManaway (288, 289) demonstrated that lowering the dam's body temperature with pentobarbital could prevent the teratogenic effects of thermal loading with microwaves.

Laskey et al. (184) exposed pregnant rats to 2,450 MHz CW microwaves, 100 mW/cm^2, for 8 to 13 minutes on days 2, 5 (pre-implantation stage), 8 (organogenesis stage), or 15 (fetal stage). These exposures produced group mean rectal temperatures ranging from 41.4 to 42.8°C (sham = 38.0°C). No changes occurred in the 5-day embryos, but there was an increased number of resorbed fetuses in the day 8 exposure and a decrease in weight of live fetuses exposed on day 8 or day 13. No obvious abnormalities were seen in any of the litters when examined on day 19 of gestation.

Dietzel et al. (97–99) exposed pregnant rats with a 27.12 MHz diathermy unit at 55, 70, or 100 W, which was sufficient to raise the animals colonic temperatures to 39, 40, or 42°C. The rats were exposed once between days 1 and 16 of gestation. The fetuses were examined near term. The peak incidence of anomalies was found to occur on gestation days 13 to 14, when 16 percent of the fetuses were abnormal. This fetal wastage, as in the studies by Rugh et al. (286, 287), are clearly associated with a general body temperature increase in the dam.

Lin et al. (195) studied the effect of repeated exposures of C3H mice to 48 MHz. The animals were exposed to 0.5 mW/cm^2 (63.25 V/m) in a TEM exposure chamber for 1 hour a day, 5 days a week, beginning on the 4th to 7th day post-partum, for 10 weeks. The formed elements in the blood were not affected by the exposure. The means of body mass of the irradiated and control animals were comparable. No significant differences in lesion onset, incidence, prevalence, extent, or type were observed when repeated RF-exposed animals were compared with sham-control groups. During the period of the study, no cataracts were noted. Fertility differences among irradiated and control animals were not detected. Body growth patterns did not differ among sham and RF-exposed animals.

Employing a multimodal cavity at 2,450 MHz, Chernovetz et al. (65) irradiated pregnant mice with a single "intense" dose of 38 mW/g for 10 minutes (22.8 J/g) on gestation day 11, 12, 13, or 14. This dose resulted in 10 percent maternal lethality. The exposure during late organogenesis or early fetal stage caused no change in fetal mortality or morbidity when compared to shams. In another study, Chernovetz et al. (66) noted an increased rate of resorption in rats after a single absorbed dose of 30 mW/g for 20 minutes on gestation days 10 to 16.

In studies of effects of in utero exposure of Long-Evans rats to 2,450 MHz CW, Michaelson et al. (232, 233) found no adverse effects on the dam or offspring when gestation length or litter size were examined. The rats were exposed at 10 or 40 mW/cm² for 1 hour on day 9 (organogenesis) or day 16 (fetal stage) of gestation. Enhanced maturation as indicated by adrenocortical response was suggested.

Jensh et al. (168) exposed pregnant rats to 10 mW/cm², 915 MHz 8 hours daily on days 1 to 14 of gestation. There were no teratogenic effects; colonic temperature was not increased.

Berman et al. (49) exposed mice to 2450 MHz at 3.4 to 28 mW/cm² 100 minutes daily throughout pregnancy. Mean live fetal weight per litter decreased with exposure at the highest power density. There was an increased incidence of cranioschisis in exposed fetuses. Estimates of the mean dose rate ranged from 2.0 to 22.2 mW/g.

Bereznitskaya (45, 46) exposed mice to 3000 MHz, 10 mW/cm² which resulted in increased fetal wastage. No definite abnormalities or inborn genetic defects were found. Neonatal mice exposed to 10.5, 19.27, or 26.6 MHz pulsed in a magnetic field of 55 amp/m and an electric field of 8000 V/m, 40 minutes per day for 5 days did not show any evidence of alteration in growth and development (322).

Boak et al. (57) administered "shortwave" radiation (10 MHz) to rabbits from the 29th day of life through several matings and pregnancies. The total exposure time ranged between 30 and 75 hours, during which the colonic temperature of the animals was raised to 41 to 42°C. There was no interference with mating, fertilization, or development of the young in utero. Litter sizes were not significantly different from those of the control animals.

A few human data are available from studies in which radiofrequency heating of the pelvic region was used in the treatment of gonorrhea, pelvic inflammatory disease, endometriosis, carcinoma of the uterus, or pelvic peritonitis (124, 298). Gellhorn (124) raised pelvic temperature in women to 115°F (46.1°C). Although he was concerned about possible harmful effects, he did not allude to specific complications. Rubin and Erdman (284) reported case histories of four women treated with microwave diathermy (2,450 MHz,

100 W output) for chronic pelvic inflammatory disease who were or became pregnant during the course of the therapy. Three women delivered normal infants; the fourth, who received eight treatments during the first 59 days of pregnancy, aborted on day 67 but delivered a normal baby following a subsequent pregnancy during which she again received microwave therapy. The authors concluded that microwaves did not interfere with ovulation, conception, and pregnancy. Daels (86, 87) used microwaves to ease parturition in women. No evidence of injury was manifested in a one-year follow-up of the children.

The reports on effects of microwave exposure on early development have been reviewed by Baranski and Czerski (28), who concluded that no serious effects are to be expected at power densities below 10 mW/cm^2 under usual exposure conditions. They further note that defects, when observed, are the result of hyperthermia. There are numerous reports of abnormalities from the induction of systemic hyperthermia of 2.5 to 5°C above the normal temperature for the species, by exposure of a pregnant animal to elevated temperatures at specific critical developmental stages of the fetus (109, 110). It would thus appear that in the reports of microwave-induced developmental abnormalities, it is the temperature rise in the fetus, irrespective of the manner in which it was produced, that caused the damage.

The Gonads

The effect of microwaves on the testes has been studied fairly extensively (112, 133, 163). Exposure of the scrotal area at high power densities (> 50 mW/cm^2) results in varying degrees of testicular damage such as edema, enlargement of the testis, atrophy, fibrosis, and coagulation necrosis of seminiferous tubules in rats and rabbits exposed to 2,450, 3,000, and 10,000 MHz. Exposure to 3,000 MHz, 8 mW/cm^2 did not affect mating of mice or rats (248). Pituitary gonadotropic function was preserved in female mice exposed to 3,000 MHz, 10 mW/cm^2, twice daily for 5 months (45).

There are reports that chronic "low-level" exposure to microwaves can result in impairment of spermatogenesis and reproductive function without measurable temperature increase of the testes (47, 104). And there is general agreement that high power density exposure can affect the testes and ovary. These responses can nevertheless be related to the heating of the organs. The sensitivity of the testes to heat is well known (348). Comparable heating of the scrotum in rats with 2,450 MHz CW microwaves or by immersion in water to temperatures of 36, 38, 40, and 42°C resulted in comparable damage at each temperature (252).

Neuroendocrine and Endocrine Effects

Response of the endocrine system of rats to whole-body exposure to microwaves has been studied in recent years, but most of the reports are based on relatively short exposures at modest to high power densities (136, 137, 157, 203, 241, 242, 342). A comprehensive review of neuroendocrine responses to microwave exposure has been presented by Lu et al. (207).

Some investigators believe that endocrine changes result from stimulation of the hypothalamic-hypophysial system due to thermal interactions at the hypothalamic or immediately adjacent levels of organization, the hypophysis itself (pituitary), or the particular endocrine gland or end-organ under study. According to other investigators, the observed changes are the result of direct microwave interactions with the central nervous system. In any case, neuroendocrine perturbations cannot be considered as necessarily pathological because the function of the neuroendocrine system is to maintain homeostasis; and hormone levels will fluctuate to maintain such organismic stability.

HYPOTHALAMIC-HYPOPHYSIAL-ADRENAL RESPONSE

Several investigators have reported biochemical and physiological changes as a result of microwave exposure, which suggest an adrenal effect. According to Petrov and Syngayevskaya (268), 3 and 24 hours after dogs were exposed to 3,000 MHz, 10 mW/cm^2, the serum corticoid content had increased by 100 to 150 percent above the original level. Serum potassium decreased 5 to 10 percent, and sodium increased by the same amount. They also noted that the susceptibility of rats to microwave exposure sharply increased one week after bilateral adrenalectomy. Chronic exposure of animals to microwaves (CW or pulsed) was accompanied by reduced cholinesterase activity and an increased amount of 17-ketosteroids in the urine, reduced ascorbic acid, and reduced weight of the adrenal glands (104).

Demokidova (93) reported increased adrenal and pituitary gland weight in rats exposed to 69.7 MHz; 12 V/m; 1 hour/day; 1.5 months and increased adrenal weight in infant rats exposed to 48 V/m; 4 hours/day; 1.5 months. The same author, however, reported decreased weight of the adrenal glands in infant rats exposed to 14.88 MHz, 70 V/m.

In female mice exposed to 3,000 MHz (10 mW/cm^2) twice daily for five months, the pituitary gland retained its gonadotropic function, although its activity was reduced in comparison with that of nonexposed animals (46). Tolgskaya and Gordon (340) noted the reversibility of changes in the neurosecretory function of the hypothalamus when exposure was terminated. Rabbits exposed to 3,000 MHz (50 to 60 mW/cm^2) 4 hours daily for 20 days tended to show a decline in the amount of urinary 17-hydrocorticosteriods (17-OHCS) at the beginning of exposure, followed by a gradual return to normal (186). No change was evident in the excretion of 17-ketosteroids in the urine.

In rats exposed to microwaves of varying intensity, no quantitative changes in corticosterone were found in the adrenals and blood plasma

(240). Prepubescent hypophysectomized rats displayed no differences in adrenal growth rate when treated with pituitary homogenates collected either from rats exposed to microwaves, or from control rats.

Rats exposed to 2,450 MHz (CW), 10 mW/cm² for 4 hours, showed no change in adrenal weight, phenylethanolamine-N-methyl transferase (PNMT) activity or epinephrine levels (263). After 16 hours of exposure, however, decrease in adrenal epinephrine (32 percent) was significant and PNMT activity was elevated (25 percent). There were no statistically significant differences (p > 0.1) in adrenal or plasma corticosterone levels between exposed and sham-exposed animals. It should be noted, however, that similar alterations in epinephrine levels can occur in rats subjected to a stress such as immobilization or acute exposure to cold.

Increased adrenal function due to microwave exposure has been correlated with colonic temperature increase in rats (203). Plasma corticosterone levels in hypophysectomized rats exposed to 60 mW/cm² for 60 minutes were below control levels; when rats were pretreated with dexamethasone before being exposed to 50 mW/cm² for 60 minutes, the corticosterone response was suppressed (204). These results suggest that the microwave-induced corticosterone response observed in intact rats depends on adrenocortico-tropic hormone secretion by the pituitary, *i.e.*, the adrenal gland is not the primary endocrine gland stimulated by microwaves. The evidence from these experiments is consistent with the hypothesis that the stimulation of the adrenal axis in microwave exposed rats is a systemic, integrative process due to a general hyperthermia (203).

HYPOTHALAMIC-HYPOPHYSIAL-THYROID RESPONSE

The literature offers comparatively few experimental studies of the effect of RF or microwaves on the thyroid. No alterations in thyroid structure or function attributable to microwave exposure were noted in rats subjected to 2,450 MHz, CW, 1 mW/cm² continuously for 8 weeks or 10 mW/cm², 8 hours/day for 8 weeks (244). On the other hand, Baranski *et al.* (34) reported a stimulatory influence of 5 mW/cm² on the trapping and secretory function of the thyroid gland of rabbits, which correlated with altered histology of the thyroids.

In rats exposed for 16 hours to 2,450 MHz (CW) at 10 to 25 mW/cm², tests of thyroid function in general showed no statistically significant devia-tions from the norm, except that in animals with a 1.0 to 1.7°C increase in colonic temperature, there was a reduction in the ability of the thyroid to concentrate iodide (263). Decreased thyroid gland weight was noted in infant rats exposed to 69.7 MHz; 48 V/m, 4 hours/day; 1.5 months (93).

Increased thyroid hormone secretion has been correlated with microwave-induced thyroid temperature increase in dogs (208, 209). Vetter (353) found that serum protein levels increased as a function of power density, indicating an alteration of protein synthesis or catabolism; levels of thyroid hormone decreased as power density of 2,450 MHz CW energy was increased from 5 to 25 mW/cm^2. This agrees with the findings of Lu *et al.* (206) who reported that serum thyroxine levels were transiently elevated after exposure of rats at 1 mW/cm^2, (2,450 MHz) and were depressed after exposure at 20 mW/cm^2. None of the reported alterations were irreversible or resulted in morbidity.

It has been reported that microwave-exposed workers have developed enlargement of the thyroid gland as well as increased radioactive iodine uptake (RAIU), but in some cases without clinical symptoms of hyperfunction (106, 316).

Perturbation of the thyroid gland may be the result of an indirect effect, the thermal stress on the body producing an hypothalmic-hypophysial response. This is consistent with microwave-induced thermal stimulation of hypothalamic-hypophysial-thyroid (HHT) activity (234). McLees and Finch (218) point out that temperature elevation and heat stress have been associated with alterations in radioactive iodine (RAI) turnover rate. The HHT axis has been shown to be sensitive to environmental temperature (74). Differences in rate of temperature change or alteration in thermal gradients could also result in qualitative differences in endocrine response.

In summary, the effects of RF exposure on endocrine function are generally consistent with both immediate and long-term responses to thermal input and to non-specific stress, which can also arise from thermal loading. Changes found in plasma levels of corticosterone and growth hormone are typical reactions of animals to non-specific stress; indeed, great care is required in performing experiments to ensure that the changes in hormone level do not result from stress caused by handling of the animals or the novelty of the experimental situation.

Metabolic Effects

Biochemical alterations have been reported to result from exposure to MW/RF energies. Such effects generally appear to be reversible; and no well-defined characteristic response pattern has been determined, nor is it known whether the changes are direct or indirect effects of exposure.

Dumansky *et al.* (104) reported a decrease in liver glycogen content together with increased lactic acid levels and phosphorylase activity, which was interpreted as evidence of impairment of glycogen synthesis in the liver of rats chronically exposed to 2.45 or 10 GHz microwaves of 5 to 20 μW/cm^2. Exposure to 2.45 or 10 GHz microwaves at 25 to 1,000 μW/cm^2 decreased the proteolytic activity of the mucous membrane of the small intestines of experimental animals, whereas the invertase and adenosine triphosphatase activity increased. Altered proteolytic activity was suggested to be due to alteration in the structure and physiocochemical characteristics of the mucous membrane. Reduced synthesis of macroglobulin and macroglobulin antibodies resulted from exposure of experimental animals to 50 $\mu W/cm^2$ (211).

Dose-dependent transient elevations in serum glucose, blood urea nitrogen, and uric acid were noted following far-field exposure of rabbits to 2.45 GHz for two hours at intensities of 5, 10, and 25 mW/cm^2 (355). There was a detectable difference between continuous wave and pulse-modulated exposures of equivalent average power density; colonic temperature increased 1.7 to 3.0°C at 10 and 25 mW/cm^2. Exposure of rats for 15 minutes to pulsed 2.86 GHz at 5, 10, 20, 50, or 100 mW/cm^2 resulted in statistically significant changes in serum albumin and phosphorous levels only at 100 mW/cm^2 (119); there was no change in serum glucose levels in rats exposed to 2.86 and 0.43 GHz pulse-modulated fields at an average power density of 5 mW/cm^2. Single or repeated exposures of rabbits to 3 or 10 GHz at 5 to 25 mW/cm^2 resulted in alterations in serum albumin/globulin ratio, an effect attributable to effects on the liver or adrenals (329, 330).

Baranski (23) found inconsistent changes in cholinesterase activity in both rabbit and guinea pig brains following 3 months of exposure 1 hour per day to pulsed fields of 25 mW/cm^2. He also found a decrease in cholinesterase activity in the brains of guinea pigs after a single 3-hour exposure to 3.5 mW/cm^2 of pulsed 2.45 GHz microwaves. Increase to 25 mW/cm^2 caused a further decrease in activity. Pulsed energy was found to produce a more severe effect than continuous wave exposures of the same average power density, suggesting that these effects are due to peak fields. Nikogosyan (253) found an increase in blood cholinesterase activity after a single 90-minute exposure to 10 cm waves at 40 mW/cm^2. Revutsky and Edelman (278) also report an increase in specific cholinesterase activity in rabbit blood exposed *in vitro* to 12.6 cm microwaves. It should be noted that what is measured in blood is "pseudocholinesterase" which has no neural-related activity.

Olcerst and Rabinowitz (255) found no effect on aqueous cholinesterase exposed to 2,450 MHz CW up to 125 mW/cm^2 for 1/2 hour or 25 mW/cm^2 for 3 hours. No effect was found on cholinesterase activity in defibrinated rabbit blood exposed for 3 hours to 21, 35, or 64 mW/cm^2, 2,450 MHz, CW or pulsed. Under similar exposure conditions, there was no effect on release of bound calcium or magnesium from rabbit red blood cells.

Ho and Edwards (156) studied oxygen consumption in mice exposed to 2.45 GHz at various SAR's in a waveguide exposure system, and found that the animals adjusted homeostatically to SAR of 10.4 mW/g or greater by a decrease in metabolic rate to compensate for thermal loading. Normal metabolic activity was resumed following cessation of exposure.

Stavinoha et al. (321) exposed mice and rats to 10 MHz energy with a magnetic field of 55 A/m and an electric field of 8,000 V/m in a near field synthesizer. There was no effect on growth of mice exposed on the 5th through the 10th days after birth. Among adult mice exposed 40 minutes a day for 5 days, a substantially higher death rate was seen in both the irradiated and thermally heated male mice as compared to similarly treated female mice and male control mice. The irradiation and thermal treatments produced an average rise in rectal temperature of approximately 1°C. After one exposure of rats for 40 minutes, the average rise in rectal temperature was approximately 1°C. No lethality was observed in either irradiated or thermally heated animals. No remarkable changes were seen in the levels of acetylcholine or catecholamines in the rats after RF or thermal exposure. No changes were seen in adenosine 5' monophasphate (AMP), but some irradiation-related changes in high energy phosphates were seen. Significant changes were seen, however, in the concentrations of several cations in the brain after exposure. Most notably, the concentration of zinc in the cerebral cortex increased from 0.28 μmole/mg to 0.53 μmole/mg after irradiation.

Changes in zinc concentration have been previously reported to be related to temperature and mw/RF radiation phenomena (138, 291). Whereas zinc was increased significantly in the cerebral cortex and liver of 19 MHz irradiated rats (321), testicular zinc uptake was decreased in rats following a 5-minute exposure to 24.5 GHz, 250 mW/cm^2 (138). Rupp et al. (291) also reported a significant loss of zinc from whole liver homogenates from rats with a core temperature increase to 45°C.

Alteration in zinc content has previously been associated with deficiency diseases in thermal environments or in surgical trauma, and is required for adequate wound healing (321). Shifts in plasma and tissue concentration of iron and probably zinc have been related to stress (42). From recent studies, it has been found that iron concentration can shift in response to a non-dialyzable factor from polymorphonuclear leukocytes. It may be that this polypeptide factor is released from lymphocytes and polymorphonuclear leukocytes in response to thermal stress.

Effects on the Nervous System

Transient changes in central nervous system (CNS) function have been reported following microwave exposure. Although some reports describe the thermal nature of microwave energy absorption, others implicate non-thermal or "specific" microwave effects at the molecular and cellular levels. The first report of the effect of microwave energy on conditional response activity in experimental animals was made by Gordon et al. (131). In subsequent years, the study of non-thermal effects of microwaves gradually occupied the central role in electrophysiological studies in the Soviet Union (254).

Yakovleva et al. (362) reported that single and repeated exposures of rats to microwaves, 5 to 15 mW/cm^2, weakened the "excitation process" and decreased the "functional mobility" of cells in the cerebral cortex. Edematous changes were most often noted throughout the cortex. The greatest number of altered cells was noted with repeated exposures at 15 mW/cm^2.

In a study with audiogenic-seizure-susceptible mice and rats, Kitsovskaya

(176, 178) found that the seizure response to noise was transiently suppressed after exposure to 3,000 MHz pulsed microwaves at an average power density of 10 mW/cm². Changes in olfactory threshold in humans following occupational exposures have also been reported (118, 126, 202).

Tolgskaya et al. (341) studied the effects on rats of pulsed and CW, 3,000 and 10,000 MHz microwaves at various intensities. More pronounced morphological changes in the CNS were found following 3,000 MHz than 10,000 MHz at 1 to 10 mW/cm². Pulsed waves were more effective than CW—an observation also made by Marha (214). Additional studies comparing pulsed and CW microwaves can be found in the monograph by Tolgskaya and Gordon (340). They noted that the microwave-induced alterations in conditioned reflex activity are functional in nature. They are reversible; they disappear at the same time the conditional reflex activity of the animals is being restored upon cessation of exposure to microwaves.

Some investigators suggest that microwave energy absorption may affect hypothalamic and midbrain function and also affect cerebral, cortical, and reticular system function (336, 365). According to Gvozdikova et al. (147), the greatest cortical sensitivity occurs in the meter-range, less in the decimeter, and least in the centimeter microwave band.

ELECTROENCEPHALOGRAPHIC CHANGES

Several investigators have reported that microwave exposure produces alterations in the electroencephalogram (EEG) (21, 30, 41, 147, 172–174, 199, 306).

Baldwin et al. (21) exposed the heads of rhesus monkeys to 225 to 440 MHz CW in a resonant cavity and noted a progressively generalized slowing and some increase in amplitude of EEG patterns accompanied by signs of agitation, drowsiness, akinesia, and nystagmus, as well as autonomic sensory and motor abnormalities. There were signs of diencephalic and mesencephalic disturbances, alternation of arousal and drowsiness, together with confirming EEG signs. The response depended on orientation of the head in the field and reflections from the surrounding enclosure.

EEG tracings in rabbits exposed to 3,000 MHz (pulsed) 5 mW/cm² showed a slight desynchronization from the motor region; at 20 mW/cm² variations in the amplitude were observed; 300 MHz had a greater effect than 3000 MHz (67, 68). Pulsed microwaves produced a greater effect than CW microwaves. Baranski and Edelwejn (30, 32) reported that rabbits exposed to 10,000 MHz (pulsed) 4 mW/cm² (single exposure) showed no changes in EEG tracings, but exposure to 3,000 MHz, 7 mW/cm² three hours a day for 60 days produced functional and morphological changes. Serdiuk (304) reported changes in the EEG and conditioned reflexes in rats and rabbits exposed to 50 MHz, 0.5 to 6 V/m, 10 to 12 hours/day for 180 days. Changes in conditional reflexes were also reported in rats exposed to 70 MHz, 150 V/m, 60 minutes/day, 4 months (201).

A review of the literature of EEG effects requires an awareness of certain deficiencies in methodology and interpretation. The EEG is difficult to quantify due to its time-varying waveform. The use of metallic electrodes either implanted in the brain or attached to the scalp also makes many of the reports on EEG or evoked responses (ER) questionable. Johnson and Guy (169) have pointed out that such metallic electrodes grossly perturb the field and produce greatly enhanced absorption of energy in the vicinity of the electrodes. Such enhancement produces artifacts in the biological material under investigation. Artifacts also result from pick-up of fields by electrodes and leads during the recording of EEG's or ER's while the animal is being exposed (344).

Bawin et al. (41) reported that electromagnetic energy at 147 MHz, amplitude-modulated at brain wave frequencies (8 and 16 Hz) influenced spontaneous and conditioned EEG patterns in cats at 1 mW/cm^2. These amplitude-modulated 147 MHz fields induced changes only when the amplitude modulation frequency approached that of physiological bioelectric function rhythms; no effects were seen at modulation frequencies either below 8 Hz or above 16 Hz. Bawin and Adey (39, 40) also reported that calcium efflux from chick brains increased 10–15 percent when exposed in vitro to 147 MHz fields, amplitude modulated at 9, 11, 16, and 20 Hz. The authors suggest that electromagnetic fields may induce conformational changes of the neuronal membrane, resulting in displacement of the surface-bound cations. Blackman et al. (53) have reported essentially similar results. Adey and Bawin (2, 39, 40) and Grodsky (135) suggest that such alterations by low-frequency modulated, low-intensity radiofrequency fields may involve field interactions with coherent membrane surface charge sites. The phenomenon is not a general property of RF energy, but depends upon the amplitude modulation of the RF energy in a narrow frequency band around 16 Hz.

HISTOPATHOLOGY

Cellular changes in the nervous systems of small animals following microexposure at 10 mW/cm^2 have been reported (337, 339, 340). Degeneration of neurons in the cerebral cortex and tissue changes in the kidney and myocardium of rabbits have been produced by exposure to 200 MHz. Head exposure of rabbits to 2,450 MHz resulted in focal lesions in the cerebral cortex; whole-body exposures of rats to 1,430 MHz produced lesions of the brain (94, 256, 338).

Exposure of cats for one hour to 10,000 MHz, 400 mW/cm^2 resulted in injury to cerebral and spinal cord nerve cells; changes occurred in the Nissl bodies and other components of nerve cells (50). On the other hand, rabbits exposed to 10,000 MHz (pulsed) 4 mW/cm^2 showed no evidence of morphological damage to the brain, but exposure to 3,000 MHz did produce such changes (30).

Tolgskaya *et al.* (341) have investigated the influence of pulsed and CW 3,000 MHz and 10,000 MHz on the morphology of nervous tissue in rats and rabbits. With exposure to 3,000 MHz (110 and 40 mW/cm^2), symptoms of overheating were observed, often leading to death. Vascular disorders such as edema and hemorrhages in the brain and internal organs were predominant. In repeated, but less prolonged exposure, vascular disorders and degenerative changes in internal organs and the nervous system were less severe. With repeated exposures, the animals were better able to withstand successive exposures; they continued to gain weight, body temperature after irradiation quickly recovered, and overheating was not evident.

At high field intensities, when death is a result of hyperthermia, the vascular changes are those of hyperemia, hemorrhage, and acute dystrophic manifestations (26, 101, 246). At lower field intensities, the changes are of a more general dystrophic character, and proliferation of the glia and vascular changes are not as prominent.

Albert and DeSantis (8) reported morphological changes in the brains of Chinese hamsters following exposure to 2,450 MHz CW microwaves at power densities of 25 and 50 mW/cm^2. Exposure durations varied from 30 minutes to 14 hours/day for 22 days. Both light and electron microscopic examination revealed alterations in the hypothalamus and subthalamic structures of exposed animals, whereas other regions of the brain appeared unaltered. It should be noted that SAR's as high as 4 W/kg per incident 1 mW/cm^2 could occur under these conditions. Peak SAR's could reach 40 to 200 W/kg in selected brain regions.

In subsequent studies at 1,760 and 2,450 MHz, 10 and 20 mW/cm^2, Albert (3, 5, 6) described similar cytoplasmic vacuolization of neurons, irregular swelling of axons and decrease in dendritic spines of cortical neurons. The axonal swelling and spine changes were seen only in chronic exposures, whereas neuronal changes were observed in acute exposure. In all studies no signs of permanent degenerative changes were recorded, and reversibility was noted 2 hours after exposure (4, 5, 6). The author concluded that while it is possible the higher exposure levels (25 and 50 mW/cm^2) could result in thermal effects, it is unlikely that 10 mW/cm^2 would result in significant thermalization of the whole brain, but they did not rule out the possibility of "hot spots." Exposure of rats at 10 mW/cm^2 to 2,450 and 2,800 MHz resulted in average hypothalmic temperature increases of 0.4°C or less. This increase is less than hypothalamic temperature increases observed during an animal's normal activity (5, 7).

EFFECTS ON THE BLOOD-BRAIN BARRIER

Sutton *et al.* (328) used 2,450 MHz to produce selective hyperthermia of the brain in rats. They then studied the integrity of the blood-brain barrier with horseradish peroxidase (HRP), a protein tracer that can be detected quantitatively. The rat brains were heated to 40, 42, and 45°C. Barrier integrity was disrupted after heating for more than 45 minutes at 40°C.

Animals with brains heated to 45°C survived for only 8 to 15 minutes. The most common site of vascular leakage was the white matter adjacent to the granular cell layer of the cerebellum. Sutton concluded that to prevent blood-brain barrier disruption, brain temperatures must not exceed 40°C in the absence of body-core hypothermia.

Albert et al. (7) also used HRP as a tracer and reported regions of leakage in the microvasculature of the brains of Chinese hamsters exposed to 2,450 MHz radiation at 10 mW/cm^2 for 2 to 8 hours. In control animals, an extravascular reaction product was found only in brain regions normally lacking a blood-brain barrier. In a later paper, Albert (4) reported that continuation of his earlier studies indicated that a partial restoration of the blood-brain barrier's impermeability may have occurred within 1 hour after exposure ceased, and that restoration was virtually complete within 2 hours. Albert believes that these changes may be clinically subacute and probably cause no lasting ill effects. It is nevertheless important to note that such leakage of the microvasculature of the brain occurs irregularly; it was observed in approximately 50 percent of exposed animals and in 20 percent of control animals studied by Albert and associates (3, 4).

Oscar and Hawkins (260) reported that a single exposure of rats to 1.3 GHz pulse-modulated microwaves for 20 minutes (0.1 to 2 mW/cm^2) induces a temporary change in the permeability of small inert polar molecules across the blood-brain barrier of rats. Increases in permeability were observed for mannitol and inulin but not for dextran, both immediately and 4 hours after exposure, but not 24 hours after exposure. The authors consider the possibility of local heating due to hot spots, since the greatest blood-brain barrier alteration occurs in the cerebellum and medulla, or close to the neck region of rats. Attempts to duplicate the findings of Oscar and Hawkins (260) have yielded equivocal results (63), or have resulted in failure (274, 319).

Merritt et al. (222), exposed rats to 1.2 GHz CW and pulsed microwaves for 30 minutes at power densities from 2 to 75 mW/cm^2, and found no alteration in the blood-brain barrier unless there was an increase of 4°C in the brain.

It is important to realize the methods used to investigate blood-brain barrier permeability are still controversial. Permeability changes in cerebral blood vessels occur under various conditions, including those that produce heat necrosis (282). Most techniques used to measure blood-brain barrier permeability, in fact, measure the net influence of several variables on brain uptake, and do not differentiate among the effects of changes in the vascular space, alterations of blood flow, and variations in membrane permeability (260).

Behavioral Effects

Studies have been conducted on the effects of MW/RF on the performance of tasks by trained rats, rhesus and squirrel monkeys (89, 90, 120, 121,

194, 296). All of the studies indicated that the radiation would suppress performance of the trained task, and that an energy power density/dose threshold for achieving the suppression existed. Depending on duration and other parameters of exposure, the threshold power density for affecting trained behavior ranged from 5 to 50 mW/cm^2.

Justesen and King (170) used a 2,450 MHz (CW) multimodal resonating cavity system to investigate conditioned operant behavior in rats with a recurrent cycle of exposure, 5 minutes on and 5 minutes off, over a 60-minute period at average absorbed energy rates of 3.0, 6.2, and 9.2 W/kg. The animal's performance usually stopped near the end of the 60-minute test period during exposure with an energy absorption rate of 6.2 W/kg; at 9.2 W/kg, this effect occurred much earlier in the test period. Hunt et al. (159), also using a multimodal resonating cavity to expose rats to 2,450 MHz (pulsed), found effects on exploratory activity, swimming, and discrimination performance of vigilance task, after a 30-minute exposure at about 6 W/kg.

Lobanova (200) exposed rats to 3,000 MHz pulsed microwaves, after which the rats were tested for swimming time. A decrease in endurance was noted after exposure to power-time combinations ranging from 100 mW/cm^2 for 5 minutes to 20 mW/cm^2 for 90 minutes.

Lin et al. (194) exposed rats to 918 MHz (CW) at levels of 10, 20, or 40 mW/cm^2 for 30 minutes. No effects on response rates were noted at the two lower levels, but at 40 mW/cm^2, the animal's performance decreased after 5 minutes of exposure and ceased after about 15 minutes of exposure. The average energy absorption rate measured thermographically was 0.21 W/kg per mW/cm^2 incident or 8.4 W/kg absorbed at 40 mW/cm^2.

Diachenko and Milroy (96) studied the effects of pulsed and CW microwaves on operant behavior in rats trained to perform a lever pressing response on a DRL (Differential Reinforcement of Low Rate) schedule. The rats were tested immediately after an one hour daily exposure to 1, 5, 10, and 15 mW/cm^2, 2,450 MHz. No behavioral effects were found at these levels, however, the subjects exposed to 10 mW/cm^2, while showing no significant decrement in performance, did show obvious signs of heat stress.

Thomas et al. (335) reported response-rate changes in rats exposed between 5 mW/cm^2 and 20 mW/cm^2 to 2,860 MHz (CW) and 9,600 MHz (pulsed) microwaves. Response rates increased in five of ten tests, which suggested to the authors that "low-level" microwaves produce effects on the CNS.

Galloway (121), studied the performance of four monkeys irradiated by means of a 2,450 MHz (CW) waveguide applicator (total absorbed power of 10, 15, or 25 W) applied to the head. The duration of exposure was 2 minutes or until convulsions began (20 W and 25 W produced convulsions). Because of skin burns, only two subjects completed this series of experiments. Even with the severe exposures, there were no performance decrements in a discrimination task the subjects performed immediately after the periodic exposures. Acquisition of a new task during the first 10 trials of training was impaired at 25 W.

Roberti et al. (279) measured the running time of rats in an electrifiable runway in which each subject was trained to peak performance. Exposure for 185 hours at 10.7 GHz (CW), 3 GHz (CW), and 3 GHz pulsed, to 1 mW/cm² caused no performance decrements. No change in baseline performance was noted when rats were irradiated with 3 GHz pulsed, for 17 days, with a power density of 25 mW/cm².

A pharmacodynamic approach has been taken by some investigators in the study of microwave exposure effects on the CNS and on behavior (31, 107, 335). Following exposure to 10 cm pulsed microwaves, altered sensitivity to neurotropic drugs was noted. Decreased tolerance of rabbits to pentylenetetrazol and increased tolerance to strychnine were observed after a single exposure to 20 mW/cm². Repeated exposures at 7 mW/cm² produced a decreased tolerance to pentylenetetrazol, strychnine, and acetophenetidin (31).

Servantie et al. (305) reported that exposure of rats to 3,000 MHz at 5 mW/cm² for several days resulted in an altered reaction to pentylenetetrazol. Using curare-like compounds, a neuromuscular site of action for this microwave effect was implicated. Edelwejn (107) observed alterations in the effects of chlorpromazine and/or D-tubocurarine on EEG recordings in rabbits repeatedly exposed to 7 mW/cm². The author concluded that synaptic structures at the level of the brain stem are affected by microwaves.

Thomas and Maitland (335) investigated the effects of pulsed 2.45 GHz at 1 mW/cm² in combination with dextro-amphetamine on behavior in rats. Both acute and repeated exposures modified the normal dose-effect function so that the maximum drug effect was obtained at lower microwave exposures.

Galloway and Waxler (122) employed a serotonin-depleting drug (Fenfluramine) to investigate the effect of 2.45 GHz CW microwaves at integral dose rates of 1 to 15 W. Combinations of the drug and microwaves at an integral dose rate of 15 W resulted in behavioral deficits, whereas the drug or microwaves alone up to 15 W failed to produce this effect. In respect to drugs such as dextro-amphetamine and Fenfluramine, their influence on thermal regulation may be significant in these results.

De Lorge (91) exposed rats, squirrel monkeys and rhesus monkeys to 2,450 MHz under far-field conditions. All animals performed on operant schedules for food reinforcement during the microwave exposures. Exposure sessions lasted 60 minutes and were repeated on a daily basis. Stable performance on the operant schedules was disrupted in all three species at power densities positively correlated with the body mass of the animals. When the averages of these power densities (28, 45, and 67 mW/cm²) were plotted as a function of body mass (0.3, 0.7, and 5 kg) a semilog relationship was evident. Extrapolation along the resulting curve could permit prediction of the power densities needed to disrupt ongoing operant behavior in larger animals. The power densities associated with behavioral disruption approximated those power densities that produced an increase in colonic temperature of at least 1°C above control levels in the corresponding animals. These data support the need for scaling factors to extrapolate from small animals to larger animals.

Most of the research on the nervous system and behavior has been carried out in rodents and other lower animals. Behavior among animal species reflects adaptive brain-behavior patterns. Behavioral thermal regulation is seen as an attempt to maintain a nearly constant internal thermal environment. Changes in body temperature bring about not only automatic drives but also behavioral drives (325). That microwaves can influence behavioral thermoregulation has been shown by Stern *et al.* (323) and Adair and Adams (1). Behavioral responses are not necessarily manifestations of specific changes in the CNS and may be a function of direct or indirect action of microwaves on other body systems. However, they do indicate the existence of alterations in the animal's behavioral response patterns. Extrapolation of brain-behavior functions from lower animals to man is thus subject to many difficulties.

In assessing the significance of the reported behavioral changes, it is important to recognize certain fundamental factors. The resting metabolic rate for rats is approximately 7 W/kg. When the power input exceeds this level, disruption of behavior can be elicited. In most of the reports, alterations in the behavior of rats were observed with exposures at average energy absorption rates of 5 to 8 W/kg or greater, *i.e.*, at similar exposure levels to those that produce increases in circulating corticosterone concentrations in rats (203). Behavioral changes may be related to more subtle heat alterations within the body. Heat may produce a generally debilitating effect or decreased motivation for food, since it has been shown that rats maintained in hot environments eat less food (148), and rats show decreased response and food reinforcement frequency on an operant schedule when the environmental temperature is 35°C, but not at 25°C (35). Behavioral responses may thus be influenced by the interaction of the organism with the environment.

The regulation of body temperature can be accomplished by complex patterns of responses of the skeletal musculature to heat and cold which modify the rates of heat production and/or heat loss (*e.g.*, by exercise, change in body conformation, change in the thermal insulation of bedding rodents and of clothing (man), and by the selection of an environment which reduces thermal stress (56).

Thermoregulation is part of a complex control system involving circulation, metabolism and respiration, as well as neural structures. Temperature signals from cutaneous thermoreceptors reach the somatosensory region of the cerebral cortex. The main processing of thermal signals and generation of a controlling signal for the effector part of thermoregulation takes place in the hypothalamus (165).

Strategies or mechanisms to maintain body temperatures in a narrow and desirable range in a complex and varying thermal environment are termed thermoregulatory, which fall into two main categories: voluntary behavioral adjustments, and involuntary physiological adjustments. The limits of effectiveness of involuntary physiological thermoregulation are rather narrow, and we must rely on behavioral thermoregulation over most of the range of environmental temperatures to which we are often exposed. Changes in body temperatures bring about not only autonomic drives, but also behavioral drives (325).

Thermal motivation arises in situations of thermal stress. The uncomfortable feeling of excessive warmth creates a desire for temperature reduction. The unpleasant feeling of being too cold elicits the desire for temperature increase. By acting in such a way as to minimize thermal discomfort and maximize thermal comfort, the organism tends to escape from situations of thermal stress, locates itself in a physiologically neutral thermal environment, thereby solving the problem of physiological temperature regulation (78).

Cardiovascular Effects

Several investigators report that exposure to microwaves may result in direct or indirect effects on the cardiovascular system. Some authors suggest that exposure to microwaves at intensities which do not produce appreciable hyperthermal effects may lead to functional changes with acute as well as chronic exposures.

Cooper et al. (76, 77) and Pinakatt et al. (271, 272) studied the influence of various drugs in pentobarbital-anesthetized rats exposed to 2,450 MHz, 80 mW/cm^2 for 10 minutes, which resulted in a 40.5°C colonic temperature. Pyridoxine and digitoxin did not alter blood pressure or heart rate. Ouabain abolished the circulatory reaction in exposed animals and increased the stroke volume in control animals, while blood pressure and heart rate remained unchanged. Reserpine, vagotomy, and pharmacological ganglioplegia diminished the reaction to microwave-induced hyperthermia.

Functional effects on the cardiovascular system indicated by hypotonia, bradycardia, delayed auricular and ventricular conductivity, decreased blood pressure, and EKG alterations in workers in RF or microwave fields has been reported (128, 261, 294). These changes do not diminish work capacity and are reversible (262), and in fact, no serious cardiovascular disturbances have been noted in man or animals as a result of microwave exposure (108).

Hematopoietic Effects

A number of investigators have stated that the blood and blood-forming system are not affected by acute or chronic microwave exposure (36, 58, 88,

102, 160, 320, 343). Effects on hematopoiesis have nevertheless been reported (22, 24, 27, 81, 82, 126, 164, 177, 234–238, 266, 292, 294, 347).

Hyde and Friedman (160) exposed anesthetized female CF-1 mice to 3,000 MHz 20 mW/cm^2 and 10,000 MHz, 17, 40, or 60 mW/cm^2 up to 15 minutes. No significant effect on total or differential leukocyte count or hemoglobin concentration was noted immediately, 2, 7, or 20 days after exposure. There were no changes in femoral bone marrow other than a variable but slight increase in the eosinophil series of the exposed animals which was not reflected in peripheral blood counts.

Kitsovskaya (177) subjected rats to 3,000 MHz, 10 mW/cm^2, 60 minutes/day for 216 days; 40 mW/cm^2, 15 minutes/day for 20 days; 100 mW/cm^2, 5 minutes/day for 6 days. At 40 mW/cm^2 and 100 mW/cm^2, total erythrocyte, leucocyte, and absolute lymphocyte counts were decreased; granulocytes and reticulocytes were elevated. At 10 mW/cm^2, total leucocyte and absolute lymphocyte counts decreased, and granulocytes increased. Bone marrow examination revealed erythroid hyperplasia at the higher power densities. Decreased leucocyte count and phagocytic activity had been reported in rats and rabbits exposed to 50 MHz, 0.5 to 6 V/m; 10 to 12 hours/day; 180 days (304).

Baranski (22, 24) exposed guinea pigs and rabbits to 3,000 MHz (pulsed or CW), 3.5 mW/cm^2 for 3 months, 3 hours daily. Increases in absolute lymphocyte counts, abnormalities in nuclear structure, and mitosis in the erythroblastic cell series in the bone marrow and in lymphoid cells in lymph nodes and spleen were observed. No alteration in the granulocyte series was noted. Baranski suggested that extrathermal complex interactions seemed to be the underlying mechanism for the changes.

Spalding et al. (320) exposed mice to 800 MHz two hours daily for 120 days in a waveguide at an incident power density of 43 mW/cm^2. Red and white blood cell count, hematocrit, hemoglobin, growth, voluntary activity, and life span remained normal.

In dogs exposed whole-body to 2,800 MHz pulsed, 100 mW/cm^2 for 6 hours, there was a marked decrease in lymphocytes and eosinophils (236). The neutrophils remained slightly increased at 24 hours post-exposure, while eosinophil and lymphocyte values returned to normal levels. Following two hours of exposure at 165 mW/cm^2, there was a slight leucopenia and decrease in neutrophils. When the exposure was of 3 hours duration, leucocytosis was evident immediately after exposure and was more marked at 24 hours, reflecting the neutrophil response. After exposure to 1,285 MHz pulsed, 100 mW/cm^2 for 6 hours, there was an increase in leucocytes and neutrophils. At 24 hours, the neutrophil level was still noticeably increased. Lymphocyte and eosinophil values were moderately depressed initially but at 24 hours, slightly exceeded their initial value. Six hours of exposure to 200 MHz (CW), 165 mW/cm^2, resulted in a marked increase in neutrophils and a mild decrease in lymphocytes. On the following day, the leucocyte count was further increased, and the lymphocytes markedly increased. Such shifts in the white blood cell picture are consistent with focal thermal lesions to be expected under these exposure conditions.

Exposure to mice to 2,450 MHz, 100 mW/cm^2 for 5 minutes resulted in a decrease followed by an increase in ^{59}Fe uptake in the spleen and bone marrow (347). Alteration in ferrokinetics was also found in rabbits and guinea pigs exposed to 3,000 MHz at 1 mW/cm^2 or 3 mW/cm^2, 2 to 4 hours daily, 14 to 79 days (81, 82). Possible alteration in the circadian rhythm of bone-marrow mitoses in guinea pigs and mice was noted. No effects were seen on precursors of granulocytes, and only minimal effects were found in the erythroid series, but pronounced phase shifts were noted in the pool of stem cells. In inbred Swiss albino mice exposed once for 4 hours at 0.5 mW/cm^2 to pulsed 3,000-MHz microwaves, the diurnal rate of proliferation of the stem-cell population was amplified and the phase shifted from that of controls (82). Of interest in this context is the phase-shift in the ciradian rhythm of body temperature observed by Lu et al. (206) in rats exposed to 2,450 MHz, CW, 1 mW/cm^2, 1 to 8 hours.

In individuals occupationally exposed to microwaves, Baranski and Czerski (27) reported a small drop in the number of erythrocytes, which was related to the length of employment. A tendency toward lymphocytosis with accompanying eosinophilia was apparent in persons employed more than five years under conditions of "low" (10 to 100 μmW/cm^2) and "medium" (0.1 to 1 mW/cm^2) microwave exposure. Leucocyte changes occurred in persons exposed to "substantial" (> 1 mW/cm^2) irradiation for more than five years. Bone marrow was found to be essentially normal. There was a tendency, however, towards reticulocytosis.

In evaluating reports of hematological changes, it is important to be aware of the relative distributions of blood cells in a population of animals or humans and the thermal influence on these alterations. Early and sustained leucocytosis in animals exposed to thermogenic levels of microwaves may be related to stimulation of the hematopoietic system, leucocyte mobilization, or recirculation of sequestered cells. Eosinopenia and transient lymphocytopenia with rebound or overcompensation, when accompanied by neutrophilia, may be indicative of increased hypothalmic-hypophysial adrenal function as a result of thermal stress (228).

Effects on the Immune Response

In recent years, considerable interest has developed on the relationship of microwave exposure and alteration of the immune response. Because of the emphasis placed on the "hazard" aspects of the reports of lymphoblastoid transformations and immunological consequences of microwave exposure, it is important to place this in perspective. In essence, the reports do not negate the thermal influences of microwave energy absorption. If the reports are confirmed, they may not be indicative of a hazard, but actually portend an exciting and important possibility for therapy of infectious diseases or cancer which have been shown to be influenced by hyperthermia.

Lymphoblastoid transformation, *in vitro*, after free field exposure to 3,000 MHz pulsed microwaves, 7 mW/cm^2 for 4 hours daily and 20 mW/cm^2 for 15 minutes daily, 3 to 5 days, has been reported (324). At this power density, the temperature of the media increased after 15 minutes by 0.5°C, and after 20 minutes, the increase was 1°C. Changes in the mitotic index depended on the exposure time. Although a 5-minute exposure did not influence the proportion of dividing cells, slight differences compared with controls were observed after 10- and 15-minute exposures, and significant differences were seen following 3- or 4-hour exposures at 7 mW/cm^2.

Czerski (80) exposed human lymphocyte suspensions to 3,000 MHz for various periods of time at several power densities. Lymphoblastoid transformations were observed, but no correlation between the cellular changes and either duration of exposure or incident power were noted.

Smialowicz (313) examined the proliferative capacity of lymphocytes that are responsible for cellular immune responses (T cells) and humoral immune responses (B cells) following 2,450 MHz exposure *in vitro*. The ability of mouse spleen lymphocytes to undergo blast transformation in response to mitogens that selectively stimulate either T or B cells was measured by the incorporation of ^{3}H-thymidine into DNA. No consistent difference was found between the blastogenic response of exposed (10 mW/cm^2, 19 W/kg, 1 to 4 hours) and control cells.

Mice exposed to 2,450 MHz (CW), 5 to 35 mW/cm^2, (SAR = 4 to 25 mW/g), for 1 to 22 consecutive days, (15 to 30 minutes/day) showed no consistent significant alterations in several parameters such as mitogen-stimulated response of T- and B-splenic lymphocytes, enumeration of the frequencies of T- and B-splenic lymphocytes, and the primary antibody response of mice to sheep erythrocytes (313).

Smialowicz *et al.* (314, 315) exposed rats *in utero* and neonatally through 40 days of age (4 hours/day, 7 days/week) in a controlled environment to either 2,450 MHz (CW, 5 mW/cm^2, SAR = 1 to 5 mW/g) or to 425 MHz (CW, 10 mW/cm^2, SAR = 3 to 7 mW/g). At 40 days of age, significant increases in the response of lymphocytes from exposed rats to *in vitro* stimulation with several mitogens was observed in several experiments. While these results have not been consistently reproduced, the trend in the results suggests that chronic exposure during fetal and neonatal development may change either the frequency or responsiveness of lymphocyte sub-populations. The biological significance of these observed changes is unknown. The mechanism by which these changes are initiated may be related to a thermally induced stress response. Similar responses have been observed in animals following prolonged exposure to non-specific stressors (251).

Hamrick (149) examined the response of mammalian lymphocytes exposed to 2,450 MHz (CW) in cultures at 20 mW/cm^2 (7 mW/g) for 48 hours. Changes in the stimulation caused by phythohemagglutinin under control and exposed conditions were tested. No effects of exposure were detected. Also, no effect on DNA was found at power densities as high as 67 mW/g to 160 mW/g (approximately 200 to 300 mW/cm^2). It was concluded that 2,450 MHz, CW microwave exposure "has very little, if any, effect other than that of heating on the secondary structure of DNA as determined by comparison of thermal denaturation curves."

Prince et al. (275) reported that 30-minutes exposure to high intensity 1.32 W/cm^2 fields at 26.6 MHz increased the mitotic potential of certain populations of circulating non-human primate lymphocytes. These findings were accompanied by substantial tissue heating, i.e., +2.4°C and 4.6°C rectal and surface temperature increases.

In an attempt to extend these observations, Lovely et al. (205) initiated a series of studies employing a temperature-controlled RF-exposure culture cup that also provides for well-defined RF-field conditions. They attempted to determine if cultured non-human primate lymphocytes exposed to intense (E = 500 V/m, H = 4.4 A/m, SAR = 400 W/kg) 30 MHz fields would yield significantly higher mitotic figures than sham-exposed control samples of cultured lymphocytes, while the temperature of the cultures under both conditions was held at 37°C ± 0.5°C. The results indicated that exposure of cultured lymphocytes, obtained from Macaca mulatta, to 500 V/m, 30 MHz provided no evidence of cell death, damage or interference with mitotic activity, whether stimulated by phytohemagglutinin (PHA) or unstimulated, immediately following, or 48 hours after exposure.

In many of the studies on microwave effects, especially in vivo, varying conditions of exposure have been used, often with sufficient power density that thermal effects may be the predominant, if not the only factor. This variation in application of microwaves may account for much of the diversity in data regarding the effects of such treatments on components of the hematopoietic system (24, 80).

Czerski and associates (81, 82) have reported that inbred Swiss mice, immunized with sheep red blood cells and exposed 2 hours/day for 6 or 12 weeks to 0.5 mW/cm^2 of 2,950 MHz, showed increased serum hemagglutinin titers and antibody-producing cells in lymph node homogenates. The increase was greater in mice exposed 6 weeks than in those exposed 12 weeks. Similar results were obtained in rabbits exposed 2 hours/day to 3 mW/cm^2 for 6 months with the maximum increase occurring after 1 or 2 months exposure, and then returning to control values. According to Czerski (80), this may indicate that after a period of response, the animals become adapted to the microwaves. The phenomenon of physiological adaptation or decreased reaction as a result of repeated exposure to microwaves has also been reported by others (28, 128, 228, 236, 266, 269).

Baranski (24) exposed adult guinea pigs 3 hours/day for 3 months to 3.5

mW/cm^2, 3,000 MHz and found an increase in lymphopoiesis over controls as indicated by increased incorporation of ^{3}H-thymidine and increased mitotic indices. No differences could be detected between pulsed or continuous wave microwaves of the same average power level. Two-fold increases in lymphocyte numbers were found in the spleen and lymph nodes.

Huang et al. (158) reported that lymphocytes from Chinese hamsters exposed from 5 to 45 mW/cm^2, 2,450 MHz CW, 15 minutes/day for 5 days showed changes in blast transformation and mitosis. No chromosomal aberrations were evident. These studies noted increased but reversible transformation of lymphocytes (without mitogenic stimulation), related to the power density, but a decreased proportion of mitogen-stimulated cells in mitoses. A thermal effect within a range that might normally be managed and dissipated by the animals could not be excluded. These investigators called attention to the changes over a range of body temperatures of less than 2°, and suggested that such limited hyperthermia might be of considerable interest to investigators of immunological effects of microwave radiation.

Microwaves have been reported to induce an increase in the frequency of complement receptor-bearing lymphoid spleen cells in mice (361). Although the significance of this is not fully assessed, it may represent a maturation of B lymphocytes to a stage with expression of an activation structure.

Wiktor-Jedrzejczak et al. (360, 361) exposed adult male mice to 2,450 MHz CW at an absorbed dose of 12 to 15 mW/g for 30 minutes in an environmentally controlled waveguide facility, and then measured the function of different classes of lymphocytes in vitro. Such exposure failed to produce any detectable changes in function of T lymphocytes or increase in DNA, RNA, or protein synthesis, as measured by incorporation of tritiated-thymidine, uridine, and leucine by spleen, bone marrow, and peripheral blood lymphocytes in vitro. However, the maturation of B lymphocytes from the spleen of exposed mice was stimulated. Consistent with this effect on B lymphocytes are the results reported by Czerski (80–82).

Microwave/radiofrequency-induced hyperthermia in mice has been associated with transient lymphopenia and neutrophilia (187, 188) with a relative increase in splenic T and B lymphocytes (189) and with decreased in vivo local delayed hypersensitivity (189). The latter was not affected by a comparable increase in core temperature produced by warm air. Reduced thymic mass and cell density (189), suppressed inflammatory response (187, 188) and suppressed allograft transplant rejection (190) have been reported. Such alterations in lymphocyte distribution and function are concomitant with a state of immunosuppression. Qualitatively similar changes can be induced by administration of synthetic gluco-corticoids or corticosterone (188). In fact, Liburdy (189), reported elevated plasma corticosterone levels in mice following exposure to MW/RF energy sufficient to cause hyperthermia. This phenomenon has been reported by Lotz and Michaelson (203) who showed a correlation between microwave-induced body heating and corticosterone levels in the blood of rats. These studies suggest that exposure to microwaves of sufficient intensity results in stimulation of the hypophysial-adrenal axis which would affect the immune system (189).

It would appear, thus, that MW/RF exposure initially causes a general stimulation of the immune system, but if the exposure continues, the stimulatory effect disappears, suggesting a phase of adaptation to continued MW/RF exposure. There is a body of literature on the influence of heat *per se* on immunity. Significant influences of microwaves on immune responsiveness would be expected on the basis of the known effects of hyperthermia. Although there has been some uncertainty whether fever enhances host resistance to infection (19, 44), recent evidence suggests that fever may enhance survival after infection in an animal model (180). Cell-mediated immunity plays a role in defense against facilitative intracellular bacteria (114), viruses (212), and certain other infectious agents. Roberts and Steigbigel (280) have shown that increased temperature (38.5°C) enhances human lymphocyte response to mitogen (PHA) and antigen (streptokinase-streptodornase) and enhances but does not accelerate certain bactericidal functions of human phagocytic leukocytes. One therefore has to be circumspect in assessing the mechanism of microwave exposure related to alterations in immune processes. It may be that if microwaves do in fact increase the proportion of lymphocytes undergoing transformation, it may not in itself be harmful but actually beneficial. The immune system has a considerable redundancy and adaptability. Perturbations of the immune system may not have clinical significance (326).

Special Senses

AUDITORY AND OLFACTORY RESPONSES

"Microwave hearing" is sensed in the head as a clicking or buzzing due to pulsed microwaves at rather low power densities. Frey (115, 116) has suggested that the acoustic response to pulsed microwaves is the result of direct cortical or neural stimulation, and is therefore indicative of a nonthermal or direct effect of microwaves on the brain. Subsequent research, however, has shown that this phenomenon is one of thermoelastic expansion (113, 142, 192, 193).

Foster and Finch (113) observed that microwave pulses in water produced acoustic pressure transients with peak amplitude within the audible frequency range of 200 Hz to 20 KHz—well above the expected threshold for perception by bone conduction. Because the calculated acoustic pressure at the surface of the head is well above the established threshold of hearing and is much higher in amplitude than that due to either radiation pressure or electrostrictive force mechanisms (69, 113, 142, 192, 193) the thermoelastic conversion mechanism has been viewed as the most probable cause of microwave-induced auditory sensation in mammals.

OCULAR EFFECTS

During the past 25 years, numerous investigations in animals and several surveys among human populations have been devoted to assessing the relationship of microwave exposure to the subsequent development of cataracts. It is significant that of the many experiments on rabbits by several investigators using various techniques, a power density above 100 mW/cm^2 for 1 hour or longer appears to be the lowest time-power threshold in the tested frequency range of 200 MHz to 10,000 MHz. In other species of animals such as dogs and non-human primates, the threshold for experimental microwave-induced cataractogenesis appears to be even higher. This threshold is a time-power threshold, that is, the higher the power density, the shorter time threshold, and vice versa down to a certain minimum power density. All of the reported effects of microwave radiation on the lens can be explained on the basis of thermal injury.

The most extensive investigations in this area were performed by Carpenter and van Ummersen (62) and Carpenter et al. (60). More recent work by Guy et al. (143, 144, 145) and Kramar et al. (181, 182) has shown that in rabbits exposed to 2,450 MHz, the threshold for cataract production is 150 mW/cm^2 for 100 minutes. The data suggest that an intraocular temperature of at least 43°C must be obtained to induce cataracts, although exceptions may be found in the literature (181). These investigators also found that single potentially cataractogenic exposures will not injure the eye under conditions of controlled general hypothermia, and exposure to 100 mW/cm^2, 2 hours/day, for 4 to 9 days produced no cataracts as evidenced by periodic examinations for 6 months after exposure. Guy et al. (144) exposed rabbits to 918 MHz, 466 mW/cm^2 for 15 minutes and 177 mW/cm^2 for 100 minutes with no evidence of cataract, and concluded that the threshold for cataractogenesis is higher for this frequency than at 2,450 MHz.

Appleton et al. (17) exposed rabbits to 3,000 MHz at 100 or 200 mW/cm^2 for 15 to 30 minutes. Examination daily for 14 days, weekly for 1 month, and monthly for a year revealed no ocular changes. At power densities of 300, 400, or 500 mW/cm^2 for 15 minutes, acute ocular changes involving especially the conjunctiva and iris occurred during exposure. In a study by Hirsch et al. (155), rabbits were exposed repeatedly once daily for a month. Clinical examinations were carried out for 1 year afterward. No changes occurred at power densities under 300 mW/cm^2.

Reports of decreased enzymatic activity (62, 175) may quite likely be due to thermal inactivation, with resultant alterations in metabolism. Decreases in ascorbic acid concentration in the lens have been cited as being the first biochemical indication of opacity formation (223, 359). Progressive clouding of the lens is associated with decreases in ascorbic acid below 60 μgm/gm of lens tissue. All of these effects could be fully repairable until the altered metabolism has produced a permanent opacification of the lens. Latent periods and time-power threshold would be in agreement with the mechanism of this nature.

Guy *et al.* (143–145), Kramar *et al.* (182), and Taflove and Brodwin (331) have computed the microwave energy deposition and induced temperatures in the eyes of rabbits and in a model of the human eye. Taflove and Brodwin (331) indicated that a distinct hot spot exceeding 40.4°C probably occurs deep within the eye at a frequency of 1.5 GHz, when the power density would be cataractogenic (*i.e.*, greater than 100 mW/cm^2).

Paulsson (264) measured the absorption of 0.915, 2.45, and 9.0 GHz microwave energy in a model of the human head. The absorbed power showed an essentially exponential decrease with the distance from the cornea at 9.0 GHz. At 2.45 GHz and 0.915 GHz, a maximum absorbed power pattern occurred within the eyeball.

The possibility of a cumulative effect on the lens from repeated "subthreshold" exposures of rabbits' eyes to microwaves has been suggested by Carpenter and associates (60). It should be noted, however, that cumulative rise in temperature can occur if the interval between exposures exceeds the time required for the tissue to return to normal temperature. The cumulative effect to be anticipated, therefore, is the accumulation of damage resulting from repeated exposures, each of which is individually capable of producing some degree of damage (171).

Analysis of available data indicates that when repeated exposures are near threshold and within the time frame of the latency, cataracts may appear. When the time interval between exposures is longer than the latency period, lesions do not appear unless the power density/time relationship is well above the threshold. The so-called "cumulative effect" is only a phenomenon confined to near threshold exposures. No one has yet been able to produce cataracts, even by repetitive exposures, when the power density is below 100 mW/cm^2.

After 25 years of studies of the effects of microwaves on the ocular lens, primarily in the rabbit, the principal conclusions are:

a) The acute thermal insult from high-intensity microwave fields is cataractogenic in the rabbit if intraocular temperatures reach 45 to 55°C;

b) The microwave exposure threshold is between 100 and 150 mW/cm^2 applied for about 60 to 100 minutes;

c) There does not appear to be a cumulative effect from microwave exposure unless each single exposure is sufficient to produce some irreparable degree of injury to the lens.

That opacity of the ocular lens can be produced in rabbits by exposure to microwaves is well-established. Extrapolating interpreted results from animal studies to humans is difficult, because the conditions, durations, and intensities of exposure are usually quite different. Several cases of alleged cataract formation in humans exposed to microwaves have been reported in the literature, but precise exposure parameters are generally impossible to determine. It is also difficult to relate cause and effect, because lens imperfections do occur in otherwise healthy individuals, especially with increasing age. Numerous drugs, industrial chemicals, and certain metabolic diseases are associated with cataracts.

CUTANEOUS PERCEPTION

Perception of microwave energy is a function of cutaneous thermal sensation or pain. The physiology of thermal sensation and pain has been the subject of several studies which suggest that a threshold sensation is obtained when the temperature of the warmth receptors in the skin is increased by a certain amount (ΔT).

Schwan et al. (301) found that if a person's forehead is exposed to 74 mW/cm^2 at 3,000 MHz, the reaction time (the time which elapses before the person is aware of the sensation of warmth) varied between 15 and 73 seconds. Warmth perception at 56 mW/cm^2 ranged between 50 seconds and 3 minutes of exposure. Hendler (151) and Hendler et al. (152) made detailed studies of the cutaneous receptor response of man to 10,000 MHz and 3,000 MHz microwaves and far infrared. Their results are shown in Table 7.1

For a 4-second exposure to 10,000 MHz over a 37 cm^2 area of the forehead, the threshold for thermal sensation was 12.6 mW/cm^2. For exposures lasting 0.5 seconds, the threshold was 25 mW/cm^2. For the entire face, assuming uniform temperature sensitivity of the facial skin, the thermal sensation threshold for 10,000 MHz was 4 to 6 mW/cm^2 for a 5-second exposure, or approximately 10 mW/cm^2 for a 0.5-second exposure.

Cook (75) investigated the pain threshold for 3,000 MHz microwaves. As far as could be judged, the sensations of warmth and pain with microwave heating differed little from those felt when heating was produced by infrared radiation. Apparently, a thermal pain sensation is evoked when end-organs located approximately 1.5 mm below the skin surface reach a temperature of about 46°C. Power density levels for pain threshold for an exposed area

TABLE 7.1. *Stimulus Intensity and Temperature Increase to Produce a Threshold Warmth Sensation*[a]

Exposure Time (sec)	3,000 MHz	10,000 MHz		Far Infrared	
	Power Density (mW/cm^2)	Power Density (mW/cm^2)	Increase in Skin Temp. (°C)	Power Density (mW/cm^2)	Increase in Skin Temp. (°C)
1	58.6	21.0	.025	4.2–8.4	.035
2	46.0	16.7	.040	4.2	.025
4	33.5	12.6	.060	4.2	

[a] 37 cm^2 forehead surface area—data from Hendler et al. (152) and Hendler (151).

of 9.5 cm^2 ranged from 3.1 W/cm^2 for a 20-second exposure to 0.830 W/cm^2 for exposures longer than 3 minutes (Table 7.2). The pain threshold was lower (0.560 W/cm^2) for an exposed area of 53 cm^2 in contrast to 0.830 W/cm^2 for a 9.5 cm^2 area.

Specific Thermal Lesions

In experiments in which rats were irradiated daily for 5 months at 10 to 150 V/m, 70 to 200 MHz, reversible morphological changes in the neural tissues and parenchyma of the heart, liver, and testis were observed (340). In another study, rats died quickly after a single exposure to high field strength (1,000 to 5,000 V/m) radio waves (70 to 200 MHz); and the animals showed marked evidence of hyperthermic stress and severe vascular disorders upon necropsy.

Investigations into microwave bioeffects indicate that for frequencies between 200 and 24,500 MHz, exposure to a power density of 100 mW/cm^2 for several minutes or hours can result in pathophysiological manifestations of a thermal nature in laboratory animals. The end result is either reversible or irreversible change, depending on the conditions of irradiation and the physiological state of the animal. Below 200 MHz, the absorbed power in exposed subjects drops sharply with frequency. In this range, magnetic fields can produce far greater absorbed power densities in man than electric fields of the same energy density, whereas the reverse is true in small animals.

Temperature elevations resulting from exposure to microwave energy may be higher in small test animals than in man. In addition, hot spots from non-uniform absorption of energy can occur in animals. Hot spots are of great importance, partly because they may not be detected without complete quantitative description of the fields induced in the tissues by the radiating energy (140). These induced fields may differ by many orders of magnitude depending on exposure conditions, even though the measured values of outside field parameters are the same. Above 200 MHz, the combination of curved surfaces and high dielectric constants of tissues can focus energy to produce very high localized internal absorption deep in the tissue with consequent steep temperature gradients.

TABLE 7.2. *Threshold for Pain Sensation as a Function of Exposure Duration (3,000 MHz, 9.5 cm^2 area)*[a]

Power Density (W/cm^2)	Exposure Time (sec)
3.1	20
2.5	30
1.8	60
1.0	120
0.83	>180

[a] Data from Cook (75).

The temperature rise depends on the cooling effect resulting from blood circulation. For an incident power density of about 10 mW/cm^2, temperature elevations in human brain tissue may be on the order of a fraction of a degree. For smaller heads, such as those of monkeys, the temperature increase can be substantially higher. Schwan (300) has noted that the data on the overall relative cross-section of man are not necessarily indicative of the energy distribution inside man or inside the phantoms which have been used to simulate man. There is still the possibility, however, that given proper excitation frequencies, selective hot spots may develop inside the body.

Health Aspects

A number of retrospective studies have been done on human populations exposed or believed to have been exposed to RF/microwave energies. An early study on U.S. Navy personnel during World War II did not reveal any conditions that could be ascribed to radar exposure (88). Ten years later, a four-year surveillance of a relatively large group of radar workers in the U.S. did not demonstrate any significant clinical or pathophysiological differences between the exposed and control groups (36, 37). On the other hand, surveys of East European workers revealed functional changes in the nervous and cardiovascular systems (128, 129, 293).

In an extensive survey (83–85, 307, 308), 841 men, aged 20 to 40 years, occupationally exposed to microwaves for various periods of time, were examined for the incidence of functional disturbances and disorders considered as contraindications for occupational exposure to microwaves according to the criteria employed in Poland. The population was involved in identical work conditions except for the exposure levels, which constituted two subgroups. Workers in the first sub-group (507 individuals) were exposed to varying power densities between 0.2 and 6 mW/cm^2; in the second subgroup, power densities were below 0.2 mW/cm^2. No dependence of incidence of disorders, such as organic lesions of the nervous system, changes in translucency of the ocular lens, primary disorders of the blood system, neoplastic diseases, or endocrine disorders on exposure level, duration, or work history could be demonstrated. The incidence of functional disturbances ("neurasthenic syndrome", gastrointestinal tract disturbances, cardiovascular disturbances with abnormal ECG) was found not to be related to the level or duration of occupational exposure. There were no instances or irreversible damage or disturbances caused by exposure to microwave energy (84).

The Medical Follow-up Agency of the National Academy of Sciences of the United States studied mortality and morbidity among personnel of the U.S. Navy. Graduates of technical schools for training in the use of radar and maintenance of equipment were compared with graduates of technical schools not involved with microwave energy. There was no indication that exposure to microwaves adversely affected mortality from all causes or from specific causes (281).

A study of employees of the U.S. Embassy in Moscow, some of whom had possibly been exposed to levels of microwaves up to 15 μW/cm^2 for variable periods of time up to 8 months revealed no differences in health status as indicated by their mortality experience and a variety of morbidity measures (191).

EASTERN EUROPEAN REPORTS

Nervous system alterations and behavioral effects of exposure of man to microwave energy have been reported mostly in Eastern European literature (127, 215, 266, 273) and have been reviewed by Michaelson (227–229), Michaelson and Dodge (231 a), Dodge and Glaser (100), Silverman (310–312), and Albrecht and Landau (10). Most of the Eastern European reports describe subjective complaints consisting of fatigability, headache, sleepiness, irritability, loss of appetite, and memory difficulties. Psychic changes that include unstable mood, hypochondriasis, and anxiety have been reported. Most of the subjective symptoms are reversible, and pathological damage to neural structures is insignificant (259). The difficulties in establishing the presence of, and quantifying the frequency and severity of "subjective" complaints cannot be stated too strongly. It should be noted that individuals suffering from a variety of chronic diseases may exhibit the same dysfunction of the central nervous and cardiovascular systems as those reported to be a result of exposure to microwaves; thus, it is extremely difficult, if not impossible, to rule out other factors in attempting to relate microwave exposure to clinical conditions.

OCULAR EFFECTS

Many cases of cataracts attributed to microwaves have been reported in the literature but substantiation has not been established.

Barron *et al.* (36, 37) and Daily (88) did not find changes in eyes of people working with radar. Zaret *et al.* (367) conducted a study on the frequency of occurrence of lenticular imperfections in the eyes of microwave workers. The number of defects showed a linear increase with age. Although an apparent statistical difference in the score of lens changes between the exposed and control groups existed, the difference was not significant from a clinical standpoint; the extent of minor lenticular imperfections did not serve as a useful clinical indicator of cumulative exposure (367).

No authentic cases of "microwave cataracts" have been described in the Polish literature, nor was this lesion found in an extensive occupational survey among microwave workers (83).

According to Zaret *et al.* (368), pre-clinical signs of microwave injury consist of roughening, thickening, and minute areas of opacification in the posterior capsule. It should be noted, however, that thickening of the posterior capsule of the lens is not a reliable criterion of microwave exposure since such changes exist in a variable manner in the population at large; they occur in many individuals with no exposure to microwaves; and they could be due to numerous other factors, *i.e.*, metabolic diseases, trauma, drugs, etc.

In a study of Appleton and McCrossen (18), 226 individuals, occupationally associated with microwaves to varying degrees, some of whom had been included in the series reported by Zaret *et al.* (368), were subjected to ophthalmological examination and were compared to a population not associated to as great an extent with microwaves. Examination was conducted in most cases semiannually over a 30-month period. Some of the workers examined were involved in this type of work for 25 years. Appleton and McCrossen (18) concluded that the available clinical evidence does not support the assumption that cataracts which develop in personnel performing duties in the vicinity of microwave-generating equipment are a result of microwave exposure, unless a specific instance or instances of severe exposure can be documented and correlated with subsequent cataract development.

Cataract formation is given special mention because this lesion has been incriminated for many years as one of the chief hazards of microwaves. A study of 2,946 patients born after 1910, who had been treated for cataracts in Veterans Administration Hospitals in the United States in the period 1950 to 1962, compared their exposure to radar with that of 2,164 controls (men with adjacent hospital register numbers). No association between exposure to radar and risk of cataracts was found (281).

Tengroth and Aurell (333) and Aurell and Tengroth (20) studied 68 workers in a factory where radar and other microwave equipment was tested. The control group of 30 was from the same factory but was not exposed to microwave radiation "as far as was known." They found a higher prevalence of lens opacities in the exposed individuals. None of the lens lesions, however, resulted in a loss of vision and, therefore, do not fit the definition of a cataract. They also reported retinal lesions in the paramacular and macular regions, which were more frequent in the exposed subjects than in the control subjects. Regrettably, the authors gave no exposure data to permit proper assessment of this material, although they did note that it was impossible to separate lens opacities due to microwave exposur from senile cataracts because no baseline data were available. Such retinal lesions had not been reliably reported previously or since this isolated report. There is no clinical or experimental evidence that lens damage due to microwave energy is morphologically different from lens abnormalities from other causes, including the aging process (14, 15, 18, 368).

Although a latency of 10 or 20 years has been claimed (368), there is no evidence in the literature that supports a long latency period for microwave cataractogenesis. Roughening and thickening of the capsule as pathognomonic or characteristic of microwave-induced cataracts has been disputed (16, 59). According to Appleton (16), the capsulopathy noted by Zaret et al. (368) is not supported by evidence in the literature nor by observations by those investigators performing microwave research. The thickness of the lens posterior capsule is such that it is almost unidentifiable under the biomicroscope or slit lamp. Based on the available evidence, both clinical and experimental, it can be concluded that lens damage probably has not occurred in humans from repeated exposure to low levels of microwave energy (13–15).

GONADS

Although studies indicate that high power density exposure can affect the testes and ovary as already mentioned, these responses can be related to the heating of the organs; the sensitivity of the testes to heat is well known (348). There are reports, however, that chronic low-level exposure can result in impairment of spermatogenesis and reproductive function without measurable temperature increase in the testes of small animals (47, 104). The power densities associated with testicular damage are generally high; Baranski's and Czerski's review (27) of more than 20 reports provides numbers that range from 10 to 400 mW/cm^2.

Reports of human sterility or infertility from exposure to microwaves are questionable. Barron et al. (36, 37) found no evidence of changes in fertility among men occupationally exposed to microwaves. Their study, however, was not designed to assess adverse effects on the testes. There is one case report of altered fertility in a man from unusually large exposures to microwaves (283). In this report, radar was implicated as being responsible for oligospermia and infertility in a young man previously demonstrated to be fecund. The difficulty in evaluating this report is that there was no pre-exposure examination of this individual, so any causal relationship is very tenuous. The authors did not designate an exposure level, but did note that the patient frequently performed maintenance on the radar antenna while the equipment was in operation; he did not wear protective clothing; and he was exposed repeatedly to microwave power densities more than 3,000 times the protection guide number (10 mW/cm^2) of the U.S. Air Force.

Lancranjan et al. (183) studied gonadal function in 31 workmen. Twenty-two of the 31 microwave technicians were reported to suffer from a loss of libido and from reduced spermatogenesis after an average of eight years of occupational exposure at "tens to hundreds of microwatts per square centimeter" to microwave frequencies between 3,600 and 10,000 MHz. Both conditions remitted in most cases three months after exposures were discontinued.

Marha (215) and Marha et al. (216) have cited decreased spermatogenesis, altered sex ratio of births, changes in menstrual patterns, retarded fetal development, congenital defects in newborn babies, and decreased lactation in nursing mothers working in RF fields. According to these authors, such effects occur at thermal microwave exposure intensities (greater than 10 mW/cm^2). The influence of intervening or co-factors such as noise, or general working conditions was not mentioned in these reports.

Five cases have been reported of inborn defects in offspring of women exposed during the early stages of pregnancy to short wave diathermy (72, 245, 284). On the other hand, neither conception nor pregnancy was disturbed by therapeutic microwave diathermy applications (284). Such therapeutic interventions by their very nature employ very high intensities. Also, the medical reason for treatment is not always clear. Assessment of these reports thus requires considerable circumspection.

In a study initiated to determine whether there was a relationship between parental exposure to ionizing radiation and the incidence of Down's syndrome, Sigler et al. (309) reported an association between Down's syndrome in children and paternal exposure to radar before conception. The association was small and not statistically significant. Subsequent investigation, however, did not find any correlation between Down's syndrome and paternal exposure to radar (73).

There is considerable difficulty in establishing the presence of, and in quantifying the frequency and severity of subjective complaints. Individuals suffering from a variety of chronic diseases may exhibit the same dysfunctions of the CNS and cardiovascular system as those reported to be a result of exposure to microwaves; thus, it is extremely difficult, if not impossible, to rule out other factors in attempting to relate microwave exposure to clinical conditions.

Although cataracts have been incriminated for many years as one of the chief hazards of exposure to microwaves, it is not possible to accept the reports as proven. There is no clinical or experimental evidence that lens damage allegedly due to microwave energy is morphologically different from lens abnormalities from other causes, including the aging process.

If the available human data are carefully reviewed, information derived from human case reports and studies actually add little to our knowledge of microwave cataractogenesis. None of these case reports of cataracts can be conclusively attributed to microwave exposure, although in some cases there may possibly be an association. The scoring methods used, both for degree of exposure and for lenticular defects, has not been particularly sound, and their validity has been questioned.

Reports of effects in man must be put in perspective. Most epidemiological and incidence studies suffer from inadequate design and examination, as well as lack of substantiation of actual power levels and duration of microwave exposure. It is essential that the multiple environmental factors be evaluated which may interact among themselves and with personal characteristics of the individual. There is always the danger that real factors may be overlooked, leading to a false association with factors of initial interest.

CRITIQUE OF EPIDEMIOLOGICAL STUDIES

An important concept of disease causation is that, in general, disease is not caused by a single factor or agent, but rather is influenced by multiple, interactive factors such as the subject and his environment. Health effects or manifestations of disease have a spectrum of intensity ranging all the way from the barely discernible and rapidly reversible symptomatic disorders, through an increasing gradient of severity to the point of irreversibility to disease states of such gravity as to ultimately cause death. For electromagnetic fields, in common with most other agents, biological or physical, the trivial end of this severity scale includes detectable physiological effects, which are well within the range of physiological adaptation and do not constitute disease in any meaningful sense. The validity of application of the epidemiological method to the study of the health impact of an agent is largely determined by the ascertainability and definition of an effect. Perhaps the main limitation of epidemiological studies of RF/MW exposure is the lack of recognized pathophysiological manifestations at realistic levels of exposure as indicators for measuring the effects of the fields on man.

Psychosocial factors were important in assessing the effects of environmental insults. Weintraub (358) found a significant overall relationship between job dissatisfaction and psychosomatic complaints.

Reports of occupational surveys of workers exposed to electromagnetic fields in the U.S.S.R. and East European countries have engendered concern regarding "safe levels" of exposure to these fields. In general, the epidemiological or incidence studies from these countries may be criticized as being inadequate in scope and detail, lacking in statistical power, and not subject to review or criticism by peer scientists. Moreover, they often appear oriented to emphasize particular preconceived end results. For example, functional disturbances of the CNS are repeatedly cited to explain a host of ill-defined symptoms and signs.

In general, one can have little confidence in these studies and the environmental standards that have emerged from them. The philosophic approaches both to science and to safety standards differ so much from those accepted in the West that it is difficult to make comparisons.

The Soviets describe such symptoms as listlessness, excitability, headache, drowsiness, and fatigue in persons occupationally exposed to electromagnetic fields. These symptoms are also caused by many other occupational factors, so it is not possible to define a cause-effect relationship. Many other factors in the industrial setting or home environment as well as psychosocial interactions can cause similar symptoms. In this context, Guskova and Kochanova (139) dispute earlier Soviet reports of the relationship of cardiovascular diseases to electromagnetic radiation. According to these authors, it is very difficult to make etiological diagnoses of pathology of the circulatory system in groups of workers who deal with sources of superhigh frequency radiations. This work involves tuning radio equipment or operating radar stations, which requires a high degree of nervous and emotional tension and involves other deleterious factors. The incidence of hypertension with chronic exposure to SHF fields coincides with the findings of a screening of the population of Moscow according to W.H.O. criteria. In addition to smoking and obesity, genetic factors and emotional stress, psychological personality factors that determine an individual's reactivity to environmental conditions are proven risk factors in the development of cardiac ischemia.

Personnel Protection

PROTECTIVE CLOTHING AND EYE SHIELDS

Although protective clothing and eye shields have been developed and demonstrated as providing effective shielding in some circumstances (70, 125, 354) their use is not recommended. Reflections can increase the hazard to the other people and faults, such as open circuits, can act as secondary sources to actually increase the hazard to the wearer. In high radiation fields, arcing problems may arise (179).

PERSONAL MONITORS

Several attempts have been made to develop devices to record individual cumulative exposures to microwaves, or to give warning when pre-determined exposure levels are exceeded (38). These are not in common use and are probably best suited to establishing whether people are being exposed to possibly significant amounts of MW/RF so that their working practices should be investigated. Because of inadequate calibration and other technical difficulties, these have not been accepted as reliable recordings of exposure.

ANCILLARY HAZARDS ASSOCIATED WITH ELECTROMAGNETIC INTERFERENCE

Aside from the primary biological hazard of direct irradiation by RF/MW energy, there is a more subtle influence which can affect users of electronic prosthetic devices such as cardiac pacemakers and diagnostic medical equipment, *i.e.*, EEG's, EKG's, electromyographs, etc. (285). This effect is termed electromagnetic interference (EMI), which may cause a variety of malfunctions. EMI occurs when signals generated by one or more electronic or electromechanical devices adversely affect the operation of other electronic devices. The offending signals can be products of intended radiation, such as radio, television, and radar transmission, or unintended signals generated by internal combustion engine ignition systems, electric razors, electrome-chanical relays, etc. The characteristic of electronic equipment that permits undesirable responses when subjected to EMI is called susceptibility; and the technology that has evolved to solve the problems of EMI is called electromagnetic compatibility (EMC). Of greatest concern has been the possibility of interference with implanted electronic cardiac pacemaker function. Improvements in pacemaker design have largely eliminated their susceptibility problems (318). Pacemakers are typically tested for EMI at least at a frequency of 450 MHz (where susceptibility is generally considered to be the greatest).

Protection Guides and Standards

EXPOSURE STANDARDS

There is a need to set limits on the amount of exposure to radiant energies individuals can accept with safety. The objective of protection is to prevent injury to man. Protection standards should be based on scientific evidence, but are quite often the result of empirical approaches to various problems reflecting current qualitative and quantitative knowledge. A numerical value for a standard implies a knowledge of the effect produced at a given level of stress, and that both effect and stress are measureable. One problem is the definition of what an "effect" is and whether it can ultimately be shown to modify man's "way of life" or that of his offspring (332).

If there were a clear-cut relationship between exposure level and patho-physiological effect, the problem of setting standards would be greatly simplified. Not only are there numerous variables to be considered, but it is often difficult or impossible to obtain the necessary data to draw valid conclusions concerning effects of exposure to noxious agents.

In most biological processes, there is a certain range between those levels that produce no effects and those that produce detectable effects. A detect-able effect is not necessarily one that is irreparable or even a sign that the threshold for damage has been reached. Ultimately, a clear differentiation has to be made between biological effects *per se* which do not result in short-term or latent functional impairment against which the body cannot maintain homeostasis and effectiveness, and injury which may impair normal body activity either temporarily or permanently.

To ensure uniform and effective control of potential health hazards from microwave exposure, it is necessary to establish uniform effect or threshold values. Ideally, effect or threshold values should be predicated on firm human data. If such data are not available, however, extrapolation from well-designed, adequately performed, and properly analyzed animal inves-tigations is required.

In considering standards, it is necessary to keep in mind the essential differences between a "personnel exposure" standard and a "performance" or "emission" standard for a piece of equipment. An exposure standard refers to the maximum level of power density and exposure time for the whole body or for any of its parts and incorporates a safety factor. An emission standard (or performance standard) refers not to people but to equipment, and specifies the maximum emission (or leakage) from a device at a specified distance. Emission standards are such that human exposure will be at levels considerably below personnel exposure limits.

Microwave exposure standards are generally based, with some variation, on those developed in the U.S., U.S.S.R., Poland, and Czechoslovakia. The U.S. Protection Guide of 10 mW/cm^2 was suggested about 20 years ago by Schwan and his associates, which was based on the "thermal load" that a standard (healthy) adult could tolerate and dissipate under usual environmental conditions without a rise in body temperature. Intensive investigation was subsequently carried out by the U.S. Department of Defense into the biological effects of microwave radiation (226). None of these investigations produced any evidence of a hazard at the proposed limit of 10 mW/cm^2. Indeed, no conclusive evidence was established for any effect below the level of 100 mW/cm^2 that could be considered hazardous for man.

Very few countries have promulgated MW/RF standards, and in those cases where standards exist, very few have legal backing. Most standards issued have been of a voluntary or consensus nature and thus provide only guidelines for exposure, *e.g.*, the U.S. ANSI standard (12).

The first standards for controlling exposure to MW/RF radiation were introduced in the 1950's in the U.S.A. and the U.S.S.R. The maximum permissible exposure levels which were proposed then have remained substantially unchanged, i.e. for continuous exposure these are respectively 10 mW/cm^2 and 10 μW/cm^2. Most countries that have developed national standards based them on either the U.S. (12) or the Soviet (346) values. Subsequently, some countries have proposed standards which are intermediate between these extremes.

The basis for the U.S. (12) and U.K. standards is the thermal consequences of exposure. Exposure to 10 mW/cm^2 is considered to result in an additional heat load comparable to basal metabolic rate. This thermal load should be readily accommodated under normal circumstances. The 10 mW/cm^2 level was felt to be about a factor of 10 or more lower than the exposure considered as a risk factor.

The U.S.S.R. standard derives from experiments on small laboratory animals and surveys of people occupationally exposed. Functional changes were reported in animals after exposure to energies in the frequency range of 1 to 10 GHz at about 1 mW/cm^2 over a period greater than 1 hour. One-tenth of this value was recommended as the safe level for exposure throughout the working day, and applying a safety factor of 10 to allow for individual variation in sensitivity, and taking into account the human studies, yielded an occupational exposure standard of 10 μW/cm^2 for the working day (28,

247, 266). The U.S.S.R. standard allows incremental increases in exposure, each by a factor of 10, for exposure durations shorter than 2 hours, and for 20 minutes, respectively.

Most of the biological investigations relevant to the development of exposure standards have been carried out over the approximate frequency range of 1 GHz to 10 GHz. There is, however, a considerable divergence in the frequency range over which the standards of individual countries apply. Reference should generally be made to the standards themselves for detailed information, but Tables 7.3 and 7.4 provide summaries of some existing standards. Table 7.3 summarizes the occupational and general public exposure standards existing in the U.S.S.R., Czechoslovakia, and Poland. Table 7.4 summarizes the standards existing in the U.S. (ANSI), Canada, U.K. and Sweden. Information on the type (general public or occupational) of standard, applicable frequency range, exposure limits, exposure duration and MW/RF source characteristics are provided for comparison purposes.

The OSHA Standard, adopted in 1972, applies to employees in the private sector. An addendum, adopted in 1975, applies to work conditions particularly in the telecommunications industry. OSHA Standards are mandatory for federal employees including the military. Maximum permissible exposure limits is 10 mW/cm^2 for durations greater than 6 min, over the frequency range 10 MHz to 100 GHz. The OSHA standard has been challenged as being unenforceable.

The "Radiation Control for Health and Safety Act of 1968" (PL 90-602), administered by HEW/FDA (BRH), provides authority for controlling radiation from electronic devices. The BRH microwave oven standard, effective October, 1971, states that microwave ovens may not emit (leak) more than 1 mW/cm^2 at time of manufacture and 5 mW/cm^2 subsequently, for the life of the product—measured at a distance of 5 cm and under conditions specified in the standard.

Additionally, there are non-government organizations which develop recommended standards and safety criteria, e.g., *American National Standards Institute (ANSI)*—A voluntary body with members from government, industry, various associations and the academic community which develops consensus standards (guides) in various areas. ANSI issued a safety standard in 1966 with maximum permissible exposures of 10 mW/cm^2 averaged over any 6-minute period for frequencies from 10 MHz to 100 GHz, which was essentially adopted by OSHA. This standard was reviewed and reissued with minor modifications in 1975. ANSI must review and withdraw, revise or reissue ANSI Standards every 5 years. Presently, Subcommittee 4 of ANSI Committee C-95, which deals with hazards to personnel, is reevaluating ANSI's radiofrequency exposure standard for adoption in 1981. The recommendations, based on frequency dependence and SAR state: For human exposure to electromagnetic energy of radiofrequency from 300 KHz to 100 GHz, the radiofrequency protection guides, in terms of equivalent

TABLE 7.3. *U.S.S.R., Polish, and Czechoslovakian Exposure Standards*

Standard	Type	Frequency	Exposure limit	Exposure duration	CW/pulsed	Antenna Stationary/Rotating	Remarks
U.S.S.R. Government 1976	Occupational	10–30 MHz	20 V/m	Working day	Both	Both	Military units and establishments of Ministry of Defense excluded
		30–50 MHz	10 V/m	Working day	Both	Both	
			0.3 A/m	Working day	Both	Both	
		50–300 MHz	5 V/m	Working day	Both	Both	
		0.3–300 GHz	10 μW/cm²	Working day	Both	Stationary	
			100 μW/cm²	Working day	Both	Rotating	
			100 μW/cm²	2 hours	Both	Stationary	
			1 mW/cm²	2 hours	Both	Rotating	
			1 mW/cm²	20 minutes	Both	Stationary	
Czechoslovakia Government 1970	Occupational	10–30 MHz	50 V/m	Working day	Both	Both	Maximum peak 1 kW/cm²
		30–300 MHz	10 V/m	Working day	Both	Both	
		0.3–300 GHz	25 μW/cm²	Working day	CW	Both	
			10 μW/cm²	Working day	Pulsed	Both	
			1.6 mW/cm²	1 hour	CW	Both	
			0.64 mW/cm²	1 hour	Pulsed	Both	
	General public	30–300 MHz	1 V/m	24 hours	Both	Both	
		0.3–300 GHz	2.5 μW/cm²	24 hours	CW	Both	
			1 μW/cm²	24 hours	Pulsed	Both	
		30–300 MHz	1 V/m	24 hours	Both	Both	
		10–30 MHz	2.5 V/m	24 hours	Both	Both	
Poland Government 1972	Occupational	0.3–300 GHz	0.2 mW/cm²	10 hours	Both	Stationary	P-power density in W/m²
			0.2–10 mW/cm²	32/P² (hours)	Both	Stationary	P-power density in W/m²
			1 mW/cm²	10 hours	Both	Rotating	
			1–10 mW/cm²	800/P² (hours)	Both	Rotating	
	General public	0.3–300 GHz	10 μW/cm²	24 hours	Both	Stationary	
			0.1 mW/cm²	24 hours	Both	Rotating	
Poland	Occupational	10–300 MHz	20 V/m	Working hours	Both	Both	E-electric field intensity in V/m
			20–300 V/m	3200/E² (hours)	Both	Both	

TABLE 7.4. *U.S., Canadian, Swedish, and U.K. Exposure Standards*

Standard	Type	Frequency	Exposure limit	Exposure duration	CW/pulsed	Antenna Stationary/Rotating	Remarks
U.S. ANSI 1966, 1974	Occupational and general public	10 MHz–100 GHz	10 mW/cm²	No limit	Both	Both	
			200 V/m				
			0.5 A/m				
			1 mW hour/cm²	0.1 hour	Both	Both	
Canada Standards Association 1966	Occupational and general public	10 MHz–100 GHz	10 mW/cm²	No limit	CW	Both	
			1 mW hour/cm²	0.1 hour	Pulsed	Both	
Canada H and W (proposed)	Occupational	10 MHz–1 GHz	1 mW/cm²	No limit	Both	Both	
	General public	1–300 GHz	5 mW/cm²	No limit	Both	Both	
		10 MHz–300 GHz	25 mW/cm² (maximum)	2.4 min	Both	Both	
			1 mW/cm²	No limit	Both	Both	
Sweden (Worker Protection Authority 1976)	Occupational	0.3–300 GHz	1 mW/cm²	8 hours	Both	Both	
		10–300 MHz	5 mW/cm²	8 hours	Both	Both	
		0.3–300 GHz	1–25 mW/cm²	60/X (minutes)	Both	Both	X = power density in mW/cm²
		10 MHz–300 GHz	25 mW/cm²	Averaged over 1 second	CW, pulsed	Both	
U.K. MRC 1971	General public	30 MHz–30 GHz	10 mW/cm²	No limit	Both	Both	
			1 mW hour/cm²	0.1 hour	Both	Both	

plane wave free space power density and in terms of the mean squared electric (E^2) and magnetic (H^2) field strengths as a function of frequency, are:

Frequency (MHz)	Power Density (mW/cm²)	E^2 (V²/m²)	H^2 (A²/m²)
0.3–3	100	400,000	2.5
3–30	$900/f^2$	4,000 ($900/f^2$)	0.025 ($900/f^2$)
30–300	1.0	4,000	0.025
300–1500	$f/300$	4,000 ($f/300$)	0.025 ($f/300$)
1500–100,000	5	20,000	0.125

Note: f is the frequency, in *megahertz* (MHz)

For near field exposure, the only applicable radiofrequency protection guides are the mean squared electric and magnetic field strengths given in columns 3 and 4. For convenience, these guides may be expressed in equivalent plane wave power density.

For both pulsed and non-pulsed fields, the power density and the mean squares of the field strengths, as applicable, are averaged over any 0.1-hour period and should not exceed the values given in the chart. For situations involving exposure of the whole body, the radiofrequency protection guide is believed to result in energy deposition averaged over the entire body mass for any 0.1-hour period of about 144 J/kg or less. This is equivalent to a SAR of about 0.40 W/kg spatially and temporally averaged over the entire body mass.

The National Institute for Occupational Safety and Health (NIOSH) is developing a criteria document with recommended standards for occupational MW/RF exposures, which is, except for certain modifications, commparable to that recommended by ANSI.

The Radiation Protection Bureau of Health and Welfare Canada is considering "Emission and Exposure Standards for Microwave Radiation." The maximum permissible levels (MPL'S) are 1 mW-hour/cm² average energy flux for whole body exposure as averaged over an hour, and a maximum exposure during any one minute of 25 mW/cm² for occupational settings. The MPL's would apply for the frequency range of 10 MHz to 300 GHz. No distinction is made between CW and pulsed waveforms. There is no lower MPL for the general population.

The State Committee on Standards of the Council of Ministers of the U.S.S.R. has promulgated "Occupational Safety Standards for Electromagnetic Fields of Radiofrquency (GOST 12.1.006–76)", effective January 1, 1977. It specifies the maximum permissible magnitudes of voltage and current density of an EM field in the workplace. It does not, however, apply to personnel of the Ministry of Defense. Maximum permissible RF fields in the workplace must not, during the course of the workday, exceed:

Frequency Range	P (mW/cm^2)	E (V/m)	H (A/m)
60 KHz–1.5 MHz		50	5
1.5 MHz–30 MHz			
3.0 MHz–30 MHz		20	
30 MHz–50 MHz		10	0.3
50 MHz–300 MHz		5	
300 MHz–300 GHz	0.01	(entire workday)	
	0.10	(2-hour period during workday)	
	1.00	(20-minute period during work-day)	

Note 1: Also applies in environments with ambient temperatures above 28°C and/or in the presence of X-ray radiation, except, under these conditions, the maximum during a 20-minute period is restricted to 0.1 mW/cm^2.

There is some indication that the U.S.S.R. Ministry of Health has endorsed guidelines for maximum exposure limits for the general population which stipulates the maximum allowable levels of electromagnetic energy in human habitation, as follows:

Frequency Range	P (W/cm^2)	E (V/m)
30–300 KHz		20
300 KHz–3.0 MHz		10
3.0–30 MHz		4
30–300 MHz		2
300 MHz–300 GHz	5	

In 1977, the Polish Ministries of Work, Wages and Social Affairs and of Health and Social Welfare promulgated a change in the Polish Standard for occupational exposure. The change extends the frequency range down from 300 to 0.1 MHz:

Frequency Range	Hazardous Zone		Intermediate Zone		Safe Zone	
		T_p		T_p		T_p
0.1–10 MHz	250 A/m	40/H	10 A/m		2 A/m	No limit
	1,000 V/m	150/E	70 V/m	Entire	20 V/m	
				Workday		
10–300 MHz	300 V/m	3200/E^2	20 V/m		7 V/m	

T_p = Permissible time of exposure/workday (minutes).
E = Electric field (volts/meter).
H = Magnetic field (amps/meter).

In 1976, the Swedish National Board of Industrial Safety promulgated a nonionizing radiofrequency standard (Worker Protection Authority Instruction No. 111) effective January 1, 1977. This regulation applies to all work which may involve exposure to radiofrequencies between 10 MHz and 300 GHz. The instruction specifically excludes applications involving the treatment of patients. Maximum permissible exposures (as averaged over a 6-minute period) are:

Frequency Range	Power Density
10 MHz–300 MHz	5 mW/cm^2
300 MHz–300 GHz	1 mW/cm^2

The maximum permissible momentary exposure is 25 mW/cm^2.

EMISSION STANDARDS

The best known emission standards concern the maximum permissible leakage from microwave ovens. The Canadian standard (95, 277) restricts the maximum leakage to 1 mW/cm^2 at 5 cm from the oven (consumer, commercial, and industrial). The U.S. standard (345) specifies a maximum emission level at 5 cm of 1 mW/cm^2 before purchase and 5 mW/cm^2 thereafter, which is consistent with standards for the general population in the U.S.S.R. and Poland (28). The standard applies to domestic and commercial ovens, but not to industrial equipment. This has been adopted in Japan and most of Western Europe.

When developing standards or regulations to control exposure levels to the general public and/or persons exposed occupationally, a number of points should be considered (277):

a) Does there or could there exist a problem where MW/RF exposure levels could rise uncontrolled to unsafe levels—if so:

b) Who is being exposed and under what conditions?

c) What are the potentially dangerous sources of MW/RF, how rapidly are these sources proliferating and how are they being controlled?

d) Would the existence and implementation of standards alleviate problems?

In order for a promulgated standard to be understood with respect to technical detail and measurement for compliance, careful consideration should be paid to the following points:

a) There should be a clear distinction between emission and exposure standards.

b) Dependent on the frequency range addressed by the standard, there should be clear definitions of electric and magnetic field strengths and power density. If possible, there should be references on how these values are measured. If this cannot be incorporated into the standard, there should be literature references where this information can be obtained.

c) The meaning of the permitted exposure duration should be described, for example, the allowed times and levels for exposure to continuous or pulsed fields. Clear explanations should be made on accepted levels for intermittent exposures and whether higher levels are allowed for short durations.

d) In general, present exposure standards refer to whole body exposure. Partial body exposures should be addressed.

e) Frequency dependence should be considered. It is generally felt that existing standards oversimplify the frequency dependence of the biological effects, health hazards, and thus, safety limits. Sufficient information is available today to expect the introduction of greater frequency dependence into future revisions of standards.

According to Gordon (130) and Gordon *et al.* (132), the criteria for setting occupational personnel exposure standards in the U.S.S.R. represent complex investigations consisting of three major components:

a) hygienic evaluation of the working conditions of persons working with sources of radiofrequency electromagnetic waves, *i.e.*, determination of the actual intensities of radiation;

b) dynamic clinical observations on the state of health of people working with sources of radiofrequency radiation over a period of several years (five or more);

c) experimental studies on the nature of the biological effects of microwaves to determine threshold values for lethal effects and potentially hazardous reactions.

Unfortunately, the concept of "threshold reaction" in the context of medical evaluation of a biological effect and, especially in the setting of standards, remains indefinite. There are as yet no clear-cut and widely applicable pathophysiological criteria for distinguishing between protective adaptive reactions and compensatory reactions, between regulatory reactions in an emergency situation, and pathological reactions at various systems levels, including the CNS. This results in significant difficulties in the analysis of homeostasis, in the analysis of the differentiated threshold characteristics of biological reactions which are determined by the general level of excitability and reactivity, and in the analysis of pathological reactions, which are determined by adaptational and compensatory capabilities existing in a biological system (130).

These concepts have enabled Soviet authorities to recommend MW/RF standards for workers, and even in recent years, to update some of them. They have also proposed a protection standard for the general population of 1 μW/cm^2 for occupational groups (130).

A search of the Soviet literature fails to reveal any basis for limiting exposure time for 2 hours or 20 minutes in a 24-hour period to levels of 100 and 1,000 μW/cm^2, respectively, although Petrov and Subbota (267) suggest the Soviet standard is based on reports noting that some disturbances occur in experimental animals at exposure levels in the vicinity of 1 mW/cm^2. Taking this value as a limiting value and considering a full work day as rounded off to 10 hours, a permissible exposure level of 0.1 mW/cm^2 seemed reasonable. Introducing an additional safety factor of 10, a level of 0.01 mW/cm^2 (10 μW/cm^2) was derived. In general, it would appear that the values obtained in this manner from experimental studies indicate a large safety factor and can be applied to the general population; but it seems that the values are too conservative for personnel subjected to periodic medical examination such as in the industrial setting (84).

It appears to a large degree that the apparent differences between U.S. and Eastern European standards are based not on actual factual information but on differences in basic philosophy. These differences appear in the areas of industrial hygiene.

The basic industrial hygiene philosophy of the U.S.S.R. can be summarized as follows (210):

a) The maximum exposure is defined as that level such that daily work in the environment will not result in *any deviation in the normal state* as well as not result in disease. Temporary changes in conditional responses are considered deviations from normal.

b) Standards are based entirely on presence or absence of biological effects without regard to the feasibility of reaching such levels in practice.

c) The values are maximum exposures rather than time-weighted averages.

d) Regardless of the value set, the optimum value and goal is zero.

e) Deviations above maximum permissible exposures "within reasonable limits" are permitted.

f) Maximum permissible exposure levels represent desirable values or ideals for which to strive.

In order to properly extrapolate the laboratory results, it is necessary to convert electromagnetic field exposure level information used for laboratory experiments into the rate of energy absorption in the bodies of the exposed test animals. In addition, it is also necessary to relate human exposure under various levels and conditions to the rate of energy absorption or SAR in the tissues. SAR rather than the exposure field is the quantity most directly related to the biological effect in the tissues of exposed subjects. Engineering work over the past several years allows easy calculation and prediction of the average SAR in man and animals exposed under various conditions and, in many cases, the actual SAR distribution over the entire body may be quantifiable (105).

The SAR is the mass-normalized rate at which the potential energy of an electromagnetic field is coupled to an absorbing body. The ultimate fate of absorbed RF energy is an increase in kinetic energy. The SAR is predicated on the axiom that it is absorbed energy and not incident energy which is responsible for biological reactions.

MW/RF safety standards in general do not take into account this extrapolation process and, as a result, many are too conservative over some portions of the frequency spectrum and not conservative enough over other portions.

In its 1979–80 recommendation, the ANSI C95.4 committee used engineering advances made over the previous decade to more accurately extrapolate laboratory data from test animals for recommending maximum incident power density or electromagnetic field strength for human exposure.

The ANSI C95.4 committee analyzed pertinent literature for thresholds of effects. There was general agreement among many of the papers reporting effects at 0.5 W/kg of average SAR and above. On the other hand, the reported thresholds for effects below 0.5 W/kg varied over a wide range with no general agreement among papers or internal consistency of results. Decrement in working ability by test animals began to occur when rats were subjected to average SAR levels of 4 to 10 W/kg. It was felt that the average SAR allowed for human exposure should be at least an order of magnitude below the threshold level of the most replicated and least controversial of the effects in the animals. This corresponds to a whole-body average SAR of approximately 0.36 W/kg which was later rounded off to one significant figure, or 0.4 W/kg. The committee then set allowable exposure levels to values that would prevent the average SAR in an exposed human from exceeding 0.4 W/kg. This resulted in the proposed standard of 1 mW/cm^2 over the frequency range of 30 to 300 MHz.

In many countries, initial and periodic medical examinations of workers is a legal requirement. In the U.S.S.R., Poland, and Czechoslovakia, for example, special requirements are mandatory for workers occupationally exposed to MW/RF energy either in periodicity of examinations or in type of medical examination. When overexposure occurs, depending on the circumstances, a medical examination may be required. In this case, the exposed person can require that a special examination be conducted.

In countries where initial and periodic medical examinations of workers are required by regulations, the type of examination to be performed is generally defined. Such exams include physical evaluation, hematology and urinalysis, and sometimes a chest X-ray examination. Some countries, Poland for example, require more specific examinations for people working with MW/RF energy, which can include electrocardiography, neurological examination with electroencephalography and ophthalmological examination using a slit lamp.

In the U.S.S.R., Poland, and Czechoslovakia, medical examinations may be used to designate people who should not work with MW/RF. As for other occupational exposures, such contraindications include neoplasia, disorders of the blood forming system, organic or pronounced functional neurological disturbances, and endocrine disorders. In certain cases such as blood diseases and gastroduodenal ulcer, the worker may be required to work in other areas for a certain period before being exposed to MW/RF energy again.

Problems and Recommendations

Elucidation of the biological effects of microwave exposure requires a careful review and critical analysis of the available literature. This requires differentiating established effects and mechanisms from speculative and unsubstantiated reports. Most of the experimental data support the concept that the effects of microwave exposure are primarily, if not only, a response to hyperthermia or altered thermal gradients in the body. There are, nevertheless, large areas of confusion, uncertainty and actual misinformation.

Although there is considerable agreement among scientists concerning the biological effects and potential hazards of microwaves, there are areas of disagreement. There also is a serious philosophical question about the definition of hazard. One objective definition of injury is an irreversible change in biological function as observed at the organ or system level. With this definition, it is possible to define a hazard as a probability of injury on a statistical basis. It is important to differentiate between the hazard levels at which injury may be sustained and effect or perception. All effects are not necessarily hazards. In fact, some effects may have beneficial applications under appropriately controlled conditions. Microwave-induced changes must be understood sufficiently so that their clinical significance can be determined, their hazard potential assessed and the appropriate benefit/risk analyses applied. It is important to determine whether an observed effect is irreparable, transient, or reversible, disappearing when the electromagnetic field is removed or after some interval of time. Of course, even reversible effects are unacceptable if they transiently impair the ability of the individual to function properly or to perform a required task.

A critical review of studies into the biological effects of microwaves shows that many of the investigations suffer from inadequacies of either technical facilities and energy measurement skills, or insufficient control of the biological specimens and the criteria for biological change. More sophisticated conceptual approaches and more rigorous experimental designs must be developed. There is a great need for systematic and quantitative comparative investigation of the biological effects, using well-controlled experiments. This should be done by using sound biomedical and biophysical approaches at the various organizational levels, from the whole animal to the sub-cellular level on an integrated basis, with full recognition of the multiple associated and interdependent variables.

It is important that research be conducted so that all aspects of the study are quantified: the type and degree of the effect; whether the effect is harmful, harmless, or merely an artifact; and how it relates to the results obtained by other investigators. For microwave bioeffects, body size of the experimental animal must be taken into account. Since body-absorption cross-sections and internal heating patterns can differ widely, an investigator may think he is observing a low-level or a non-thermal effect in one animal because the incident power is low, while in actuality the animal may be exposed to as much absorbed power in a specific region of the body as another larger animal is with much higher incident power. In performing experimental studies on animals for extrapolation to man, interspecies scaling factors must be considered.

The question of whether reported CNS changes in man (if they are validated) would be important enough to affect his performance should be resolved. Better understanding of local, regional, and whole-body thermal regulation is required. More precise and better controlled long-term, low-level laboratory studies have been suggested. But, these have to be rigidly controlled to obviate circadian rhythm and biological drift over time, which will influence responses.

Particular attention should be paid to instrumentation problems, such as developing more adequate probes for making measurements in the presence of electromagnetic fields. Field strength, electrophysiological, and thermal probes are essential which will give artifact-free readings, which will not distort the field in any way, and which will not give rise to inadvertent stimulation of the tissue due to induced currents.

Well-designed and appropriately controlled epidemiological and clinical investigations of groups of workers and others exposed to microwaves should be encouraged. Studies of workers and individuals exposed to MW/RF energies, along with appropriate control groups, should include a thorough analysis of the exposure environment, including co-factors as well as electromagnetic fields. Epidemiological study is applicable not only to disorders in which there may be a major, definable, etiological agent, but is also useful in evaluating disorders in which multiple environmental factors may interact. There is always the danger that real factors may be overlooked, leading to false associations with factors included in the study. Such interacting factors could be heat, cold, toxic agents, hypoxia, noise, other radiant energy such as X-rays, chronic disease state and/or medication.

Above all, there is a need for scientific competence and integrity. It is important to maintain a proper perspective and assess realistically the biomedical effects of microwave exposure, so that the worker or the general public will not be unduly exposed, nor will research, development, and beneficial utilization of this energy be hampered or unnecessarily restricted.

REFERENCES

1. ADAIR, E. R. AND ADAMS, B. W. Microwaves modify thermoregulatory behavior in squirrel monkey. *Bioelectromagnetics, 1:* 1–20, 1980.
2. ADEY, W. R. AND BAWIN, S. M. (Eds). Brain interactions with weak electric and magnetic fields. *Neurosci. Res. Program Bull., 15:* 129, 1977. MIT Press.
3. ALBERT, E. N. Light and electron microscopic observations on the blood brain barrier after microwave irradiation. *Symp. Biol. Eff. and Measurements of Radiofrequency/Microwaves.* D. S. Hazzard, (Ed). HEW Publ. (FDA) 77–8026, Rockville, pp. 294–304, 1977.

4. ALBERT, E. N. Reversibility of the blood brain barrier. *URSI/USNC Int. Symp. Biol. Eff. Electromagnetic Waves Airlie* (Abstract), 1977.
5. ALBERT E. N. Ultrastructural pathology associated with microwave induced alterations in blood-brain barrier permeability. *Proc. Biol. Eff. E. M. Waves.* XIX Gen. Assembly. Int. Union Radio Sci., Helsinki, August, 1978, Wash. D.C., Nat. Acad. Sci., 1978.
6. ALBERT, E. N., BRAINARD, D. L., RANDALL, J. D., AND JANNATTA, F. S. Neuropathological observations on microwave-irradiated hamsters. *Proc. Biol. Eff. E. M. Waves.* XIX Gen. Assembly. Int. Union Radio Sci., Helsinki, August, 1978, Wash., D. C., Nat. Acad. Sci., 1978.
7. ALBERT, E. N., GRAU, L., AND KERNS, J. Morphologic alterations in hamster blood-brain barrier after microwave irradiation. *J. Microwave Power, 12:* 43–44, 1977.
8. ALBERT, E. N. AND DeSANTIS, M. Do microwaves alter nervous system-structure? *In: Biologic Effects of Nonionizing Radiation.* Tyler, P. E. (Ed). *Ann. N.Y. Acad. Sci., 247:* 87–108, 1975.
9. ALBERT, E. N., McCULLARS, G., AND SHORT, M. The effect of 2450 MHz microwave radiation on liver adenosine triphosphate (ATP). *J. Microwave Power, 9:* 205–211, 1974.
10. ALBRECHT, R. M. AND LANDAU, E. Microwave radiation: An epidemiologic assessment. *Rev. Envir. Hlth., 3:* 44–58, 1979.
11. ALLIS, J. W. Irradiation of bovine serum albumin with a crossed-beam exposure-detection system. *In: Biologic Effects of Nonionizing Radiation.* P. E. Tyler (Ed). *Ann. N.Y. Acad. Sci., 247:* 312–322, 1975.
12. ANSI *Safety Level of Electromagnetic Radiation with Respect to Personnel,* American National Standards Institute, C95.1–1966, C95.1, 1974, New York.
13. APPLETON, B. *Results of clinical surveys of microwave ocular effects.* DHEW Publication No. (FDA) 73–8031. BRH/DBE 73–3, 1972.
14. APPLETON, B. Experimental microwave ocular effects. *In: Biologic Effects and Health Hazards of Microwave Radiation.* P. Czerski, et al (Eds). Polish Medical Publishers, Warsaw, pp. 186–188, 1974.
15. APPLETON, B. Microwave cataracts. *J.A.M.A., 229:* 407, 1974.
16. APPLETON, B. Comment. *In: Biological Effects of Non-Ionizing Radiation.* Tyler, P. E. (Ed). *Ann. N.Y. Acad. Sci., 247:* 133, 1975.
17. APPLETON, B., HIRSCH, S., AND BROWN, P. V. K. Investigation of single-exposure microwave ocular effects at 3000 MHz. *In: Biologic Effects of Nonionizing Radiation.* Tyler, P. E. (Ed). *Ann. N. Y. Acad. Sci., 247:* 125–134, 1975.
18. APPLETON, B. AND McCROSSEN, G. C. Microwave lens effects in humans. *Arch Opthal., 88:* 259, 1972.
19. ATKINS, E. AND BODEL, P. Fever. *N. Engl. J. Med., 286:* 27, 1972.
20. AURELL, E., AND TENGROTH, B. Lenticular and retinal changes secondary to microwave exposure. *Acta Ophthal., 51:* 764, 1973.
21. BALDWIN, M. S., BACH, S. A., AND LEWIS, S. A. Effects of radio frequency energy on primate cerebral activity. *Neurol., 10:* 178–187, 1960.
22. BARANSKI, S. Effect of chronic microwave irradiation on the blood forming system of guinea pigs and rabbits. *Aerospace Med., 42:* 1196–1199, 1971.
23. BARANSKI, S. Histological and histochemical effects on microwave irradiation on the central nervous system of rabbits and guinea pigs. *Amer. J. Phys. Med., 51:* 192–191, 1972.
24. BARANSKI, S. Effect of microwaves on the reactions of the white blood cell system. *Acta Physiol. Pol., 23:* 685, 1972.
25. BARANSKI, S., BAL, J., DEBIEC, H., KWARECKI, K., AND MEZYKOWSKI, T. The influence of microwaves on genetic apparatus functions. *Proc. Biol. Eff. E. M. Waves.* XIX Gen. Assembly. Int. Union Radio Sci., Helsinki, August, 1978.
26. BARANSKI, S., CZEKALINSKI, C., CZERSKI, P., AND HADUCH, S. Experimental research on fatal effect of micrometric wave electromagnetic radiation. *Rev. Med. Aeronaut.,* (Paris) *2:* 108, 1963.
27. BARANSKI, S. AND CZERSKI, P. Investigations of the behavior of corpuscular blood

constituents in persons exposed to microwaves. *Lek. Woisk.*, *42:* 903, 1966.

28. BARANSKI, S. AND CZERSKI, P. *Biological Effects of Microwaves.* Dowden, Hutchinson & Ross, Stroudsburg, PA, 234 pp., 1976.

29. BARANSKI, S., DEBIEC, H., KWARECKI, K., AND MEZYKOWSKI, T. Influence of microwaves on genetical processes of Aspergillus nidulans. *J. Microwave Power*, *11:* 146–147, 1976.

30. BARANSKI, S. AND EDELWEJN, Z. Electroencephalographic and morphological investigations on the influence of microwaves on the central nervous system. *Acta Physiol. Pol.*, *18:* 423, 1967.

31. BARANSKI, S. AND EDELWEJN, Z. Studies on the combined effect of microwaves and some drugs on biolelectric activity of the rabbit CNS. *Acta Physiol. Pol.*, *19:* 37–50, 1968.

32. BARANSKI, S. AND EDELWEJN, Z. Experimental morphologic and electroencephalographic studies of microwave effects on the nervous system. *In: Biologic Effects of Nonionizing Radiation.* Tyler, P. E. (Ed). *Ann. N. Y. Acad. Sci., 247:* 109–116, 1975.

33. BARANSKI, S., SZMIGIELSKI, S., AND MONETA, J. Effects of microwave irradiation *in vitro* on cell membrane permeability. *In: Biological Effects and Health Hazards of Microwave Radiation.* Czerski, P., et al. (Eds). Polish Medical Publishers, Warsaw, pp. 173–177, 1974.

34. BARANSKI, S., OSTROWSKI, K., AND STODOLNIK-BARANSKA, W. Functional and morphological studies of the thyroid gland in animals exposed to microwave irradiation. *Acta Physiol. Pol., 23:* 1029, 1972.

35. BAROFSKY, I. The effect of high ambient temperature on timing behavior of rats. *J. Exp. Anal. Bev., 12:* 59, 1969.

36. BARRON, C. I. AND BARAFF, A. A. Medical considerations of exposure to microwaves (radar). *J.A.M.A., 168:* 1194, 1958.

37. BARRON, C. I., LOVE, A. A., AND BARAFF, A. A. Physical evaluation of personnel exposed to microwave emanations. *J. Aviat. Med., 26:* 442, 1955.

38. BASSEN, H. A limited evaluation of CICOIL personal EM radiation hazard detector. *Health Physics, 37:* 171–174, 1979.

39. BAWIN, S. M. AND ADEY, W. R. Sensitivity of calcium binding in cerebral tissue to weak environmental electric fields oscillating at low frequency. *Proc. Natl. Acad. Sci., 73:* 1999–2003, 1976.

40. BAWIN, S. M. AND ADEY, W. R. Calcium binding in cerebral tissue. *In: Symposium on Biological Effects and Measurement of Radio Frequency/Microwaves*, Washington, D. C., HEW Publication (FDA) 77–8026, 1977.

41. BAWIN, S. M., GAVALAS-MEDICI, R. J., AND ADEY, W. R. Effects of modulated very high frequency fields on specific brain rhythms in cats. *Brain Res., 48:* 365–384, 1973.

42. BEISEL, W. R. AND PEKAREK, R. S. Neurobiology of the trace metals zinc and copper. *Internat. Rev. Neurobiol. Suppl., 1:* 53–82, C. C. Pfeiffer (Ed). N. Y., Academy Press. 1972.

43. BELKHODE, M. L., JOHNSON, D. L. AND MUC, A. M. Thermal and athermal effects of microwave radiation on the activity of glucose-6-phosphate dehydrogenese in human blood. *Hlth. Phys., 26:* 45, 1974.

44. BENNETT, I. L. JR. AND NICASTRI, A. Fever as a mechanism of resistance. *Bact. Rev., 24:* 16–24, 1960.

45. BEREZNITSKAYA, A. N. The effect of 10-centimeter and ultrashort waves on the reproductive function of female mice. *Gig. Tr. Prof. Zabol., 9:* 33, 1968.

46. BEREZNITSKAYA, A. N. Research on the reproductive function in female mice under the impact of low-intensity radio waves of different ranges. *In: Industrial Health and Biological Effects of Radio Frequency Electromagnetic Waves.* Material of the Fourth All-Union Symposium, 17–19 October 1972, Moscow, 51 pp., 1972.

47. BEREZNITSKAYA, A. N. AND KAZBEKOV, I. M. Studies on the reproduction and testicular microstructure of mice exposed to microwaves. *In: Biological Effects of Radiofrequency Electromagnetic Fields*, Gordon, Z. V. (Ed). No. 4, Moscow 221–229, JPRS63321, 1974, 1973.

48. BERMAN, E. AND CARTER, H. Mutagenic and reproductive tests in male rats exposed to

425 or 2450 MHz (CW) microwaves. *Proc. Biol. Eff. E. M. Waves.* XIX Gen. Assembly. Int. Union Radio Sci., Helsinki, August 1978 (Abstr.), 1978.

49. BERMAN, E., KINN, J. B., AND CARTER, H. B. Observations of mouse fetuses after irradiation with 2.45 GHz microwaves. *Hlth. Phys., 35:* 791–801, 1978.

50. BILOKRYNYTSKIY, V. S. Changes in the tigroid substance of neurons under the effect of radio waves. *Fiziol. Zh., 12:* 70, 1966.

51. BINI, M., CHECCUCCI A, IGNESTI, A., MILLANTA, L., RUBINO, N., CAMICI, S., MANAO, G., AND RAMPONI, G. Analysis of the effects of microwave energy on enzymatic activity of lactate dehydrogenase (LDH). *J. Microwave Power, 13:* 96–99, 1978.

52. BLACKMAN, C. F., BENANE, S. G., WEIL, C. M., AND ALI, J. S. Effects of nonionizing electromagnetic radiation on single-cell biologic systems. *In: Biologic Effects of Nonionizing Radiation.* Tyler, P. E. (Ed). *Ann. N.Y. Acad. Sci., 247:* 352–365, 1975.

53. BLACKMAN, C. F., ELDER, J. A., WEIL, C. M., BENANE, S. G., EICHINGER, D. C., AND HOUSE, D. E. Induction of calcium ion efflux from brain tissue by radio-frequency radiation: Effects of modulation frequency and field strength. *Radio Sci., 14:* 93–98, 1979.

54. BLACKMAN, C. F., SURLES, M. C., AND BENANE, S. G. The effects of microwave exposure on bacteria mutation reduction. *Symp. Biol. Eff. of E.M. Waves.* USDHEW Publ. (FDA) 77–8010 Vol. 1 406–413, 1976.

55. BLIGH, J. Physiologic responses to heat. *In: Fundamental and Applied Aspects of Nonionizing Radiation.* Michaelson, S. et al. (Eds). Plenum, New York, pp. 143–154, 1975.

56. BLIGH, J. AND JOHNSON, K. G. Glossary of terms for thermal physiology. *J. Appl. Physiol., 35:* 941, 1973.

57. BOAK, R. A., CARPENTER, C. M., AND WARREN, S. L. Studies on the physiological effects of fever temperatures. II. The effect of repeated short wave (30 Meter) fevers on growth and fertility of rabbits. *J. Exp. Med., 56:* 725–739, 1932.

58. BUDD, R. A., LASKEY, J., AND KELLY, C. Hematological response of fetal rats following 2450 MHz microwave irradiation. *In: Radiation Bio-effects.* Summary Report, Hodge, D. M. (Ed). USDHEW, PHS, BRH/DBE 70-7, p. 161, 1970.

59. CARPENTER, R. L. Comment. *In: Biological Effects of Non-Ionizing Radiation.* Tyler, P. E. (Ed). *Ann. N.Y. Acad. Sci., 247:* 154, 1975.

60. CARPENTER, R. L., BIDDLE, D. K., AND VAN UMMERSEN, C. A. Biological effects of microwave radiation with particular reference to the eye. *Proc. Third Int. Conf. Med. Electronics (London), 3:* 401, 1960.

61. CARPENTER, R. L. AND LIVSTONE, E. M. Evidence for nonthermal effects of microwave radiation: abnormal development of irradiated insect pupae. *IEEE Trans., MTT-19:* 173, 1971.

62. CARPENTER, R. L. AND VAN UMMERSEN, C. A. The action of microwave radiation on the eye. *J. Microwave Power, 3:* 3, 1968.

63. CHANG, B. K., HUANG, A. T., JOINES, W. T. AND DRAMER, R. S. The effect of microwave radiation (1.0 GHz) on the blood-brain barrier in dogs. *Proc. Biol. Eff. E.M. Waves.* XIX Gen. Assembly. Int. Union Radio Sci., Helsinki, August, 1978.

64. CHEN, K. M., SAMUEL, A. AND HOOPINGAVNER, R. Chromosomal abberrations of living cells induced by microwave radiation. *Envir. Lett., 6:* 37–46, 1974.

65. CHERNOVETZ, M. E., JUSTESEN, D. R., KING, N. W. AND WAGNER, J. E. Teratology, survival, and reversal learning after fetal irradiation of mice by 2450 MHz microwave energy. *J. Microwave Power, 10:* 391, 1975.

66. CHERNOVETZ, M. E., JUSTESEN, D. R. AND OKE, A. F. A teratologic study of the rat: Microwave and infrared radiations compared. *Radio Sci., 12(6S):* 191, 1977.

67. CHIZENKOVA, R. A. Brain biopotentials in the rabbit during exposure to electromagnetic fields. *Fiziol. Zh. SSR (Moscow), 53:* 514, 1967.

68. CHIZENKOVA, R. A. Background and induced activity of neurons of the optical cortex of a rabbit after the action of a SHF field, *Zh. Vysshey Nervnoy Deyatel'nosti, 19:* 495, 1969.

69. CHOU, C. K., GALAMBOS, R., GUY, A. W. AND LOVELY, R. H. Cochlear microphonics generated by microwave pulses. *J. Microwave Power*, *10:* 361, 1975.

70. CHRISTIANSON, C. AND RUTKOWSKI, A. *Electromagnetic Radiation Hazards in the Navy*. Naval App. Sci. Lab. Tech. Memo No. 3 AD 645–696, 1967.

71. CLEARY, S. F. Biological effects of microwaves and radiofrequency radiation. *In: CRC Critical Reviews in Environmental Control*. Straub, C. (Ed). *7:* 121–165, 1977.

72. COCCORRA, G., BLASIO, A. AND NUNCIATA, B. Remarks on embryopathies induced by shortwaves. *La Pediatria-Riv. Igiene. Med. Chir Infantia*, *68:* 7, 1960.

73. COHEN, B., LILIENFELD, A. M., KRAMER, S. AND HYMAN, L. C. Parental factors in Down's syndrome. Results of the second Baltimore case-control study. *In: Population Cytogenetics: Studies in Humans*. Hook, E. B. and Porter, I. H. (Eds). Academic Press, Inc., New York, p. 301, 1977.

74. COLLINS, K. J. AND WEINER, J. S. Endocrinological aspects of exposure to high environmental temperatures. *Physiol. Rev.*, *48:* 785, 1968.

75. COOK, N. F. The pain threshold for microwave and infra-red radiations. *J. Physiol.*, *118:* 1, 1952.

76. COOPER, T., JELLINEK, M., PINAKATT, T. AND RICHARDSON, A. W. The effects of pyridoxine and pyridoxal on the circulatory reponses of rats to microwave radiation. *Experientia*, *21:* 28, 1965.

77. COOPER, T., PINAKATT, T., JELLINEK, M. AND RICHARDSON, A. W. Effects of adrenalectomy, vagotomy and ganglionic blockade on the circulatory response to microwave hyperthermia. *Aerospace Med.*, *33:* 794, 1962.

78. CORBIT, J. D. Thermal motivation. *In: Neural Control of Motivated Behavior*. A report based on a NRP work session. *Neurosci. Res. Program Bull.*, 11(4), 1973.

79. CORRELLI, J. C., BUTMANN, R. J., KOHAZI, S. AND LEVY, J. Effects of 2.6–4.0 GHz microwave radiation on E.-coli B. *J. Microwave Power*, *12:* 141, 1977.

80. CZERSKI, P. Microwave effects on the blood-forming system with particular reference to the lymphocyte. *In: Biologic Effects of Nonionizing Radiation*. Tyler, P. E. (Ed). *Ann. N.Y. Acad. Sci.*, *247:* 232–242, 1975.

81. CZERSKI, P., PAPROCKA-SLONKA, E., SIEKIERZYNSKI, M. AND STOLARSKA, A. Influence of microwave radiation on the hematopoietic system. *In: Biologic Effects and Health Hazards of Microwave Radiation*. Czerski, et al. (Eds). Warsaw, Polish Medical Publishers, pp. 67–74, 1974.

82. CZERSKI, P. E., PAPROCKA-SLONKA, E. AND STOLARSKA. Microwave irradiation and the circadian rhythm of bone marrow cell mitosis. *J. Microwave Power*, *9:* 31–37, 1974.

83. CZERSKI, P. E., SIEKIERZYNSKI, M. AND GIDYNSKI, A. Health surveillance of personnel occupationally exposed to microwaves. I. Theoretical considerations and practical aspects. *Aerospace Med.*, *45:* 1137, 1974.

84. CZERSKI, P. AND PIOTROWSKI, M. Proposals for specification of allowable levels of microwave radiation. *Medycyna Lotnicza (Polish)*, *39:* 127–129, 1972.

85. CZERSKI, P. AND SIEKIERZYNSKI, M. Analysis of occupational exposure to microwave radiation. *In: Fundamentals and Applied Aspects of Non-Ionizing Radiations*. Michaelson, S. M., Miller, M. W., Magin, R. and Carstenesen, E. L. (Eds). Plenum Press, New York, pp. 367, 1975.

86. DAELS, J. Microwave heating of the uterine wall during parturition. *Obstet. Gynecol.*, *42:* 76–79, 1973.

87. DAELS, J. Microwave heating of the uterine wall during parturition. *J. Microwave Power*, *11:* 166–168, 1976.

88. DAILY, L. A clinical study of the results of exposure of laboratory personnel to radar and high frequency radio. *U.S. Nav. Med. Bull.*, *41:* 1052, 1943.

89. D'ANDREA, J. A., GANDHI, O. P. AND LORDS, J. L. Behavioral and thermal effects of microwave radiation at resonant and nonresonant wave lengths. *Radio Sci.*, *12(6S):* 251–256, 1977.

90. DE LORGE, J. *Operant Behavior and Colonic Temperature of Squirrel Monkeys (Saimiri sciureus) During Microwave Irradiation.* NAMRL-1236 Naval Aerospace Medical Res. Lab., Pensacola, FL, 32508, 1977.

91. DE LORGE, J. Disruption of behavior in mammals of three different size exposed to microwaves: extrapolation to larger mammals. *In: 1978 Symposium on Electromagnetic Fields in Biological Systems.* Stuchly, S. S. (Ed). Ottawa, p. 215–228, 1978.

92. DE LORGE, J. Operant behavior and rectal temperature of squirrel monkey during 2.45 GHz microwave irradiation. *Radio Sci., 14:* 217–225, 1979.

93. DEMOKIDOVA, N. K. The effects of radiowaves on the growth of animals. *In: Biological Effects of Radiofrequency Electromagnetic Fields*, Gordon, Z. V. (Ed). Arlington, VA., U.S. Joint Publications Research Service No. 63321, pp. 237–242, 1974.

94. DE SEGUIN, L. AND CASTELAIN, G. Action of ultrahigh frequency radiation (wavelength 21 cm) on temperature of small laboratory animals. *Compt. Rend. Acad. Sci. (Paris), 224:* 1662, 1947.

95. DHEW Canada. *Radiation Emitting Devices Regulations.* SOR/74-601 23 October 1974. Part III Microwave Ovens Canada Gazette Part V *108*, pp. 2822–2825, 1974.

96. DIACHENKO, J. A. AND MILROY, W. C. The effects of high power pulsed and low level CW microwave radiation on an operant behavior in rats. Naval Surface Weapons Center, Dahlgren Laboratory, Dahlgren, VA, 1975.

97. DIETZEL, F. Effects of non-ionizing electro-magnetic radiation on the development and intrauterine implantation of the rat. *In: Biologic Effects of Nonionizing Radiation.* Tyler, A. E. (Ed). *Ann. N.Y. Acad. Sci., 247:* 367, 1975.

98. DIETZEL, F. AND KERN, W. Abortion following ultra-shortwave hyperthermia animal experiments. *Arch. Gynakol., 209:* 445, 1970.

99. DIETZEL, F., KERN, W. AND STECKENMESSER, R. Deformity and intrauterine death after short-wave therapy in early pregnancy in experimental animals. *Munch. Med. Wschr., 114:* 228, 1972.

100. DODGE, C. H. AND GLASER, Z. R. Trends in nonionizing radiation bioeffects research and related occupational health aspects. *J. Microwave Power, 12:* 319, 1977.

101. DOLINA, L. A. Morphological changes in the central nervous system due to the action of centimeter waves on the organism. *Arkh. Patol., 23:* 51, 1961.

102. DROGICHINA, E. A., SADCHIKOVA, M. N., SNEGOVA, M. N., KONCHALOVSKAYA, G. V. AND GLOTOVA, K. T. Autonomic and cardiovascular disorders during chronic exposure to super-high frequency electromagnetic fields. *Gig. Tr. Prof. Zabol. (USSR), 10:* 13, 1966.

103. DUMANSKY, Y. D. AND RUDICHENKO, V. F. Dependence of the functional activity of liver mitochondria on the super-high frequency radiation. *Hyg. and Sanit.*, pp. 16–19 April, Moscow, 1976.

104. DUMANSKY, YU. D., SERDYUK, A. M., LITVINOVA, C. I., TOMASHEVSKAYA, L. A. AND POPOVICH, V. M. Experimental research on the biological effects, of 12-centimeter low-intensity waves. *In: Health in Inhabited Localities*, Edition II, Kiev, p. 29, 1972.

105. DURNEY, C. H., JOHNSON, C. C., BARBER, P. W., MASSOUDI, H., ISKANDER, M. F., LORDS, J. L., RYSER, D. K., ALLEN, S. J. AND MITCHELL, J. C. *Radiofrequency Radiation Dosimetry Handbook.* 2nd edition. USAF Report SAM-TR-78-22, Brooks Air Force Base, TX, 1978.

106. D'YACHENKO, N. A. Changes in thyroid function with chronic exposure to microwave radiation. *Gig. Tr. Prof. Zebol., 14:* 51, 1970.

107. EDELWEJN, Z. An attempt to assess the functional state of the cerebral synapses in rabbits exposed to chronic irradiation with microwaves. *Acta. Physiol. Pol., 19:* 897–906, 1968.

108. EDELWEJN, Z., ELDER, R. L., KLIMKOVA-DEUTSCHOVA, E. AND TENGROTH, B. Occupational exposure and public health aspects of microwave radiation. *In: Biologic Effects and Health Hazards of Microwave Radiation.* Czerski, P., et al. (Eds)., Warsaw, Polish Medical Publishers, pp. 330–331, 1974.

109. EDWARDS, M. J. Congenital malformations in the rat following induced hyperthermia during gestation, *Teratology, 1:* 173–178, 1968.
110. EDWARDS, M. J. Congenital defects in guinea pigs: fetal resorption, abortions, and malformations following induced hyperthermia during early gestation. *Teratology, 2:* 313–328, 1969.
111. ELDER, J. A., ALI, J. S., LONG, N. D. AND ANDERSON, G. E. A coaxial air line microwave exposure system: Respiratory activity of mitochondria irradiated at 2-4 GHz. *In: Biological Effects of Electromagnetic Waves.* Rockville, Md. HEW Publication (FDA) 77–8010, 1976.
112. ELY, T. S., GOLDMAN, D., HEARON, J. Z., WILLIAMS, R. B. AND CARPENTER, H. M. *Heating Characteristics of Laboratory Animals Exposed to Ten Centimeter Microwaves.* Bethesda, Md., US Nav. Med. Res. Inst. (Res. Rep. Proj. NM 001–056. 13.02), *IEEE Trans. Biomed. Eng., 11:* 123–137, 1964.
113. FOSTER, K. R. AND FINCH, E. E. Microwave hearing; Evidence for thermoacoustical auditory stimulation by pulsed microwaves. *Science, 185:* 256, 1974.
114. FRENKEL, J. K. AND CALDWELL, S. A. Specific immunity and nonspecific resistance to infection: Listeria, protozoa, and viruses in mice and hamsters. *J. Infect. Dis., 131:* 201, 1975.
115. FREY, A. H. Auditory system response to rf energy, *Aeropsace Med., 32:* 1140, 1961.
116. FREY, A. H. Human auditory system response to modulated electromagnetic energy. *J. Appl. Physiol., 17:* 689, 1962.
117. FRÖHLICH, H. The extraordinary dielectric properties of biological materials and the action of enzymes. *Proc. Nat. Acad. Sci., 72:* 4211, 1975.
118. FUKALOVA, P. P. The sensitivity of olfactory and optic analyzers in persons exposed to the effect of constantly-generated SW and USW, *Tr. Gig. Prof. AMN SSR (Moscow), 2:* 144, 1964.
119. FULK, D. W. AND FINCH, E. D. *Effects of Microwave Irradiation In Vivo on Rabbit Blood Serum.* Report No. 5 Project MF 51.524.015–0001BD7X, Naval Medical Research Institute, Bethesda, MD, 1972.
120. GAGE, M. Behavior in rats after exposure to various power densities of 2450 MHz microwaves. *Neurobehav. Toxicol., 1:* 137–143, 1979.
121. GALLOWAY, W. D. Microwave dose-response relationships in two behavioral tasks. *In: Biological Effects of Non-Ionizing Radiation.* Tyler, P. E. (Ed). *Ann. N.Y. Acad. Sci., 247:* 410, 1975.
122. GALLOWAY, W. D. AND WAXLER, M. Interaction between microwave and neuroactive compounds. *In: Symp. on Biol. Eff. and Measurement of Radio Frequency/Microwaves.* Hazzard, D. (Ed). pp. 62–66 HEW Publ. (FDA) 77–8026, Rockville, MD, 1977.
123. GANDHI, O. P., HUNT, E. L. AND D'ANDREA, J. A. Deposition of electromagnetic energy in animals and in models of man with and without grounding and reflector effects. *Radio Sci., 12(S):* 39–48, 1977.
124. GELLORN, G. Diathermy in gynecology, *J.A.M.A., 90:* 1005–1008, 1928.
125. GLASER, Z. R. AND HEIMER, G. M. Determination and elimination of hazardous microwave fields aboard naval ships. *IEEE Trans. Microwave Theory and Tech., MTT-19:* 232, 1971.
126. GONCHAROVA, N. N., KARAMYSHEV, V. B. AND MAKSIMENKO, N. V. Occupational hygiene problems in working with ultrashort-wave transmitters used in TV and radio broadcasting. *Gig. Tr. Prof. Zabol., 10:* 10, 1966.
127. GORDON, Z. V. The problem of the biological action of UHF. *Tr. Gig. Tr. Prof. AMN SSR, 1:* 5, 1960.
128. GORDON, Z. V. *Biological Effect of Microwaves in Occupational Hygiene,* Izd. Med., Leningrad (TT 70–50087, NASA TT F-633, 1970) 164 pp., 1966.
129. GORDON, Z. V. Occupational health aspects of radio-frequency electromagnetic radiation. *In: Ergonomics and Physical Environmental Factors.* Occupational Safety and Health

Series, No. 21, Geneva, International Labour Office, p. 159, 1970.

130. GORDON, Z. V. New results of investigations on the problems of work hygiene and the biological effects of radiofrequency electromagnetic waves. *In: Biological Effects of Radiofrequency Electromagnetic Fields*, Gordon, Z. V. (Ed). 4, Moscow, pp 7–14, 1973.

131. GORDON, Z. V., LOBANOVA, Y. A. AND TOLGSKAYA, M. S. Some data on the effect of centimeter waves (experimental studies). *Gig. Sanit. (USSR)*, *12:* 16, 1955.

132. GORDON, Z. V., ROSCIN, A. V. AND BYCKOV, M. S. Main directions and results of research in the USSR on the biologic effects of microwaves. *In: Biologic Effects and Health Hazards of Microwave Radiation. Proceedings of an International Symposium.* Warsaw, 15–18 October 1973. Warsaw, Polish Medical Publishers, 22–35, 1974.

133. GORODETSKAYA, S. F. The effect of centimeter radio waves on mouse fertility. *Fiziol. Zh.*, *9:* 394, 1963.

134. GRANT, E. Determination of bound water in biologic materials from dielectric measurements. *In: The Physical Basis of Electromagnetic Interactions with Biological Systems.* Taylor, L. S. and Chung, A. Y. (Eds). Rockville, MD. DHEW pp. 113–119, Publ. No. (FDA) 78–8055, 1978.

135. GRODSKY, I. T. Possible physical substrates for the interaction of electromagnetic fields with biologic membranes. *In: Biological Effects of Nonionizing Radiation.* Tyler, P. A. (Ed). *Ann. N.Y. Acad. Sci.*, *247:* 117, 1975.

136. GUILLET, R., LOTZ, W. G. AND MICHAELSON S. M. Time-course of adrenal response in microwave-exposed rats. *In: Proc. of the 1975 Annual Meeting of USNC/URSI.* University of Colorado, Boulder, CO. National Academy of Sciences, Washington, D.C., pp. 316, 1975.

137. GUILLET, R. AND MICHAELSON, S. M. The effect of repeated microwave exposure on neonatal rats. *Radio Sci. 12 6(S):* 125–130, 1977.

138. GUNN, S. A., GOULD, T. C. AND ANDERSON, W. A. D. The effect of microwave radiation (24000 Mc) on the male endocrine system of the rat. *In: Biological Effects of Microwave Radiation.* Vol. 1. Peyton, M. F. (Ed). Plenum Press, New York, pp. 99–115, 1961.

139. GUSKOVA, A. K. AND KOCHANOVA, YE. H. Some aspects of etiological diagnostics of occupational diseases as related to the effects of microwave radiation. *Gig Truda i Prof. Zabol.* (Moscow) 3: 14, 1975; JPRS L/6135, June, 1976.

140. GUY, A. W. Quantitation of induced electromagnetic field patterns in tissue and associated biologic effects. *In: Biologic Effects and Health Hazards of Microwave Radiation.* Czerski, P. et al. (Eds). Warsaw, Polish Medical Publishers, p. 203, 1974.

141. GUY, A. W. A method for exposing cell cultures to electromagnetic fields under controlled conditions of temperature and field strength. *Radio Sci. 12 6(S):* 87–96, 1977.

142. GUY, A. W., CHOU, C. K., LIN, J. C. AND CHRISTENSEN, D. Microwave induced acoustic effects in mammalian auditory systems and physical materials. *Ann N.Y. Acad. Sci.*, *247:* 194–215, 1975.

143. GUY, A. W., LIN, J. C., KRAMAR, P. O. AND EMERY, A. F. Measurement of absorbed power patterns in the head and eyes of rabbits exposed to typical microwave sources. *In: Proceedings of 1974 Conference on Precision Electromagnetic Measurements.* London, England, p. 255, 1974.

144. GUY, A. W., LIN, J. C., KRAMAR, P. O. AND EMERY, A. F. *Quantitation of Microwave Radiation Effects on the Eyes of Rabbits at 2450 MHZ and 918 MHz.* Scientific Report No. 2, Jan. 1974, Univ. Washington, Seattle, WA, 1974.

145. GUY, A. W., LIN, J. C., KRAMAR, P. O. AND EMERY, A. F. Effect of 2450 MhZ Radiation on the rabbit eye. *IEEE Trans., MIT 23:* 492, 1975.

146. GUY, A. W., WEBB, M. D. AND SORENSEN, C. C. Determination of power absorption in man exposed to high frequency electromagnetic fields by thermographic measurements on scale models. *IEEE Trans. Bio. Med. Eng. BME 23:* 361–371, 1976.

147. GVOZDIKOVA, Z. M., ANAN'YEV, V. M., ZENINA, I. N. AND ZAK, V. I. Sensitivity of the

rabbit central nervous system to a continuous (non-pulsed) ultrahigh frequency electromagnetic field. *Biul. Eksp. Biol. Med. (Moscow)*, *58*: 63, 1964.

148. HAMILTON, C. L. Interactions of food intake and temperature regulation in the rat. *J. Comp. Physiol. Psychol.*, *56*: 476, 1963.

149. HAMRICK, P. E. Thermal denaturation of DNA exposed to 2450 MHz CW microwave radiation. *Radiat. Res.*, *56*: 400, 1973.

150. HELLER, J. H. Cellular effects of microwave radiation. *In: Biological Effects and Health Implications of Microwave Radiation, Symposium Proceedings*. Cleary, S. F. (Ed). U.S. DHEW, Public Health Service BRH/DBE 70-2, pp. 116–121, 1970.

151. HENDLER, E. Cutaneous receptor response to microwave irradation. *In: Thermal Problems in Aerospace Medicine*. Hardy, J. D., (Ed). Surrey, Unwin, Ltd., pp 149–161, 1968.

152. HENDLER, E., HARDY, J. D. AND MURGATROYD, D. Skin heating and temperature sensation produced by infra-red and microwave irradiation. *In: Temperature Measurement and Control in Science and Industry*. Part 3, Biology and Medicine, Hardy, J. D., (Ed). New York, Reinhold, pp. 221–230, 1963.

153. HERSHBERGER, W. D. Microwave transmission through normal and tumor cells. *IEEE Trans. Microwave Theory Tech.*, *MTT-26*: 618–619, 1978.

154. HILL, D. W., HAGMANN, M. J., RIAZI, A., GANDHI, O. P., PARTLOW, L. M. AND STENSAAS, L. J. Effect of millimeter waves on bacteria and viruses. *Proc. Biol. Eff. EM Waves*. XIX Gen. Assembly. Int. Union Radio. Sci., Helsinki, August 1978.

155. HIRSCH, S. E., APPLETON, B., FINE, B. S. AND BROWN, P. V. K. Effects of repeated microwave irradiations to the albino rabbit eye. *Invest. Opthalmol. Vis. Sci. 16*: 315, 1977.

156. HO, H. S. AND EDWARDS, W. P. Oxygen-consumption rate of mice under differing dose rates of microwave radiation. *Radio Sci.*, *126(S)*: 131, 1977.

157. HOUK, W. M., MICHAELSON, S. M. AND BEISCHER, D. E. The effects of environmental temperature on thermoregulatory, serum lipid, carbohydrate, and growth hormone responses of rats exposed to microwaves. *In: Proc. of the 1975 Annual Meeting of USNC/ URSI*. pp. 309. University of Colorado, Boulder, CO. National Academy of Sciences, Washington, D.C., 1975.

158. HUANG, A. T., ENGLE, M. E., ELDER, J. A., KINN, J. B. AND WARD, T. R. The effect of microwave radiation (2450 MHz) on the morphology and chromosomes of lymphocytes. *Radio Sci.*, *12(S)*: 173, 1977.

159. HUNT, E. L., KING, N. W. AND PHILLIPS, R. D. Behavioral effects of pulsed microwave radiation. *In: Biological Effects of Nonionizing Radiation*. Tyler, P. E. (Ed). *Ann. N.Y. Acad. Sci.*, *247*: 440–453, 1975.

160. HYDE, A. S. AND FRIEDMAN, J. J. Some effects of acute and chronic microwave irradiation of mice. *In: Thermal Problems in Aerospace Medicine*. Hardy, J. D., (Ed). Surrey, Unwin, Ltd., pp. 163–175, 1968.

161. ILLINGER, K. The attenuation function for biological fluids at millimeter and far-infrared wavelengths. *In: Biological Effects of Electromagnetic Waves*. Johnson, C. L. and Shore, M. L. (Eds). Vol II. pp. 169–183. USDHEW Publication (FDA) 77–8011, December 1976.

162. ILLINGER, K. Millimeter wave and far-infrared absorption in biological systems. *In: The Physical Basis of Electromagnetic Interaction with Biological Systems*. pp. 43–64, Taylor, L. S. and Cheung, A. Y. (Eds). USDHEW Publication (FDA) 78–8055, Rockville, MD, 1978.

163. IMIG, C. J., THOMSON, J. D. AND HINES, H. M. Testicular degeneration as a result of microwave irradiation. *Proc. Soc. Exp. Biol.*, *69*: 382–386, 1948.

164. IVANOV, A. I. Changes of phagocytic activity and mobility of neutrophils under the influence of microwave fields. *In: Summaries of reports, questions of the biological effect of a SHF-UHF electromagnetic field*. Leningrad, Kirov Order of Lenin Military Medical Academy, p. 24, 1962.

165. IVANOV, K. P. Temperature signalization and its processing in an organism (Temperatur-

naia signalizatsiia i ee obrabotka v organizme). *In: Mechanisms of Information Processing in Sensory Systems*. Izdatel'stvo Nauka, Leiningrad, p. 7, 1975.

166. JANES, D. E., LEACH, W. M., MILLS, W. A., MOORE, R. T. AND SHORE, M. L. Effects of 2450 MHz microwaves on protein synthesis and on chromosomes in Chinese hamsters. *Non. Ioniz. Radiat., 1:* 125–130, 1969.

167. JANIAK, M. AND SZMIGIELSKI, S. Injury of cell membranes in normal and SV40-virus transformed fibroblasts exposed *in vitro* to microwave (2,450 MHz) or water-bath hyperthermia (43 deg C). *In: Abstracts of 1977 International Symposium on the Biological Effects of Electromagnetic Waves*. Airlie, VA, 1977.

168. JENSH, R. P., LUDLOW, J., WEINBERG, W. H., VOGEL, RUDDER, T., AND BRENT, R. L. Teratogenic effects on rat offspring of non-thermal chronic prenatal microwave irradiation. *Teratology, 15(2):* 14A, 1977.

169. JOHNSON, C. C. AND GUY, A. W. Non-ionizing electromagnetic wave effects in biological materials and systems. *Proc. IEEE, 60:* 692–718, 1972.

170. JUSTESEN, D. R. AND KING, N. W. Behavioral of low level microwave irradiation in the closed space situation. *In: Biological Effects and Health Implications of Microwave Radiation*. Cleary, S. F. (Ed). Symposium Proceedings, USDHEW, PHS, BRH/DBE 70-2, p. 154, 1970.

171. KALANT, H. Physiological hazards of microwave radiation, survey of published literature, *Canad. Med. Assoc. J., 81:* 575, 1959.

172. KHOLODOV, YU. A. Changes in the electrical activity of the rabbit cerebral cortex during exposure to a UHF-HF electromagnetic field. Part 2. The direct action of the UHF-HF field on the central nervous system. *Biul. Eksp. Biol. Med. (Moscow). 56:* 42, 1963.

173. KHOLODOV, YU. A. The influence of a VHF-HF electromagnetic field on the electrical activity of an isolated strip of cerebral cortex. *Biul. Eksp. Biol. Med. (Moscow), 57:* 98, 1964.

174. KHOLODOV, YU. A. *The Effect of Electromagnetic and Magnetic Fields on the Central Nervous System*. Moscow, Nauka Press, 283 pp. NASA TT-F-465, 1966.

175. KINOSHITA, J. H., MEROLA, L. D., DIKMAK, E. D. AND CARPENTER, R. L. Biochemical changes in microwave cataracts. *Doc. Ophthalmol., 20:* 91, 1966.

176. KOTSOVSKAYA, I. A. An investigation of the interrelationships between the main nervous processes in rats on exposure to SHF fields of various intensities. *Tr. Gig. Tr. Prof.* AMN SSSR, *1:* 75, 1960.

177. KOTSOVSKAYA, I. A. The effect of centimeter waves of different intensities on the blood and hemopoietic organs of white rats *Gig. Tr. Prof. Zabol., 8:* 14, 1964.

178. KITSOVSKAYA, I. A. The effect of radiowaves of various ranges on the nervous system (sound stimulation method). *In: On the Biological Effect of Radio-Frequency Electromagnetic Fields*. Moscow, p. 81, 1968.

179. KLASCIUS, A. F. Microwave radiation protective suit. *Am. Ind. Hyg. Assoc. J., 32:* 771–774, 1971.

180. KLUGER, M. J., RINGLER, D. H. AND ANVER, M. R. Fever and survival. *Science, 188:* 166–168, 1975.

181. KRAMAR, P. O., EMERY, A. F., GUY,.A. W. AND LIN, J. C. The ocular effects of microwaves on hypothermic rabbits: A study of microwave cataractogenic mechanisms. *Ann. N.Y. Acad. Sci., 247:* 155–165, 1975.

182. KRAMAR, P. O., GUY, A. W., EMERY, A. F., LIN, J. C. AND HARRIS, C. A. Quantitative of microwave radiation effects on the eyes of rabbits and primates at 2450 MHz and 918 MHz. University of Washington Bioelectromagnetics Research Laboratory Scientific Report No. 6, Seattle, WA, 1976.

183. LANCRANJAN, I., MAICANESCU, M., RAFAILA, E., KLEPSCH, I. AND POPESCU, H. I. Gonadic function in workmen with long-term exposure to microwaves. *Hlth. Phys., 29:* 381, 1975.

184. LANSKEY, J., DAWES, D. AND HOWES, M. Progress report on 2450 MHz irradiation of

pregnant rats and the effect on the fetus. *In: Radiation Bioeffects Summary Report PHS.* USDHEW, BRH/DBE-70, Rockville, MD, pp. 167–173, 1970.

185. LEACH, W. M. On the induction of chromosomal aberrations by 2450 MHz microwave radiation. *J. Cell Biol. 70 (S):* 387a, (Abstract), 1976.

186. LENKO, J., BOLATOWSKI, A., GRUSZECKI, L., KLAJMAN, S. AND JANUSZKIEWICZ, L. Effect of 10-cm radar waves on the level of 17-ketosteroids and 17-hydroxycorticosteroids in the urine of rabbits. *Przeglad Lekarski, 22:* 296, 1966.

187. LIBURDY, R. P. Effects of radiofrequency radiation on peripheral vascular permeability. *Ann. Meet. Internat. Union of Radio Science,* Amherst, MA (Abstract), 1976.

188. LIBURDY, R. P. Effects of radio-frequency radiation on inflammation. *Radio Sci., 12(S):* 179–183, 1977.

189. LIBURDY, R. P. Radiofrequency radiation alters the immune system: modulation of *in vivo* lymphocyte circulation. *Rad. Res., 83:* 66–73, 1980.

190. LIBURDY, R. P. Suppression of allograft rejection by whole-body microwave hyperthermia. *Fed. Proc., 37:* 1281 (Abstract), 1978.

191. LILIENFELD, A. M., TONASCIA, J., TONASCIA, S., LIBAUER, C. H., CANTHEN, G. M., MARKOWITZ, J. A. AND WEIDA, S. *Foreign Service Health Status Study: Evaluation of Health Status of Foreign Service and other Employees from Selected Eastern European Posts Final Report* July 31, 1978 Contract No. 6025–619073 Dept. of Epidemiol., Johns Hopkins Univ., Baltimore, MD, 1978.

192. LIN, J. C. Microwave auditory effect—a comparison of some possible transduction mechanisms. *J. Microwave Power, 11:* 77, 1976.

193. LIN, J. C. On microwave-induced hearing sensation. *IEEE Trans., MTT 25:* 605, 1977.

194. LIN, J. C., GUY, A. W. AND CALDWELL, L. T. Thermographic and behavioral studies of rats in the near field of 918 MHz radiations. *Trans. IEEE, MTT 25:* 833–836, 1977.

195. LIN, J. C., NELSON, J. C. AND EKSTROM, M. E. Effects of repeated exposure to 148 MHz radiowaves on growth and hematology of mice. *Radio Sci., 14:* 173–179, 1979.

196. LINDAUER, G. A., LIU, L. M., SKEWES, G. W. AND ROSENBAUM, F. J. Further experiments seeking evidence of nonthermal biological effects of microwave radiation. *IEEE Trans. Microwave Theory Tech., 22:* 790–793, 1974.

197. LIU, L. M., NICKLES, F. G. AND CLEARY, S. F. Effects of microwave radiation on erythrocyte membranes. *Radio Sci., 14:* 109–115, 1979.

198. LIU, L. M., ROSENBAUM, F. J. AND PICKARD, W. F. The relation of teratogenesis in *Tenebrio molitor* to the incidence of low level microwaves. *IEEE Trans. Microwave Theory and Tech., 23:* 929–931, 1975.

199. LIVANOV, M. N., TSYPIN, A. B., GRIGORIEV, G. YU, KRUSCHEV, V. G., STEPANOV, S. M. AND ANAN'YEV, V. M. The effect of electromagnetic fields on the bioelectric activity of cerebral cortex in rabbits. *Byull. Eksp. Biol. i Med., 49:* 63–67, 1960.

200. LOBANOVA, YE. A. Survival and development of animals at various intensities and duration of SHF action. *Tr. Gig. Prof. AMN SSSR, 1:* 61, 1960.

201. LOBANOVA, E. A., AND GONCHAROVA, A. V. Investigation of conditioned-reflex activity in animals (albino rats) subjected to the effect of ultrashort and short radio-waves. *Gig. Tr. Prof. Zabol., 15:* 29–33, 1971.

202. LOBANOVA, YE. A. AND GORDON, Z. V. The study of olfactory sensitivity in persons exposed to SHF. *Tr. Gig. Prof. AMN SSR., 1:* 52, 1960.

203. LOTZ, W. G. AND MICHAELSON, S. M. Temperature and corticosterone relationship in microwave exposed rats. *J. Appl. Physiol., 44:* 438–445, 1978.

204. LOTZ, W. G. AND MICHAELSON, S. M. Effects of hypoplysectomy and dexamethasone on rat adrenal response to microwaves. *J. Appl. Physiol., 47:* 1284–1288, 1979.

205. LOVELY, R. H., SPARKS, T. J., GUY, A. W. AND CHOU, C. K. Radiofrequency field exposure of cultured lymphocytes from Macaca Mulatta. Final Report SAM-TR-79-25. USAF School Aerospace Med. Brooks AFB, TX, 1979.

206. LU, S. T., LEBDA, N. A., MICHAELSON, S. M., PETTIT, S. AND RIVERA, D. Thermal and endocrinological effects of protracted irradiation of rats by 2450 MHz microwaves. *Radio Sci.*, *12(6S)*; 147–156, 1977.

207. LU, S. T., LOTZ, W. G. AND MICHAELSON, S. M. Advances in microwave-induced neuroendocrine effects: the concept of stress. *Proc. IEEE 68*: 73–77, 1980.

208. MAGIN, R. L., LU, S. T. AND MICHAELSON, S. M. Stimulation of dog thyroid by local application of high intensity microwaves. *Am. J. Physiol.*, *233*: E363–368, 1977.

209. MAGIN, R. L., LU, S. T. AND MICHAELSON, S. M. Microwave heating effect on the dog thyroid. *IEEE Trans. Biomed. Eng.*, *24*: 522–529, 1977.

210. MAGNUSON, H. J., FASSETT, D. W., GARARDE, H. W., ROWE, V. K., SMYTH, H. F. AND STOKINGER, H. E. Industrial toxicology in the Soviet Union—theoretical and applied. *Amer. Indust. Hyg. Ass. J.*, *25*: 185–197, 1964.

211. MALYSHEV, V. T. AND TKACHENKO, M. I. Activity of ferments on the mucous membrane of the small intestine under the influence of an SHF field. *In: Physiology and Pathology of Digestion*, Kishenev, p. 186, 1972.

212. MANDELL, G. L. Effect of temperature on phagocytosis by human polymorphonuclear neutrophils. *Infect. Immun.*, *12*: 221, 1975.

213. MANIKOWSKI, E., LUCIANI, J. M., SERVANTIE, B., CZERSKI, P., OBRENOVITCH, J. AND STAHL, A. Effects of 9.4 GHz Microwave exposure on meiosis in mice. *Experientia*, *35*: 388, 1979.

214. MARHA, K. Biological effects of rf electromagnetic waves. *Pracovni Lekarstvi (Prague)*, *15*: 387, 1963.

215. MARHA, K. Maximum admissible values of HF and UHF electromagnetic radiation at work places in Czechoslovakia. *In:* Cleary, S. F. (Ed). *Biological Effects and Health Implications of Microwave Radiation*. Symposium Proceedings, USDHEW, PHS, BRH/DBE 70–2, p. 188, 1970.

216. MARHA, K., MUSIL, J. AND TUHA, H. *Electromagnetic Fields and the Living Environment*. 1968. Prague, State Health Publishing House (Transl. SBN 911302-13-7, San Francisco Press, 1971).

217. MASSOUDI, H. *Long Wavelength Analysis of Electromagnetic Power Absorption by Prolate Spheroidal and Ellipsoidal Models of Man*. Salt Lake City: University of Utah, Ph.D. Thesis, pp. 1–217, 1976.

218. MCLEES, B. D. AND FINCH, E. D. *Analysis of the Physiologic Effects of Microwave Radiation*. US Nav. Med. Res. Inst., (Rep. No. 3 Proj. MF12. 524.015–0001B) Bethesda MD, 1971.

219. MCLEES, B. D., FINCH, E. D. AND ALBRIGHT, M. L. *An Examination of Hepotic Tissue Following in vivo Exposure to RF Radiation*. US Naval Med. Res. Inst. Report No. 1, Project M.F. 12.524.015–0001B Bethesda, MD, 1971.

220. MCREE, D. I. AND HAMRICK, P. E. Exposure of Japanese Quail embryos to 2.45 GHz microwave radiation during development. *Radiat. Res.*, *71*: 355–366, 1977.

221. MCREE, D. I., HAMRICK, P. E., ZINKL, J. E., THAXTON, P. AND PARKHYRST, C. R. Some effects of exposure of the Japanese quail embryo to 2.45 GHz microwave radiation. *In: Biologic Effects of Nonionizing Radiation*. Tyler, P. E. (Ed). *Ann. N.Y. Acad. Sci.*, *247*: 377–390, 1975.

222. MERRITT, J. H., CHAMNESS, A. F. AND ALLEN, S. J. Studies on blood-brain barrier permeability after microwave-radiation. *Rad. Envir. Bioph.*, *15*: 367–377, 1978.

223. MEROLA, L. O. AND KINOSHITA, H. H. Changes in the ascorbic acid content in lenses of rabbit eyes exposed to microwave radiation. *In:* Peyton, M. F. (Ed). *Biological Effects of Microwave Radiation*. Vol. 1. New York, Plenum Press, p. 285, 1961.

224. MICHAELSON, S. M. Biological effects of microwave exposure. *In: Biological Effects and Health Implications of Microwave Radiation, Symposium Proceedings*. Cleary, S. F. (Ed). USDHEW, PHS BRH/DBE 70–2, p. 35, 1970.

225. MICHAELSON, S. M. Discussion following the paper: Effects of 2,450 MHz microwave radiation on cultivated kangaroo rat cells. *In: Biological Effects and Health Implications of Microwave Radiation.* Cleary, S. F. (Ed). HEW Publication No. BRH/DBE 70-2, p. 133, 1970.

226. MICHAELSON, S. M. The tri-service program—a tribute to George H. Kanuf, USAF (MC), *IEEE Trans. Microwave Theory and Techniques, MTT-19:* 131–146, 1971.

227. MICHAELSON, S. M. Human exposure to non-ionizing radiant energy—potential hazards and safety standards. *Proc. IEEE, 60:* 389–421, 1972.

228. MICHAELSON, S. M. Effects of exposure to microwaves: Problems and perspectives. *Envir. Hlth. Perspec., 8:* 133–156, 1974.

229. MICHAELSON, S. M. Radiofrequency and microwave energies, magnetic and electric fields. *In: The Foundations of Space Biology and Medicine.* Chap. 1, Vol. II, Book 2. pp. 409–452 Calvin, M. and Gazenko, O. G. (Eds). NASA, Washington, D.C., 1975.

230. MICHAELSON, S. M. Biologic and pathophysiologic effects of exposure to microwaves. *In: Microwave Bioeffects and Radiation Safety. Trans IMPI Vol. 8.* Stuchly, M. A. (Ed). The International Microwave Power Institute, Edmonton, Alberta, Can. pp. 55–94, 1978.

231. MICHAELSON, S. M. Microwave biological effects: An overview. *Proc. IEEE, 68:* 40–49, 1980.

231a. MICHAELSON, S. M. AND DODGE, C. H. Soviet views on the biologic effects of microwaves: an analysis. *Hlth. Phys., 21:* 108–111, 1971.

232. MICHAELSON, S. M., GUILLET, R., CATALLO, M. A., SMALL, J., INAMINE, G. AND HEGGENESS, F. W. Influence of 2450 MHz microwaves on rats exposed in utero. *J. Microwave Power, 11:* 165, 1976.

233. MICHAELSON, S. M., GUILLET, R. AND HEGGENESS, F. W. The influence of microwave exposure on functional maturation of the rat. Proc. 17th Hanford Biology Symposium: *Developmental Toxicology of Energy—Related Pollutants.* Department of Energy Symposium Series 47. Mahlum, D. et al. (Eds). pp. 300–316, CONF 771017 TIC. USDOE NTIS Springfield, VA, 1978.

234. MICHAELSON, S. M., THOMSON, R. A. E. AND HOWLAND, J. W. Physiologic aspects of microwave radiation of mammals. *Am. J. Physiol., 201:* 351, 1961.

235. MICHAELSON, S. M., THOMSON, R. A. E. AND HOWLAND, J. W. Comparative studies on 1285 and 2800 mc/sec pulsed microwaves. *Aerospace Med., 36:* 1059, 1965.

236. MICHAELSON, S. M., THOMSON, R. A. E. AND HOWLAND, J. W. *Biologic Effects of Microwave Exposure.* Griffiss Air Force Base, Rome Air Development Ctr., Rome, New York (ASTIA Doc. No. AD 824–242), 138 pp., 1967.

237. MICHAELSON, S. M., THOMSON, R. A. E., TAMAMI, M. Y. E., SETH, H. S. AND HOWLAND, J. W. Hematologic effects of microwave exposure, *Aerospace Med., 35:* 824–829, 1964.

238. MICKEY, G. H. Electromagnetism and its effect on the organism. *N.Y. State J. Med., 63:* 1935, 1963.

239. MICKEY, G. H., ADLER, J. H. AND SNYDER, E. Nonthermal hazards of exposure to radiofrequency fields. Final Report. The New England Instit., Ridgefield, CT, 1975.

240. MIKOLAJCZYK, H. Hormone reactions and changes in endocrine glands under influence of microwaves. *Medycyna Lotnicza, 39:* 39, 1972.

241. MIKOLAJCZYK, H. Microwave irradiation and endocrine functions. *In: Biologic Effects and Health Hazards of Microwave Radiation,* Czerski, P. et al. (Eds). Polish Medical Publishers, Warsaw, p. 46, 1974.

242. MIKOLAJCZYK, H. Microwave-induced shifts of gonadotrophic activity in anterior pituitary gland of rats. *In: Biological Effects of Electromagnetic Waves.* Vol. I. Johnson, C. C. and Shore, M. L. (Eds). DHEW (FDA) 77–8010, Rockville, MD, pp. 377–383, 1977.

243. MILROY, W. C., AND MICHAELSON, S. M. Biological effects of microwave radiation. *Hlth. Phys., 20:* 567, 1971.

244. MILROY, W. C. AND MICHAELSON, S. M. Thyroid pathophysiology of microwave radiation.

Aerospace Med., 43: 1126, 1972.

245. MINECKI, L. High frequency electromagnetic radiation. *In: Biological Effect and Health Protection.* Wydawnictwo Zwiazkowe CRZZ Press, Warsaw, 1967.

246. MINECKI, L. AND BILSKI, R. Histopathological changes in internal organs of mice exposed to the action of microwaves. *Medcyna Pracy (Poland), 12:* 337, 1961.

247. MININ, B. A. Microwaves and Human Safety—Part I and II. JPRS 65506–1 and 2, 1975. (Transl. from Russian "Svch i Bezopasnost Cheloveka" Ivol. 342 pp. Izdatel'stvo Sovetskoye Radio, Moscow, 1974).

248. MIRO, L., LOUBIERE, R. AND PFISTER, A. Studies of visceral lesions observed in mice and rats exposed to UHF waves. A particular study of the effects of these waves on the reproduction of these animals. *Rev. Med. Aeronaut. (Paris), 4:* 37, 1965.

249. MIRO, L., LOUBIERE, R. AND PFISTER, A. Effects of microwaves on the cell metabolism of the reticulo-endothelial system. *In: Biologic Effects and Health Hazards of Microwave Radiation.* Czerski, P. et al. (Eds). pp. 89–97. Polish Medical Publishers, Warsaw, 1974.

250. MITTLER, S. Failure of 2 and 10 meter radio waves to induce genetic damage in Drosophila melanogaster. *Environmental Res., 11:* 326–330, 1976.

251. MONJAN, A. A. AND COLLECTOR, N. I. Stress-induced modulation of the immune response. *Science, 197:* 307–308, 1977.

252. MURACA, G. J., JR., FERRI, E. S. AND BUCHTA, F. L. A study of the effects of microwave irradiation of the rat testes. *In: Biological Effects of Electromagnetic Waves.* Johnson, C. C. and Shore, M. (Eds). Vol. I. pp. 484–494. DHEW (FDA) 77–8010. Rockville, MD, 1977.

253. NIKOGOSYAN, S. V. Influence of UHF on the cholinesterase activity in the blood serum and organs in animals. *In: The Biological Action of Ultrahigh Frequencies.* Letavet, A. A. and Gordon, Z. V. (Eds). JPRS 12471, p. 83, 1962.

254. NOVITSKIY, YU. I., GORDON, Z. V., PRESMAN, A. S. AND KHOLODOV, YU. A. *Radio Frequencies and Microwaves, Magnetic and Electrical Fields.* Washington, D.C., NASA (NASA TT F–14.021), 1971.

255. OLCERST, R. B. AND RABINOWITZ, J. R. Studies on the interaction of microwave radiation with cholinesterase. *Rad. Environm. Biophys. 15:* 289, 1978.

256. OLDENDORF, W. H. Focal neurological lesions produced by microwave irradiation. *Proc. Soc. Expt. Biol. Med., 72:* 432, 1949.

257. OLSEN, R. G. Insect teratogenesis in a standing-wave irradiation system. *Radio Sci., 12(6S):* 199–208, 1977.

258. OLSEN, R. G. Constant dose microwave irradiation of insect pupae. *Proc. Biol. Eff. E.M. Waves.* XIX Gen. Assembly. Int. Union Radio Sci., Helsinki, August 1978.

259. ORLOVA, T. N. Clinical aspects of mental disorders following protracted human exposure to super-high frequency electromagnetic waves. *In: Cerebral Mechanisms of Mental Illnesses.* Kazan', pp. 16–18, 1971.

260. OSCAR, K. J. AND HAWKINS, T. D. Microwave alteration of the blood-brain barrier system of rats. *Brain Res., 126:* 281–293, 1977.

261. OSIPOV, YU. A. The effect of VHF-HF under industrial conditions, *Gig. Sanit, USSR, 6:* 22, 1952.

262. OSIPOV, YU. A. *Occupational Hygiene and the Effect of Radio-frequency Electromagnetic Fields on Workers,* Leningrad, Izd. Meditsina Press, p. 78–103, 1965.

263. PARKER, L. N. Thyroid suppression and adrenomedullary activation by low-intensity microwave radiation. *Am. J. Physiol., 224:* 1388, 1973.

264. PAULSSON, L. E. Measurements of 0.915, 2.45, and 9.0 GHz absorption in the human eye. Presented at the 6th European Microwave Conference, Rome, Italy, 1976.

265. PAY, T. L., BEYER, E. C. AND REICHELDERFER, C. F. Microwave effects on reproductive capacity and genetic transmission in Drosophila melanogaster. *J. Microwave Power, 7:* 75, 1972.

266. PETROV, I. R., (Ed). *Influence of Microwave Radiation on the Organism of Man and Animals,* Leningrad, Meditsina Press (NASA TT F-708), 1970.
267. PETROV, I. R., AND SUBBOTA, A. G. Conclusion. *In: Influence of Microwave Radiation on the Organism of Man and Animals.* Petrov, I. R. (Ed). Leningrad, Meditsina Press, NASA TT F-708, 1970.
268. PETROV, I. R. AND SYNGAYEVSKAYA, V. A. Endocrine glands. *In: Influence of Microwave Radiation on the Organism of Man and Animals.* Petrov, I. R. (Ed). Meditsina Press, Leningrad, p. 31 (NASA TT F-708), 1970.
269. PHILLIPS, R. D., HUNT, E. L., CASTRO, R. D. AND KING, N. W. Thermoregulatory, metabolic and cardiovascular response of rats to microwaves. *J. Appl. Physiol., 38:* 630–635, 1975.
270. PICKARD, W. F. AND OLSEN, R. G. Developmental effects of microwaves in Tenebrio molitor: Experiments to detect possible influences of radiation frequency and of culturing protocols. *In: Abstracts of the 1977 USNC/URSI Symposium on Biological Effects of Electromagnetic Waves.* National Academy of Sciences, Washington D.C., p. 66, 1977.
271. PINAKATT, T., COOPER, T. AND RICHARDSON, A. W. Effect of ouabain on the circulatory response to microwave hyperthermia in the rat. *Aerospace Med., 34:* 497, 1963.
272. PINAKATT, T., RICHARDSON, A. W. AND COOPER, T. The effect of digitoxin on the circulatory response of rats to microwave irradiation. *Arch. Int. Pharmcodyn. Ther., 150:* 151, 1965.
273. PRESMAN, A. S. *Electromagnetic Fields and Life.* Izd-vo Nauka, Moscow, 1968 (Transl. Plenum Press, New York, 1970).
274. PRESTON, E., VAVASOUR, E. J. AND ASSENHEIM, H. M. Permeability of the blood-brain barrier to mannitol in the rat following 2450 MHz microwave irradiation. *Brain Res., 174:* 109–117, 1979.
275. PRINCE, J. E., MORI, L. H., FRAZER, J. W. AND MITCHELL, J. C. Cytologic aspects of RF radiation in the monkey. *Aerosp. Med., 43:* 759–761, 1972.
276. PROHOFSKY, E. Microwave frequencies and the structure of the double helix. *In: The Physical Basis of Electromagnetic Interactions with Biological Systems.* pp. 133–140, USDHEW Publication (FDA) 78–8055, 1978.
277. REPACHOLI, H. H. Proposed exposure limits for microwave and radiofrequency radiations in Canada. *J. Microwave Power, 13:* 199–277, 1978.
278. REVUTSKY, E. L. AND EDELMAN, F. M. Effects of centimeter and meter electromagnetic waves in the content of biologically active substances in human blood. *Philosophical J. Ukr. Acad. Sci., 10:* 379, 1964.
279. ROBERTI, B., HEEBELS, G. H., HENDRICX, J. C. M., DE GREEF, A. H. A. M. AND WOLTHUIS, O. L. Preliminary investigations of the effects of low-level microwave radiation on spontaneous motor activity in rats. *In: Biological Effects of Nonionizing Radiation.* Tyler, P. E. (Ed). *Ann. N.Y. Acad. Sci., 247:* 417–423, 1975.
280. ROBERTS, N. J., JR. AND STEIGBIGEL, R. T. Hyperthermia and human leukocyte functions: Effects on response of lymphocytes to mitogen and antigen and bactericidal capacity of monocytes and neutrophils. *Infect. Immun., 18:* 673–679, 1977.
281. ROBINETTE, C. D., SILVERMAN, C. AND JABLON, S. Effects upon health of occupational exposure to microwave radiation. (Radar). *Am. J. Epidemiol., 112:* 39–53, 1980.
282. RODZILSKY, B. AND OLSZEWSKI, J. Permeability of cerebral blood vessels studied by radioactive iodinated bovine albumin. *Neurology, 7:* 279, 1957.
283. ROSENTHAL, D. S. AND BEERING, S. C. Hypogonadism after microwave radiation, *J.A.M.A., 205:* 245, 1968.
284. RUBIN, A. AND ERDMAN, W. J. Microwave exposure of the human female pelvis during early pregnancy and prior to conception. *Am. J. Phys. Med., 38:* 219–220, 1959.
285. RUGGERA, P. S. AND ELDER, R. L. Electromagnetic Radiation Interference with Cardiac Pacemakers. USDHEW Publ. (BRH/DEP) 71–5, 25 pp., 1971.

286. RUGH, R., GINNS, E. I., HO, H. S. AND LEACH, W. M. Are microwaves teratogenic? *In: Biological Effects and Health Hazards of Microwave Radiation.* Czerski, P. et al. (Eds). Polish Medical Publishers, Warsaw, p. 98, 1974.

287. RUGH, R., GINNS, E. I., HO, H. S. AND LEACH, W. M. Responses of the mouse to microwave radiation during estrous cycle and pregnancy. *Radiation Res., 62:* 225, 1975.

288. RUGH, R. AND MCMANAWAY, M. Can electromagnetic waves cause congenital anomalies? *International IEEE/AP-S USNC/URSI Symposium, Amherst, Mass.,* p. 143, 1976.

289. RUGH, R. AND MCMANAWAY, M. Anesthesia as an effective agent against the production of congenital anomalies in mouse fetuses exposed to electromagnetic radiation. *J. Exp. Zool., 197:* 363, 1976.

290. RUGH, R. AND MCMANAWAY, M. Mouse fetal sensitivity to microwave radiation. *Congen. Anom., 17:* 39–45, 1977.

291. RUPP, T., MONTET, J. AND FRAZER, J. W. A comparison of thermal and radiofrequency exposure effects on trace metal content of blood plasma and liver cell fractions of rodents. *Ann. N.Y. Acad. Sci., 247:* 282–290, 1975.

292. SACCHITELLI, F. AND SACCHITELLI, G. Protection of personnel exposed to radar microwaves. *Folia Med. (Naples), 43:* 1219, 1960.

293. SADCHIKOVA, M. N. Clinical manifestations of reactions to microwave irradiation in various occupational groups. *In: Biologic Effects and Health Hazards of Microwave Radiation.* Czerski, P. et al. (Eds). Warsaw, Polish Medical Publishers, p. 261, 1974.

294. SADCHIKOVA, M. N. AND ORLOVA, A. A. Clinical picture of the chronic effects of electromagnetic centimeter waves. *Ind. Hyg. Occupat. Dis. (USSR), 2:* 16–22, 1958.

295. SAITO, M., AND SCHWAN, H. P. The time constants of pearl-chain formation. *In: Biological Effects of Microwave Radiation.* Vol. 1. Peyton, M. F. (Ed). Plenum Press, New York, p. 85, 1961.

296. SANZA, J. N. AND DE LORGE, J. Fixed interval behavior of rats exposed to microwaves at low power densities. *Radio Sci., 12(6S):* 273–277, 1977.

297. SAVAGE, J. R. K. Use and abuse of chromosomal aberrations as an indicator of genetic damage. *Intern. J. Envir. Stud., 1:* 233–240, 1971.

298. SCHUMACHER, P. H. Kurzwellentherapie in der Gynakologie. *Zentralbl. Gynaekol., 60:* 1923–1924, 1936.

299. SCHWAN, H. P. Radiation biology, medical applications and radiation hazards. *In: Microwave Power Engineering.* Vol. 2. Okress, E. C. (Ed). Academic Press, New York, pp. 213–243, 1968.

300. SCHWAN, H. P. Interaction of microwave and radio frequency radiation with biological systems. *IEEE Trans. Microwave Theory and Techniques, MTT-19:* 146, 1971.

301. SCHWAN, H. P., ANNE, A. AND SHER, L. *Heating of Living Tissues.* Report NAEC-ACEL-534, US Naval Air Engineering Center, Philadelphia, PA, 1966.

302. SCHWAN, H. P. AND PIERSOL, G. M. The absorption of electromagnetic energy in body tissues, a review and critical analysis, Part I, Biophysical aspects. *Am. J. Phys. Med., 33:* 371–404, 1954.

303. SCHWAN, H. P. AND PIERSOL, G. M. The absorption of electromagnetic energy in body tissues, a review and critical analysis, Part II, Physiological and clinical aspects. *Am. J. Phys. Med., 34:* 425–448, 1955.

304. SERDIUK, A. M. Biological effect of low-intensity ultrahigh frequency fields. *Vrach. Delo 11:* 103–111, 1969.

305. SERVANTIE, B., BERTHARION, G., JULY, R., SERVANTIE, A. M., ETIENNE, J., DREYFUS, P. AND ESCOUBET, P. Pharmacologic effects of a pulsed microwave field. *In: Biologic Effects and Health Hazards of Microwave Radiation.* Czerski, P. et al. (Eds). pp. 36–45. Polish Medical Publishers, Warsaw, 1974.

306. SERVANTIE, B., SERVANTIE, A. M. AND ETIENNE, J. Synchronization of cortical neurons by a pulsed microwave field as evidenced by spectral analysis of EEG from the white rat.

In: Biological Effects of Nonionizing Radiation. Tyler, P. E. (Ed). *Ann. N.Y. Acad. Sci., 247:* 82, 1975.

307. SIEKIERZYNSKI, M. A study of the health status of microwave workers. *In: Biologic Effects and Health Hazards of Microwave Radiation.* Czerski, P. et al. (Eds). Polish Medical Publishers, Warsaw, p. 273.

308. SIEKIERZYNSKI, M., CZERSKI, P., MILCZAREK, H., GIDYNSKI, A., CZARNECKI, C., DZIUK, E. AND JEDRZESCAK, W. Health surveillance of personnel occupationally exposed to microwaves. II. Functional disturbances. *Aerospace Med., 45:* 1143, 1974.

309. SIGLER, A. T., LILIENFELD, A. M., COHEN, B. H. AND WESTLAKE, J. E. Radiation exposure in parents of children with mongolism. *Bull. Johns Hopkins Hosp., 117:* 374, 1965.

310. SILVERMAN, C. Nervous and behavioral effects of microwave radiation in humans. *Am. J. Epidemiol., 97:* 219, 1973.

311. SILVERMAN, C. Epidemiologic approach to the study of microwave effects. *Bull. N. Y. Acad. Med., 55:* 1106–1181, 1979.

312. SILVERMAN, C. Epidemiologic studies of microwave effects. *Proc. IEEE, 68:* 78–84, 1980.

313. SMIALOWICZ, R. J. The effect of microwaves (2450 MHz) on lymphocyte blast tranformation in vitro. *In: Biological Effects of Electromagnetic Waves.* Johnson, C. C. and Shore, M. L. (Eds). HEW Publ. (FDA) 77–8010, Rockville, MD, pp. 472–483, 1976.

314. SMIALOWICZ, R. J., KINN, J. B. AND ELDER, J. A. Perinatal exposure of rats to 2450 MHz (CW) microwave radiation: Effects on lymphocytes. *Radio Sci., 14:* 147–153, 1979.

315. SMIALOWICZ, R. J., WEIL, C. M., KINN, J. B. AND ELDER, J. A. Exposure of rats to 425 MHz (CW) microwave radiation: Effects on lymphocytes. *J. Microwave Power,* (in press).

316. SMIRNOVA, M. I. AND SADCHIKOVA, M. N. Determination of the functional activity of the thyroid gland by means of radioactive iodine in workers with UHF generators. *In: The Biological Action of Ultrahigh Frequencies.* Letavet, A. A. and Gordon, Z. V. (Eds). Moscow, p. 50, 1960.

317. SMOLYANSKAYA, A. Z. AND VILENSKAYA, R. L. Effects of millimeter-band electromagnetic radiation on the functional activity of certain genetic elements of bacterial cells (Trans.). *Usp Fiz. Nauk., 110:* 571–572, 1973.

318. SMYTH, H. The pacemaker patient and the electromagnetic environment. *J.A.M.A., 227:* 1412, 1974.

319. SPACKMAN, D. H. AND RILEY, V. Studies of RF radiation effects on blood-brain barrier permeability using fluorescein and amino acids. *Proc. Biol. Eff. E. M. Waves.* XIX Gen. Assembly. Int. Union Radio Sci., Helsinki, August, 1978.

320. SPALDING, J. F., FREYMAN, R. W. AND HOLLAND, L. M. Effects of 800 MHz electromagnetic radiation on body weight, activity, hematopoiesis and life span in mice. *Hlth. Phys., 20:* 421–424, 1971.

321. STAVINOHA, W. B., MEDINA, M. A., FRAZER, J., WEINTRAUB, S. T., ROSS, D. H., MODAK, A. T. AND JONES, D. J. The effects of 19 megacycle irradiation on mice and rats. *In: Biological Effects of Electromagnetic Waves.* Vol. I. Johnson, C. C. and Shore, M. L. (Eds). HEW Publ. (FDA) 77–8010, Rockville, MD, pp. 431–448, 1976.

322. STAVINOHA, W. B., MODAK, A., MEDINA, M. A. AND GASS, A. E. *Growth and Development of Neonatal Mice Exposed to High-Frequency Electromagnetic Fields,* Report SAM–TR–75–51, School of Aerospace Medicine, Brooks Air Force Base, TX, 1975.

323. STERN, S., MARGOLIN, L., WEISS, B., LU, S. T. AND MICHAELSON, S. M. Microwaves: effect on thermoregulatory behavior in rats. *Science, 206:* 1198–1201, 1979.

324. STODOLNIK-BARANSKA, W. The effects of microwaves on human lymphocyte cultures. *In: Biologic Effects and Health Hazards of Microwave Radiation.* Czerski, P., et al. (Eds). Warsaw, Polish Medical Publishers, p. 189–195, 1974.

325. STOLWIJK, J. A. J. Responses to the thermal environment. *Fed. Proc. 36:* 1655–1658, 1977.

326. STOSSEL, T. P. Introductory overview/tutorial on immunology. *In: Fifth Report In Program for Control of Electromagnetic Pollution of the Environment: The Assessment*

of Biological Hazards of Nonionizing Electromagnetic Radiation. NTIA Report 79–19, p. C–23, March 1979.

327. STRAUB, K. D. AND CARVER, P. Effects of electromagnetic fields on microsomal ATPase and mitochondrial oxidative phosphorylation. In: Biological Effects of Nonionizing Radiation. Tyler, P. E. (Ed). Ann. N. Y. Acad. Sci., 247: 292–300, 1975.

328. SUTTON, C. H., NUNNALLY, R. L. AND CARROLL, F. B. Protection of the microwave-irradiated brain with body-core hypothermia. Cryobiology 10: 513, 1973.

329. SWIECICKI, W. AND EDELWJN, Z. The influence of 3 cm and 10 cm microwave irradiation on blood proteins in rabbits. Med. Lotnicza, 11: 54, 1963.

330. SWIECICKI, W. AND EDELWEIJN, Z. Electrophoresis of blood protein in rabbits exposed to acute irradiation with very high frequency electromagnetic waves. Farmacja Polska, 19: 189, 1963.

331. TAFLOVE, A. AND BRODWIN, M. E. Computation of the electromagnetic fields and induced temperatures within a model of the microwave-irradiated human eye. IEEE Transactions on Microwave Theory and Techniques, MTT-23: 888–896, 1975.

332. TAYLOR, L. S. Radiation protection trends in the United States. Hlth. Phys., 20: 499–504, 1971.

333. TENGROTH, B. AND AURELL, E. Retinal changes in microwave workers. In: Biologic Effects and Health Hazards of Microwave Radiation. Czerski, P. C. et al. (Eds). Warsaw, Polish Medical Publishers, p. 302, 1974.

334. THOMAS, J. R., FINCH, E. D., FULK, D. W. AND BURCH, L. S. Effects of low level microwave radiation on behavioral baselines. In: Biologic Effects of Nonionizing Radiation. Tyler, P. E. (Ed). Ann. N.Y. Acad. Sci., 247: 425, 1975.

335. THOMAS, J. R. AND MAITLAND, G. Microwave radiation and dextroamphetamine: Evidence of combined effects on behavior of rats. Radio Sci., 14: 253–258, 1979.

336. THOMPSON, W. D. AND BOURGEOIS, A. E. Effects of Microwave Exposure on Behavior and Related Phenomena. Primate Behavior Lab., Aeromedical Research Lab. Report, Wright-Patterson AFB, OH (ARL-TR-65–20; AD 489245), 1965.

337. TOLGSKAYA, M. S. Morphological changes in animals exposed to 10 cm microwaves. Voprosy Kurortologi i Fizioterapii i Lechebnoy Fizicheskoy Kul'tury, 1: 21, 1959.

338. TOLGSKAYA, M. S. AND GORDON, Z. V. Changes in the receptor and interoreceptor apparatuses under the influence of UHF. In: The Biological Action of Ultrahigh Frequencies. Letavet, A. A. and Gordon, Z. V. (Eds). Moscow, Academy of Medical Science, p. 104, 1960.

339. TOLGSKAYA, M. S. AND GORDON, Z. V. Comparative morphological characterization of action of microwaves of various ranges. Tr. Gig. Tr. i Prof. AMN., 2: 80, 1964.

340. TOLGSKAYA, M. S. AND GORDON, Z. V. Pathological Effects of Radio Waves. Moscow Meditsina Press (Consultants Bureau, Plenum Press, New York, 1973 Transl.).

341. TOLGSKAYA, M. S., GORDON, Z. V. AND LOGANOVA, YE. A. Morphological changes in experimental animals under the influence of pulsed and continuous waves SHF-UHF radiation. Tr. Gig. Tr. i Prof. AMN SSSR., 1: 90, 1960.

342. TRAVERS, W. D. AND VETER, R. J. Low intensity microwave effects on the synthesis of thyroid hormones and serum proteins. In: Proc. of the 1976 Annual Meeting of USNC/URSI, p. 91. University of Masachusetts, Amherst, MA. National Academy of Sciences, Washington, D.C., 1976.

343. TYAGIN, N. V. Change in the blood of animals subjected to a SHF-UHF field. Voyenno-Medit. Akad. Kirov, Leningrad, 73: 116–126, 1957.

344. TYAZHELOV, V. V., TIGRANIAN, R. E. AND KHIZHNIAK, E. P. New artifact-free electrodes for recording of biological potentials in strong electromagnetic fields. Rad. Sci., 12: 121–123, 1977.

345. USDHEW Regulations for Administration and Enforcement of the Radiation Control of Health and Safety Act of 1968 paragraph 1030.10 Microwave Ovens DHEW Publ. No. (FDA) 75–8003 pp. 36–37, July, 1974.

346. USSR *Temporary Sanitary Rules for Working with Centimeter Waves.* Ministry of Health Protection of the USSR, 1958.

347. VACEK, D. R. A. Effect of high-frequency electromagnetic field upon haemopoietic stem cells in mice. *Folia Biologica (Praha), 18:* 292, 1972.

348. VANDEMARK, W. R. AND FREE, J. R. Temperature effects. *In: The Testis.* Vol. III. Johnson, A. D., Gomes, W. R. and VanDemark, M. K. (Eds). Academic Press, New York, 1973, p. 233–312, 1973.

349. VAN UMMERSEN, C. A. The effect of 2450 mc radiation on the development of the chick embryo. *In: Biological Effects of Microwave Radiation.* Peyton, M. F. (Ed). Vol. 1, Plenum Press, New York, p. 201, 1961.

350. VAN UMMERSEN, C. A. *An Experimental Study of Developmental Abnormalities Induced in the Chick Embryo by Exposure to Radio Frequency Waves.* Ph.D. Dissertation, Tufts University, Medford, MA, 1963.

351. VARMA, M. M., DAGE, E. L. AND JOSHI, S. R. Mutagenicity induced by nonionizing radiation in Swiss male mice. *In: Biological Effects of Electromagnetic Waves.* Johnson, C. C. and Shore, M. L. (Eds). Vol. 1, pp. 397–405. U.S. Department of Health, Education, and Welfare, Food and Drug Administration, Rockville, MD, HEW Publication (FDA) 77–8010, 1976.

352. VARMA, M. M. AND TRABOULAY, E. A. JR. Evaluation of dominant lethal test and DNA studies in measuring mutagenicity caused by non-ionizing radiation. *In: Biological Effects of Electromagnetic Waves,* Johnson, C. C. and Shore, M. L. (Eds). Vol. 1, pp. 386–396. U.S. Department of Health, Education, and Welfare, Food and Drug Administration, Rockville, MD. HEW Publication (FDA) 77–8010, 1976.

353. VETTER, R. J. Neuroendocrine response to microwave irradiation. *Proc. Nat. Electron. Conf., 30:* 237–238, 1975.

354. WADEY, W. G. Magnetic shielding with multiple cylindrical shells. *Rev. Sci. Instrum., 27:* 910–916, 1956.

355. WANGEMANN, R. T. AND CLEARY, S. F. The *in vivo* effects of 2.45 GHz microwave radiation on rabbit serum components. *Radiat. Environ. Biophys., 13:* 89–103, 1976.

356. WARD, T. R., ALLIS, J. W. AND ELDER, J. A. Measure of enzymatic activity coincident with 2450 MHz microwave exposure. *J. Microwave Power, 10:* 315–320, 1975.

357. WEBB, S. J. Genetic continuity and metabolic regulation as seen by the effects of various microwave and black light frequencies on these phenomena. *In: Biologic Effects of Nonionizing Radiation.* Tyler, P. E. (Ed). *Ann. N.Y. Acad. Sci., 247:* 327–351, 1975.

358. WEINTRAUB, J. R. The relationship between job satisfaction and psychosomatic disorders. Presented at the Western Psychological Association convention, Sacramento, April, 1975.

359. WEITER, J. J., FINCH, E. D., SCHULTZ, W. AND FRATTALI, V. Ascorbic acid changes in cultured rabbit lenses after microwave irradiation. *In: Biologic Effects of Nonionizing Radiation.* Tyler, P. E. (Ed). *Ann. N.Y. Acad. Sci., 247:* 175–181.

360. WIKTOR-JEDRZEJCZAK, W., AHMED, A., CZERSKI, P., LEACH, W. M. AND SELL, K. W. Immunologic response of mice of 2450 MHz microwave radiation: Overview of immunology and empirical studies of lymphoid spleen cells. *Radio Sci., 12 (6S):* 209–219, 1977.

361. WIKTOR-JEDRZEJCZAK, W., AHMED, A., SELL, K. W., CZERSKI, P. AND LEACH, W. M. Microwaves induce an increase in the frequency of complement receptor-bearing lymphoid spleen cells in mice. *J. Immunol., 118:* 1499–1502, 1977.

362. YAKOVLEVA, M. I., SHLYAFER, T. P. AND TSVETKOVA, I. P. On the question of conditioned cardiac reflexes, and the functional and morphological state of cortical neurons under the action of superhigh-frequency electromagnetic fields. *Zh. Vysshei Nervnoi Deyatel'nosti Imeni i Pavlova* (USSR), *18:* 973, 1968.

363. YAO, K. T. S. Cytogenetic consequences of microwave incubation of mammalian cells in culture. *Genetics, 83 (Suppl): 584* Abstract, 1976.

364. YAO, K. T. S. Microwave radiation-induced chromosomal aberrations in corneal epithelium of Chinese hamsters. *J. Heredit., 69:* 409–412, 1978.

365. YERMAKOV, YE. V. On the mechanism of developing astheno-vegetative disturbance under the chronic effect of a SHF-field, *Voyenno Medit. Zh. (USSR)*, *3:* 42, 1969.
366. ZABLUBOVSKAYA, N. P. Reactions of living organisms to exposure to millimeter-band electromagnetic waves. *Trans. Usp. Fiz. Nauk. 110:* 574–575, 1973.
367. ZARET, M. M., CLEARY, S., PASTERNACK, B., EISENBUD, M. AND SCHMIDT, H. *A Study of Lenticular Imperfections in the Eyes of a Sample of Microwave Workers and a Control Population.* New York University, New York Final Rep. RADC-TDR-63-124, ASTIA Doc. AD 413-294, 1963.
368. ZARET, M. M., KAPLAN, I. T. AND KAY, A. M. Clinical microwave cataracts. *In: Biologic Effects and Health Implications of Microwave Radiation.* Cleary, S. (Ed). USDHEW, PHS, BRH/DBE 70-2, p. 82, 1970.

8

Biophysics of Ultrasound

LEON A. FRIZZELL
FLOYD DUNN[1]

Introduction

Ultrasound is acoustic energy beyond the audible range (*viz.*, frequencies above 20 kHz). This form of energy is used extensively in medical diagnosis as well as in therapeutic applications. In this chapter, a) the physical characteristics of ultrasonic fields are presented, including discussion of the acoustic variables; b) information is provided on ultrasonic sources and measurement methods; and c) ultrasonic propagation in, and interaction with, tissues is described. It was considered essential to include the mathematical expressions which relate the various acoustic field variables and quantities which characterize the state of a system for a quantitative understanding of ultrasonic methods. While these equations are discussed in sufficient detail to be used to compute quantities of interest, their derivations have not been included. Readers desiring a deeper knowledge of the origin of these expressions are urged to consult the references provided. For the purpose of this discussion, only infinitesimal amplitude (linearized relations) acoustic disturbances are presented.

Physical Characteristics of Ultrasonic Fields

Initial discussion of acoustic relationships and transmission phenomena is confined to plane acoustic waves, *i.e.*, those for which the wave fronts are plane surfaces. More complex beam profiles originating from typical unfocused sources and focusing systems are discussed later.

FUNDAMENTAL ACOUSTIC RELATIONSHIPS

The fundamental acoustic relationships are the same whether ultrasound or audible sound is discussed. For either, changes occur in a number of

[1] The authors acknowledge gratefully support for the portions of the work, described in this chapter, accomplished at this laboratory in recent years, by the National Institutes of Health and the National Science Foundation.

physical variables which describe the state of a system or medium. Changes occur, for example, in the pressure and density of an elastic medium in which an acoustic field exists. For a sinusoidal plane traveling wave (traveling in the positive direction of the x-axis) with no attenuation of acoustic energy occurring in the medium (*i.e.*, no loss of energy from the waves as they travel along the x-axis), the changes in each of these (and other) physical parameters can be expressed as follows for the "linear range":

$$m = M \cos \omega(t - x/c) \tag{1}$$

where m designates any one of the variables which undergoes change during the presence of the disturbance in the medium, and M is the amplitude of the cyclic changes in the variable. The quantity c is the free field sound velocity for the medium (the speed with which a plane wave disturbance propagates in a medium of infinite extent); t and x are the time and space variables, respectively; and ω is the angular frequency, which is equal to $2\pi f$, where f is the frequency.

That Equation *1* describes a wave traveling in the positive x-direction is apparent upon examination of the argument of the cosine function. The argument is a constant when a time increase by an amount Δt is coupled with a positive shift in distance of $\Delta x = c\Delta t$ (see Figure 8.1*a*). It is equally apparent that if the minus sign in the argument of the cosine function were made a plus sign, Equation *1* would describe a wave traveling in the negative x-direction.

Acoustic propagation is characterized by adiabatic changes in the state of the medium; that is, heat transfer does not occur to any great extent during the changes in pressure. It follows, therefore, that the free field velocity can be expressed as

$$c = \sqrt{\frac{1}{\rho_0 K_{ad}}} \tag{2}$$

where ρ_0 designates the undisturbed density of the medium (density of the medium in the absence of an acoustic disturbance); and K_{ad} designates its adiabatic compressibility (1). That is, for the linearized case (small amplitude acoustical disturbances) with negligible absorption, the velocity of acoustic wave transmission is independent of frequency and amplitude, and is determined solely by the density and adiabatic compressibility of the medium. Hence, waves of arbitrary shape travel without change in form.

In the presence of an acoustic wave, the molecules of a liquid and the particles of other materials in the liquid undergo periodic excursions from their undisturbed positions, termed the particle displacement. The amplitudes of the resulting particle velocity and particle acceleration, which are the first and second time derivatives of displacement, respectively, depend upon the amplitude of this excursion and the frequency of the acoustic waves. The frequency is equal to the reciprocal of the period τ of the wave

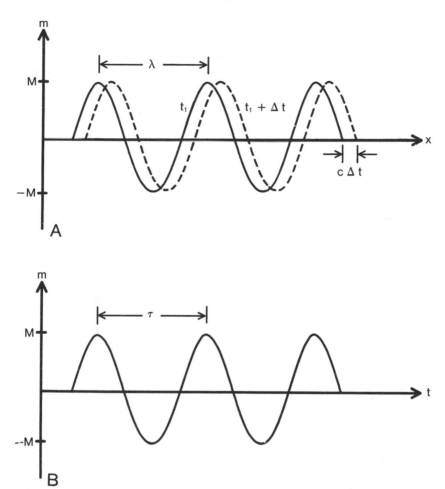

Fig. 8.1. (a) Instantaneous spatial distribution of a sinusoidally varying acoustic field variable at two instants of time. (b) Temporal distribution of an acoustic variable at a specific point in the field.

(see Figure 8.1b). The wavelength λ, which is defined by the relationship

$$c = f\lambda \tag{3}$$

is the distance separating adjacent planes of equal phase, *e.g.*, the distance from crest to crest (see Figure 8.1a). The interaction of ultrasound and biological systems may involve any of a number of physical parameters which undergo changes in the field. It is, therefore, desirable to summarize the relationships between the more important parameters. For a plane traveling wave, the variations in pressure, particle velocity and particle acceleration all satisfy Equation 1, where m designates any one of the parameters and M designates its amplitude. The relationships between the

TABLE 8.1 *Relationships Between Amplitudes of Acoustic Parameters*[a]

Parameter	Parameter Symbol	Amplitude Symbol	P (Pa)[b]	D (m)	U (m/s)	A (m/s²)	I (W/m²)
Acoustic Pressure	p	P	± 1	$\pm j\omega\rho_0 c$	$\pm \rho_0 c$	$\pm \dfrac{\rho_0 c}{j\omega}$	$\pm \sqrt{2\rho_0 c I}\,\dfrac{1}{I}$
Particle Displacement	ξ	D	$\pm \dfrac{1}{j\omega\rho_0 c}$	$\substack{+\\+}1$	$\substack{+\\+}\dfrac{1}{j\omega}$	$=\dfrac{1}{\omega^2}$	$\substack{+\\+}\sqrt{\dfrac{2I}{\rho_0 c\omega^2}}\,\dfrac{1}{I}$
Particle Velocity	$\dot\xi$	U	$\pm \dfrac{1}{\rho_0 c}$	$\substack{+\\+}j\omega$	$\substack{+\\+}1$	$\substack{+\\+}\dfrac{1}{j\omega}$	$\pm\sqrt{\dfrac{2I}{\rho_0 c}}\,\dfrac{1}{I}$
Particle Acceleration	$\ddot\xi$	A	$\pm \dfrac{j\omega}{\rho_0 c}$	$\substack{+\\+}\omega^2$	$\substack{+\\+}j\omega$	$\substack{+\\+}1$	$\substack{+\\+}\sqrt{\dfrac{2\omega^2 I}{\rho_0 c}}\,\dfrac{1}{I}$
Intensity		I	$\substack{+\\+}\dfrac{1}{2}\dfrac{P}{\rho_0 c}$	$\substack{+\\+}\dfrac{1}{2}\rho_0 c\omega^2$	$\substack{+\\+}\dfrac{1}{2}\rho_0 c U$	$\substack{+\\+}\dfrac{1}{2}\dfrac{\rho_0 c}{\omega^2}A$	$\substack{+\\+}1$

[a] Multiply expressions in table by column heading to obtain the amplitude quantities tabulated in the Amplitude Symbol column. ($j = \sqrt{-1}$). The *upper sign* applies to waves traveling in the positive direction, while the *lower sign* applies to waves traveling in the negative direction.

[b] $1\,P_a = 1\,N/m^2$.

amplitudes of these parameters are listed in Table 8.1, where all quantities are expressed in *SI* units. The symbol $j = \sqrt{-1}$ in Table 8.1 indicates a 90° phase difference. A positive j indicates that the parameter in the left-most column *leads* the parameter in question by 90°, a negative j is associated with a 90° phase *lag*, while a minus sign only indicates 180° in phase difference. The product $\rho_0 c$, which appears in a number of these equations, is defined entirely in terms of constants characteristic of the medium, and is called the characteristic acoustic impedance of the medium. For plane waves in lossless media the specific acoustic impedance, defined as the ratio of the acoustic pressure amplitude to the particle velocity amplitude, is equal to the characteristic acoustic impedance. Impedance ratios are used for determining the reflection at interfaces between media, as discussed later.

The intensity of a sound wave is defined as the time average of the rate of propagation of energy through a unit area normal to the direction of propagation (unit area perpendicular to the x-axis for waves designated by Equation *1*). It is desirable to consider numerical examples to develop a feeling for the magnitudes of the changes which occur in the various physical parameters. Accordingly, some values are listed in Table 8.2. For convenience, the technology of ultrasound developed using a mixed system of units, where intensity is expressed in watts per square centimeter while acoustic pressure amplitude is in atmospheres; this is found throughout the literature. Therefore, the values in Table 8.2 are presented in the more-commonly used units as well as in *SI* units. However, because workers in the field cling to the more commonly used units as being more useful and meaningful, these will be used in the rest of the chapter.

The propagation of a plane traveling wave in an absorbing medium is

TABLE 8.2. *Numerical Examples of Acoustical Parameters for Water.*
Frequency = 1 MHz, Temperature = 30° C, Ambient pressure = 1 Atm $\simeq 10^5$ Pa[a]

Parameter	I	P	D	U	A
For common units of	$\dfrac{W}{cm^2}$	Atm	cm	cm/s	$\dfrac{cm}{s^2}$
Multiply figures in table by	1	1	10^{-6}	1	10^6
For SI units of	$\dfrac{W}{m^2}$	Pa	m	m/s	m/s^2
Multiply figures in table by	10^4	10^5	10^{-8}	10^{-2}	10^4
	0.01	0.171	0.183	1.15	7.22
	1	1.71	1.83	11.5	72.2
	100	17.1	18.3	115	722

[a] 1 Pa = 1 N/m^2

described as

$$m = Me^{-\alpha x}\cos \omega\left(t - \frac{x}{c}\right) \tag{4}$$

where α is the amplitude absorption coefficient, absorption per unit path length. The amplitude $Me^{-\alpha x}$ of the wave decreases exponentially as it progresses in the positive x-direction. The intensity I of a plane progressive wave moving in the positive direction, at any position x in the medium, can be expressed in terms of the intensity I_0 at $x = 0$ as

$$I = I_0'e^{-2\alpha x} \tag{5}$$

Absorption is the conversion of the mechanical energy of an ultrasonic wave into heat. In an inhomogeneous medium (*i.e.*, one whose properties vary with position) other processes occur which may redirect the acoustic energy out of the main beam and prevent its being received by a suitable detector. One such process is the scattering of energy in all directions because of reflections at interfaces of structures which are small compared with the wavelength of sound and which have different acoustic properties from those of the surrounding medium. These processes, including absorption, contribute to the attenuation of the ultrasonic wave as it propagates; their combined effect can be described by an equation such as Equation 5 where an attenuation coefficient is substituted for the absorption coefficient. The absorption coefficient, however, determines the heat generated by the passage of ultrasound through tissue, and is thus of primary importance in ultrasound therapy. The values of the acoustic parameters for tissues will be given later.

Wave phenomena can produce steady forces on interfaces between media which have different values of acoustic velocity and/or density and within homogeneous absorbing media. The radiation force at a plane interface depends on the relative amount of incident energy reflected versus the amount transmitted or absorbed, and is equal to the difference in energy densities in the two media. The energy density E, or total energy per unit volume, of the plane wave is given by

$$E = I/c \tag{6}$$

where I is the acoustic intensity and c is the acoustic velocity. The use of the phenomenon of radiation force to determine total acoustic power and intensity is discussed later in this chapter.

REFLECTION, REFRACTION AND MODE CONVERSION

In order to understand the characteristics of transmission of ultrasound through tissue it is important to be familiar with certain quantitative relationships which describe the reflection and transmission of acoustic waves at boundaries. The amplitudes of waves reflected and/or refracted (redirection upon transmission past an interface) at an interface between media are determined by the acoustic velocities and densities of the respective media and by the angle at which the wave is incident on the interface.

The acoustic disturbances described by Equation 1 represent unattenuated traveling plane waves. For this type of wave, the magnitude of the change in each physical parameter is the same at all positions in the field. However, if reflection of acoustic energy takes place, the simple traveling wave equation no longer describes the acoustic conditions. Four relevant cases are described:

Case 1: Consider first the case of partial reflection at normal incidence (1), defined by a 90° angle between the direction of the incident wave and the boundary (see Figure 8.2). The acoustic pressure variation in the medium of incidence, Medium 1, can be represented analytically as

$$p = P_+\cos \omega\left(t - \frac{x}{c}\right) + P_-\cos \omega\left(t + \frac{x}{c}\right) \tag{7}$$

where P_+ is the pressure amplitude of the wave traveling in the positive x-direction (the incident wave), and P_- is the pressure amplitude of the wave traveling in the negative x-direction (the reflected wave). The two waves

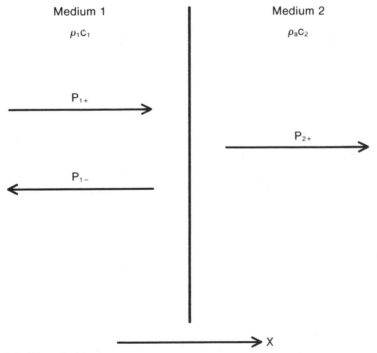

Fig. 8.2. Wave in Medium 1 incident normal to plane interface between Medium 1 and Medium 2. No energy returned to interface in Medium 2 and no absorption within media.

combine to produce a standing wave having maxima and minima of acoustic pressure, and of the other acoustic quantities, at fixed distances from the boundary. The pressure amplitude of the reflected wave P_- is given by the product of the pressure amplitude of the incident wave P_+ and the pressure reflection coefficient R_P which is a function only of the ratio of the characteristic acoustic impedances of the two media,

$r_{21} = \dfrac{\rho_2 c_2}{\rho_1 c_1}$, as follows

$$R_P = \frac{r_{21} - 1}{r_{21} + 1} \tag{8}$$

The pressure amplitude of the transmitted wave, P_{2+} in Figure 8.2, is given by the product of the pressure amplitude of the incident wave and the pressure transmission coefficient T_p where

$$T_p = \frac{2r_{21}}{1 + r_{21}} \tag{9}$$

It is assumed that there is no reflector or source in Medium 2.

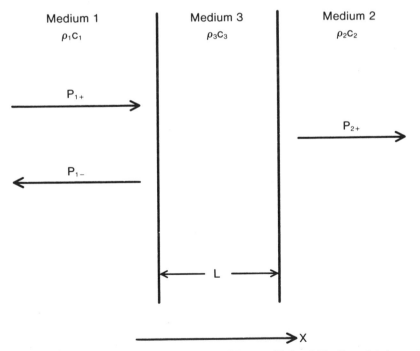

Fig. 8.3. Wave in Medium 1 at normal incidence. Slab of Medium 3 interposed between Medium 1 and Medium 2. No energy returned to interface in Medium 2 and no absorption within media.

The intensity reflection coefficient R_I and the intensity transmission coefficient T_I are given by

$$R_I = R_p{}^2 = \left[\frac{r_{21} - 1}{r_{21} + 1} \right]^2 \qquad (10)$$

$$T_I = T_p{}^2 / r_{21} = \frac{4r_{21}}{(r_{21} + 1)^2} \qquad (11)$$

A number of points should be noted from Equations 8 through 11. First, if the impedances are equal in the two media ($r_{21} = 1$), the incident wave is totally transmitted beyond the interface. If $r_{21} > 1$ the pressure amplitude reflected at the interface adds to the incident pressure amplitude, increasing the value at that point in the field. Where $r_{21} < 1$, the opposite effect occurs, and the pressure amplitude at the interface is decreased below that of the incident wave. For the two extremes, $r_{21} = 0$ and $r_{21} = \infty$, all incident energy is reflected (i.e., none is transmitted).

Case 2: Consider normal incidence again, but with a slab of a third medium of thickness L interposed between the two media (see Figure 8.3). The pressure reflection coefficient R_P and the pressure transmission coefficient T_P are functions of the ratios of the characteristic impedances of the three media and of the quantity $\omega L / c_3$ (equal to $2\pi L / \lambda_3$), which is determined by the ratio of the thickness L to the wavelength in Medium 3. For normally incident continuous waves, these coefficients are

$$R_P = \frac{P_{1-}}{P_{1+}} = \left[1 - \frac{4r_{21}}{(r_{21} + 1)^2 \cos^2 \dfrac{\omega L}{c_3} + (r_{31} + r_{23})^2 \sin^2 \dfrac{\omega L}{c_3}} \right]^{1/2} \qquad (12)$$

$$T_P = \frac{P_{2+}}{P_{1+}} = \left[\frac{4r_{21}^2}{(r_{21} + 1)^2 \cos^2 \dfrac{\omega L}{c_3} + (r_{31} + r_{23})^2 \sin^2 \dfrac{\omega L}{c_3}} \right]^{1/2} \qquad (13)$$

where

$$r_{21} = \frac{\rho_2 c_2}{\rho_1 c_1}, \qquad r_{31} = \frac{\rho_3 c_3}{\rho_1 c_1}, \quad \text{and} \quad r_{23} = \frac{\rho_2 c_2}{\rho_3 c_3}$$

The intensity reflection coefficient R_I and the intensity transmission coefficient T_I are given by the following:

$$R_I = R_P{}^2 = 1 - \frac{4r_{21}}{(r_{21} + 1)^2 \cos^2 \dfrac{\omega L}{c_3} + (r_{31} + r_{23})^2 \sin^2 \dfrac{\omega L}{c_3}} \qquad (14)$$

$$T_I = T_p{}^2 / r_{21} = \frac{4r_{21}}{(r_{21} + 1)^2 \cos^2 \dfrac{\omega L}{c_3} + (r_{31} + r_{23})^2 \sin^2 \dfrac{\omega L}{c_3}} \qquad (15)$$

Several situations are of interest: if the characteristic impedance of Medium 3 is intermediate between those of Media 1 and 2, transmission of energy T_I can be maximized by choosing the thickness L to satisfy the equation

$$L = (2n - 1)\lambda/4, \qquad n = 1, 2, 3, \ldots. \tag{16}$$

The intensity transmission coefficient then becomes

$$T_I = \frac{4r_{21}}{(r_{31} + r_{23})^2} \tag{17}$$

That is, the best choice of thickness for maximum transmission for any interposed material (if its characteristic acoustic impedance is anywhere between the values of the other media) is an odd number of quarter wavelengths. In addition, if it is possible to choose the interposed material so that its characteristic acoustic impedance is optimum for transmitting acoustic energy, the reflected wave in Medium 1 can be completely eliminated by choosing the intermediate material so that

$$\rho_3 c_3 = \sqrt{(\rho_1 c_1)(\rho_2 c_2)} \tag{18}$$

If the characteristic acoustic impedance of Medium 3 is not between those of the other two media, the optimum choice of thickness for the slab (to obtain the maximum value of the transmission coefficient) is an integral multiple of a half-wavelength (*i.e.*, $L = n\lambda/2$, $n = 1, 2, 3, \ldots$). The transmission coefficient then becomes the same as that for Case 1.

If Media 1 and 2 have nearly equal characteristic acoustic impedances, and if the thickness of the interposed slab satisfies

$$L \leq \frac{\lambda}{20\pi r_{31}} \tag{19}$$

then the transmission coefficient will not differ from that of Case 1 by more than one percent, *i.e.*, Medium 3 acts largely as a transparent acoustic window. If the characteristic acoustic impedance of Medium 3 is less than that of Media 1 and 2, r_{23} should be used in place of r_{31} in Equation 19.

Case 3: A plane wave is incident at any angle θ_1 to the normal of the plane interface between two media (see Figure 8.4). The angle of refraction θ_2 is a function of the angle of incidence and the ratio of the velocity of sound in the two media as follows

$$\sin \theta_2 = \frac{c_2}{c_1} \sin \theta_1 \tag{20}$$

and the angle of reflection is equal to the angle of incidence. The pressure transmission and reflection coefficients, and the intensity transmission and reflection coefficients, further involve the ratio of the characteristic imped-

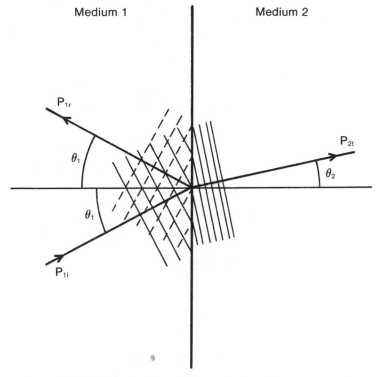

Fig. 8.4. Wave in Medium 1 incident at an angle θ_1, with respect to the normal to the interface between two media. No energy returned to the interface in Medium 2 and no absorption within media.

ances as shown in the following equations:

$$R_P = \frac{r_{21} - \dfrac{\cos \theta_2}{\cos \theta_1}}{r_{21} + \dfrac{\cos \theta_2}{\cos \theta_1}} \tag{21}$$

$$T_P = \frac{2r_{21}}{r_{21} + \dfrac{\cos \theta_2}{\cos \theta_1}} \tag{22}$$

$$R_I = R_P{}^2 = \frac{\left(r_{21} - \dfrac{\cos \theta_2}{\cos \theta_1}\right)^2}{\left(r_{21} + \dfrac{\cos \theta_2}{\cos \theta_1}\right)^2} \tag{23}$$

$$T_I = \frac{4r_{21}}{\left(r_{21} + \dfrac{\cos \theta_2}{\cos \theta_1}\right)^2} \tag{24}$$

If $\sin \theta_1 > (c_1/c_2)$, the incident wave is totally reflected, and there is no propagation of a reflected wave in Medium 2.

Case 4: This case is very similar to that of Case 3 except that the two media are considered to be viscoelastic solids capable of propagating transverse (shear) waves. Shear waves (waves with particle displacement perpendicular to the direction of propagation) may exist in solids or very viscous liquids. A longitudinal wave incident on an interface between two such materials will generate reflected and refracted shear waves in addition to longitudinal waves, i.e., mode conversion from longitudinal waves to shear waves occurs (see Figure 8.5). The angles are defined in terms of the appropriate velocities and the angle of incidence θ_1 as follows:

$$\sin \theta_2 = \frac{c_{2L}}{c_{1L}} \sin \theta_1 \tag{25a}$$

$$\sin \beta_1 = \frac{c_{1S}}{c_{1L}} \sin \theta_1 \tag{25b}$$

$$\sin \beta_2 = \frac{c_{2S}}{c_{2L}} \sin \theta_1 \tag{25c}$$

where c_{1L} and c_{1S} are the longitudinal and shear velocities in Medium 1, and c_{2L} and c_{2S} are the longitudinal and shear velocities in Medium 2. If $\sin \theta_1 > (c_{1L}/c_{2L})$, there is no transmitted longitudinal wave. Further, if $\sin \theta_1 > (c_{1L}/c_{2S})$, there is no transmitted shear wave, i.e., neither wave is transmitted since $c_{2L} > c_{2S}$ is always true. Since the reflection and transmission coefficients for each wave are quite complex, further discussion of mode conversion is delayed until later, where related heating phenomena are discussed.

DIFFRACTION AND BEAM PROFILES

In the previous sections only the idealized case of plane wave propagation was considered. The acoustic field distribution from a real source will approximate a plane wave in very limited regions only. In general, it will be a rather complex distribution depending on a) the dimensions of the radiator relative to the wavelength of sound in the transmitting medium; b) the shape of the radiator; c) the displacement amplitude distribution over the surface of the radiator; and d) the acoustic absorption coefficient of the medium at the frequency of the acoustic field. The acoustic field produced by non-focusing sources is considered in this section; focusing is discussed separately in the next section.

It is convenient to discuss acoustic fields produced by non-focusing radiators by considering first the field near the radiator (the Fresnel region) and then the far field (the Fraunhofer region) (1). The dependence of the

Medium 1   Medium 2

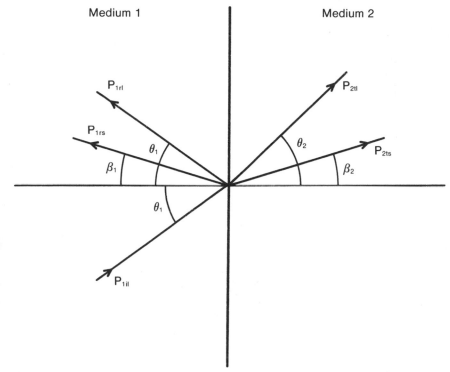

Fig. 8.5. Wave in Medium 1 incident at angle θ_1 with respect to the normal to the interface between two viscoelastic solids. Both shear waves and longitudinal waves are reflected and refracted.

field configuration on the factors listed previously is illustrated by discussing the fields produced by plane circular vibrating surfaces. The formulas given can be used to estimate the effects of varying the dimensional parameters.

The Near Field

The near field, or Fresnel region, distribution exhibits a number of maxima and minima along the axis of the radiator (1). The positions and amplitudes of these depend greatly on the velocity amplitude distribution over the source and on the ratio of source diameter to wavelength.

Figure 8.6 shows, for a plane circular vibrating element, the calculated axial field distribution of the near field for a 6.67 ratio of radius a to wavelength λ. The velocity amplitude distribution is uniform over the radiating element, and the vibrating surface is at $x/a = 0$. At distances beyond the farthest maximum, the pressure amplitude decreases monotonically and inversely with the distance from the vibrating surface. The extent of the near field and the number of maxima and minima along the axis are determined by the quantity a/λ. If $a/\lambda \gg 1$, the distance to the maximum

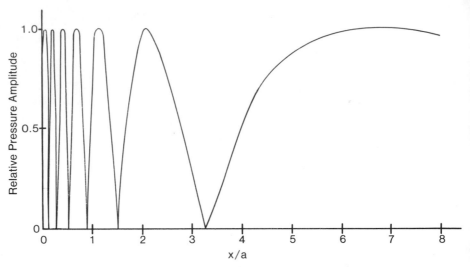

Fig. 8.6. Axial pressure amplitude distribution in the near field produced by a uniformly vibrating plane circular element.

farthest from the vibrating surface is given by

$$(X_0)_{\max} = \frac{a^2}{\lambda} \qquad (26)$$

The quantity $(X_0)_{\max}$ is the distance from the face of the radiator to the point where the transition from near to far field approximately occurs, the last axial maximum. The number of maxima N in the near field can be obtained from

$$\frac{a}{\lambda} + \frac{1}{2} > N \qquad (27)$$

That is, N is the nearest integer which is less than the numerical value of the left hand term of this equation. It should be noted that when $a/\lambda \gg 1$, the extent (in radii of the element) and number of maxima in the near field region are both nearly equal to the number of wavelengths of sound contained in the radius of the vibrating element exposed to the medium. The distance between adjacent maxima or minima decreases as one moves from the transition region toward the radiating element. It is clear from Equations 26 and 27 that for any element, as the operating frequency increases (the wavelength in the medium decreases), the distance to the transition to the far field recedes farther from the radiating element, and the number of extrema (maxima and minima) increases. These changes are proportional to the first power of the frequency.

The field distribution normal to the axis of the beam also exhibits a fairly complex structure in the near field. The number of extrema in the transverse field pattern changes with position along the axis of the beam (2). Such pattern shifts occur in increments of distance along the axis corresponding to positions of adjacent extrema.

When non-uniform vibration amplitude distributions exist over the radiating face of the element, some shifting of the positions of the various extrema in the near field occurs. Drastic modifications of the amplitude of the swing from maximum to minimum of the extrema also occur (2). The position of the last axial maximum and the number of extrema, however, are still given approximately by Equations 26 and 27. Instead of the constant amplitude shown in Figure 8.6, the axial field distribution exhibits swing amplitudes which are completely different in magnitude for some extrema. An interesting feature of non-uniform amplitude distributions is that the ratios of maxima to minima in the axial distribution are not nearly as large as with uniform distributions. Thus, by appropriate choice of amplitude distribution, it is possible to "flatten out" the axial distribution over a considerable distance (2).

If the medium has an acoustic absorption coefficient sufficiently large at the frequency of the field such that an appreciable fraction of the acoustic energy is absorbed in traversing the distance from the element to the position in the near field under attention, then the swing of the extrema at that position is modified compared with that characteristic of the field produced in a non-absorbing medium having the same value of the sound velocity. This effect increases in importance as the frequency increases, since the absorption per unit path length increases with frequency.

The Far Field

The far field, or Fraunhofer region, may be considered to begin at the position of the last axial maximum of the near field (see Equation 26). Beyond this position, the axial acoustic pressure amplitude varies inversely with the distance from the source; the intensity varies as the inverse square of the distance; and the cross section of the acoustic beam increases.

Figure 8.7 provides a useful though very simplified representation of the field from a circular source with a uniform velocity amplitude distribution. The near field is shown as a region of uniform cross-section, whereas the cross-section in the far field increases with distance from the source.

The structure of the far field for a circular source, having a uniform velocity amplitude distribution, can be described more completely in terms of the pressure amplitude as follows (1)

$$|p| = \left(\frac{P}{x}\right) \left| \frac{2J_1\left(\frac{2\pi a}{\lambda}\sin\phi\right)}{\frac{2\pi a}{\lambda}\sin\phi} \right| \qquad (28)$$

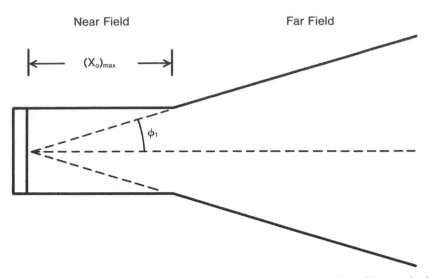

Fig. 8.7. Conception of field distribution for a circular source with uniform velocity amplitude distribution.

The first factor of this expression describes the decrease in pressure amplitude which occurs with increasing distance from the source. The second factor, in which J_1 designates the Bessel function of the first kind of order one (3) and ϕ is the azimuth angle measured from the axis of the radiating element, describes the angular width of the beam and the number and magnitude of the side lobes. This is called the directivity function and is shown graphically in Figure 8.8. For a radiator of a specified radius operating at a fixed frequency, there exists a minimum angular width of the main beam which cannot be reduced regardless of the vibration amplitude distribution over the radiating surface. The radius of the source (measured in wavelengths) affects the width of the main beam and the number of the side lobes (2). The minimum width of the main beam, as measured between the zeros on either side (which can be derived from Equation 28), is given by

$$\sin \phi_1 = 0.61 \frac{\lambda}{a} \qquad (29)$$

where ϕ_1 is the half-width, in angular measure, of the beam (see Figure 8.7).

If the vibration amplitude is non-uniformly distributed ("shading" of the vibration amplitude) over the radiator face, the beam characteristics can be greatly altered (2). That is, the amplitudes of one or more side lobes can be decreased; however, the width of the main beam increases.

FOCUSING

Ultrasonic waves can be focused, according to the same principles as light waves, allowing for higher concentrations of energy, narrower beams, and

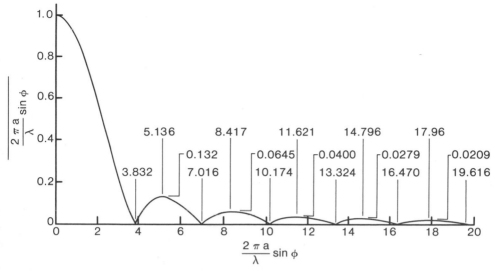

Fig. 8.8. Directivity function for a circular source with a uniform velocity amplitude distribution. See Equation 28.

control of field distributions as the experimenter wishes. This allows small, circumscribed volumes of tissue to be treated hyperthermically (4). Various types of focusing techniques are available including lens, formed vibrating element, and electronic focusing systems. Reflector focusing systems have also been used in the past (5).

Lens Focusing Systems

A typical lens focusing system is shown in Figure 8.9, consisting of a piezoelectric vibrating element which may be directly bonded to the lens, or separated from it by an appropriate thickness of acoustic coupling material. Other lens focusing systems might consist of an array of vibrating elements with a single lens, or might use several of the systems pictured in Figure 8.9, all arranged to have a common focal region. Since solids are commonly used in fabricating lenses for precision transducers, and since the velocity of sound in most solids is greater than that in water or in non-mineralized physiological media, the lens shape is plano-concave. The index of refraction n (n = speed of sound in lens material/speed of sound in propagating medium) of the lens material, relative to the medium of interest, is greater than unity so that plane waves incident normally on the plane surface of the lens are refracted toward the principal axis when emerging at the concave surface and thus, for a properly shaped lens, are brought to a focus. Referring to Figure 8.9a, the focal length F of the lens is defined as the distance from the point on the curved surface on the axis to the midpoint of the region of convergence (*i.e.*, the center of the focal region). The working distance H is the distance from the plane containing the peripheral boundary

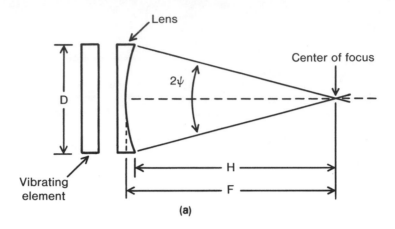

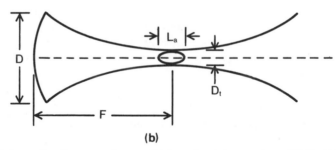

Fig. 8.9. (a) Schematic diagram of acoustic lens focusing system. (b) Illustration of the focal region of the lens.

of the curved surface of the lens to the center of the focal region. In many cases, this distance is the maximum working depth for the radiation of biological systems, since these systems are in general too large to be brought into the region bounded by the peripheral plane and the concave surface. The aperture angle 2ψ (hereafter referred to as simply the aperture) of the lens is the angle of the right cone with its apex at the center of the focal region and an altitude equal to the working distance.

If R designates the radius of curvature of the concave surface of a spherical lens of small aperture, the focal length F is

$$F \simeq \frac{R}{1 - (1/n)} \qquad (30)$$

where it is assumed that the aperture D is small and that the angles of incidence and refraction are small enough so that the sine function can be approximated by the tangent function. The working distance H is given by

$$H \simeq F\left(1 - \frac{F \tan^2\psi}{2R} \right) \tag{31}$$

Large aperture lens systems may be designed using elliptical refracting surfaces (5).

The design of lens focusing systems requires knowledge of the relationships between the dimensions of the focal region, which depend on the wavelength of sound in the medium and on the lens parameters. The size and shape of the focal region determine the *minimum* volume of material which can be irradiated and the geometric shape which can be treated without affecting surrounding structures. It is convenient to describe the size of the focal region in terms of a transverse diameter and an axial length (see Figure 8.9b). The transverse diameter D_t is the distance across the focal region, perpendicular to the direction of propagation, at which the intensity of the acoustic field is reduced to one half the peak value. It may be expressed as

$$D_t \simeq q_t \, (F/D)\lambda \tag{32}$$

where D is the diameter of the lens (as shown in Figure 8.9b), F is the focal length, and λ is the wavelength in the medium. The quantity q_t is dimensionless and depends somewhat on the half-aperture angle ψ. For values of $\psi \leq 50°$, an average value of q_t which permits calculation of D_t to within about 20 percent, is 1.0. Similarly, the axial length L_a of the focal region, the distance between points along the direction of propagation at which the intensity is reduced to one-half the peak value, is given by

$$L_a \simeq q_a D_t \tag{33}$$

The quantity q_a depends on the half-aperture angle ψ as shown in Figure 8.10. From Equation 33 and Figure 8.10, it can be seen that the ratio of axial length to transverse diameter decreases as the aperture angle increases. Further, since q_a is always greater than unity, the focal region will always be ellipsoid-like with its major axis along the axis of the sound beam.

The gain of the lens is defined as the ratio of the intensity at the center of the focal region I_F to that at the surface of the lens in contact with the medium I_o when the lens is driven uniformly. This lens gain G_1 can be expressed for lenses with small aperture angles ($2\psi \leq 38°$) approximately in terms of the lens diameter and the transverse diameter of the focal region as

$$G_1 = I_F/I_o \simeq 0.8(D/D_t)^2 \tag{34}$$

The spacing between the vibrating element and the lens, and the change in thickness of the lens material, modify the total gain of the lens system (5,6).

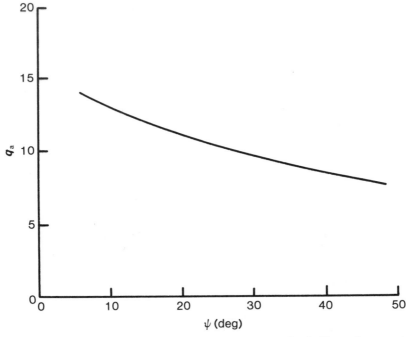

Fig. 8.10. The dimensionless lens parameter q_a versus the half-aperture angle Ψ.

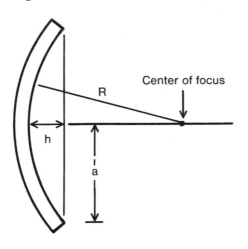

Fig. 8.11. Schematic of a section of a spherical shell used as a focusing transducer.

Formed Focusing Systems

Curved or "bowl"-shaped focusing systems can be fabricated from polycrystalline materials by casting ceramic material into the desired shape and then polarizing the material. If the concave surface is spherical, the transducer may be called a spherical shell, and the sound wave produced will converge to a focus (see Figure 8.11). The focal region is located near the center of curvature of the shell, and is closer to the exact center for larger values of h/λ, where h is the depth of the shell (2). The lateral width D_t of the focal region is expressed as

$$D_t \simeq 1.22 \frac{R\lambda}{a} \qquad (35)$$

where a is the radius of the disk and R is the radius of curvature (2,7), see Figure 8.11. The gain of this system is given by

$$G = \frac{I_F}{I_o} \simeq \left(\frac{2\pi h}{\lambda}\right)^2 \qquad (36)$$

where I_F is the intensity at the focus and I_o is the intensity at the shell surface (2,7).

Electronic Focusing Systems

Both one- and two-dimensional arrays of piezoelectric elements may be used, with varied delays of the electrical signal to the elements, to achieve dynamic focusing (8). This principle is illustrated for a linear array in Figure 8.12 where the delay to each element is adjusted so that the signals reach a common point at distance F on axis at the same time, i.e., the system focuses at this point. By changing the delays, the focal region may be moved in range and azimuth. A two-dimensional array of elements would allow movement of the focus in three dimensions.

Another common type of electronic focusing system consists of an annular

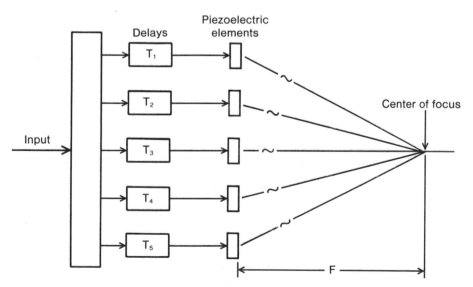

Fig. 8.12. Linear array with electrical delays adjusted for on axis focus at focal distance F.

array which can be formed by creating an annular electrode pattern on a piezoelectric element or by using separate elements as illustrated in Figure 8.13. This allows movement of the focal region along the transducer axis. The transverse dimension of the focal region of an annular array is given by an equation similar to Equation 35, where a is the radius of the active portion of the array and R is the focal length. The aperture of any of the electronic focusing systems may be varied to adjust the dimensions of the focal region, *i.e.*, the larger the aperture the smaller the focal dimensions.

Comparing the various focusing systems, plastic materials such as plexiglass possess appropriate values for the speed of sound and impedance to focus sound into water, but they also have appreciable absorption coefficients and are subject to failure at high continuous power levels. The ceramic shell represents a convenient focusing system since it is compact and free from the problems associated with lens systems. Since the shells are formed from ceramic materials, however, they may suffer from failure at high acoustic outputs, and their response may change over long periods of time. The electronic or dynamic focusing systems provide a means of changing focal position and size, but suffer from the need for much more complex electronic driving circuitry and for complex mechanical mounting of the elements into an array.

Instrumentation

This section provides basic information about sources of ultrasound, various receivers, and measurement devices. The discussion of sources ignores radio frequency electrical drive circuitry, but covers the fundamentals of piezoelectric elements which convert electrical energy into acoustical energy (and vice versa). A number of measurement methods which are used to determine ultrasonic field distributions and to determine the absolute magnitude of the acoustic power and/or energy flux from a given source are discussed.

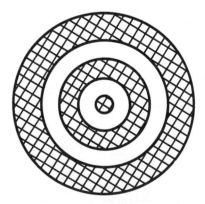

Fig. 8.13. Arrangement of active elements to form an annular array.

SOURCES, PIEZOELECTRIC ELEMENTS

Materials which exhibit the piezoelectric effect are used to generate continuous ultrasonic waves for therapeutic applications. It is the inverse piezoelectric effect which describes the linear relationship between the change in geometry of the material and the applied electric field (see Figure 8.14). A disk of a piezoelectric material of proper crystallographic orientation will change its thickness when a voltage is applied to the electrodes on the faces of the disk. The inverse piezoelectric effect, in this example, manifests itself as relative motion of the two disk faces toward and away from each other in response to the applied alternating voltage. Thus, a material in contact with one of these oscillating faces experiences a periodic disturbance which propagates away from the face at the speed of sound in that medium. The frequency of the ultrasonic wave propagating in the medium is the same as the frequency of the applied sinusoidal voltage. For a useful output, however, this frequency must correspond to one of the resonant frequencies f_n of the transducer given by

$$f_n = n \frac{c}{2d} \qquad n = 1,3,5,7,\ldots \qquad (37)$$

where d is the thickness of the disk, and c is the ultrasonic velocity in the transducer material. Equation 37 can be rearranged to give the thickness

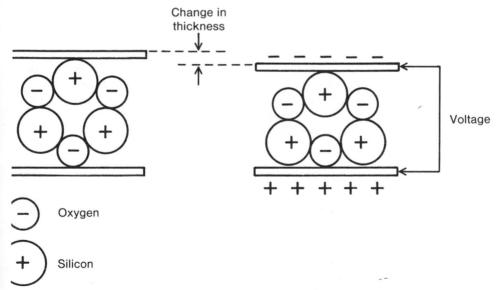

Fig. 8.14. Schematic representation of the piezoelectric effect in quartz. The change in thickness of a disk is related to the voltage between its faces.

for a given resonance frequency as

$$d = n \frac{c}{2f_n} = n \frac{\lambda_n}{2} \qquad (38)$$

where λ_n is the wavelength in the transducer material at the frequency f_n. It is apparent that the resonant thicknesses are equal to odd multiples of a half-wavelength, though the first resonant or fundamental frequency is generally used for efficient and convenient operation. As a sample calculation, a PZT-4 ceramic disk can be cut to a thickness of 2.0 mm (c = 4000 m/s) for a fundamental resonant frequency of 1 MHz. Although several natural piezoelectric materials exist and are used in ultrasonic applications, the typical therapeutic unit uses transducers of polycrystalline ceramic materials. These materials are formed into appropriate shapes, e.g., a disk, and are then polarized to make them piezoelectric. These piezoelectric ceramics have been formulated to provide stronger coupling of the electrical and acoustical energies than is provided by natural crystals such as quartz. Although they have high internal losses compared to quartz, they are also more convenient to use since they may be excited with lower driving voltages. The amount of energy radiated from the transducer depends upon the properties of the transducer material, the loading material (the material into which the energy is radiated), any loading applied to the back of the transducer, and the losses within the transducer material itself.

MEASUREMENT METHODS

For effective application of therapeutic ultrasound, it is important to know the beam profile of the source and the peak intensity and/or total acoustic power output over the range of output level adjustment. Figure 8.15 shows a typical intensity profile transverse to the transducer axis. From such a distribution and knowledge of the attenuation characteristics, absorption coefficients and thermal properties of tissue, it is possible to determine the heating rate at various locations within a specimen. The following four methods have been found to be very effective in providing the above information under free field conditions:

Piezoelectric Probe

A piezoelectric probe is fabricated from a piezoelectric material, usually a ceramic material, and uses the direct piezoelectric effect to convert the mechanical energy of the acoustic wave into electrical energy for measurement. Such probes produce a voltage output proportional to the acoustic pressure on a surface(s) (see Figure 8.16). Provided that it has dimensions which are small compared to the distances over which significant changes in the pressure field occur, the hydrophone probe (so called because it is used to detect sound underwater) may be used to determine the relative

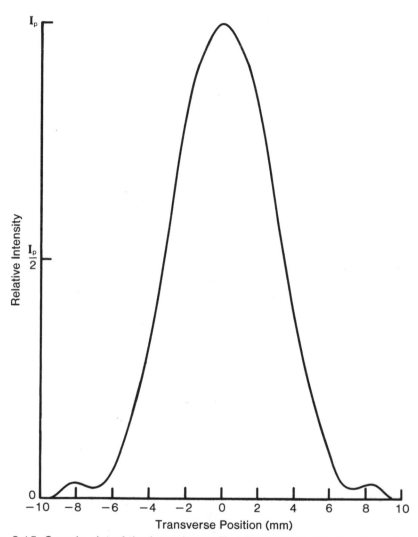

Fig. 8.15. Sample plot of the intensity profile transverse to the direction of propagation in the far field of a circular source.

pressure distribution of a source. If such a probe is calibrated, it can be used to determine the pressure amplitude in a field directly; and assuming a plane wave field, the intensity distribution can be calculated (see Table 8.1).

Transient Thermoelectric Probe

A transient thermoelectric probe consists of a small diameter thermocouple junction embedded in an absorbing material. The absorbing material converts a portion of the incident acoustical energy into heat, causing a

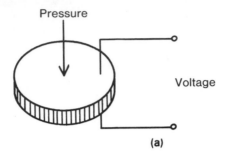

Fig. 8.16. Piezoelectric transducer elements: (*a*) disk. (*b*) section of cyclindrical probe.

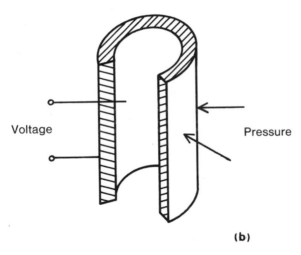

(b)

temperature rise at a rate which is given by

$$\left(\frac{dT}{dt}\right)_o = \frac{2\alpha I}{\rho C_p} \tag{39}$$

where $\left(\dfrac{dT}{dt}\right)_o$ is the initial rate of temperature rise (*i.e.*, before diffusion becomes significant), α is the absorption coefficient, I is the acoustic intensity, and ρC_p is the product of the material density and its heat capacity at constant pressure. This initial rate of temperature rise can be determined experimentally by monitoring the emf output of the embedded thermocouple. If α and ρC_p are known for the embedding material, the intensity at the thermocouple junction can be determined in an absolute manner at points of interest within the field by Equation 39. If these properties are not known, the probe can be calibrated by another standard absolute method or can simply be used to determine relative intensity levels.

A number of factors affect the observed temperature rise dT of Equation 39. In the presence of an acoustic wave, relative motion occurs between the thermocouple wire and the surrounding medium, producing heating in addition to that from absorption. This additional viscous heating tends toward an equilibrium value in a short time (on the order of 0.1 to 0.3 seconds) and can be minimized by making the thermocouple wire very small in diameter. Thus, for small wire sizes (on the order of 15 μm diameter or less), the rate of temperature rise may be determined from the slope of the thermal emf at approximately 0.5 seconds after the sound is turned on. The accuracy of Equation 39 is also reduced by any diffusion of heat toward or away from the point of measurement. The importance to this technique of heat diffusion and other artifacts has been discussed previously (9–12). Since the thermocouple wire and junction are small compared to distances over which field variations occur, and are in fact small compared to a wavelength, this probe may be used to measure the fine detail of an ultrasonic field.

Radiation Force Power Meter

The two methods just discussed are used to determine pressure or intensity at various points in an acoustic field. On the other hand, a radiation force power detector may be used to determine the total acoustic power output, which is the integrated intensity over the entire beam area. A knowledge of the relative beam profile, such as that shown in Figure 8.15, would allow the total acoustic power to be calculated from the absolute intensity at one point, or vice versa, the absolute intensity at any point to be calculated from the total acoustic power.

A radiation force power detector simply measures the force exerted on a target by a sound beam. This may be accomplished using various mechanical systems or electromechanical balances. The force (F_r) per unit area on a given target (i.e., the radiation pressure P_r) can be expressed as

$$P_r = GE = G\left(\frac{I}{c}\right) \tag{40}$$

where E is the energy density given as I/c, and G is a parameter which depends on the target type and physical configuration (7) as shown in Table 8.3. The force exerted on a target large compared to the sound beam is the integration (summation) of the radiation pressure (related to the intensity by Equation 40) over the beam. The average intensity I_{ave} in a beam of known cross-section A (often taken as the transducer area) can be determined from the measurement of the force F_r. In this case, the average

TABLE 8.3. *The Constant G of Equation 40 for Various Physical Configurations*

Physical Configuration	G
Perfect absorber, normal incidence	1
Perfect reflector, normal incidence	2
Perfect reflector, incident at angle θ_1 to surface normal	$2 \cos^2 \theta_1$

radiation pressure would be expressed as

$$P_{r_{ave}} = \frac{F_r}{A} \qquad (41)$$

Using Equation *40*, the average intensity is given by

$$I_{ave} = \frac{c}{G} P_{r_{ave}} = \frac{c}{G} \frac{F_r}{A} \qquad (42)$$

For example, if the force from a source of cross-sectional area 5 cm² on a perfect absorber in water at 37°C was measured to be 0.01 Newtons, the average intensity of the acoustic field producing the force was 3 W/cm².

The average intensity I_{ave} is equal to the integration of the intensity distribution transverse to the beam divided by the area of the field:

$$I_{ave} = \frac{2\pi \int_{o}^{x_o} I(x)\, x\, dx}{A} \qquad (43)$$

where $I(x)$ is the intensity as a function of distance off axis x, and x_o is the limit of the lateral extent of the beam. For example, if $I(x) = I_p(1 - 7x^2)$ where I_p is the peak intensity, then for $x_0 = 0.4$ cm

$$I_{ave} = \frac{2\pi I_p \int_{0}^{0.4} (1 - 7x^2)\, x\, dx}{\pi(0.4)^2} = 0.44\, I_p \qquad (44)$$

Ball Radiometer

The radiation force exerted on a small sphere suspended in an ultrasonic field is used as an absolute measure of the intensity averaged over the cross section of the sphere. The sphere is typically made of a rigid material such as stainless steel, *i.e.*, a stainless steel ball bearing, and can be small (1 mm diameter or less) compared to the distance for field variations. This technique is an absolute method for determining intensities, and requires no previous calibration.

The steel ball of a typical radiometer is suspended by a bifilar arrangement of very small diameter nylon monofilament. The radiation force F_r deflects the sphere; the magnitude of the deflection d permits evaluation of the force exerted by the ultrasonic irradiation field according to

$$F_r = \frac{mgd}{(L^2 - d^2)^{1/2}}$$ (45)

where L is the length of the suspension; m is the mass of the sphere plus the mass of the suspension structure involved, both corrected for buoyancy; and g is the gravitational constant (see Figure 8.17). The intensity is related to the force by

$$I = \frac{F_r c}{\pi a^2 Y}$$ (46)

where a is the radius of the sphere; c is the speed of sound in the fluid medium; and the dimensionless quantity Y is known as the acoustic radiation force function. This function is known to have a complex dependence on the ratio of the wavelength in the fluid to the ball radius. For accurate determination of intensity, the rather detailed plots of this function for 440C stainless steel have been published (13). As an example, consider a 1/16 inch diameter (a = 0.79 mm) stainless steel (440 C) ball suspended in water and

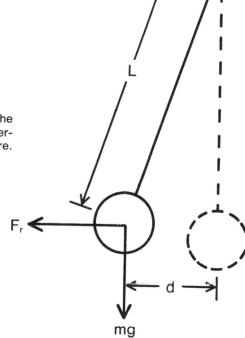

Fig. 8.17. Schematic illustration of the experimental arrangement for determining the radiation force on a sphere.

exposed to 1 MHz sound. For this case, $Y = 0.886$ such that for $d = 1$ cm, $m = 0.0133$ gm, $L = 11$ cm and $c = 1500$ m/s, an intensity of approximately 1 W/cm^2 is calculated.

Propagation in and Interaction with Tissues

A knowledge of the propagation properties of ultrasound in tissues and of the interaction of ultrasound with tissues are both fundamental to the safe and effective use of therapeutic ultrasound.

PROPAGATION PROPERTIES OF ULTRASOUND IN TISSUES

A substantial body of literature is available which reports results of ultrasonic propagation property measurements in tissues (14–16). However, the usefulness of these measurements to clinical applications is limited because most of them were not made in freshly excised tissues, the temperatures varied over a broad range, the conditions of measurement were not always specified, and the bulk of the measurements were made in the same limited number of tissues (17). These limitations exist in part because measurements are often made to gain a basic understanding of the interaction between ultrasound and tissues, rather than to provide data for development of, and application to, clinical instrumentation.

As is evident from the two earlier parts of this chapter, the propagation parameters of interest include the speed of propagation (velocity), the attenuation coefficient, the absorption coefficient, and the characteristic impedance. Table 8.4 contains a listing, ordered by increasing attenuation coefficient, of the results of measurements at 1 MHz compiled from the literature for a few tissues relevant to therapeutic ultrasound (15, 16). The entries in Table 8.4 represent averages over a broad range of reported measurements. Within experimental error, the velocity and characteristic impedance are independent of frequency. In the frequency range 0.5 to 10 MHz, the attenuation and absorption coefficients for tissues other than bone can be assumed to have a power dependence on frequency (18) expressed as

$$\alpha = \alpha_1 f^{1.1} \tag{47}$$

where f is the frequency in MHz, α_1 is the loss coefficient (attentuation or absorption coefficient) at 1 MHz, and α is the loss coefficient at the specified frequency. Only a slight reduction in accuracy results if a linear dependence on frequency is assumed. In Table 8.4, the attenuation coefficient is specified in both decibels per centimeter and nepers per centimeter since this parameter may be used with instrument adjustments in decibels and also in the equations describing attenuation which require the attenuation coefficient in nepers per centimeter. The absorption coefficients for a number of tissues have been reported (18) and are about ⅓ to ½ of the attenuation coefficient for the same tissues. The attenuation coefficient has been found to increase with structural protein content and with decreasing water content (19), as

TABLE 8.4. *Listing, by Increasing Attenuation Coefficient, of Propagation Properties of some Relevant Tissues at 1 MHz*

Tissue	Attenuation Coefficient		Velocity	Density	Impedance	Trends
	$\left(\dfrac{dB}{cm}\right)$	$\left(\dfrac{Np}{cm}\right)$	$\left(\dfrac{m}{s}\right)$	$\left(\dfrac{g}{cm^3}\right)$	$(10^5$ rayls)	
Blood	0.12	0.014	1566	1.04	1.63	Increasing structural protein content / Decreasing water content
Fat	0.61	0.07	1478	0.92	1.36	
Nerve	0.88	0.10				
Muscle	1.2	0.14	1552	1.04	1.62	
Blood Vessel	1.7	0.20	153.0	1.08	1.65	
Skin	2.7	0.31	1519			
Tendon	4.9	0.56	1750			
Cartilage	5.0	0.58	1665			
Bone	13.9	1.61	3445	1.82	6.27	

indicated in Table 8.4. The speed of sound in the medium also seems to follow the same pattern. It has recently been shown that ultrasonic properties depend on the collagen and noncollagenous protein contents of tissues (20, 21). It appears that tissues of greater protein content have higher velocities and absorption coefficients, and thus, greater heating rates than tissues of lesser protein content.

INTERFACIAL HEATING

The use of ultrasound for therapeutic heating necessarily involves several tissue types or organs; thus, phenomena associated with the surfaces between tissues become important. The phenomenon of mode conversion at an interface was introduced previously, and its relevance to therapeutic ultrasound will now be considered.

The contribution to heating in bone from energy converted to the shear mode at the bone interface has been examined (22). While it was considered that shear waves do not propagate in soft tissues, bone exhibits a shear stiffness that supports the propagation of shear waves. Measurement of the shear properties of soft tissues (23), and an examination of generation of shear waves by mode conversion in these tissues (24), support these views. Since the amount of shear wave generation at an interface depends strongly on the angle of incidence, a number of angles of incidence for a fat-muscle-bone layered system have been studied (22). The results show that, for angles of incidence in the range 45 to 60°, the heating within the bone due to shear energy is greater than that due to energy in the longitudinal mode, due in part to the higher absorption coefficient of the shear waves over that for longitudinal waves.

The results demonstrating additional heating due to mode conversion in mineralized tissues suggest that heating by this mechanism also may be important in other rigid tissues such as cartilage, although this has not yet been studied.

It is also known that increased heating occurs at interfaces in the absence of mode conversion, e.g., normal incidence, when a significant amount of energy is reflected (24). For total reflection, the heating rate is increased by a factor of two for plane waves normally incident on plane interfaces.

REFERENCES

1. KINSLER, L. E. AND FREY, A. R. *Fundamentals of Acoustics.* 2nd edition, John Wiley & Sons, New York, 1962.
2. KIKUCHI, Y. Transducers for ultrasonic systems. *In: Ultrasound: Its Applications in Medicine and Biology.* Fry, F. J. (Ed). Elsevier, New York, pp. 289–342, 1978.
3. McLACHLAN, M. W. *Bessel Functions for Engineers.* 2nd Edition, Oxford University Press, London, 1955.
4. KREMKAU, F. W. Cancer therapy with ultrasound: a historical review. *J. Clin. Ultrasound,* 7: 287–300, 1979.
5. FRY, W. J. AND DUNN, F. Ultrasound: Analysis and experimental methods in biological research. *In: Physical Techniques in Biological Research.* Nastuk, W.L. (Ed). Vol. 4. Academic Press, New York, pp. 261–394, 1962.
6. FRY, W. J. AND DUNN, F. Ultrasonic intensity gain by composite transducers. *J. Acoust. Soc. Am., 34:* 188–192, 1962.
7. HUETER, T. F. AND BOLT, R. H. *Sonics.* John Wiley & Sons, New York, 1955.
8. WELLS, P. N. T. *Biomedical Ultrasonics.* Academic Press, New York, 1977.
9. FRY, W. J. AND FRY, R. B. Determination of absolute sound levels and acoustic absorption coefficients by thermocouple probes—Theory. *J. Acoust. Soc. Am., 26:* 294–310, 1954.
10. FRY, W. J. AND FRY, R. B. Determination of absolute sound levels and acoustic absorption coefficients by thermocouple probes—Experiment. *J. Acoust. Soc. Am., 26:* 311–317, 1954.
11. GOSS, S. A., COBB, J. W. AND FRIZZELL, L. A. Effect of beam width and thermocouple size on the measurement of ultrasonic absorption using the thermoelectric technique. *1977 Ultrasonic Symposium Proceedings,* IEEE Cat. #77CH1264–1SU, pp. 206–211, 1977.
12. GOSS, S. A., FRIZZELL, L. A. AND DUNN, F. Frequency dependence of ultrasonic absorption in mammalian testis. *J. Acoust. Soc. Am., 63:* 1226–1229, 1978.
13. DUNN, F., AVERBUCH, A. J. AND O'BRIEN, W. D., JR. A primary method for the determination of ultrasonic intensity with the elastic sphere radiometer. *Acustica, 38:* 58–61, 1977.
14. CHIVERS, R. C. AND PARRY, R. J. Ultrasonic velocity and attenuation in mammalian tissues. *J. Acoust. Soc. Am., 63:* 940–953, 1978.
15. GOSS, S. A., JOHNSTON, R. L. AND DUNN, F. Comprehensive compilation of empirical ultrasonic properties of mammalian tissues. *J. Acoust. Soc. Am., 64:* 423–457, 1978.
16. GOSS, S. A., JOHNSTON, R. L. AND DUNN, F. Compilation of empirical ultrasonic properties of mammalian tissues. II. *J. Acoust. Soc. Am., 68:* 93–108, 1980.
17. GOSS, S. A., JOHNSTON, R. L. AND DUNN, F. Ultrasound mammalian tissue properties literature search. *Acoust. Lett., 1:* 171, 1978.
18. GOSS, S. A., FRIZZELL, L. A. AND DUNN, F. Ultrasonic absorption and attenuation in mammalian tissues. *Ultrasound Med. Biol., 5:* 181–186, 1979.

19. JOHNSTON, R. L., GOSS, S. A., MAYNARD, V., BRADY, J. K., FRIZZELL, L. A., O'BRIEN, W. D., JR. AND DUNN, F. Elements of tissue characterization Part I. Ultrasonic propagation properties. *In: Ultrasonic Tissue Characterization II.* Linzer, M. (Ed). National Bureau of Standards, Spec. Publ. 525, 1979.

20. O'BRIEN, W. D., JR. The role of collagen in determining ultrasonic propagation properties in tissue. *In: Acoustical Holography.* Vol. 7. Kessler, L. W. (Ed). Plenum Press, New York, pp. 37–50, 1977.

21. GOSS, S. A., FRIZZELL, L. A. AND DUNN, F. Dependence of the ultrasonic properties of biological tissue on constituent proteins. *J. Acoust. Soc. Am., 67:* 1041–1044, 1980.

22. CHAN, A. K., SIGELMANN, R. A. AND GUY, A. W. Calculations of therapeutic heat generated by ultrasound in fat-muscle-bone layers. *IEEE Trans. Biomed. Eng., BME-21:* 280–284, 1974.

23. FRIZZELL, L. A., CARSTENSEN, E. L. AND DYRO, J.F. Shear properties of mammalian tissues at low megahertz frequencies. *J. Acoust. Soc. Am., 60:* 1409–1411, 1977.

24. FRIZZELL, L. A. Ultrasonic heating of tissues. Ph.D. Thesis, University of Rochester, Rochester, N. Y., 1975. (Same as: Frizzell, L. A. and Carstensen, E. L. Ultrasonic heating of tissues. Elec. Eng. Tech. Report No. GM09933–20, University of Rochester, Rochester, NY, 1975.)

9

Bioeffects of Ultrasound

FLOYD DUNN
LEON A. FRIZZELL[1]

Introduction

In the beginning of Chapter 8, the inherent non-linear equations of acoustics were linearized to obtain a tractable approach to sound wave propagation in fluid media. This led to a benign interaction between the wave process and the propagating medium, where neither was affected by the other. The attenuation (absorption) factor was then introduced to the wave equation to describe the decrease in amplitude of the acoustic parameters as the wave process propagates through the medium. At the extreme in non-linear phenomena are the strong shock waves characterized by discontinuities at the wave front. The interest here, however, is in the intermediate range of non-linear acoustic fields, where a number of distinct phenomena which are not observed in low-amplitude acoustic fields become apparent. These may account for both the reversible and irreversible biological effects produced by ultrasound.

Mechanisms of Interaction

In this chapter, phenomena associated with thermal effects, radiation force, and cavitation events are described briefly, and quantitative relations are presented which are useful for obtaining estimates of the magnitudes of the effects.

THERMAL PHENOMENA

As shown in Chapter 8, the decrease in intensity of a plane acoustic wave in a free field may be approximated by

$$I = I_0 e^{-2\alpha x} \tag{1}$$

[1] The authors acknowledge gratefully support for the portions of the work, described in this chapter, accomplished at this laboratory in recent years, by the National Institutes of Health and the National Science Foundation.

where I is the acoustic intensity at the position x, I_0 is the intensity at $x = 0$, and α is the ultrasonic absorption coefficient of the propagating medium, provided that $\alpha \ll k$, where the wave number $k = \dfrac{\omega}{c} = 2\pi/\lambda$. The coefficient α is often expressed in nepers (Np) per unit length. For example, if $\alpha = 1$ Np/cm, the intensity is reduced in each centimeter of propagation to $e^{-2} = 0.135$ of its previous value (note that the wave amplitude is reduced to $e^{-1} = 0.37$ of its value, see Equation 4, Chapter 8. Depending upon the experimental measuring schema, it is often convenient to express α in decibels (dB) per unit length; the conversion is that 1 Np/cm = 8.686 dB/cm.

Equation 1 suggests that if α represents the portion of attenuation ascribed to absorption processes (energy irreversibly converted to heat in the body of the propagating medium), the rate of energy transfer per unit volume from the sound field is

$$-\frac{dI}{dx} = 2\alpha I \tag{2}$$

For the situation where heat conduction or radiation processes are unimportant, the rate of heat production per unit volume results in an initial time rate of increase of temperature in the medium

$$\left(\frac{dT}{dt}\right)_0 = \frac{2\alpha I}{\rho CK} \tag{3}$$

where (ρC) is the heat capacity per unit volume of the medium (ρ is the density and C is the heat capacity per unit mass per °C), and K is the mechanical equivalent of heat, equal to 4.2 J/cal. As an example of the use of this equation, consider that muscle tissue, for which α (at 1 MHz) is 0.15 Np/cm and $\rho C \simeq 1$ cal/cc°C, is exposed to a 1 MHz ultrasonic field of intensity 1 W/cm^2. The initial time rate of temperature increase is approximately 0.07°C/s, and will remain so throughout the exposure, until thermal conduction processes work to establish thermal equilibrium with the surrounding tissue.

Where heat conduction plays a significant role, the following equation is used instead of Equation 3:

$$2\alpha I = \rho CK \frac{dT}{dt} + \kappa \frac{d^2T}{dx^2} \tag{4}$$

where κ is the thermal conductivity of the medium. It is typical of therapeutic ultrasound that the dimensions of the acoustic field are always small in comparison with the specimen being irradiated, so that heat is conducted away from the center of the heated region. This results in a temperature increase lower than that calculated from Equation 3, and which approaches an equilibrium value. Additionally, blood perfusion affects the flow of heat and may be considered, to a first approximation, to have the effect of increasing the value of κ in Equation 4.

Boundary Layer Heat Generation

In addition to heat being generated in the body of a medium due to absorption of ultrasonic energy, it is also possible for heat to develop in boundary layers, and thus preferentially heat small regions dispersed throughout an exposed volume. Very small "hot spots" could then develop which may not be revealed by macroscopic temperature measurements. These result from particle velocity gradients and associated viscous shear effects. Suppose the particle velocity along x to be u_x and to vary primarily with z. The particle velocity gradient is $\frac{\partial u_x}{\partial z}$; let its magnitude be G. Heat is generated by this motion at the time-averaged rate per unit volume of $\eta(G_{av})^2$, where η is the coefficient of viscosity of the fluid medium and G_{av} is the time average value of the magnitude of the particle velocity gradient (1). For the situation where the boundary layer is established near a rigid surface, *e.g.*, by a plane wave at grazing incidence in the x-direction, it can be shown that on the surface $G = u_a/B_L \cos \omega t$ and $G_{av}^2 = \frac{1}{2}\left(\frac{u_a}{B_L}\right)^2$. Here u_a is the amplitude of the particle velocity and $B_L = \left(\frac{2\eta}{\rho\omega}\right)^{1/2}$, where ω is the angular frequency (1). The boundary layer is characterized by the thickness B_L and has the value of approximately 0.6 μm at 1 MHz for water. Using the previous relations (recalling also that for a plane wave $I = \frac{1}{2}\rho c u_a^2$) the rate of heat deposition is $\eta G_{av}^2 = \frac{k}{2} I$, where k is the wave number, which would substitute for $2\alpha I$ in Equations 3 and 4. Since $k \gg \alpha$ for most biological media at megahertz frequencies, the heat generation rate at a boundary layer with a rigid surface is much greater than the heating rate due to absorption within the medium. Boundary heating, however, occurs in a very small volume so that the resultant temperature elevation is drastically reduced by heat conduction, governed by Equation 4. In the human body these conditions (a boundary layer near a rigid surface) will likely only exist at bone-tissue interfaces, and it may be only there that such significant heat generation rates occur. For interfaces between soft tissues, the rigid surface condition does not obtain such that G, and consequently the heat produced by this particle velocity gradient are appreciably reduced.

Heating Due to Mode Conversion

The contribution to heating in bone by energy converted to the shear propagation mode is discussed in Chapter 8. A quantitative example of this phenomenon is developed here.

In Figure 9.1, the ratio of energy in the wave of interest to the energy of the incident wave is plotted for each of the waves leaving a muscle-bone

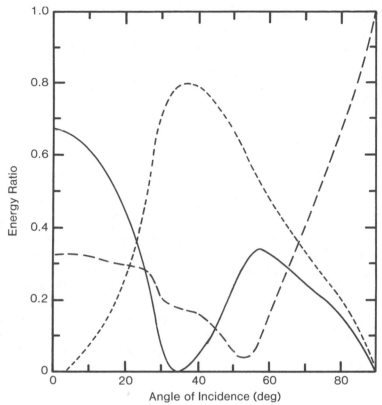

Fig. 9.1. Energy ratios (energy in wave of interest/energy in incident wave) versus angle of incidence for a longitudinal wave incident upon a muscle-bone interface (transmitted longitudinal——, reflected longitudinal— —, transmitted shear – – – – – –).

interface for a 1 MHz longitudinal wave incident from the muscle (2) (see Table 9.1 for the values used in the calculations). The energy ratio for the reflected shear wave is always less than 0.01 so that it does not appear in the figure, and the contribution to heating from the wave is neglected. It is apparent from Figure 9.1 that over a significant range of angles of incidence, the energy in the transmitted shear wave exceeds the energy in the transmitted longitudinal wave. Additionally, Table 9.1 shows that the absorption coefficient for shear waves in bone is almost twice that for longitudinal waves. As an example of the relative contribution to heating by these two waves, the ratio of heating rates at the interface, $2\alpha_s E_s/2\alpha_L E_L$, is 4.3 for an angle of incidence of 50°. Here, E_s and E_L are the energy fluxes normal to the interface for the shear and longitudinal waves, respectively, and α_s and α_L are the absorption coefficients for the shear and longitudinal waves, respectively. Details of the heating rates in a three layer, fat-muscle-bone system can be found in the literature (3).

TABLE 9.1. *Properties of Tissues at 1 MHz Used for the Mode Conversion Computations (3)*

Tissue	Longitudinal Velocity (m/s)	Longitudinal Absorption Coefficient (Np/cm)	Shear Velocity (m/s)	Shear Absorption Coefficient (Np/cm)	Density $\left(\dfrac{g}{cm^3}\right)$
Muscle	1530	0.12	22^a	5000^a	1.07
Bone	3380	1.52	1940	2.6	1.79

[a] Data from Frizzell *et al.* (26).

RADIATION FORCE

Radiation force results when the momentum transported by the acoustic wave process changes with position in the medium. It can occur at an interface between two media of different acoustic properties and also within an absorbing homogeneous medium. The rate at which momentum per unit volume is transported along the direction of propagation of the wave is the product of the momentum per unit volume (in the medium traversed by the plane traveling wave) and the particle velocity, viz. $\rho U \times U = \rho U^2$. For a traveling wave of intensity I and cross-sectional area A, the time-average rate of momentum transport is IA/c, where c is the velocity of propagation of the wave. The force on a material object is the rate at which momentum is transported to it. Thus, for a perfectly absorbing object, all the momentum of the sound wave is transferred to the object, which experiences a force

$$F_r = \frac{IA}{c} \tag{5}$$

For a perfect reflecting object, the sound wave is reversed in direction at the interface, its momentum is changed by $2IA/c$ per unit time, and

$$F_r = \frac{2IA}{c} \tag{6}$$

Radiation force also produces flow of a homogenous viscous medium. This occurs because absorption of sound in the medium results in a spatial gradient of the acoustic energy and conservation of momentum requires that the momentum disappearing from the field manifest itself as a steady force in the medium. The gradient of the radiation force is

$$\frac{dF_r}{dx} = -\frac{2\alpha IA}{c} \tag{7}$$

which produces streaming in the fluid medium. For the case where $2L \leq 3$, where L is the "length" of the acoustic beam (L can be taken as several times the axial length of the focal region for a focused field and at least ten times the beam diameter for an unfocused beam), the streaming speed v_{ST} can be computed (1) from

$$v_{ST} \simeq \frac{\alpha \rho a^2 U_a^2}{2\eta} \tag{8}$$

Here U_a is the acoustic particle velocity amplitude (axial value for a focused beam and average value for an unfocused beam), a is the beam radius and α, ρ, and η are the pressure absorption coefficient, the density and the shear viscosity coefficient of the medium, respectively. For example, consider a 1 MHz focused beam in water at room temperature for $a = 0.2$ cm, $\rho = 1$ gm/cm^3, $\alpha = 2 \times 10^{-4}$ cm^{-1}, $\eta = 0.01$ poise, and $U_a = 11.5$ cm/s (approximately 1 W/cm^2). This yields a streaming speed $v_{ST} = 0.05$ cm/s.

CAVITATION

Cavitation phenomena are produced in liquid media subjected to acoustic disturbances when the acoustic pressure during the rarefaction phase of the cycle reduces the hydrostatic pressure to a specific "threshold" value. This threshold value of the acoustic pressure amplitude is a function of a number of physical parameters which describe the state of the medium. These include temperature, pressure, frequency, kind and amount of dissolved gas, and previous history of the medium. Two types of cavitation phenomena can be distinguished, stable and transient cavitation, each of which exhibits different kinds of behavior of a gas or vapor bubble in response to an acoustic field. Stable cavitation of a medium containing dissolved or entrained gas prevails when a bubble(s) oscillates in a radial mode about a resonance size for a number of cycles without leaving the field. Transient cavitation occurs during the compression phase, in media experiencing a tension stress during a portion of the rarefaction phase of the acoustic disturbance, following growth of the bubble over several cycles to an unstable size. Here, the bubble collapse is very rapid and the bubble disintegrates, possibly by surface instability, and is thus of transient existence.

Transient cavitation is known to occur in tissues, but only at the highest intensities attainable in the frequency range of 1 to 10 MHz. Cavitation-mediated lesions have been produced in cat brain at 1 MHz at a peak intensity of 5,000 W/cm^2 and exposure times of at least 2 ms (4). Subsequent studies have implied that transient cavitation may occur at intensities beyond about (1,000 W/cm^2, related to the time of exposure by $It^{1/2} = 200$. Here, I is the acoustic intensity in W/cm^2 delivered to the site in the tissue, and t (s) is the exposure time.

Evidence for the existence of stable cavitation in tissues is lacking, except for blood (5) *in vitro*. This suggests a relatively high threshold level, 130 to 260 W/cm^2, although details of the extraction and handling of the specimen material are insufficient to determine the gas content relative to that expected *in vivo*. Stable cavitation has been associated with the production of irreversible effects on cells in suspension, macromolecules in solution, etc.

Discussion of Biological Effects

That ultrasound could produce effects in biological systems became apparent at its inception near the end of World War I, when techniques for locating submarines were being developed. An acoustic method was investigated in which a piezoelectric transducer was shock excited to vibrate at the resonant frequency of the structure and emit ultrasound into the bay at Toulon. As the electric potentials applied to the quartz plate at times were as high as 40,000 V, the amplitude of the acoustic wave was appreciable and small fish and other marine animals were found dead in the vicinity of the transducer (6).

The first extensive investigation of these phenomena had to await the development of the vacuum-tube oscillator. The destruction of *Spirogyra* and the killing of small fish and frogs exposed to 300 kHz ultrasound for several minutes at an intensity believed to be in the neighborhood of 10 W/ cm^2 was observed (6). Subsequently, streaming within cells and cellular destruction were observed at 406 kHz, when viewed with an optical microscope. These events were also accompanied by an increase in temperature (7).

The early observation that ultrasound provided an opportunity for true deep heating in tissues, and not simply the superficial heating that attended irradiation with infrared and the like (8), spawned attempts to understand the interaction of ultrasound with biological materials. Consequently, experimental studies were conducted at various levels of biological complexity. Some attention has been devoted to interaction studies in solutions of macromolecules and suspensions of microorganisms and cells, with the hope that these would provide simpler models. Herein, a principal question deals with the necessity for the presence of cavitation to affect the biological endpoint. By experimental design, thermal mechanisms are generally minimized in these systems. Interest in the interaction of ultrasound with biological tissues, organs, and whole animals was dominated by investigations of the role of thermal events in the production of irreversible structural changes and by determinations of threshold levels for such effects. The motivation for these pursuits was, of course, the probable application to medical problems. The choice of central nervous tissue as an often-employed tissue specimen was promoted by its relatively static acoustic and biological properties.

In the following, findings are identified that have emerged from these kinds of studies, progressing from whole organism studies, through tissues and organs, to cellular and molecular levels. The attempt has not been made to be exhaustive, but rather to illustrate the nature of the studies undertaken and the types of results obtained at the low megahertz frequencies. Studies were carried out for a variety of purposes, satisfying specialized interests in specific topics, and leading to a very scattered literature. Thus, crucial questions directed toward a specified purpose may not be answerable simply because the pertinent experiments and measurements have never been carried out.

WHOLE BODY RADIATION

In the low megahertz frequency range the wavelength of sound in soft tissues is on the order of a millimeter; and the half-power beam width of transducers designed for clinical purposes is approximately a centimeter. Thus, it is apparent that whole body exposure of animals to ultrasound will be limited to a few cases. Foremost among these is the mammalian fetus, though model studies have included insects and microorganisms.

Pregnant mice irradiated for 5 hours at 40 mW/cm^2, 2.25 MHz ultrasound on the 9th day of gestation, and sacrificed on Day 18, exhibited a significant increase in fetal mortality (9). Some increase in fetal abnormalities were also observed, but there was no significant alteration in fetal weight. It has been suggested that the unusual irradiation conditions could have resulted in a uterine temperature increase sufficient to produce the observed abnormalities (10). Others were unable to detect differences in abnormality rates in fetuses between Days 8 and 20 of gestation, as well as in subsequent brother-sister cross-matings, of mice irradiated for as much as 60 minutes per day, for as many as 5 days, for up to 1 W/cm^2 with 2.25 MHz ultrasound (11). Early chick embryos (corresponding to approximately three weeks human development) were affected by 5 minutes of exposure to pulsed 1 MHz ultrasound of 2.5 W/cm^2 average intensity, but not to 1 W/cm^2 average intensity (12). More advanced embryos (corresponding to approximately 6 weeks human development) were unaffected at 10 W/cm^2 average intensity. Further, no effects were found on developing embryos exposed for 24 hours to irradiation from a 2.25 MHz Doppler diagnostic instrument having an electrical input power of 100 mW/cm^2. Others have reported finding no effects on mice (13–15), nor on rats (16–18), nor on rabbits (19).

More recently (20), it has been shown that the mean weight per fetus is reduced significantly when pregnant mice are exposed to 1 MHz ultrasound for 5 minutes at an average intensity as low as 1 W/cm^2. Another study (21) found irradiation of pregnant mice with 1 MHz, 0.35 W/cm^2 average intensity for 3 minutes resulted in a significant increase in mortality in litters observed at 21 days post-partum; however, others (22) found no such increase. This discrepancy may be related to the day of gestation on which exposure to the ultrasound was perpetrated and to other differences in specimen strain, specimen preparation and procedure. A report of work-in-progress suggests that neuromuscular development in the rat is delayed on exposure to 5 minutes of CW ultrasound at 10 mW/cm^2 (23).

An early study with insects involved exposure of Drosophila eggs to 1 MHz, 0.5 W/cm^2 ultrasound. This demonstrated a variety of developmental abnormalities, most likely associated with undetected cavitation (24). A more recent study involved large scale breeding experiments with Drosophila. Those surviving the irradiation procedure exhibited no significant increase in the frequency of recessive lethal mutations and chromosomal non-disjunction, even under exposure conditions sufficient to kill a substantial portion of the flies (25).

TISSUES AND ORGANS

Much activity has occurred in identifying specific effects to selected tissues and organs irradiated by particular ultrasonic exposure regimes and in the quantitative determination of threshold levels at which unique events occur. The following illustrates the considerable range of interests of the investigators and the breadth of their findings.

The mammalian CNS provides an acoustically static organ for study in that the ultrasonic propagation properties remain largely unchanged in response to physiological and behavioral stimuli. Remarkable agreement has been reached in determining the relationship between the acoustic intensity in the tissue and the single-pulse duration necessary to produce threshold lesions in the brain (4, 27, 28). The relationship $It^{1/2} = 200$, where I is the acoustic intensity at the site of interest in the tissue in (W/cm^2), and t is the time duration of the single-pulse exposure in (s), defines the threshold. That is, exposures greater than 200 W/cm^2 $s^{1/2}$ always produce lesions identifiable under the optical microscope, while those less than this value do not. This relation has been determined experimentally to describe threshold events over the range of exposure from 100 μs to 10 minutes, beyond which it alters to approach an infinite time exposure condition. Thermal processes have been shown to dominate in the low intensity-long pulse exposure region (29), while transient cavitation events are believed to be of greatest importance at the highest intensity-shortest pulse exposure region. In the mid-intensity region, about 700 to 1500 W/cm^2, other mechanical mechanisms are believed to occur. Histologically, white matter exhibits a lesser threshold than does gray matter, with the vascular structures being most resistant (30). The observed lack of frequency dependence (31) of the threshold boundary may be due, at least in the thermal region, to the combined effects of the nearly linear dependence of the absorption coefficient on frequency and the inverse dependence of focal volume on frequency. These tend to balance each other, maintaining a relatively constant lesion volume independent of frequency (29). A study involving exposure of the lumbar enlargement of the spinal cord of neonatal mice (maintained at 37°C), a preparation permitting temperature variation of the specimen, and involving a functional rather than structural endpoint, yielded threshold levels approximately one-eighth of the above for the mature brain (32, 33).

Rat spinal cords were exposed to ultrasonic frequencies in the range 0.5 to 6 MHz at 25 W/cm^2 using 10-μsecond pulses with a 10 percent duty factor (34). A decrease in damage with increase in frequency and increased damage under hypoxic conditions were observed. Recent studies show the threshold for irreversible structural changes in cat liver to be about twice that for brain (35) and thresholds for kidney and testis to be higher still (36). A significant reduction in the frequency of mitotic cells has been reported in surgically stimulated rat liver in response to exposure to 60 mW/cm^2, 1.9 MHz ultrasound (37). However, others (38) were not able to confirm these findings with surgically stimulated rat liver irradiated 1 and 5 minutes with 2.2 MHz ultrasound in the range 0.06 to 16 W/cm^2. One major difference in the procedures employed by these two groups was that the latter used a circular motion of the transducer over the animal's ventral surface, while the former maintained the transducer stationary. Negative results were also obtained for exposure of regnerating rat liver to 2.5 MHz ultrasound pulsed at 10 to 50 kHz prf and 33 W/cm^2 peak intensity (39). However, an increase was noted in the frequency of hemorrhage at the lower frequencies, in the range 0.5 to 6 MHz, in surgically exposed liver to 56 W/cm^2 peak intensity ultrasound for 5 minutes where 10-ms pulses were used with a 10 percent duty factor (40). Although the temperature rise did not exceed 5°C, damage was particularly severe in the neighborhood of the central vein.

Conflicting reports have resulted from animal studies of the ultrasonic effects on testes, viz., effects on spermatogenesis and fertility (41, 42), while others failed to make such observations (43, 44). In a more recent study, mouse testes were exposed sequentially for 30 s at a spatial peak ultrasonic intensity of 25 W/cm^2 at 1 MHz. The testes were removed at varying times post-irradiation from immediately to 19 days, and were then examined histologically. The results suggest that two types of ultrasonically induced damage occur for different specimens under identical exposure conditions: either seminiferous tubule disruption occurs with a suggestion of minor intertubule space involvement or a more severe form of tubule damage occurs with significant interstitial tissue involvement (45). Spermatocytes appear to be affected earlier than spermatogonia, contrary to the situation following ionizing radiation.

Blood cell stasis has been demonstrated in the vessels of chick embryos exposed to ultrasound in the range of 1 to 5 MHz (46). Both CW and pulsed ultrasound were found to be effective; the intensity necessary to produce stasis may be as low as 0.5 W/cm^2 (at 3 MHz), depending upon blood vessel size, type, and orientation. The stasis is reversible upon cessation of the sound exposure, although electron microscopy has revealed damage to some endothelial cells lining the embryonic vessels in which stasis is produced. As the production of stasis is associated with standing waves, it can be avoided by either continually moving the sound source or by using sufficiently short irradiation pulses (47).

Tissue regeneration in response to ultrasonic irradiation has been studied (48). The rate of repair of 10 mm square holes in rabbit ears exposed to 3.6 MHz ultrasound for 5 minutes three times per week, under either 0.1 W/cm^2 CW application or various pulse regimes with the intensity in the range 0.25 to 8 W/cm^2, was significantly more rapid than the untreated control ear. The attending temperature rise was considered to be too small to be responsible for these effects. Subsequently, patients with chronic varicose ulceration were treated with 3 MHz ultrasound at 1 W/cm^2 for 10 minutes, three times per week for 4 weeks with encouraging results (49). Other reports of inhibited tissue regeneration in response to ultrasonic irradiation have also appeared. In one, slightly slower tissue renewal of the amputated prelimb of a newt occurred, following ultrasound exposure, compared to that of the opposite amputated prelimb, although details were sparse and conditions were complicated for identifying the crucial dosages (50).

The effects of ultrasound on neoplastic tissues has involved at least two lines of inquiry: a direct effect on tissue possibly involving hyperthermic effects, and a synergistic involvement with other modalities. A recent example of the former deals with the irradiation of subcutaneously implanted Rat Wilm's tumors. The use of 1 MHz ultrasound at 1.5 W/cm^2 resulted in a reduction in tumor volume and weight, and an increase in mean rat survival time (51). Histological observation revealed nuclei with condensed chromatin patterns. Substantial temperature increases also occurred. In regard to synergism, it was noted that the X-ray dosage required to produce regression in an experimental tumor was substantially reduced when simultaneously irradiated with 1 MHz ultrasound at 8.4 W/cm^2; the effect was believed to be due to heating resulting from sound absorption (52). Marked improvement in the treatment of human superficial cancer was reported from the simultaneous use of ultrasound and X-rays (53). However, synergistic effects were not observed with either cultured mouse lymphoma cells or implanted tumors in rats (54). It has been reported that a preliminary irradiation of transplanted sarcoma 37 tumors in mice with 1 MHz ultrasound in the range 0.5 to 2.5 W/cm^2 for periods of 1 to 5 minutes enhances the sensitivity of the tumor cells to subsequent gamma radiation (55). A synergism with chemotherapy has been suggested (56), where malignant brain tumors were irradiated simultaneously, through a bone flap, with 1 MHz ultrasound at 3 W/cm^2. Although the patient population was small, they believed the effectiveness of chemotherapy improved.

Enhanced DNA synthesis has been reported in neonatal mouse tibiae exposed for 5 minutes, three times in 24 hours, to 1.8 W/cm^2, 1 MHz ultrasound (57). Observations revealed that growth, protein accumulation, and ^{3}H-proline incorporation remained unaffected. The DNA synthesis may have been affected by the substantial temperature rise which accompanied absorption of the ultrasonic energy in the highly absorbing bone tissue, though the authors are not so convinced.

CELLS AND MICROORGANISMS

Cells and microorganisms in suspension provide model systems of tissues and organs. They have the advantage of being composed of single cell lines, possibly even in mitotic synchrony, but with the disadvantage of not being constrained by tissue architectural features, though gel-caging can reduce the importance of this. Such systems have been attractive for studies dealing with the physical mechanisms by which ultrasound can produce alterations in more complex structures. Thus, it has emerged that ultrasonic exposure of cells and microorganisms in suspension can lead to cell death, and that cavitation is important to the process. Indeed, some investigators (58) have been able to associate the destruction of an amoeba with the specific number of discrete cavitation events occurring during the irradiation procedure. This apparent relationship of cavitation to cell destruction is important in attempts to determine risk in the clinical use of ultrasound, especially since virtually nothing is known of cavitation phenomena in tissues. It appears that cell disintegration occurs preferentially, at least when cavitation is allowed to occur, during the mitotic phase of the cell cycle. Mouse leukemia cells in aqueous suspension were most susceptible to damage in M-phase when exposed to 1 MHz ultrasound having a spatial peak intensity of 15 W/cm^2 for 10 seconds (59). It has been suggested that the mechanical strength of the cell membrane may vary during the cell cycle. In one interesting case, gel-caged suspensions of an amoeba were exposed to 1 MHz ultrasound sufficient to produce irreversible alterations in mammalian tissues (60). They employed samples from logarithmically growing and synchronous cultures treated in free field and standing wave field conditions in both CW and pulsed regimes. The treated samples, however, failed to show differences in growth patterns compared to controls.

Non-lethal effects on cells have also been investigated. A reduction in the electrophoretic mobility of Ehrlich ascites cells was observed following exposure to low megahertz ultrasound, implying alteration of the electric charge density of the cellular surface (61, 62). Ultrasonic irradiation at 1.8 MHz with intensities greater than 1 W/cm^2 of rat thymocytes was followed by an immediate decrease in potassium content, suggesting a sublethal alteration in the structures intimate to permeability (63). Additionally, investigations of ultra-structural details has revealed mitochondrial modifications in cells exposed to ultrasound (64).

Microorganisms have been employed in genetic studies without positive results. An increase was not found in the back-mutation of an auxotrophic strain of *Bacillus subtilis* in response to 2 MHz ultrasonic irradiation for 5 minutes at intensities up to 60 W/cm^2, in a pulsed regime (65). Also, abnormal genetic effects did not occur in ultrasonically irradiated yeast cells, even when treated in such a manner that the cells were killed to 0.1 percent of the survival rate of the controls (66).

BIOMACROMOLECULES AND THEIR ASSEMBLAGES

The response of large molecules of biological importance to ultrasonic exposure has been studied in aqueous solution to determine details of tissue interaction mechanisms. The findings showing that ultrasonic absorption is largely attributable to tissue protein content (67) and that tissue interactions resulting in irreversible structural changes must occur at levels of structure below that identifiable with the light microscope (32) encouraged some of these inquiries.

For molecules having molecular weights below about 10^4, *i.e.*, proteins, in aqueous solution, degradation appears to occur only in the presence of cavitation in the ultrasonic frequency range of 1 to 27 MHz (68). For larger molecules in aqueous solution, *e.g.*, DNA with molecular weights greater than about 10^6, it has been possible to demonstrate degradation in the absence of any phenomena suggesting the presence of cavitation (69). Using intensities as high as 30 W/cm^2, essentially monodisperse fragments were produced with the limiting value depending upon intensity, *i.e.*, greater intensities of exposure produced smaller fragments. This sequential halving of the molecules with continued irradiation time is also a characteristic feature of the much more prevalent studies of degradation of DNA in the presence of cavitation (70). The breaking of DNA molecules preferentially at the midpoints of their extended conformation in solution suggests a mechanical mechanism being responsible. However, chemical effects, largely due to free radical production in the presence of cavitation, have been described extensively (71), in particular in the low megahertz frequency range (72). Nonetheless, while it is an easy task to degrade nucleic acid molecules in solution, it has not been possible to produce mutagenic lesions following *in vitro* irradiation of transforming DNA (65). The apparent necessity for the extended conformation of DNA molecules in solution for degradation to occur implies a much lesser opportunity for denaturation of cellular DNA to occur.

An interesting finding from two laboratories is that the order of ultrasonic reactivity obtained by observing spectral changes (73) in nucleic acid bases in solution at 1 MHz and less than 5 W/cm^2 (viz., Thy > Ura > Cyt > Gua > Ade) seems to be the same as that obtained by chromatography (74) in dilute solutions of nucleic acids at 800 kHz and approximately 10 W/cm^2. No information exists about the occurrence of such events intracellularly. A recent study of the effect of 1 MHz ultrasound in the range 15 to 36 W/cm^2 for 10 minutes on human leucocytes failed to increase sister chromatid exchange frequency, implying no effects to chromosomes (75).

Considerable attention has been devoted to possible ultrasonic effects on chromosomes. Much of this interest has been associated with studies involving human lymphocyte chromosomes from cultured preparations, with the overwhelming result that ultrasound does not produce an increase in aberrations even at much greater exposure intensities and longer irradiation times than are likely to occur during medical diagnositic procedures (76–81), though such a synergistic effect with X-rays may occur (82).

A few studies have treated membranes and membrane models. The permeability of membranes formed from oxidized cholesterol was increased by exposure to 1 MHz ultrasound (83) at intensities greater than 1.5 W/cm^2. Liver plasma membranes exhibited decreased 5′ nucleotidase activity and altered morphology in response to 0.87 MHz ultrasound in the range 0.75 to 3 W/cm^2 for exposures ranging from 2 to 10 minutes (84). An unlinking of the membrane potential and short circuit current was found to occur in that their time courses in response to ultrasound differed, *i.e.*, the short circuit current increased continuously for exposures of 0.5 seconds and longer while the membrane potential reached its maximum within 0.5 seconds and did not alter with increased duration of exposure (85). This occurred at 1 MHz in the intensity range 1 to 100 W/cm^2 for isolated frog skin preparations. Alteration of the recalcification time of platelet-rich plasma occurs with 1 MHz ultrasound at approximately 0.2 W/cm^2 (spatial peak) in 5 minutes (86).

Summary of Biological Effects

From the investigations that have been conducted, it appears that ultrasound can be considered a very inefficient mutagenic agent. Chromosome damage in response to ultrasonic irradiation is most likely to be lethal. Because of the particular molecular conformation necessary to bring about effects *in vitro*, it does not appear likely that selective effects can be produced in cellular nucleic acids.

As ultrasound appears to induce embryological effects, the treatment of pregnant women in the abdominal area., *e.g.*, possibly for lower back pain, should be avoided.

A systematic analysis of existing reliable data for mammalian tissues has led to the following two summary statements (87)

a) No substantial bioeffects have been demonstrated for spatial peak-temporal average intensities less than 100 mW/cm^2.

b) No substantial bioeffects have been demonstrated for which the product I·t is less than 50 J/cm^2 where, for pulsed operation, t is the total ("on" + "off") time.

(It should be noted that the spatial peak intensities referred to in the statement are typically very much greater than the spatial average values of intensity used in the specification of ultrasonic instrumentation.) The statements may need to be modified as new data appear, since a) most of the data are from mammals other than man, and the extrapolation to man is not always a clear procedure, b) the influence of exposure factors such as pulsing conditions and acoustic frequency are not included, and c) the most sensitive biological tests may not have been used yet.

No fully satisfactory epidemiological study has as yet been performed. However, a retrospective survey which was not case-controlled of more than 1000 apparently normal women examined diagnostically with ultrasound during various stages of pregnancy exhibited only a 2.7 percent incidence of congenital abnormalities on newborn physical examination. This is to be compared with the figure of 4.8 percent from a separate and unmatched survey of women who did not receive ultrasonic diagnosis (88). Neither the gestation period at which the first ultrasonic examination occurred nor the number of examinations appeared to increase the risk of fetal abnormality. A smaller study has also yielded no indication of either congenital malformations or chromosomal aberrations in the fetus (89).

Finally, although not scientifically objective, it must be noted that a substantial number of persons receiving ultrasonic diagnosis also undergo subsequent clinical examinations; undesirable effects from such procedures, or suspicions thereof, have not been reported (33).

REFERENCES

1. NYBORG, W. L. *Intermediate Biophysical Mechanics.* Cummings Publishing Co., Inc., Menlo Park, CA, 1975.
2. FRIZZELL, L. A. Ultrasonic Heating of Tissue. Ph.D. Thesis, University of Rochester, Rochester, N.Y., 1975. (Same as Frizzell, L.A. and Carstensen, E. L. Ultrasonic Heating of Tissues. Elec. Eng. Tech. Report No. GM09933-20, University of Rochester, Rochester, NY, 1975.)
3. CHAN, A. K., SIGELMANN, R. A. AND GUY, A. W. Calculations of therapeutic heat generated by ultrasound in fat-muscle-bone layers. *IEEE Trans. Biomed. Eng., BME-21:* 280–284, 1974.
4. FRY, F. J., KOSSOFF, G., EGGLETON, R. C. AND DUNN, F. Threshold ultrasonic dosage for structural changes in the mammalian brain. *J. Acoust. Soc. Am., 48:* 1413–1417, 1970.
5. ESCHE, R. Untersuchung der Schwingungskavitation in Flüssigkeiten. *Akust. Beih., 4:* 208–218, 1952.
6. WOOD, R. W. AND LOOMIS, A. L. The physical and biological effects of high-frequency sound waves of great intensity. *Phil. Mag., 4:* 417–436, 1927.
7. HARVEY, E. N. AND LOOMIS, A. L. High frequency sound waves of small intensity and their biological effects. *Nature, 12:* 622–624, 1928.
8. DUNN, F. AND O'BRIEN, W. D., JR. (eds) *Ultrasonic Biophysics.* Dowden, Hutchinson, and Ross, Stroudsburg, 1976.
9. SHOJI, R., MOMMA, E., SHIMIZU, T. AND MATSUDA, S. Experimental studies on the effect of ultrasound on mouse embryos. *Teratology, 6:* 119, 1972.
10. LELE, P. P. Ultrasonic teratology in mouse and man. *In: Proc. 2nd European Congress on Ultrasonics in Medicine.* Excerpta Medica, Amsterdam, pp. 22–27, 1976.
11. MANNOR, S. M., SERR, D. M., TAMARI, I., MESHOREV, A. AND FREI, E. H. The safety of ultrasound in fetal monitoring. *Am. J. Obstet. Gynec., 113:* 653–661, 1972.
12. TAYLOR, K. J. W. AND DYSON, M. Toxicity studies on the interaction of ultrasound on embryonic and adult tissues. *In: Ultrasonics in Medicine.* deVlieger, M, White, D. N. and McCready, V. R. (Eds). Excerpta Medica, Amsterdam, pp. 353–359, 1974.
13. KIRSTEN, E. G., ZINSSLER, H. H. AND REID, J. M. Effect of 1 mc ultrasound on the genetics of mouse. *IEEE Trans. Ultrason. Engr., UE-10:* 112–116, 1963.
14. SMYTH, M. G. Animal toxicity studies with ultrasound at diagnostic power levels. *In: Diagnostic Ultrasound.* Grossman, C. C., Holmes, J. H., Joyner, C. and Purnell, E. W. (Eds). Plenum Press, New York, pp. 296–299, 1966.
15. WARWICK, R., POND, J. B., WOODWARD, B., AND CONNOLLY, C. C. Hazards of diagnostic ultrasonography—a study with mice. *IEEE Trans. Sonics Ultrason., SU-17:* 158–164, 1970.
16. MCCLAIN, R. M., HOAR, R. M. AND SALTZMAN, M. B. Teratologic study of rats exposed to ultrasound. *Am. J. Obstet. Gynec., 114:* 39–42, 1972.
17. TAKEUCHI, H. Experimental studies on ultrasonic doppler method in obstetrics. *Acta Obstet. Gynec. Jap., 17:* 11–16, 1970.
18. WOODWARD, R., WARWICK, R. AND POND, J. B. How safe is diagnostic sonar? *Br. J. Radiol., 43:* 719–725, 1970.
19. HOLMES, J. Ultrasonic visualization of living tissues. (Abstracts) *Fed. Proc., 21:* 304, 1962.
20. O'BRIEN, W. D., JR. Ultrasonically induced fetal weight reduction in mice. *In: Ultrasound in Medicine.* White, D. and Barnes, R. (Eds). Plenum Press, New York, pp. 531–532, 1976. Vol. 2.
21. CURTO, K. Early postpartum mortality following ultrasound radiation. *In: Ultrasound in*

Medicine. White, D. and Barnes, R. (Eds). Plenum Press, New York, pp. 535–536, 1976. Vol. 2.

22. EDMONDS, P. D., STOLZENBERG, S. J., TORBIT, C. A., MADAN, S. M. AND PRATT, D. C. Post partum survival of mice exposed *in utero* to ultrasound. *J. Acoust. Soc. Am., 66:* 590–593, 1979.

23. SIKOV, M. R., HILDEBRAND, B. P. AND STEARNS, J. D. Postnatal sequalae of ultrasound exposure at fifteen days of gestation in the rat. (work in progress). Presented before the First Meeting of the World Federation for Ultrasound in Medicine and Biology, San Francisco, August, 1976.

24. SELMAN, G. G. AND COUNCE, S. J. Abnormal embryonic development in Drosophila induced by ultrasonic treatment. *Nature, 172:* 503–504, 1953.

25. THACKER, J., AND BAKER, N. V. The use of Drosophila to estimate the possibility of genetic hazard from ultrasound irradiations. *Br. J. Radiol., 49:* 367–371, 1976.

26. FRIZZELL, L. A., CARSTENSEN, E. L. AND DYRO, J. F. Shear properties of mammalian tissues at low megahertz frequencies. *J. Acoust. Soc. Am., 60:* 1409–1411, 1977.

27. POND, J. B. The role of heat in the production of ultrasonic focal lesions. *J. Acoust. Soc. Am., 47:* 1607–1611, 1970.

28. ROBINSON, T. C. AND LELE, P. P. An analysis of lesion development in the brain and in plastics by high-intensity focused ultrasound at low-megahertz frequencies. *J. Acoust. Soc. Am., 51:* 1333–1351, 1972.

29. LERNER, R. M., CARSTENSEN, E. L. AND DUNN, F. Frequency dependence of thresholds for ultrasonic production of thermal lesions in tissue. *J. Acoust. Soc. Am., 54:* 504–506, 1973.

30. FRY, W. J. Intense ultrasound in investigations of the central nervous system. *In: Advances in Medical and Biological Physics.* Vol. 6. Lawrence, J. H. and Tobias, C. A. (Eds). Academic Press, New York, pp. 281–348, 1958.

31. JOHNSTON, R. L. AND DUNN, F. Influence of subarachnoid structures on transmeningeal ultrasonic propagation. *J. Acoust. Soc. Am., 60:* 1225–1227, 1976.

32. DUNN, F. Physical mechanisms of the action of intense ultrasound on tissue. *Am. J. Phys. Med., 37:* 148–151, 1958.

33. DUNN, F., AND FRY, F. J. Ultrasonic Threshold Dosages for the Mammalian Central Nervous System. *IEEE Trans. Biomed. Engr., BME-18:* 253–256, 1971.

34. TAYLOR, K. J. W. AND POND, J. B. A study of the production of haemorrhagic injury and paraplegia in rat spinal cord by pulsed ultrasound of low megahertz frequencies in the context of safety for clinical usage. *Br. J. Radiol., 45:* 343–353, 1972.

35. CHAN, S. AND FRIZZELL, L. A. Ultrasonic thresholds for structural changes in the mammalian liver. *Proc. IEEE Ultrasonic Symp.* (Cat. #77CH1264–ISU), pp. 153–156, 1977.

36. FRIZZELL, L. A., LINKE, C. A., CARSTENSEN, E. L. AND FRIDD, C. W. Thresholds for focal ultrasonic lesions in rabbit kidney, liver, and testicle. *IEEE Trans. Biomed. Eng., BME-24:* 393–396, 1977.

37. KREMKAU, F. W. AND WITKOFSKI, R. L. Mitotic reduction in rat liver exposed to ultrasound. *J. Clin. Ultrasound, 2:* 123–126, 1974.

38. MILLER, M. W., KAUFMAN, G. E., CATALDO, F. L. AND CARSTENSEN, E. L. Absence of mitotic reduction in regenerating rat livers exposed to ultrasound. *J. Clin. Ultrasound, 4:* 169–172, 1976.

39. BARNETT, S. AND KOSSOFF, G. Negative effect of long duration pulsed ultrasonic irradiation on the mitotic activity in regenerating rat liver. *In: Ultrasound in Medicine.* White, D. and Brown, R. (Eds). Plenum Press, New York, pp. 2033–2044, 1977.

40. TAYLOR, K. J. W. AND POND, J. B. The effects of ultrasound of varying frequencies on rat liver. *J. Pathol., 110:* 287–293, 1970.

41. KAMOCSAY, D., RONA, G. AND TARNOCZY, T. Effects of ultrasonics on testicles. Experimental studies on white rats. (in German) *Arztliche Forschung, 9:* 389–395, 1955.

42. FAHIM, M. S., FAHIM, Z., DER, R., HALL, D. G. AND HARMAN, J. Heat in male contraception (hot water 60°C, infrared, microwave, and ultrasound). *Contraception, 11:* 549–562, 1975.

43. LYON, M. F. AND SIMPSON, G. H. An investigation into the possible genetic hazards of ultrasound. *Br. J. Radiol., 47:* 712–722, 1974.

44. URRY, R. L., DOUGHERTY, K. A., CHILD, S., FERNANDEZ, F., COCKETT, A. T. K., LINKE, C. AND CARSTENSEN, E. L. Ultrasound and spermatogenesis in the rat. *Andrology,* in press.

45. O'BRIEN, W. D., JR., BRADY, J. K. AND DUNN, F. Morphological changes to mouse testicular tissue from *in vivo* ultrasonic irradiation (preliminary report). *Ultrasound Med. Biol., 4:* 35–43, 1979.

46. DYSON, M., POND, J. B., WOODWARD, B. AND BROADBENT, J. The production of blood cell stasis and endothelial damage in blood vessels of chick embryos treated with ultrasound in a stationary wave. *Ultrasound Med. Biol., 1:* 133–148, 1974.

47. TER HAAR, G. AND WYARD, S. J. Blood cell banding in ultrasonic standing wave fields: A physical analysis. *Ultrasound Med. Biol., 4:* 111–123, 1978.

48. DYSON, M., POND, J. B., JOSEPH, J. AND WARWICK, R. The stimulation of tissue regeneration by means of ultrasound. *Clin. Sci., 35:* 273–285, 1968.

49. DYSON, M. AND SUCKLING, J. Stimulation of tissue repair by ultrasound: A survey of the mechanisms involved. *Physiotherapy, 64:* 105–108, 1978.

50. PIZZARELLO, D. J., WOLSKY, A., BECKER, M. H. AND KEEGAN, A. F. A new approach to testing the effect of ultrasound on tissue growth and differentiation. *Oncology, 31:* 226–232, 1975.

51. LONGO, F., TOMASHEFSKY, P., RIVIN, B. D., LONGO, W. E., LATTIMER, J. K. AND TANNENBAUM, M. Interaction of ultrasound with neoplastic tissue. *Urology, 6:* 631–634, 1975.

52. LEHMANN, J. F. AND KRUSEN, F. H. Biophysical effects of ultrasonic energy on carcinoma and their possible significance. *Arch. Phys. Med. Rehabil., 36:* 452–459, 1955.

53. WOEBER, K. The effect of ultrasound in the treatment of cancer. *In: Ultrasonic Energy.* Kelly, E. (Ed). Univ. of Illinois Press, Urbana, IL, pp. 137–147, 1965.

54. CLARKE, P. R., HILL, C. R. AND ADAMS, K. Synergism between ultrasound and X-rays in tumor therapy. *Br. J. Radiol., 43:* 97–99, 1970.

55. GAVRILOV, L. R., KALENDO, G. S., RYABUKHIN, V. V., SHAGINYAN, K. A. AND YARMONENKO, S. P. Ultrasonic enhancement of the gamma radiation of malignant tumors. *Sov. Phys. Acoust., 21:* 119–121, 1975.

56. HEIMBURGER, R. F., FRY, F. J., FRANKLIN, T. D. AND EGGLETON, R. C. Ultrasound potentiation of chemotherapy for brain malignancy. *In: Ultrasound in Medicine.* White, D. N. (Ed). Vol. 1. Plenum Press, New York, pp. 273–281, 1975.

57. ELMER, W. AND FLEISCHER, A. Enhancement of DNA synthesis in neonatal mouse tibial epiphyses after exposure to therapeutic ultrasound. *J. Clin. Ultrasound, 2:* 191–195, 1974.

58. COAKLEY, W. T., HAMPTON, D. AND DUNN, F. Quantitative relationships between ultrasonic cavitation and effects upon amoebae at 1 MHz. *J. Acoust. Soc. Am., 50:* 1546–1553, 1971.

59. CLARKE, P. R. AND HILL, C. R. Biological action of ultrasound in relation to the cell cycle. *Expl. Cell Res., 58:* 443–444, 1969.

60. BROWN, R. C. AND COAKLEY, W. T. Unchanged growth patterns of *Acanthamoeba* exposed to intermediate intensity ultrasound. *Ultrasound Med. Biol., 2:* 37–41, 1975.

61. REPACHOLI, M. H., WOODCOCK, J. P., NEWMAN, D. L. AND TAYLOR, K. J. W. Interaction of low intensity ultrasound and ionizing radiation with the tumor cell surface. *Phys. Med. Biol., 16:* 221–227, 1971.

62. TAYLOR, K. J. W. AND NEWMAN, D. L. Electrophoretic mobility of Ehrlich suspensions exposed to ultrasound of varying parameters. *Phys. Med. Biol., 17:* 270–276, 1972.

63. CHAPMAN, I. V. The effect of ultrasound on the potassium content of thymocytes *in vitro. Br. J. Radiol., 47:* 411–413, 1974.

64. HRAZDIRA, I. Changes in cell ultrastructure under direct and indirect action of ultrasound. *In: Ultrasonographia Medica.* Bock, J. et al. (Eds). Academy of Medicine, Vienna, pp. 457–463, 1970.

65. COMBES, R. D. Absence of mutation following ultrasonic treatment of *Bacillus Subtilis* cells and transforming deoxyribonucleic acid. *Br. J. Radiol., 48:* 306–311, 1975.

66. THACKER, J. An assessment of ultrasonic radiation hazard using yeast genetic systems. *Br.*

J. Radiol., 47: 130–138, 1974.

67. CARSTENSEN, E. L., LI, K. AND SCHWAN, H. P. Determination of the acoustic properties of blood and its components. *J. Acoust. Soc. Am., 25:* 286–289, 1953.

68. MACLEOD, R. M. AND DUNN, F. Effects of intense noncavitating ultrasound on selected enzymes. *J. Acoust. Soc. Am., 44:* 932–940, 1968.

69. HAWLEY, S. A., MACLEOD, R. M. AND DUNN, F. Degradation of DNA by intense, noncavitating ultrasound. *J. Acoust. Soc. Am., 35:* 1285–1287, 1968.

70. PEACOCKE, A. R. AND PRITCHARD, N. J. The ultrasonic degradation of biological macro-molecules under conditions of stable cavitation. II, Degradation of deoxyribonucleic acid. *Biopolymers, 6:* 605–623, 1968.

71. EL'PINER, I. P. *Ultrasound: Physical, Chemical, and Biological Effects.* Consultants Bureau, New York, 1964.

72. HILL, C. R. Ultrasonic exposure thresholds for changes in cells and tissues. *J. Acoust. Soc. Am., 52:* 667–672, 1972.

73. MCKEE, J. R., CHRISTMAN, C. L., O'BRIEN, W. D., JR. AND WANG, S. Y. Effects of ultrasound on nucleic acid bases. *Biochem., 16:* 4651–4654, 1977.

74. BRAGINSKAYA, F. I. AND EL'PINER, I. Y. Metachromatic reaction of nucleic acids (DNA and RNA) native and irradiated with ultrasonic waves. *Biofizika, 9:* 31–40, 1964.

75. MORRIS, S. M., PALMER, C. G., FRY, F. J. AND JOHNSON, L. K. Effect of ultrasound on human leucocytes. Sister chromatid exchange analysis. *Ultrasound Med. and Biol., 4:* 253–258, 1978.

76. COAKLEY, W. T., SLADE, J. S., BRAEMAN, J. M. AND MOORE, J. L. Examination of lymphocytes after exposure to ultrasonic irradiation. *Br. J. Radiol., 45:* 328–332, 1972.

77. HILL, C. R., JOSHI, G. P. AND REVELL, S. H. A search for chromosome damage following exposure of Chinese hamster cells to high intensity, pulsed ultrasound. *Br. J. Radiol., 45:* 333–334, 1972.

78. WATTS, D. L., HALL, A. J. AND FLEMING, J. E. E. Ultrasound and chromosome damage. *Br. J. Radiol., 45:* 335–339, 1972.

79. BUCTON, K. E. AND BAKER, N. V. An investigation into possible chromosome damaging effects of ultrasound of human blood cells. *Br. J. Radiol., 45:* 340–342, 1972.

80. ROTT, H. D. AND SOLDNER, R. The effect of ultrasound on human chromosomes *in vitro. Humangenetik, 20:* 103–112, 1973.

81. MACINTOSH, I. J. C., BROWN, R. C. AND COAKLEY, W. T. Ultrasound and *in vitro* chromosome aberrations. *Br. J. Radiol., 48:* 230–232, 1975.

82. KUNZE-MÜHL, E. Chromosome damage in human lymphocytes after different combinations of X-ray and ultrasonic treatment. *In: Ultrasonics in Medicine.* Kazner, E. et al. (Eds). Excerpta Medica, Amsterdam, pp. 3–9, 1975.

83. ROHR, K. AND ROONEY, J. Effect of ultrasound on a bilayer lipid membrane. *Biophys. J., 23:* 33–40, 1978.

84. MONTMORY, E. AND POURHADI, M. Action d'ultra-sons sur des plasmalemmes isolés á partir de foies de souris adultes: Étude biochimique et cytochimique. *C. R. Acad. Sci., Paris, 283:* 1743–1745, 1976.

85. COBLE, A. J. AND DUNN, F. Ultrasonic production of reversible changes in the electrical parameters of isolated frog skin. *J. Acoust. Soc. Am., 60:* 225–229, 1976.

86. WILLIAMS, A. R., O'BRIEN, W. D., JR. AND COLLER, B. S. Exposure to ultrasound decreases the recalcification time of platelet-rich plasma. *Ultrasound Med. Biol., 2:* 113–118, 1976.

87. NYBORG, W. L. *Physical Mechanism for Biological Effects of Ultrasound.* (HEW Publ. FDA 78-8062), U.S. Government Printing Office, Washington, D.C., 1977.

88. HELLMAN, L. M., DUFFUS, G. M., DONALD, I. AND SUNDEN, B. Safety of diagnostic ultrasound in obstetrics. *Lancet, 1:* 1133–1135, 1970.

89. KORANYI, G., FALUS, M., SOBEL, M., PESTI, E. AND VAN BAO, T. Follow-up examination of children exposed to ultrasound *in utero. Acta Paed. Acad. Scient. Hungar., 13:* 231–238, 1972.

10

Therapeutic Heat[1]

JUSTUS F. LEHMANN
BARBARA J. DE LATEUR

Introduction

This chapter will be limited to local thermotherapy: general body heating, hyperthermia, will not be included. The rationale for heat application, indications and contraindications, will be developed on the basis of experimental evidence that desirable physiological responses can be produced by heat and on the basis of controlled clinical studies as much as they are available. The rationale for using different heating modalities is primarily based on the fact that they produce different heating patterns, with the peak temperatures in different locations. Heat will be discussed in the context of other therapeutic interventions, medical and surgical. It is not considered a cure for any of the disease entities discussed. It is, rather, a valuable adjunct which is helpful in management of specific symptoms.

Generally, it is accepted that heat produces the following desirable therapeutic effects:
a) it increases the extensibility of collagen tissues;
b) it decreases joint stiffness;
c) it produces pain relief;
d) it relieves muscle spasms;
e) it assists in resolution of inflammatory infiltrates, edema, and exudates;
f) it increases blood flow; and
g) more recently, it has been used as part of cancer therapy.

Physiological Effects as a Basis for Therapy

CHANGES IN EXTENSIBILITY OF COLLAGEN AS A BASIS FOR TREATMENT OF JOINT CONTRACTURES

Most joint contractures are due to a limitation in the range of motion resulting from shortened structures which cross the joint. These frequently

---

[1] This chapter is in part based on research supported by Research Grant # G008003029 from the National Institute of Handicapped Research, Department of Education, Washington, D.C. 20202.

404

include a tight joint capsule, a scarred and thickened synovium, fibrotic muscles, and scars such as occur in burns. In most of these cases, the tightness of the offending structure is the result of deposition of fibrous, that is collagenous, tissue. Thus, any therapy which will increase the extensibility of these tissues is advantageous to the treatment of joint contractures.

In 1955, Gersten (132) found an increase in extensibility of tendons after ultrasound exposure which he related to the temperature rise in the tendon during treatment. It has been shown that collagen shrinks and then melts at temperatures above 50°C (107, 290, 404). When tendons were subjected to temperatures within the therapeutic range (from 41 to 45°C), they showed a different behavior (262). At normal tissue temperatures, determination of a length-tension diagram shows that the tendon has essentially elastic behavior, that is, a reversible proportionality between stress and strain over the stress-strain elongation curve (see Figure 10.1). Once a specific elongation is obtained and the tension continuously recorded, the tension at normal tissue temperatures can be observed to deteriorate, gradually and slightly. The viscous properties of the tendon are thus revealed. However, if a specimen is exposed to a therapeutic temperature of 45°C, the viscous properties became dominant and the tension deteriorates, rapidly and substantially. If different loads (stresses) are applied to tendons at 45°C, it is noted that with increasing load application an increasing residual elongation (one which persists after the stretch is removed) occurs (see Figure 10.2). By comparison, the same load levels do not produce any residual elongation if the material is maintained at normal tissue temperature. If the temperature is elevated, but no load (stress) applied, no residual elongation is observed either. Therapeutically, this implies that it is necessary to

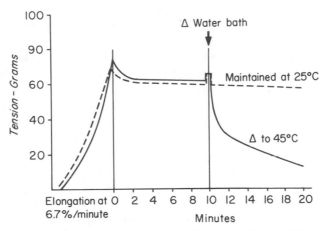

Fig. 10.1. Relaxation of tension in tendon (initial load, 73 g), 25°C for 10 minutes and at 45°C for another 10 minutes. From Lehmann *et al.* (262).

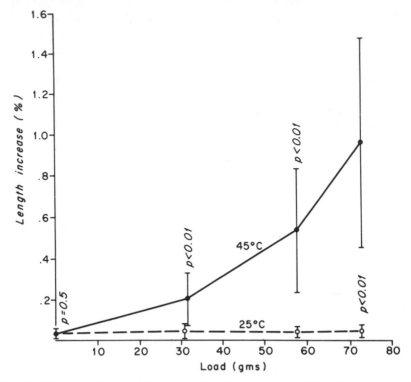

Fig. 10.2. Percent increase in tendon length as function of load in grams at 45°C and at 25°C. From Lehmann *et al.* (262).

stretch the tight structures during or immediately after heating. Without application of stretch, no elongation and therefore no therapeutic effect on the contracted tissues can be anticipated. These experiments clearly demonstrate that less force is required to get a significant residual elongation when heat is applied together with the stretch or range of motion exercise. The next investigation (see Figure 10.3) was of the structural soundness of the material after the combined heat and stretch application. A constant stretch was applied to the tissues at temperatures of 39, 41, 43, and 45°C until a strain (elongation) of 2.6 percent was obtained. The load was removed for 10 minutes. Subsequently, the material thus treated was elongated at a constant rate until rupture occurred. The elongation and the stress at rupture were compared with controls not treated.

It was found that the time needed to get an elongation of 2.6 percent decreased with increasing temperature. Since the elongation was limited to 2.6 percent, the residual length increase was the same at all temperatures. At 45°C, the strain at rupture was 70 percent of that of the untreated control. At 39°C, the strain at rupture was slightly less than 30 percent of that of the untreated control. A similar result was observed when the load

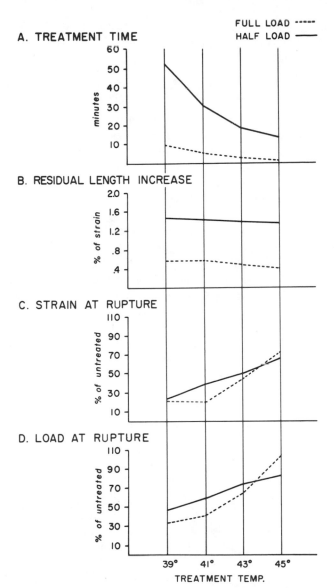

Fig. 10.3. *A–D*, Effect of load level and temperature in the therapeutic range on rat tail tendon. *A*, Time to achieve an elongation of 2.64 percent. *B*, Length increase produced by the treatment procedures. *C*, Strain at rupture expressed as a percent of untreated tendon. *D*, Load at rupture expressed as a percent of untreated tendon. From Lehmann *et al.* (273) and Warren *et al.* (410).

at rupture was measured and compared with the untreated control. At 45°C, the values of the load at rupture were very close to those of the untreated control. At 39°C, the load at rupture ranged from 30 to 50 percent of that of the untreated control. One must conclude from these experiments that stretch producing a prescribed residual elongation alters the strength of the material less when heat is applied at higher temperatures within the therapeutic range (272, 410, 411).

EFFECTS ON VISCO-ELASTIC PROPERTIES OF TISSUES AS A BASIS FOR THE TREATMENT OF JOINT STIFFNESS IN RHEUMATOID ARTHRITIS

Hunter *et al.* (190) showed that joint temperature influences the resistance to movement and the maximum speed with which the joint can be moved. Low temperatures increase the resistance and decrease the speed. Higher temperatures produce the opposite effect. The authors attributed the changes to an increased drag imposed by increased viscosity of the synovial fluid. Wright and Johns (431) developed a crank which moved the second metacarpophalangeal joint through the full range of extension and flexion. Strain gages attached to the lever moving the finger measured the resistance to the motion. In addition, displacement and velocity were measured. A hysteresis loop was obtained which showed that the resistance to motion on the upstroke was different from that of the downstroke (see Figure 10.4). From these measurements they were able to calculate the relationships among the components of stiffness of the normal joints (see Figure 10.5). Wright and Johns determined that elastic, viscous, and frictional stiffness bear the same mutual relationships in the arthritic as in the normal joint. They found that elastic stiffness was significantly decreased on warming the joint (see Figure 10.6). In untreated rheumatoid patients, the elastic stiffness was greatly increased. After steroid therapy, it was markedly decreased. Some other connective tissue disorders showed a similar behavior of joint stiffness (197). There was a 20 percent decrease in stiffness at 45° as

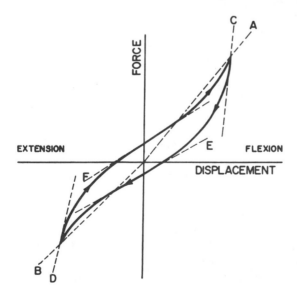

Fig. 10.4. Diagram of joint stiffness showing the slopes measured (*broken lines*). A, Stiffness at full flexion. B, Stiffness at full extension. C, Maximum stiffness during extension. D, Maximum stiffness during flexion. E, Minimum stiffness during extension. F, Minimum stiffness during flexion. From Wright *et al.* (431)

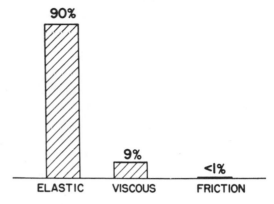

90%

9%

<1%

ELASTIC   VISCOUS   FRICTION

Fig. 10.5. Relationship between the components of stiffness in the normal joint. The maximum torque required to overcome elastic, viscous, and frictional stiffness (total torque = 100 percent). Inertial stiffness was less than 1 percent. From Wright *et al.* (431).

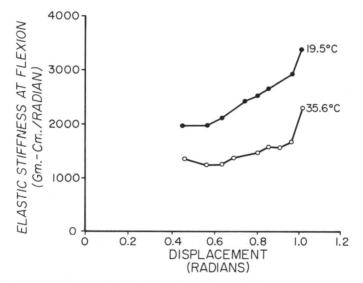

Fig. 10.6. Alteration of elastic stiffness with temperature. *A,* Elastic stiffness at full flexion at different amplitudes of rotation, skin temperature 35.6°C (*open circles*). Increased stiffness at high amplitude is apparent. *B,* same experiment with joint cooled (*closed circles* with skin temperature 19.5°C). Stiffness was clearly increased. From Wright *et al.* (431).

compared with the 33°C when the joint was treated selectively with infrared radiation (432). The findings of Wright and Johns were confirmed by Bäcklund and Tiselius (27). They too found an increased stiffness in their series of rheumatoid patients. The subjective complaint of stiffness correlated with the objective measurements of the stiffness of the finger joint. They confirmed that elevated temperatures of 43°C decreased stiffness and that lowered temperatures of 10°C increased joint stiffness in the rheumatoid patient. All of the previous findings are consistent with the fact that rheumatoid patients usually feel better with relief of morning stiffness after heat application (158)

THE PHYSIOLOGICAL BASIS FOR TREATMENT OF MUSCLE SPASMS

Clinically, it is commonly observed that muscle spasms secondary to underlying skeletal, joint, or neuropathology can be relieved by heat (158, 413); the physiological underpinnings of these observations are extremely limited. From the bits of information pertinent, one can perhaps glean some possible underlying mechanisms. Spindle afferents from nuclear chain and nuclear bag fibers, as well as the secondary afferents and gamma efferents are shown in Figure 10.7 (129). The response of the I-A primary afferents is greater to phasic stretch than to tonic stretch, whereas the secondary afferents respond more to the tonic than to the phasic changes (see Figure 10.8).

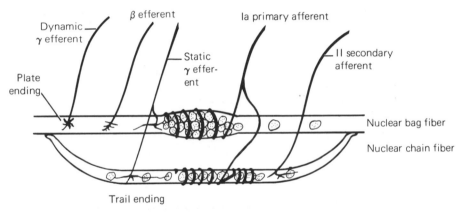

Fig. 10.7. Diagram of muscle spindle. From Ganong (129), modified from Stein (373).

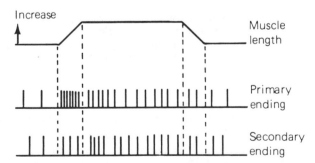

Fig. 10.8. Response of spindle afferents to muscle stretch. The bottom two lines represent the number of discharges in afferent nerves from the primary and secondary endings as the muscle is stretched and then permitted to return to its original length. From Ganong (129).

Mense (294) studied the effect of temperature on the spindles and found that in a pre-stretched muscle at a tension of 100 pounds, the rate of firing of the group I-A afferents was increased by warming and depressed by cooling. The effect of warming was much more pronounced than that of cooling (see Figures 10.9 and 10.10). Those secondary afferents which had a high background discharge responded in a manner similar to the I-A afferents, whereas those with a low initial discharge rate showed an activation by cooling and a depression or cessation of firing by warming (see Figure 10.11).

The majority of the secondary endings showed a cessation of firing when heated (see Figure 10.12). In addition, Mense subjected the Golgi tendon

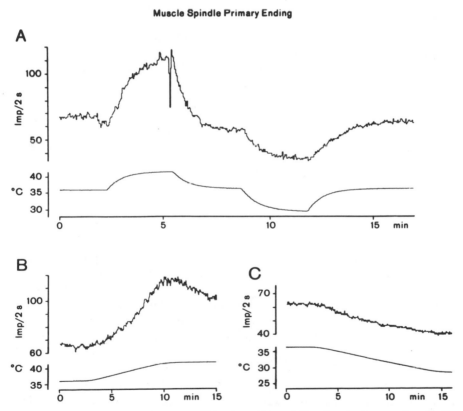

Fig. 10.9. Effect of temperature on the impulse activity of a single muscle spindle primary ending, conduction velocity 84.0 m/second. *Upper traces*: time histogram of fiber activity, dwell time 2 seconds. The ordinates indicate the frequency of the discharges in Imp/2 seconds. *Lower traces*: intramuscular temperature. *A*, Response to fast temperature changes ("steps"). *B*, Response to a slowly rising warming "ramp." *C*, Response to a slowly falling cooling "ramp." From Mense (294).

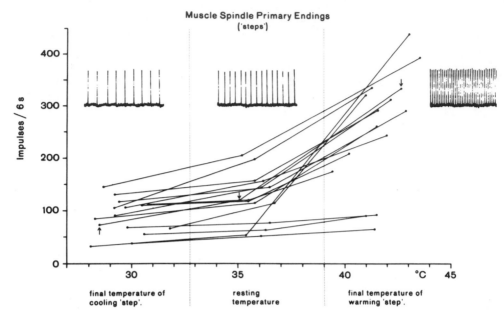

Fig. 10.10. Impulse activity of 15 primary spindle ending afferents under resting conditions and following temperature "steps." In each curve, the three measuring points indicate the activity at the end of a cooling "step" (*left*), under resting conditions (35 to 37°C, muscle prestretched to 100 p) (*middle*) and at the end of a warming "step" (*right*). *Arrows* indicate the unit which is shown in the original registrations. From Mense (294).

organs to heating and found that the rate of firing from this organ was increased by warming (see Figure 10.13). In all cases, the temperature elevations which produced these changes to a maximal extent were within the therapeutic range.

On the basis of these findings, one could speculate that, assuming secondary muscle spasm is to a large degree a tonic phenomenon, the selective cessation of the firing from the secondary endings may reduce the muscle tone. This effect would be supplemented by the greater inhibitory impulses from the Golgi tendon organs.

In addition, it has been demonstrated (105) that stimulation of the skin in the neck region decreases γ fiber activity resulting in a decreased spindle excitability. This may explain why superficial heating devices that primarily raise the skin temperature may also decrease muscle spasms.

Finally, Petajan and Eagan (327) showed that when heat was applied by external means with the resultant rise in muscle temperature the relaxation time of the ankle jerk was decreased and there was little change in the rise time. However, these observations extended only to temperatures below

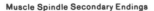

Muscle Spindle Secondary Endings

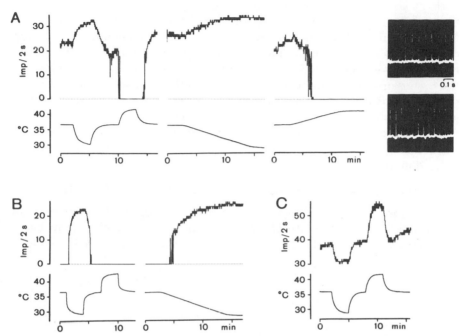

Fig. 10.11. Effects of temperature on the discharges of single secondary spindle ending afferents. *Upper traces*: time histogram of fiber activity, dwell time 2 seconds. The ordinates indicate the frequency of the discharges in Imp/2 second. *Lower traces*: intramuscular temperature. *A*, Cold-responsive unit with background discharge, conduction velocity 48.5 m/second. *Left panel*: response to temperature "steps." *Middle panel*, response to a cooling "ramp." *Right panel*, response to a warming "ramp." Original registrations: *upper trace*: impulse activity before start of cooling "ramp"; *lower trace*: activity at the end of cooling "ramp." *B*, Cold-responsive unit without background discharge, conduction velocity 54.1 m/second. *Left panel*: response to temperature "steps." *Right panel*: response to cooling "ramp." *C*, Warm-responsive unit, conduction velocity 45.6 m/second, stimulation by temperature "steps." From Mense (294).

40°C and were, therefore, below the therapeutic range; it is doubtful how far they are applicable to therapeutic phenomena.

PAIN RELIEF FROM HEAT APPLICATION

There is a widespread, empirically based, use of heat to relieve pain in a large variety of musculo-skeletal conditions. In some of these, pain may be relieved by reducing the secondary muscle spasms. In tension syndromes, pain allegedly is related to ischemia, which, in turn, can be improved by the hyperemia heat application produces. Heat has also been applied as a "counter-irritant", that is, the thermal stimulus may affect the pain sensation as explained by the gate theory of Melzack and Wall (293). It could perhaps also be explained through the action of endorphins. Gammon and Starr (128) furnished limited support for the use of heat as a counter-irritant. Heat ranked third in providing relief, as compared with other counter-irritants. In pain produced artificially by injection of sodium chloride, there is evidence that heat, when applied to the free nerve endings in the tissues or to the peripheral nerve, reduced the pain sensation. Lehmann *et al.* (234) measured the pain threshold with the Hardy *et al.* (153) method and before and after heat application. The pain threshold was elevated after heating. In contrast to the almost universal empirical application of heat for the relief of pain, the physiological data as a basis for this therapeutic indication are limited.

EFFECTS ON BLOOD FLOW AND RESOLUTION OF INFLAMMATION

In the past, much emphasis was placed on the heat-induced increase of blood flow in the musculature, without clearly tying the change in blood flow to therapeutic effects (2). At the present time, such an increase in blood

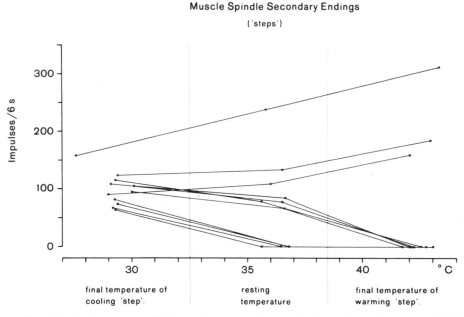

Fig. 10.12. Impulse activity of 11 secondary spindle ending afferents under resting conditions and following temperature "steps." In each curve the three measuring points indicate the activity at the end of a cooling "step" (*left*), under resting conditions (35 to 37°C, muscle prestretched to 100 p) (*middle*), and at the end of a warming "step" (*right*). Note that in the cooled muscle all the secondary endings were active whereas in the warmed muscle the majority of the units was silent. From Mense (294).

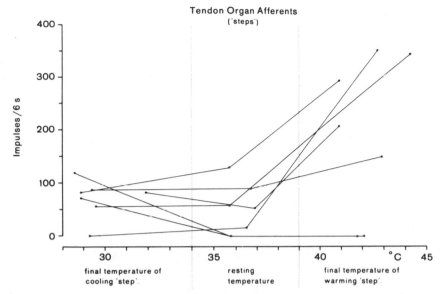

Fig. 10.13. Impulse activity of seven afferent units from tendon organs (conduction velocities between 73.6 and 102.2 m/second) under resting conditions and following temperature "steps." In each curve, the three measuring points indicate the activity at the end of a cooling "step" (*left*), under resting conditions (35 to 37°C, muscle prestretched to 100 p) (*middle*), and at the end of a warming "step" (*right*). From Mense (294).

flow is considered to be beneficial in muscle spasm or sustained contractions as they occur in tension states; in such conditions, ischemia may contribute to the pain and perpetuate the abnormal muscle contractions.

Infections

Superficial heat application, in the form of hot compresses and soaks, is a time-honored treatment of skin and soft tissue infections such as folliculitis, furuncles, carbuncles, and paronychia. The intent of this treatment is to localize the inflammation and accelerate abscess formation. Because of superficial location, the abscess is readily drained, spontaneously or surgically (368).

However, the use of the diathermy to promote abscess formation in deep tissues might be catastrophic. Yet, in chronic pelvic inflammatory disease, diathermy may be used to promote blood flow and assist in the resolution of the process. Prior to the ready availability of antibiotics, Krusen and associates used heating of the pelvic organs as an adjunct to other therapy, and observed that in 86.5% percent of a series of 37 patients with gonorrheal pelvic inflammatory disease the cultures became negative and remained so. This success may have been, in part, due to the temperature sensitivity of the gonococci (23, 61, 209, 210, 335).

Heat itself may produce an inflammatory reaction in higher temperatures of the tissues. As part of this process, the capillary permeability is increased to protein and cell migration. Proteins may be denatured and polypeptides and histamine-like substances produced. Vascular alterations may be due directly to heat, but are also chemically mediated by such vaso-active compounds as histamine and bradykinin (342).

Reflex Phenomena

The temperature regulatory mechanism, in response to elevation of the body core temperature and thus hypothalamic warming, is basically as follows (see also Chapter 5) (1, 5, 67, 136, 328, 400): the cutaneous blood flow is increased; if necessary, sweating also occurs. Blood flow to active organs such as the exercising musculature is increased. Blood flow to the resting organs is reduced. The response to local heating without core temperature elevation is consistent with the phenomena involved in core temperature maintenance. Only fragments of the total response are observed (see Chapter 5).

Thus, when heat is applied to the skin, blood flow to inactive organs is reflexly reduced. The underlying musculature, if not heated directly (1, 3, 67, 147, 193, 328) will show either a reduction in blood flow or a maintenance of the resting level unless the muscle is actively exercised. The term "consensual reaction" (105) refers to the fact that heating the skin of one extremity not only produces local blood flow change, but also increases the blood flow in the contralateral extremity; however, the latter occurs to a lesser degree. The contralateral reflex response depends upon the intensity of the heat applied to the arm treated and also upon the area of skin thus affected, implying that a reflex response is greater in proportion to the greater neural input at the site of temperature elevation. Similarly, Gibbon and Landis (136) demonstrated vasodilatation of the lower extremities in response to immersing the forearm in warm water. Kerslake and Cooper (204) observed vasodilatation of the hand in response to heating the skin elsewhere. They demonstrated that this reflex vasodilatation occurred without core temperature elevation. These authors heated the front of the trunk and measured the blood flow to the skin of the hand and found that the latency was so short that the vasodilatation could have been produced only through a reflex phenomenon. These authors observed no rise in core temperature as measured in the esophagus, mouth, and rectum. In some cases, they found even a fall of core temperature.

If the muscle itself is heated, the vascular responses observed are similar to those occurring during exercise. Blood flow increases of up to 30 ml/100 gm tissue/minute have been documented (147, 269). These blood flow changes have been observed irrespective of which deep heating modality was used to elevate muscle temperature. Guy *et al.* and Lehmann *et al.* (147, 269) used microwaves. Abramson and associates (1, 2, 4, 6), Imig *et al.*

(193) and Paul and Imig (324) used other modalities, including shortwaves and ultrasound. Lehmann *et al.* (238, 248) applied shortwaves with a helical induction coil applicator, the monode.

Some of the reflex phenomena described previously have been used in an attempt to increase the collateral flow in peripheral arterial occlusive disease by heating above the level of the lesion (98).

Although this has been clearly shown to be possible in normals, the effectiveness in diseased vessels is yet to be demonstrated. Furthermore, the increase which has been demonstrated is that of skin blood flow; whether an increase in muscle blood flow occurs as a result of indirect heating has yet to be documented (3).

Of practical significance is the fact that if the skin of the abdominal wall is heated, there is a reflex reduction in blood flow to the mucous membranes of the stomach and intestines (40, 105, 300). The evidence of this blood flow reduction is blanching of the mucous membranes. It is associated with a simultaneous relaxation of the smooth musculature and a reduction or abolition of peristalsis. It is further associated with a reduction of gastric acidity (see Figure 10.14).

Local Mechanisms

The local rise of temperature produces a vasodilatation and increase in blood flow by various mechanisms (430). The temperature elevation appears to have a direct effect on the state of dilatation of the capillaries, arterioles,

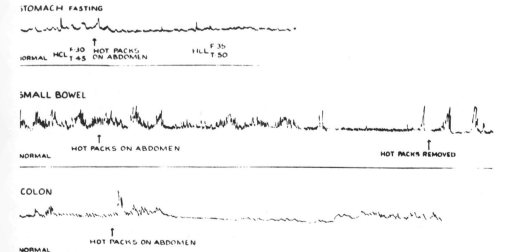

Fig. 10.14. Recordings of motor activity of the stomach, small bowel, and colon before and after covering the abdominal wall with hot water bottles. After an interval of 5 to 10 minutes, tonus became slightly diminished and peristalsis greatly inhibited in all three segments. Note that the acidity of the gastric contents remained unchanged. From Bisgard *et al.* (40).

and venules. Crockford *et al.* (68) observed that patients with cervical sympathectomy or complete brachial plexus tears showed the same vaso-dilatation in heated skin as did normal subjects. They concluded that an axon reflex or any other neural mechanism is thus unlikely and that the findings suggested that the temperature elevation in the tissue acts directly on the smooth musculature of the vessels. Consistent with these observations, Hales and Iriki (150) found that when skin is heated directly the capillary flow is significantly increased, in contrast to the temperature regulatory mechanism where flow through arteriovenous anastomoses is markedly increased by reduction in sympathetic vasoconstrictor tone. In addition, heat, by denaturing proteins, may produce an inflammatory reaction resulting from release of histamine-like substances and bradykinin, which, in turn, produce vasodilatation. Vasodilatation is also produced by axon reflexes and by reflexes changing the vasomotor output. In skin and mucosa, α receptors respond to adrenergic impulses by vasoconstriction. In skeletal muscle, α receptors in blood vessels also produce constriction, whereas β receptors produce vasodilatation; the parasympathetic impulses produce vasodilatation (129). In the abdominal viscera, adrenergic impulses upon α receptors produce vasoconstriction; adrenergic impulses upon β receptors produce vasodilatation. In addition, heat may raise the metabolic rate and the quantity of metabolites. Reduction of oxygen tension, lowering of pH, accumulation of carbon dioxide, and other metabolites may produce vasodilatation by acting directly on the vessels.

The vasodilatation in the skin of the human forearm produced by indirect heating may not be due to the release of vasoconstrictor tone but may be the result of an active vasodilator mechanism (94, 140, 343).

Following their experiments, Fox and Hilton (113) concluded that the active vasodilatation in human skin accompanying body heating is produced in the main by bradykinin resulting from sweat gland activity. In addition, Fox and Hilton showed that vasodilatation of the skin of the human forearm has several features in common with vasodilatation associated with sweat gland activity and the appearance of bradykinin-forming enzymes.

HEAT AS AN ADJUNCT IN THE RESOLUTION OF TRAUMA

Heat in the form of packs, whirlpool, shortwave diathermy, microwave diathermy, and ultrasound has been advocated by numerous practitioners dealing with sports injuries (31, 47, 51, 194, 318, 319, 321, 419, 425).

These authors recommended the use of heat no sooner than several days after the injury and felt that early application of heat would increase edema and hemorrhage and would therefore be contraindicated. There are a few experimental papers where a hemorrhage was produced either by a controlled, quantifiable, mechanical trauma or by injection of a measured quantity of blood into a specified location. The resolution of this hemorrhage after some form of diathermy or superficial heat was compared with that of a control. Fenn (103) injected blood into rabbit ears and treated one group with shortwave diathermy at a frequency of 27.12 MHz and an average output of up to 38 Watts. The rate of pulsing was 400 per second. It was applied daily for 30 minutes. The photographically measured area of the hematoma was significantly reduced at a greater than 5 percent level of significance on the 6th through the 9th day. Hustler et al. (191) used quantified mechanical traums to produce bruises in the pinnae of guinea pigs. The pinnae were then treated with ultrasound in an effort to inhibit bruise formation by increasing hemostasis. Ultrasound frequency was 0.75 MHz; other characteristics of ultrasonic treatment were a non-uniform beam applied with stationary technique and an average intensity of 0.61 Watts per square centimeter. This dose uniformly produced a central tissue necrosis of 5 mm in diameter and inflammatory reaction and edema. The results fell into two categories. One group of the guinea pigs showed an accelerated resolution of the bruise. The others healed at a slower rate than the controls. Thus his results were equivocal and may be related to the dosage and technique of application. Lehmann et al. (242) injected red cells labeled with radioactive chromium (Cr^{51}) into the gluteal musculature of 128-pound pigs and treated them daily for 120 minutes with microwaves at a frequency of 915 MHz with a direct contact applicator which allowed skin cooling and produced temperatures in the 43 to 45°C range in the musculature at a forward output of 40 W with an incident intensity of 236.7 mW/cm². The clearance of radioactive material in the treated side was compared with that of the contralateral, non-treated side where an equal amount of labeled blood had been injected at the corresponding site (see Figure 10.15). No difference was found in the clearance of the hematomas thus treated.

While clinicians advocate the use of heat for hematoma resolution after the acute phase of trauma, the experimental results are equivocal. Differences in results may be related to the differences in the modalities used or the technique of application or the different sites of the hematoma studied. Further investigations will be needed to clarify whether or not heat significantly contributes to an increased rate of resorption of the hematoma. Brown (47) advocated the heat treatment of subacute and chronic stages of trauma where the resolution of hemorrhage and swelling is desired. He advocated application of heat in conjunction with exercise and massage. Heat in his opinion facilitates the resolution of these signs of musculoskeletal injury. Pasila et al. (321) suggested that diathermy application may reduce the swelling after the acute phase following ankle and foot sprains. On the other hand, Stillwell (374) suggested that non-inflammatory edema is aggravated by the use of either local or remote heating. Marek et al. (286) studied the effect of various types of heat application to traumatic edema produced in the rat's hind paws by a quantified mechanical insult. They applied cold water (16°C), tepid water (25°C), warm water (36 to 38°C), and "Plumbin" Aluminum Acetate Solution compresses at a temperature of 25°C 1 hour

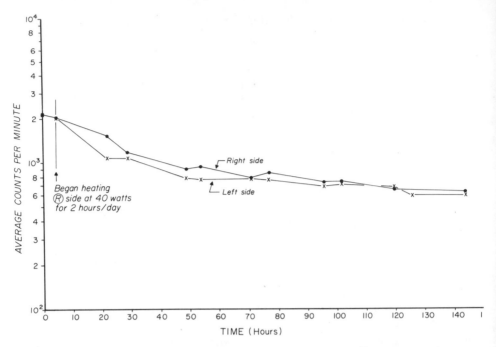

Fig. 10.15. Clearance of radioactivity after injection of Cr^{51}-labeled red cells in right and left gluteal musculature. The right side was heated daily for 2 hours with microwaves at 40 W forward power into the tissues; a 915 MHz direct contact applicator with air cooling of the skin was used. From Lehmann *et al.* (242).

after the trauma for a period of 4 hours with a renewal of the application every 30 minutes. They found that the edema was temporarily reduced as compared with the controls (see Figure 10.16). However, after 24 hours, no significant difference was found in the edema, irrespective of treatment. On the other hand, Marek *et al.* (287) found no improvement of the edema when treated with radiant heat. In fact, there was a tendency toward increasing the edema.

EFFECT ON ENZYME SYSTEMS

The rate of any chemical reaction is increased with an increase in temperature (see Figure 10.17). According to van't Hoff's law, the rate of a chemical reaction increases two- or three-fold for each rise of 10°C (Q_{10}). Components of enzyme systems such as proteins are usually heat-sensitive and are increasingly destroyed with the rise of temperature beyond some threshold value. The addition of these two phenomena produces at first an increase of the enzyme activity to a peak value and then a decline and finally abolition of the enzyme activity. Thus, tissue metabolism may be increased or decreased depending on the temperature. For instance, Abram-

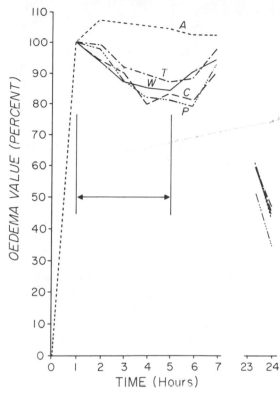

Fig. 10.16. Effects of cold, warm, lepid, and Plumbin compresses on the course of traumatic edema of the rat paw. Edema values are expressed as percentages of the first hour (=100 percent). Segment indicated with arrows shows the intervals in which compresses were applied. C=cold compress (16.1%C); W=warm compress (37.9°C); T-tepid compress (25.4°C); P=Plumbin compress (25.3°C); A=Control. From Marek et al. (286).

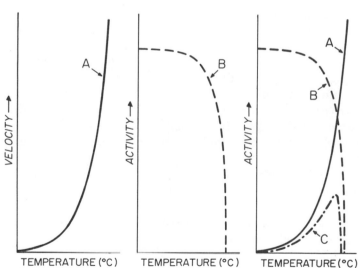

Fig. 10.17. A, The relationship between activity rate of chemical reaction and temperature. B, The relationship between temperature and the amount of intact heat-sensitive component of enzyme system. C, The relationship between rate of enzyme activity and temperature as a result of interaction of A and B. From Fischer et al. (105).

son *et al.* (7) demonstrated an increase in oxygen uptake in the human forearm with muscle temperature averaging 38.6°C (bath temperature 45°C), 35.8°C (bath temperature 32°C), and 28.3°C (bath temperature 17°C), whereas Lehmann and associates observed a decrease in muscle metabolism at muscle temperatures of 46.5°C (218, 221, 255).

Specific destructive enzymes, such as collagenase, found to play an important role in rheumatoid arthritis, have been investigated by Harris and McCroskery (156) and Harris and Krane (155). These authors found an increase of collagenolysis at 36°C as compared with 30°C. They related this increase in enzyme activity to the increased destruction occurring in a rheumatoid joint, since Hollander and Horvath and associates (177, 178, 181) demonstrated that normal knee joints had a temperature of 30.5°C to 33°C, whereas joints with active synovitis had temperatures between 34 and 37.6°C.

Castor and Yaron (57) studied the effect of temperature elevation on two normal and two rheumatoid human synovial cell cultures. The cultures showed an increased rate of hyaluronate synthesis and glycolysis as temperature was increased from 30 to 39°C. Cultures which were stimulated by a connective-tissue-activating peptide showed a striking increase in hyaluronic acid synthesis, glucose uptake, and lactate formation at these temperatures. It is intersting to note that at temperatures of 39 to 41°C in the cultures stimulated by the addition of the peptide, the rate of activity dropped markedly after an initial increase which peaked at about 38°C. These observations raise a question of what would have happened to the collagenase activity as observed by Harris and McCroskery (156) if the temperature had been increased to the range of 40 to 45°C. It can be anticipated that enzyme activities are reduced at higher temperatures when their protein component is denatured. From these experimental results, further clarification is needed as to what therapeutic temperatures would do to destructive enzyme substances in various arthritides; however, one should remember that vigorous heating can produce an inflammatory reaction by itself. It is therefore doubtful that it is therapeutically desirable to impose the heat-produced inflammatory reaction upon the already existing synovitis. On the other hand, vigorous heating which brings the joint temperature into the 41 to 45°C range may in fact inactivate the destructive collagenase, whereas the temperature produced by mild heating may actually accelerate the activity of the collagenase. The net effect of these opposing forces, *in vivo*, is not known at present.

EFFECT ON BONE GROWTH

Nelson and associates (313) showed that ultrasound selectively raises the temperature in bone with an average rise of 5.9°C in dogs. Barth and Kellner (30) demonstrated that exposure to high ultrasound intensities was more damaging to bone when the circulation was shut off, preventing the cooling effect of the blood flow. Nelson and associates stated that the bone damage was due to the heating effect of ultrasound. Since treatment of joint contractures often results in exposure of joints to ultrasound, the question arose as to what heating would do to the epiphyses in the growing bone. Buchtala (48) found that ultrasound applied with stationary technique with high dosage (1 MHz, from 0.8 W/cm^2 to 3.6 W/cm^2) would destroy bone when applied for 5 to 10 minutes. Lower doses (0.4 W/cm^2) produced no change. Barth and Bülow (29) used ultrasound at a frequency of 0.8 MHz, and with an applicator with a radiating surface diameter of 8 cm. They applied ultrasound with a semistationary technique (10 mm movement), to the epiphyseal growth lines of 5-week-old dogs. The contralateral extremity was used as a control. At ultrasonic intensities of 2.5 W/cm^2, applied for 3 to 15 minutes, either once or repeatedly up to 10 times, they found no damage or growth inhibition, even though some of these exposures produced some discomfort. Exposures to high intensities such as 4.0 W/cm^2 applied for 3 minutes produced noticeable strong pain and produced damage, as did intensities of 3.25 W/cm^2. These authors concluded that a threshold intensity, and probably temperature, which produces significant pain is necessary to destroy the epiphyseal lines. The dosages which do not produce pain or which produce minimal temporary pain are safe even when applied repeatedly. There is no cumulative effect.

Hutchison and Burdeaux (192), in animal experiments showed that shortwave diathemy produced delay in healing of fractures in non-human bone grafts.

On the other hand, Doyle and Smart (85) exposed growing rats to temperatures above the normal tissue temperature, but below a temperature which would produce any signs of burns such as edema. On this basis, they selected a temperature of 40°C. Shortwave diathermy was used to elevate the temperature of one limb. The contralateral limb was used as a control. In contrast to the previous experiments with ultrasound, animals were treated for a prolonged period of time, that is, 0.5 to 1 hour daily on alternating days. Treatment was given from the 21st to the 27th day of life. Total duration of diathermy was 25 hours. With these mild and prolonged temperature elevations, the authors found that the epiphyseal growth was stimulated with corresponding lengthening of the limb. Similarly, an increase in growth was observed with increasing temperature elevation around the knee in conditions such as arteriovenous fistula, hemangioma, and osteomyelitis near the epiphysis in children. These physiological experiments suggest that short-term therapeutic joint temperature elevations, used as part of the treatment of contractures, are not harmful to bone growth, provided that no thermal damage is done and no pain is observed. On the other hand, low level temperature elevation applied over a prolonged period of time may accelerate bone growth.

General Contraindications to Heat Therapy

Heat is generally contraindicated or should be used with special precaution over an anesthetic area or in an obtunded patient. The reason for this precaution is that in most of the heat application dosimetry is not exact and therefore, one has to rely on the ability of the patient to perceive pain as a warning that injury threshold levels are exceeded. Heating of tissues with inadequate vascular supply is contraindicated since the elevation of the temperature increases metabolic demand without associated vascular adaptations. The result may be an ischemic necrosis. Heat is not applied in hemorrhagic diatheses, since any bleeding is enhanced when blood flow and vascularity are increased. Heat should not be applied to malignancies without exact tissue temperature monitoring since sub-therapeutic temperatures may accelerate tumor growth. It is also conceivable that hyperemia and blood flow increase may increase the likelihood of formation of metastases (83, 84, 95, 96, 97, 135, 160, 165, 295, 299, 307, 369). Similarly, heat therapy should not be applied to gonads or the developing fetus.

Factors Determining the Extent of the Biological Reaction

LOCAL HEATING VERSUS DISTANT HEATING

When the temperature is elevated locally, a variety of reactions can be observed. These reactions include most of the physiological responses discussed previously, and include changes in the extensibility of collagen tissue, changes in neuromuscular activity, changes in pain threshold, blood flow, capillary permeability, tissue metabolism, and enzymatic activity. These reactions can be produced to varying degrees, depending on the conditions of heating. They are produced in part by direct action of the temperature elevation on tissue and cellular function, by the production and accumulation of metabolites and carbon dioxide, by the reduction of oxygen tension, and by the production of histamine-like substances and bradykinin. They are also produced by reflex mechanisms, ranging from the simple axon reflex to complex phenomena occurring as part of core temperature control. Thus, a very vigorous local response may be produced. In contrast, heating distant from the site of the physiological response produces only a limited number of reflexogenic reactions. These are always milder than those produced locally at the site of the temperature elevation. These distant reactions of therapeutic significance include blood flow changes in skin (*e.g.,* the consensual reaction), muscle, and gastrointestinal mucous membranes. They include reflexogenic changes in muscle activity such that relaxation occurs both in striated muscle and in the smooth muscle of the gastrointestinal tract and uterus. They include reflex reduction of gastric acidity. Thus heating distant from the site of the observed reaction may produce effects limited in number, type, and extent. In summary, when vigorous responses are desired, local heating is essential.

In addition, the factors determining the range and intensity of the physiological reactions are as follows:

a) Level of tissue temperature (approximate range 40 to 45°C) (see Figure 10.18).

b) Duration of tissue temperature elevation (approximate therapeutic range: 5 to 30 minutes) (see Figure 10.19).

In addition, for reflex mechanism, the neural input is dependent on the rate of temperature rise in tissue and the size of the area heated.

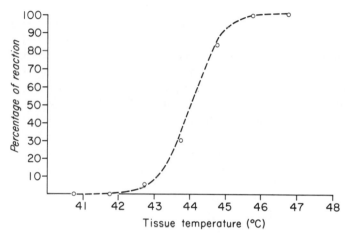

Fig. 10.18. Dependence of hyperemia on tissue temperature. From Lehmann, *et al.* (221).

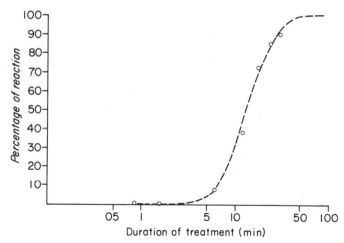

Fig. 10.19. Dependence of hyperemia on duration of treatment. From Lehmann *et al.* (221).

Heating for Vigorous versus Mild Effects

In general, if vigorous response is to be produced it is necessary to a) attain the highest temperature at the site of the tissue pathology to be treated: b) elevate the tissue temperature close to the maximally tolerated level; c) maintain the effective temperature elevation for an adequate period of time. In addition, it may be desirable to raise the tissue temperature rapidly. The modality which raises the temperature rapidly may be more effective because of its greater capability for reflex stimulation. It is also more effective because for a given treatment period the tissue temperature will be in the effective range for a greater portion of the time.

This concept of obtaining vigorous responses is illustrated in Figure 10.20. If the temperature effect on the extensibility of a contracted joint capsule is supposed to be used, it is necessary to select a modality which will selectively raise the temperature to its highest point at the site of the pathology. By increasing the output of the appropriate modality, this temperature must be raised to the maximally tolerated level. In this way, a vigorous effect is obtained without exceeding the tolerance level in the more superficial or deeper tissues.

If, in contrast, a modality with a different temperature distribution is applied, for instance, a surface heating agent, the highest temperature will be found in the most superficial tissues. If this temperature is maintained within tolerance limits, no effective rise of temperature is obtained at the site of the deeply situated pathology. If, on the other hand, the output of

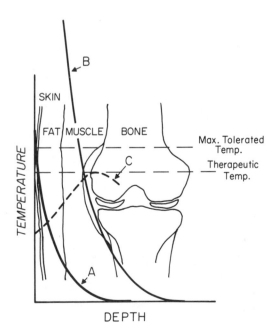

Fig. 10.20. Temperature distributions of superficial (*A* and *B*) and deep (*C*) heating agents. *A*, Temperatures stay within tolerance limits but joint capsule is not heated. *B*, Joint capsule is heated, but superficial temperatures exceed tolerance levels. *C*, Selective heating of joint capsule without exceeding temperature levels. From Lehmann *et al.* (241).

the modality is increased to raise the temperature to effective levels at the site of the tissue pathology, a severe burn will occur in the superficial tissues. In summary, in order to obtain vigorous responses, one must select that type of modality which will produce the highest temperature at the site of the pathology to be treated. For this reason, in spite of the fact that all heating modalities produce their effect through tissue temperature elevation, it is advantageous to have different modalities available since the location of the pathology to be treated varies considerably.

If mild heating effects are desired, either of the following two approaches can be used: a) one selects a modality which produces the highest temperature throughout the tissues at the site of the pathology, but one reduces the output so that only relatively low temperatures are obtained in the target tissues; b) one chooses a superficial heating agent to obtain a limited response at the site of the deeply located pathology. For instance, this method is used to reduce muscle spasms. The superficial heating agents used in this way usually produce a slow rise in temperature: even though the direct effect on the skin may be vigorous, the remote (deep) effect is mild.

Vigorous heating is required to produce certain therapeutic responses, such as the increase in extensibility of connective tissue in capsular contractures. Vigorous heating is necessary if maximal blood flow increase is to be obtained. Vigorous heating may be needed in a chronic inflammatory process where stimulation of body defense mechanisms and resolution of the process is desired. Vigorous heating is usually contraindicated in acute processes. Mild heating effects are obtained by a limited temperature elevation locally or by heating vigorously at a distance from the pathology, usually by heating the body surface. Mild heating is commonly used in an acute or relatively acute process. In highly acute processes, any form of heat is usually contraindicated.

The following may serve as examples for the use of vigorous and mild heating. Assume a patient is suffering from a herniated intervertebral disk encroaching upon the intervertebral foramen and the contained nerve root and producing a secondary pain and muscle spasm. Selective and vigorous heating of this area will produce hyperemia and edema in a confined space and aggravate the condition. In contrast, application of superficial heat may reflexly produce a reduction in muscle spasm and alleviation of the secondary symptomatology without influencing the underlying pathology.

In acute pelvic inflammatory disease, selective and vigorous heating of the pelvic organs may aggravate the situation, potentially precipitating abscess formation with perforation into the peritoneal cavity. On the other hand, in chronic, low-grade pelvic inflammatory disease, vigorous heating may markedly increase blood flow and thus, help resolve the inflammation. It may improve vascularity and thus delivery of antibiotics to the infected area.

In an acute rheumatoid joint, vigorous and selective heating is likely to aggravate the inflammatory reaction, whereas mild superficial heating may decrease secondary muscle spasm and stiffness. In contrast, vigorous heating can be used in a contracted, burnt-out rheumatoid joint. Vigorous heat is needed to produce increased extensibility of the contracted collagenous tissues, and is a useful adjunct to other forms of therapy.

Factors Determining Tissue Temperature Distribution

In any application of heat, the temperature distribution in the tissues depends on three factors. First, it depends on the amount of energy converted into heat at any tissue depth. This is called the pattern of relative heating. Second, it depends on the thermal properties of the tissues, such as specific heat, and, if heating continues for a relatively long period of time, on thermal conductivity. These factors determine the temperature rise produced by the calories absorbed. Third, it depends on the technique of application of a given modality which will modify the temperature distribution. Finally, it must be recognized that any temperature distribution thus obtained is modified by biological factors and superimposed upon the pre-existing temperature distribution with its gradient from low temperatures on the outside to high temperatures at the core. When tissue temperatures trigger physiological responses such as blood flow increases, the cool blood rushing into heated tissue may cool those areas selectively.

The available heating modalities are subdivided according to the primary mode of heat transfer into the tissues and according to their ability to selectively heat superficial or deep tissues (see Table 10.1). Heat transfer rarely occurs exclusively through one mode; however, one type of heat transfer is usually dominant.

In case of heat transfer by conversion, a non-thermal form of energy penetrates the tissues where it is converted into heat by absorption.

TABLE 10.1. *Heating Modalities Subdivided According to Primary Mode of Heat Transfer*

Primary Mode of Heat Transfer	Modality	
Conduction	Hot packs Paraffin bath	Superficial heat
Convection	Fluidotherapy Hydrotherapy Moist air	
Conversion	Radiant heat	
	Microwaves Shortwaves Ultrasound	Deep heat

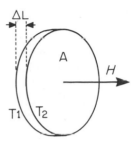

Fig. 10.21. Heat conduction through a thin plate. From Lehmann *et al.* (236), modified from Weber *et al.* (412).

Superficial Heat

Superficial heat is commonly applied with hot packs, paraffin bath, "fluidotherapy", hydrotherapy, hot moist air, and radiant heat.

HYDROCOLLATOR PACKS

Technique of Application

The commercially available Hydrocollator packs contain silicate gel in a cotton bag. The purpose of the gel is to absorb and hold a large amount of water with its high heat-carrying capacity. These packs are immersed in a thermostatically controlled tank filled with water at a temperature of 160 to 175°F (71.1 to 79.4°C). Application is done drip-dry over layers of terry cloth for 20 to 30 minutes (99).

Physics of Heat Transfer and Dosimetry

The main transfer of heat from the hot pack to the patient is by conduction. This does not exclude some heat transfer by infrared radiation and convection (see Figure 10.21). The amount of heat (H) which flows through a body by conduction is directly proportional to the time of flow (t), the area through which it flows (A), the temperature gradient (ΔT), and the thermal conductivity (k) and is inversely proportional to the thickness of the layer (ΔL) across which the temperature gradient is measured.

$$H = k\, At(\Delta T/\Delta L)$$

Thus, an increased thickness of towelling will reduce heat flow and produce less temperature rise. To avoid potential burns, the patient should not lie on the pack, since body weight squeezes the water out of the pack into the terry cloth, which when wet conducts the heat rapidly to the tissues. Even if plastic is placed between the hot pack and the terry cloth to avoid wetting, the terry cloth is compacted to the point that it also accelerates heat conduction.

Temperature Distribution

The temperature distribution for this modality is shown in Figure 10.22. The highest temperature is obtained in the skin after approximately 8 minutes with subsequent reduction of these temperatures because of increase in blood flow. That this reduction of the temperature occurs as a result of blood flow cooling can be demonstrated by applying a tourniquet with resulting increase in the temperature. Repeated packing may prolong the period of temperature elevation; however, it does not significantly alter the temperature distribution (see Figure 10.23).

As in all other superficial heating modalities, the deeper tissues, including the musculature, are usually not significantly heated because the heat transfer from the skin surface into the deeper tissues is inhibited by the subcutaneous fat, which acts as a thermal insulator, and by the increased skin blood flow which cools and carries away the heat externally applied.

Other Packs

Another form of hot pack is the so-called Kenny pack (415). A piece of woolen cloth is steam heated, wrung out by hand or in a spin dryer, and rapidly applied so that the pack temperature is 140°F (60°C). Since the contained water (and therefore its heat-carrying capacity) is minimal, the

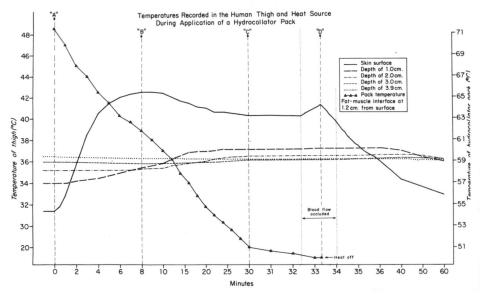

Fig. 10.22. Temperatures recorded in the human thigh during application of Hydrocollator hot packs. A, Temperature distribution before heat is applied. B, Peak temperature at skin surface. C, Temperature equilibrium approached throughout specimen. D, Blood flow obstructed by tourniquet just before heat is discontinued. From Lehmann *et al.* (267).

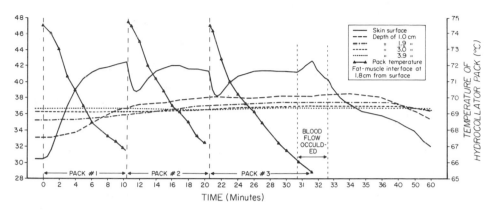

Fig. 10.23. Temperatures recorded in the human thigh during application of Hydrocollator hot pack, repeating application every 10 minutes. From Lehmann *et al.* (267).

temperature drops to about 100°F (37.8°C) within 5 minutes. Thus, this application produces a vigorous but short-term therapeutic stimulation and may produce a reflex response to a greater degree than obtained otherwise. Another mode of pack application is the rubber hot water bottle. Temperatures should be approximately the same as in the Hydrocollator pack. Towelling should be used for slowing the heat transfer in the same fashion. Finally, the electrical heating pad can be used either dry or in conjunction with a moist cloth (154). Again, towelling should be used for controlling the rate of heat transfer. The heat output of the pad can be regulated by a switch controlling the wattage. These packs have a potential electric shock hazard if not properly insulated, especially when used with moist towelling. They also have the disadvantage that the heat output steadily increases over a long period of time until equilibrium is reached. In therapeutic situations, they are therefore one of the most common causes of significant burns, especially when the patient falls asleep and lies on the pad. Therefore, pads which are heated by circulation of a thermostatically controlled fluid are preferable for hospital use.

Common Indications

Hot packs are commonly used in secondary painful muscle spasms (374). The Kenny pack, when applied repeatedly, seems to be effective in the muscle soreness associated with poliomyelitis. In polio patients, Fountain *et al.* (112) measured the force required to initiate movement about the joints and found that the resistance to movement was reduced significantly more by hot packs than by other heat applications.

Hot packs are applied for abdominal cramps resulting from gastrointestinal upset. Peristalsis and gastric acidity are reduced (40). Hot packs are used also for the relaxation of smooth musculature in menstrual cramps.

Finally, hot moist compresses, but not usually Hydrocollator or Kenny packs, are used in superficial thrombophlebitis with an evident inflammatory component and in localized infections of the skin such as furuncles. Hot water has also been advocated to relieve itching from a variety of causes such as mosquito bits and poison ivy (376). In the absence of proof and side effects, it is suggested that this treatment method may be tried.

PARAFFIN BATH

Technique

Paraffin wax, when heated and mixed with liquid paraffin, may be kept molten in a range of temperatures depending upon the proportion of each. For therapeutic purposes, it is usually maintained at its melting point of 125 to 130°F (51.7 to 54.4°C) (209,374) in a thermostatically controlled container. Two methods of application are used. In the dip method, the patient inserts his hand or foot into the liquid paraffin and withdraws it when a thin layer of adherent solid paraffin is formed and covers the skin. Dipping is repeated until a thick glove is formed. The heat then can be retained by wrapping with terry cloth for a period of approximately 20 minutes. At the end of this time, the glove of solid paraffin is peeled off. The other method continues the immersion in the paraffin bath while a glove of solid paraffin is formed around the skin. Immersion is maintained up to 20 to 30 minutes.

Physics of Heat Transfer

In either the dip or the immersion method, heat transfer is primarily by conduction from the layer of solid paraffin into the skin.

Dosimetry

Since paraffin has a low heat-carrying capacity, the dip method makes available only a limited amount of heat to be transferred to the skin, and therefore this method is considered a mild heat application. The immersion method allows the transfer of heat not only from the solid paraffin in contact with the skin, but also from the liquid paraffin through the solid glove into the skin. The rate of transfer from the liquid paraffin into the skin is appropriately slowed by the fact that the solid paraffin is a poor thermal conductor. Nevertheless, this method is considered a vigorous heat application. According to Abramson (9), it produces a marked increase in tissue temperature up to 46°C at the skin with a marked drop-off in the subcutaneous tissues. Water of the same temperature, applied in the same fashion, could not be tolerated, because of its high specific heat and thermal conductivity. The temperature of the paraffin should be 125 to 130°F (51.7 to 54.4°C) (209, 374). For safety, the temperature should also be monitored by a thermometer.

Temperature Distribution

The temperature distribution produced by paraffin application has a skin temperature which exceeds that of core.

Common Indications

Paraffin baths are used primarily for conditions of hands and feet, specifically to combat joint stiffness in rheumatoid arthritis. In such cases, the dip method is commonly used. The dip method is also used in degenerative joint disease with acute inflammation of Heberden's nodes (9). In chronic degenerative joint disease, the submersion method may be used. Both methods are used in scleroderma with subsequent use of physical therapy to increase range of motion. It is also used in early development of Dupuytren's contractures. As part of mobilization after hand trauma, paraffin baths may be used preceding appropriate exercise programs.

FLUIDOTHERAPY

Technique of Application

Fluidotherapy is a bed of finely divided solids (*e.g.*, glass beads with average diameter 0.0165 inch, at a density of 155 lb/ft^3) (45) through which thermostatically controlled, heated air is blown to produce a warm semifluid mixture into which hand, foot, or part of an extremity can be immersed. Sterilization of the particles can be obtained by an auxiliary 300-W heater, which is added to the 200-W heater in the air line.

Physics of Heat Transfer

The heat transfer occurs by convection.

Dosimetry

Dosimetry is governed by the temperature of the air which is blown into the bed of beads. This is a dry application of heat where elimination of heat through sweating can occur.

Temperature Distribution

Borrell *et al.* (46) applied fluidotherapy at 118°F (47.8°C). Temperature rises of 16.2°F(9°C) were obtained in the capsules of the small joints of the hands and feet; temperature rises of 9.5°F (5.3°C) occurred in hand muscle. They compared these rises with those produced by the mild heat application with a dip method of the paraffin bath and found a rise of 13.5°F (7.5°C) and 8.1°F (4.5°C), respectively., With a water bath treatment at a temperature of 102°F (38.9°C), a rise of 10.8°F (6°C) and 7.7°F (4.3°C), respectively, occurred. The authors' conclusion that fluidotherapy is a more effective heating therapy than the other methods, based on the previous comparison is not valid. The described temperature differences are related to the fact that the authors used a mild paraffin application (dip method) and they selected relatively low water bath temperatures. At higher temperatures of the water bath, and with immersion paraffin technique, it is likely that different results would have been obtained.

Common Indications

These are the same as those for paraffin bath. Common indications would include the treatment of arthritides of small joints as in the paraffin bath and the remobilization of these joints after trauma (45, 46).

HYDROTHERAPY

Technique of Application

For total immersion, hydrotherapy is usually applied as a hot tub or Hubbard tank. For partial immersion, whirlpool baths are available for legs and arms. The water is usually agitated. the configuration of the tanks allows limited arm and leg exercises. Since infected wounds may be treated, it is essential that the equipment be readily sterilized. Whereas the Hubbard tank itself is easy to clean, the commercially available agitators often have to be diassembled for cleansing and sterilization. Without this precaution, they represent a ready source of infection. Agitators using a specially designed tube through which air is forced have the advantage that only the tube is in contact with the contaminated water, and it is readily cleansed. The use of compressed air prevents back flow of infected water (see Figure 10.24). For cost-effective use of the expensive therapy equipment, it is desirable to have available large volumes of hot water with large inlets for rapid filling and large outlets of the tank for rapid emptying. Some tanks are of sufficient depth to allow ambulation in the water.

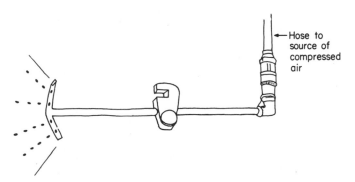

Hose to source of compressed air

Fig. 10.24. Compressed air agitator for whirlpool or Hubbard tank. Detachment of tube allows easy sterilization.

Physics of Heat Transfer

Heat transfer with this type of equipment occurs primarily by convection. The heat transfer is controlled by the water temperature.

Dosimetry

For total immersion in the Hubbard tank or hot tub, water temperatures not exceeding 105°F (40.6°C) are used. For partial immersion, that is immersion of a limb, temperatures up to 115°F (46.1°C) are applied. Duration of treatment is usually 20 to 30 minutes. With total body immersion, oral temperatures should be monitored at water temperatures over 100°F (37.8°C) to prevent an inadvertent rise of body temperature. In these cases, the body's heat regulatory mechanism is essentially disabled, since heat losses can occur only in the area of the uncovered skin of head and neck, and in man (unlike dogs), to a very limited degree by panting.

Temperature Distribution

The temperature distribution produced by hydrotherapy, as in any other superficial heating agent, shows the highest temperature in the skin. However, if the total body is immersed in water of higher temperatures, core temperature elevation and artificial fever can be produced (210).

Common Indications

The Hubbard tank is commonly used in the arthritides involving multiple joints of the upper and lower extremities or the large proximal joints alone (102). The heat application may relieve stiffness, including morning stiffness. In addition, tank therapy produces some non-thermal therapeutic effects. In bone and joint diseases, exercise can be done not only under the influence of heat, but also with elimination of the stresses from gravity. The agitation of the water can be used for cleansing of open wounds, including the undermined edges. This is frequently used for the debridement of decubiti. In addition, a spray or douche table is used for debridement of the skin in thermal burns. The temperature of 102°F (38.8°C) is chosen to prevent cooling of the body rather than to apply heat therapy. In the Hubbard tank, the cleansing action can be used in conjunction with additives such as pHisohex, Betadine, or detergents. A wading tank or large pool also allows ambulation training with elimination of gravity. In these cases, tepid water temperatures are used. The indications of the use of arm and leg tanks (whirlpool baths) are the same as for the Hubbard tank except that the treatment is limited to the submersed parts.

MOIST AIR CABINET

The moist air cabinet covers part or all of the body. Water vapor-saturated air of a thermostatically controlled temperature is blown over the patient.

The temperatures recommended are the same as for Hubbard tank therapy. Heat transfer occurs primarily through convection and dosimetry through adjustment of the temperature. The temperature distribution, as in all superficial heating agents, shows the selective heating of the skin and more superficial tissues. The most common indications are back muscle spasm with underlying skeletal or joint pathology, including root irritation through herniated intervertebral disks. In addition, the moist air cabinet is commonly used for arthritides with multiple joint involvement as with Hubbard tank therapy. The precautions taken with Hubbard tanks in order to avoid fever also apply to the moist air cabinet.

CONTRAST BATH

The contrast bath provides a simple method for producing hyperemia and has been advised for rheumatoid arthritis of the fingers, wrists, feet, and ankles (289, 330, 428). The "hot" water of the contrast bath is between 105 and 110°F (40.6 and 43.3°C), the "cold" water between 59°F (15°C) and 68°F (20°C). The most effective rhythm for increasing hyperemia is to start with submersion in hot water for 10 minutes, then cold water for 1 minute. This temperature cycle is continued by immersion in hot water for 4 minutes and cold water for 1 minute for a total of 30 minutes. Subjective relief of stiffness and pain have been reported following such a regimen.

RADIANT HEAT

Technique of Application

Radiant heat application is dry and non-contact. The spectrum of light producing the temperature rise in tissues ranges from the far-infrared to the visible yellow. In this area of the spectrum, the photons primarily produce biological effects through heating. This is in contrast to the photons in the range from green to ultraviolet, which primarily produce photochemical reactions at absorbed energy levels which do not significantly raise the tissue temperature. Common commercially available radiant heat sources include lamps which primarily produce infrared with some visible light (see Figure 10.25).

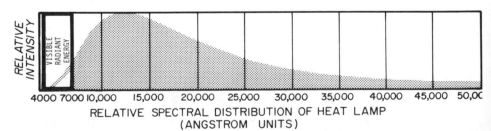

Fig. 10.25. Relative spectral distribution of heat lamp in Ångstrom units. From *Burdick Syllabus* (50).

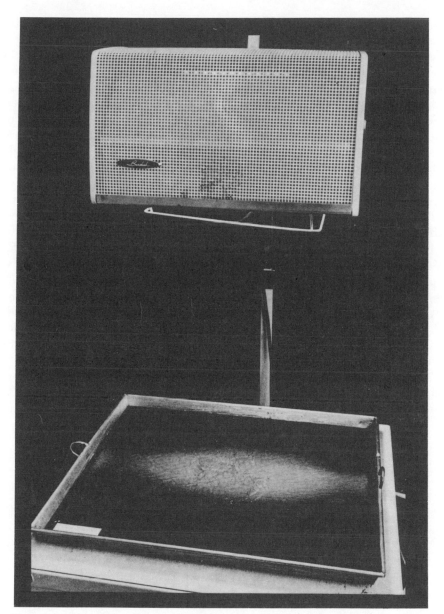

Fig. 10.26. Heating pattern of lamp as demonstrated by melting of blackened paraffin.

The heating elements of such lamps may be made of Carborundum, special quartz tubes, or metal alloys. In other heat lamps, such as the 250 W clear bulb Mazda lamp, the filament is tungsten, which gives off more light in the visible range; carbon filaments take an intermediate position. The energy content and wavelength of the photon emitted will depend upon the material heated and upon its temperature. The higher the temperature the higher the energy content of the photons and therefore the shorter the wavelength. Consistent with the Stefan-Boltzmann law, the output of a heat lamp will depend on the temperature of the element and its radiating area. For practical purposes, the output of the lamp can be gauged by its electrical wattage rating. The effectiveness of the equipment also depends on the quality of the reflector. Its design should allow irradiation of a large area of the body surface with even even distribution of the incident light intensity. A simple test will allow a check of the evenness of the intensity distribution the lamp produces. Carbon-blackened paraffin is melted and poured into a pan. Once it has cooled and is rigid, it is exposed to the lamp's radiation. One may then observe the area which begins to melt. The area which melts simultaneously is that which is evenly heated (see Figure 10.26).

Many commercial lamps are adequate by these criteria, whereas the 250-W bulb with a built-in reflector produces a small focal area. The quality of a lamp should also be gauged by the stability, extensibility and adaptability of the lamp stand, since it is preferred to have a perpendicular incidence of the light, and dosimetry is done by raising the lamp away from the body surface. An alternate application device is the so-called heat cradle which contains a number of bulbs with either tungsten or carbon filaments and a switch which dials the number of bulbs lit.

The cradle provides even covering of a large portion of the body (see Figure 10.27. Two cradles can be used to cover the entire body from neck to toes.

Physics of Heat Transfer

Radiant heat therapy is a form of conversion heating, since the photons penetrate the tissues, are absorbed there, and converted to heat. A photon

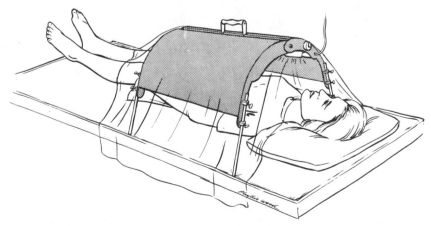

Fig. 10.27. Heat cradle. From Lehmann *et al.* (236).

TABLE 10.2. *Percentage of Energy Available at Depths of 1 mm and 1 cm in the Tissue from Common Radiant Sources*[a]

Percent of Incident Energy at a Depth of	Iron Heater (1000°K)	Carbon Filament Lamp (2150°K)	Tungsten Filament Lamp (2970°)	Sun
1 mm flesh (percent)	0.58	15.0	30.0	29.0
1 cm flesh (percent)	0.02	0.9	1.9	2.3

[a] From Forsythe *et al.* (111)

is a quantum of electromagnetic radiation, the energy of which is expressed as $E = hF$, where h is a constant proposed by Planck and F is the frequency of radiation. Thus, the wavelength of the photon is dependent upon the frequency, which is determined by the energy content of the photon ($\lambda = c/F$ where λ = wavelength, c = velocity of light, F = frequency). In therapeutic equipment, the heating unit is excited by passing a current through a resistor to increase its temperature. The level of current will determine both the total photon output and the energy content and thus, the wavelength of the photon. The far infrared includes wavelengths from 14,000 Å to approximately 120,000 Å, the near infrared from 7,000 Å to 14,000 Å, and the visible light used for heating from approximately 5,500 Å to 7,000 Å. Since the photons of longer wave length have less energy content, they penetrate less deeply into the tissue. As a result (236), photons produced by different heat lamps penetrate to different depths of the tissue (see Table 10.2). The percentage of energy available at a depth of 1 mm and 1 cm of tissue is shown.

Dosimetry

All radiant heat applications have in common that the heat output increasses over a long period of time. The output of the heating element increases while, in addition, the heated envelope of the bulb and reflector progressively augment the radiant heat output. Evans *et al.* (100) found that the output of the heat cradle was three times as great at the end of an hour as it was at the beginning. To modify the incident intensity of the heat lamp, a modified version of the so-called inverse square law is used. With a point source of light, doubling the distance from the source results in quadrupling the area covered. Therefore, the intensity drops of 1/4 per unit area. The reflectors greatly modify the rate of dilution of the light beam with distance; however, increasing distance is still used to reduce the light intensity incident on the skin. Also, the so-called cosine law applies in that a light beam incident at an acute angle will cover a larger area of the skin than a light beam of perpendicular incidence. The intensity is reduced by the cosine of the angle. Therapeutically, it is therefore preferred to have the light beam incident perpendicular to the skin. With the heat cradle, the dosage can be greatly modified by turning on more bulbs. If total body coverage with one or two heat cradles is used, one should keep in mind that the amount of heat which the human body can transfer to the outside is, under normal circumstances, about 0.01 W/cm^3 body surface. This may be raised about 10-fold under favorable circumstances (*e.g.*, evaporative cooling by sweating). This means that the human body's ability to absorb radiant energy without causing a core temperature rise is limited to somewhere between 100 and 1,000 W. It, therefore, is unlikely that a heat cradle with an output of approximately 300 would raise body temperature. However, this possibility has to be kept in mind and the same precautions should be taken as in tank therapy, especially if a double cradle is used.

Temperature Distribution

Although photons of different energy content penetrate to different tissue depths before they are absorbed, none of them penetrates to any great depth. As a result, irrespective of the energy content of photons emitted by the lamp, the temperature distribution in the human volunteers is the same (see Figure 10.28). This also shows that red colored glass envelopes of heat bulbs do not change the therapeutic effect and eliminate only the glare at a significant increase in cost.

Common Indications

The common indications include the reflexogenic relief of the muscle spasms resulting from underlying joint or skeletal pathology; muscle ache in

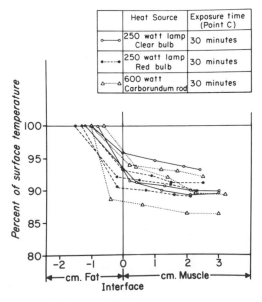

Fig. 10.28. Comparison of temperature distribution in the human thigh during exposure to infrared radiation in nine individuals using three modalities. From Lehmann *et al.* (267).

tension states, relieved by radiant heat through muscle relaxation; the treatment of "myofibrositis", and the treatment of rheumatic joints, where direct temperature elevation of the joint is contraindicated, but where the relief of secondary muscle spasm is desired. Mild infrared application is used to treat superifical skin breakdown as it occurs frequently in the inguinal and perineal areas and the gluteal folds. To dry the area, radiant heat is applied with a 40-W bulb at at a minumum of 18 inches. According to Freeman (116), Starr (372), and Sevringhaus (363), superifical heat via cradle can be applied in patients with peripheral arterial occlusive disease. The goal is to maintain an optimal blood flow rate to the affected part, avoiding vasoconstriction resulting from sympathetic reflex action in response to cold, and avoiding too much temperature elevation which would increase metabolic demand (3, 7, 8), potentially precipitating gangrene. Therefore, only moderate temperatures are used which should be carefully controlled. In general, the temperature should be maintained at the highest level which does not increase the circulatory discrepancy as shown by cyanosis and pain.

CONTRAINDICATIONS TO SUPERFICIAL HEAT

Beyond the general contraindications to heat, there are some conditions where superficial heat per se should be used with special precaution if at all. Paraffin should not be used in open wounds, clean or infected; the same applies to fluidotherapy. Hydrotherapy should not be used immediately post-surgery as the wound is healing. In a patient with a tracheostomy, precautions should be taken in using a Hubbard tank. In a patient with an ostomy, the stoma should be shielded for sanitation reasons; or, an extremity whirlpool, such a leg whirlpool, may be used if this is sufficient. Radiant heat is not used in the presence of light sensitivity. In Hubbard tank treatment, core temperature elevations should be avoided in sensitive patients, such as those with adrenal suppression, systemic lupus erythematoisus, and multiple sclerosis (unless this is used as a diagnostic test) (86). Total body immersion in hydrotherapy is relatively contra-indicated in pregnancy since Smith et al. (369) showed that developmental abnormalities apparently evolve during the first trimester if the body temperature is elevated to or above $38.9°C$ irrespective of the cause of the fever. Core temperatures were taken vaginally (see Figure 10.29) (160,369). It is, therefore, suggested that if tank therapy is used the oral temperature be kept well below this level and that water temperatures (according to the Consumer Product Safety Commission) (399) be kept at $100°F$ or below. Smith and co-workers' findings are consistent with animal experiments of Narendranath and Kiracofe (311, 312). Finally, in any type of superifical heat, specifically in the case of radiant heat, heat- or photo-sensitivity should be considered. Reactions such as heat-induced urticaria have been observed (297, 414, 420).

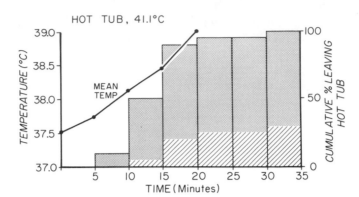

Fig. 10.29. Hot tub, 41.1°C. The *line graph* depicts the average temperature levels achieved by two or more subjects at 5-minute intervals. The *bar graph* shows the cumulative percentage of participants who left the hot environment. The *stippled area* of the bars indicates those who left because of discomfort before reaching 38.9°C and the *diagonally striped* area represents those who left after reaching a temperature of 38.9°C or more. From Harvey *et al.* (160).

Deep Heating

In any deep heating modality, heat results from conversion of the energy into heat as it penetrates into the tissues of the body. The forms of energy used are high frequency currents (short-wave diathermy), electromagnetic radiation (microwaves), and ultrasound (acoustic waves). As in any heating modality, the justification of having the three diathermy modalities available for therapeutic purposes is that each selectively heats different areas of the body. The indications for usage will depend on the site of the pathology to be treated. The distribution of the temperature throughout the tissues in any of these three modalities depends primarily on the relative amount of energy converted into heat at any given point throughout the tissues (pattern of "relative heating"). Once the energy is delivered to the tissues the rise of temperature will depend on the thermal properties of the tissues, such as specific heat and, if the modality is applied for a longer period of time, thermal conductivity. The temperature rise and distribution produced by the modality are superimposed upon the physiological temperature distribution in tissues prior to diathermy exposure. The normal temperature distribution of the organism shows low temperatures at the skin and high temperatures at the core. If the temperature elevation in some parts of the exposed tissue reaches a point where increase in blood flow is triggered, cooling occurs selectively in that area, since the blood rushing into this area is of a lower temperature than the temperature of the tissues heated. Thus, the ultimate temperature may again be altered by physiologic factors.

Definition and Biophysics

Definition. The term diathermy comes from the Greek words $\delta\iota\alpha$ (through) and $\Theta\epsilon\rho\mu\eta$ (heat). It was first used by Nagelschmidt in 1907 (309, 310) to describe the tissue heating resulting from application of high-frequency currents. It is now used to refer not only to shortwave but also to microwave and ultrasonic diathermy.

Shortwave diathermy is the therapeutic application of high frequency currents. It utilizes radiofrequency electromagnetic fields, usually at the frequency of 27.12 MHz with a wavelength of 11.06 meters for the purpose of therapeutic heating of tissues. An elevation of tissue temperature into the therapeutic range of 40 to 45°C is considered to be necessary for therapy to be effective (219). Currently used equipment generally applies energy to the tissues either by capacitive coupling using a pair of electrode plates or by inductive coupling using various configurations of coils. For both types of application, the power absorption density or specific absorption rate (H) is proportional to the square of the induced electrical current (i) and inversely proportional to the electrical conductivity of the tissue (G) (353).

$$H = \frac{i^2}{G}$$

Biophysics: Propagation and Absorption in Tissues. Guy, et al. (147) discussed some problems and characteristics of shortwave diathermy applicators. It was shown theoretically in this reference that many capacitor-electrode therapeutic heating arrangments recommended by shortwave diathermy manufacturers appear to have the fundamental characteristic of inducing greater power absorption in subcutaneous fat than in deeper muscle tissues, especially in situations where capacitive fields must pass through a thick layer of fat. In some situations, however, capacitor electrodes can be effective in heating deeper tissue. By judicious choice of electrode design, fields in the subcutaneous fat can be made significantly smaller in amplitude than fields in the region to be treated. For example, capacitive applicators for therapeutically heating the pelvic region using an internal electrode of small diameter and an external electrode of large surface area over the abdomen can produce internal fields which are much greater than those in subcutaneous fat over the abdomen because of the concentration of fields at the small electrode. The heating patterns of most capacitive applicators have not yet been determined. Also, for other situations where

---

[2] Largely based on Lehmann *et al.* (251), Review of evidence for indications techniques of application, contraindications, hazards, and clinical effectiveness for shortwave diathermy. Contract Number FDA 74-32. Report Dates: January 1, 1974 to December 31, 1974.

subcutaneous fat thickness is negligible, conventional capacitive plate applicators may be used. For example, cylindrical, spherical, and ellipsoidal tissue shapes with negligibly thin fat layers placed in uniform time-varying electric fields can receive relatively uniform heating due to the induced internal fields, providing the objects are small compared to a wavelength. One can envision many diathermy treatment situations which may satisfy these geometric conditions. For example, the hands, the wrists, the ankles, the feet, and associated joints could be effectively heated by such arrangements. The high heating in what little subcutaneous fat may exist could be easily dissipated in many cases by blood flow to the skin and by surface condition. Also, bony or joint regions buried within muscle tissue of high water content could conceivably be selectively heated by capacitor electrode configurations for the same reasons that subcutaneous fat at the surface is selectively heated. The dielectric properties of bone are nearly identical to those of subcutaneous fat, so that if fields are set up in muscle and bone tissue, the fields in bone will be increased by the ratio of the dielectric constant of bone to that of muscle. Unfortunately, very little has appeared in the literature providing quantitative information on heating patterns set up under these conditions. Clearly, additional reaserch is needed in this area.

Inductive applicators, on the other hand, with proper design have been shown both theoretically and experimentally to produce higher power absorption in the deeper, high water content tissues (*e.g.*, muscle) than in the subcutaneous fat. This is accomplished by the induction of circular electric fields or eddy currents in the tissues by the applied magnetic fields. If magnetic fields from the applicator are directed normal to the tissue interfaces, the induced electric fields are tangential to tissue interfaces and are not greatly modified by tissue boundaries as in the case of the capacitive electrode applicators. Since the electrical conductivity of muscle is an order of magnitude greater than fat, the power absorption density will be an order of magnitude greater in muscle for the same electric field strength (356, 357). This is a strong argument for the use of inductive applicators over the capacitive electrode applicators if muscle heating is desired. Under certain conditions, however, where the diameter and spacing of coil turns are excessive, or when the coil is placed too close to the tissue, more power may be coupled to subcutaneous fat than to deeper tissues. This is caused by the sharp decrease of magnetic fields as a function of distance from the coil and the high electric field between coil turns.

The heating in fat can be minimized while maintaining maximum relative heating and depth of penetration in the muscle by controlling a) the magnitude of the applied magnetic field; b) the cross-sectional area of the magnetic field, and c) the gradient of the magnetic field in the direction perpendicular to the surface of the tissues. Guy *et al.* (147) discussed in detail the interplay between these various parameters and the heating of tissues by means of typical inductive diathermy applicators. The cross-sectional area of the field determines the ratio of muscle to fat heating and the depth of tissue which may be heated. The magnitude of the magnetic field determines the maximum power absorption density in the tissue, which in turn determines the rate of increase of tissue temperature. There are indications, however, that the final temperature attained in treated vascular tissue is controlled principally by blood flow, which seems to limit the temperature to below 45°C regardless of the applied power within the operating range of the diathermy modality (239). Only the rate of change of temperature in reaching this maximum value seems to be governed by the applied power. In poorly vascularized tissues, however, the final temperature would indeed be determined by both the applied power or field level and the thermal conductivity characteristics of the tissues (407).

Equipment

In spite of many variations, shortwave diathermy machines have three basic components which are common to all. They are the power supply with full wave rectification with moderate filtering; the oscillating circuit; and the patient circuit. Some machines insert an amplifier circuit between the oscillating circuit and the patient circuit. Inductive coupling is generally used. Output control uses, among others, variable inductive coupling between amplifier and patient circuit or bias-level control on the amplifier. Some machines allow the application of pulsed high-frequency currents of high intensity. Such equipment produces pulses of the duration of 65 to 95 microseconds with adjustable pulse rate from 80 to 7,000/second. For instance, in some equipment the instantaneous energy level of the pulses is adjustable up to 1025 W with a pulse rate of 600/second at a duty cycle of 3.9 percent and, therefore, the average power is 40 W. Equipment which produces continuous wave output usually has a power several times greater than the 40-W value. This is necessary to raise temperatures in the tissues high enough to produce vigorous therapeutic effects.

The frequency of the oscillating current and, thus, of the patient circuit is rigorously controlled to comply with tolerance specified by the Federal Communications Commission. Frequencies allowed for medical applications are 13.56, 27.12, and 40.68 megahertz (101). The wavelength is dependent on frequency as follows: $\lambda = c/F$ where c is the velocity of light and F the frequency of oscillation. The corresponding wavelengths in air are therefore 22, 11, and 7.5 meters. Most of the commercially available equipment operates at a frequency of 27.12 MHs. It is important to recognize that the patient's electrical impedance becomes part of the impedance of the patient's circuit and, therefore, it is necessary for the given application to tune the patient's circuit to resonance with the oscillating circuit, which is usually done by adjusting a variable capacitor in the patient circuit. This assures maximum flow of current through the patient and, therefore, avoids any possible surge of the current in the patient circuit by movement of the patient tuning himself to maximal flow. Some machines are equipped with automatic tuning devices eliminating a manual adjustment, or tuning can be eliminated by designing the patient circuit so that the patient's electrical impedance has a negligible effect on the overall impedance of the patient circuit. If the machine is equipped with a meter on the control panel this serves only for tuning of maximal flow in the circuit.

Most existing shortwave diathermy equipment has no means whatsoever of indicating the actual power being coupled to the patient, or what the peak power absorption or relative heating values may be in the exposed tissues. The difficulty in providing this information is inherent in the design of the applicator, which is part of a high Q parallel resonant circuit (32). This is also due to the relatively low efficiency of power coupling to biological tissues by radiofrequency magnetic fields. The tissues are practically transparent to these fields, thus a very high magnetic field strength is required to produce any significant heat in them. In producing these high magnetic field strengths, a considerable part of the generator power is lost in the induction coil and associated wiring through resistance losses. The relationship between coil losses and tissue heating is a function of the spacing between the applicator and the tissue.

Technique of Application and Temperature Distribution

The technique of application greatly influences the heating pattern (132).

As discussed in biophysics, there are various methods of applying shortwave diathermy, using capacitor plates or inductive coil applicators (77, 219, 236, 250, 360, 374). Both applicator design and technique of application will modify the induced current in the organism and therefore produce variations of the heating pattern (146, 264). The electrical properties and geometry of the tissues will influence the temperature distribution (18–20, 142, 143, 173–175, 198, 351, 354, 355, 364). For vigorous heating effects, the technique of application should be selected to produce the highest tissue temperature in the area to be treated.

The technique of application greatly influences the distribution of current densities throughout the tissue. According to Kirchhoff's law, heating occurs in proportion to the square of the current and in direct proportion to the resistance. Thus, if the tissues are arranged in parallel with a given technique of application, the greatest current flow will occur through the tissue with the least resistance. In the extremity, this is likely to be the muscle, and thus, this tissue will be heated most. If the technique of application is arranged so that the tissues are in series, an equivalent circuit can be given where the capacitance and resistance for each tissue are parallel (see Figure 10.30). Since the ratio, resistance to capacitance, for the tissues is essentially the same for all tissues of the extremity, simplification of the schematic equivalent circuit is allowed to consider only the resistances in series.

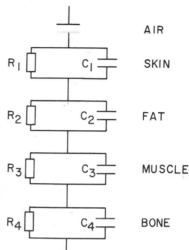

Fig. 10.30. Current distribution between R and C depends on the resistance (R) and capacitance (C). This ratio is similar for fat and muscle. However, R for fat is greater than R for muscle. Therefore, R_2 will be heated more than R_3.

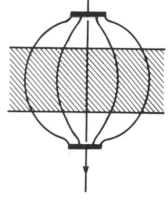

Fig. 10.31. Schematic field pattern that might be expected with spacing between tissue and electrodes. From Lehmann (219), modified from Schwan (353).

Therefore, the current flow is the same through all the tissue layers and as a result the tissue with the greatest resistance, *i.e.*, the subcutaneous fat, is heated most.

Capacitor Applications. In any capacitor application, to avoid overloading of the superficial tissues, spacing of the plates, as pointed out under biophysics, is essential. This is done in order to avoid exposure of the skin close to the electrode where the field is diluted at the maximal rate (see Figure 10.31). The spacing is usually provided either by plastic or glass spacers or by the use of terry cloth. None of these materials does interfere with the electrical field significantly.

An example of shortwave diathermy given to the back is shown in Figures 10.32 and 10.33. As can be predicted, the highest temperatures will be achieved in the subcutaneous fat under the electrodes where the tissues are in series. Between the electrodes, the superficial musculature will be heated more than the other tissues. The highest current density is found in this area because the tissues are in parallel between the plates. If a limb is put between the two capacitor plates, it can be assumed that the highest temperatures will be found in the subcutaneous fat when the two capacitor plates face each other. There is no evidence that the deep-seated joints such as the hip can be adequately or vigorously heated. On the other hand, the small joints of hand and foot may be vigorously heated. Also, a large joint such as the knee joint with little subcutaneous fat cover may be vigorously heated. It may even be heated selectively if there is an effusion (406). Finally, this technique has also been used to apply shortwave diathermy to the elbow.

As pointed out in the paragraph on biophysics, concentration of the field and therefore, selective heating can be produced if electrodes of uneven size are used. The practical technique of application based on this concept is the application of shortwave diathermy to the pelvic organs. The small internal rectal or vaginal electrodes are used in conjunction with a large belt-like electrode applied to the abdominal wall (see Figures 10.34 and 10.35).

It is important to use the largest internal electrode that will fit so that total tissue contact is assured, since partial contact may lead to selective concentration of the current at the areas of contact and to burns. It is also important that the concave part of the vaginal electrodes fit under the

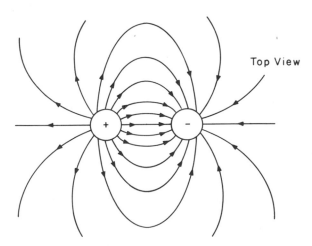

Fig. 10.32. Schematic drawing of current flow in uniform tissues when shortwaves are applied with capacitor plates, *top view*. Current density is proportional to the current flow line density. From Lehmann (219).

Side View

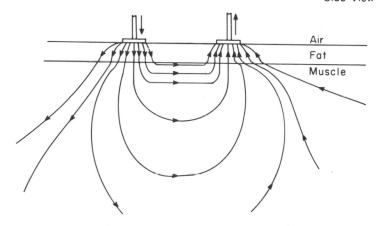

Fig. 10.33. Schematic drawing of current flow lines in tissue layers when short-waves are applied with capacitor plates in one plane to fat-muscle layers, *side view.* From Lehmann (219).

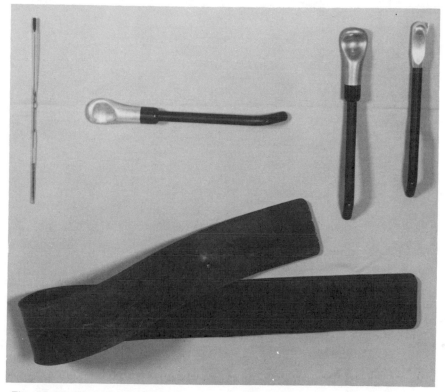

Fig. 10.34. Internal vaginal and rectal electrodes with external belt and thermometer. From Lehmann (219).

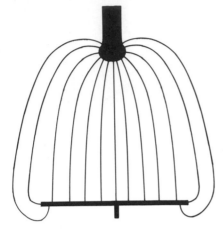

Fig. 10.35. Field pattern which might be expected with the use of an internal electrode. From Scott (360).

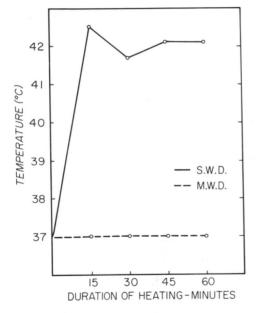

Fig. 10.36. Mean rectal temperature during intrapelvic heating with shortwave diathermy or low abdominal heating with microwave diathermy. Redrawn from Kottke (205).

cervix and the external orifice of the uterus, and that the concavity of the rectal electrodes fit over the prostate of the male. This method allows selective heating of the pelvic organs.

The selective temperature rise cannot be reproduced by microwave diathermy or by the standard methods of ultrasound application (see Figure 10.36). This method of application allows temperature measurement within the electrode. A thermometer is inserted into the metal portion of the internal electrode and records the temperature of the metal electrode which, because of the high thermal conductivity of the metal, assumes the sur-

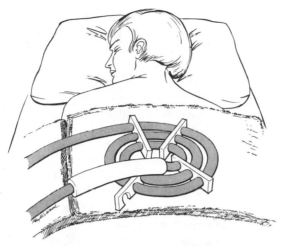

Fig. 10.37. Shortwave diathermy application to back with induction coil (pancake coil). Spacing between coil and skin is provided by layers of terry cloth. From Lehmann *et al.* (236).

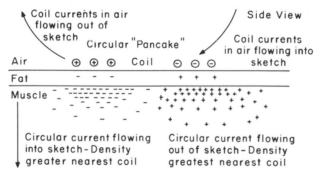

Fig. 10.38. Schematic drawing of current flow in tissue with superficial induction (pancake) coil applicator. Current density and direction of flow indicated by + and −. From Lehmann (219).

rounding tissue temperature. The location of the thermometer inside the electrode shields it from the high frequency field, and therefore Mercury thermometers can be used.

Coil Applications. Induction coils can be applied in many forms; as pancake coil, wrap-around coil, with a drum, the "monode", and a variety of specially designed coil applicators. In general, from the discussion of the biophysics it can be anticipated that the induction coil applicators will produce more current in the musculature and less in the subcutaneous fat than the capacitor applicators. As an example, the pancake coil application to the back may be used (see Figure 10.37).

Proper spacing from the skin is as important in these applicators as in the capacitor pad applicators. The maximal rate of dilution of the alternating magnetic field occurs in the close proximity of the coil. Terry cloth is used as a spacer. The anticipated current distribution in the pancake coil application is shown in Figure 10.38.

The wrap-around coil application also requires terry cloth for spacing and produces the maximal current density in the superficial musculature (see Figures 10.39 and 10.40).

The drum applicator (see Figure 10.41) is a coil encased in a plastic housing which can be folded to accommodate the contour of the body. Special induction coils have been developed. Among these is the monode (see Figure 10.42). The coil is also covered by a plastic housing. It should be noted, however, that in any one of the applicators which are covered by a housing, the latter should not be applied directly to the skin, since it interferes with the heat exchange. The result of direct contact application in human volunteers is shown in Figure 10.43 where the deep heating agent is converted into an agent producing the highest temperature in the skin,

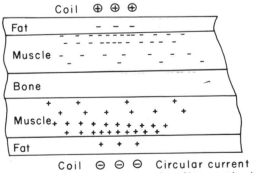

Fig. 10.39. Induction coil application to knee with spacing provided by layers of terry cloth. From Lehmann *et al.* (236).

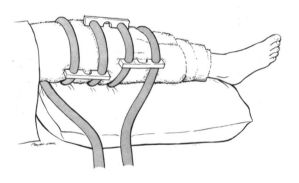

Fig. 10.40. Longitudinal cross-section of thigh with wrap-around coil showing current flow at coil near fat-muscle interface. Current density and direction of flow indicated by + and −. From Lehmann (219).

whereas the same applicator with appropriate air space of 2 cm between skin and plastic housing produces the highest temperatures in the superficial musculature (see Figure 10.44).

In conclusion, all the induction coil applicators, if properly used, heat the superficial musculature selectively unless they are applied to joints with little soft tissue cover (403). Applications are commonly made to the posterior neck, the back, the knees, the ankles, and the musculature covering the hip or the shoulder.

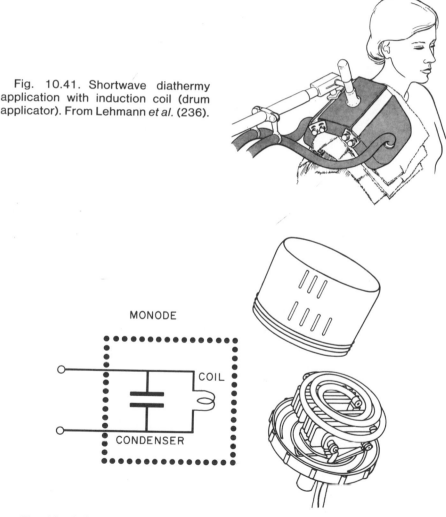

Fig. 10.41. Shortwave diathermy application with induction coil (drum applicator). From Lehmann *et al.* (236).

MONODE

COIL

CONDENSER

Fig. 10.42. Monode applicator with wiring diagram. From Lehmann (219).

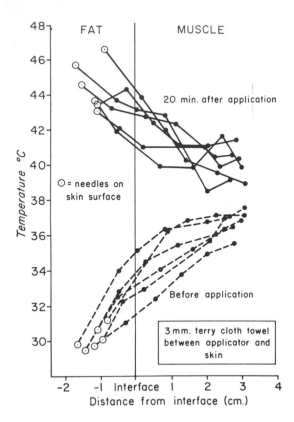

Fig. 10.43. Temperature distribution in the human thigh at the completion of 20 minutes of exposure to shortwave (27.12 MHz) applied with the monode with 3 mm terry cloth inserted between applicator and skin. From Lehmann *et al.* (239).

Dosimetry

The only technique of application where accurate dosimetry is available is in the use of internal electrodes for pelvic diathermy. As mentioned, the temperature of the internal electrodes and thus, of the surrounding tissue can be readily measured. Therefore, the time of the effective temperature elevation in the tissues can be determined, and thus, the two most important factors affecting the biologic and therapeutic results can be controlled (205). For the reasons given, it is not possible to measure the output to the patient and even less feasible to measure tissue temperature elevations in common clinical practice.

Therefore, dosimetry for use in other clinical indications does not exist. At the present time, semi-quantitative dosimetry is based on the physiological responses of the patient and relies primarily on the feeling of warmth or the feeling of pain of tolerance levels are exceeded. The following guidelines can be used:

a) For mild treatment, the shortwave diathermy application is used to produce a feeling of warmth in the patient.

b) For vigorous treatment, not only a feeling of warmth should be

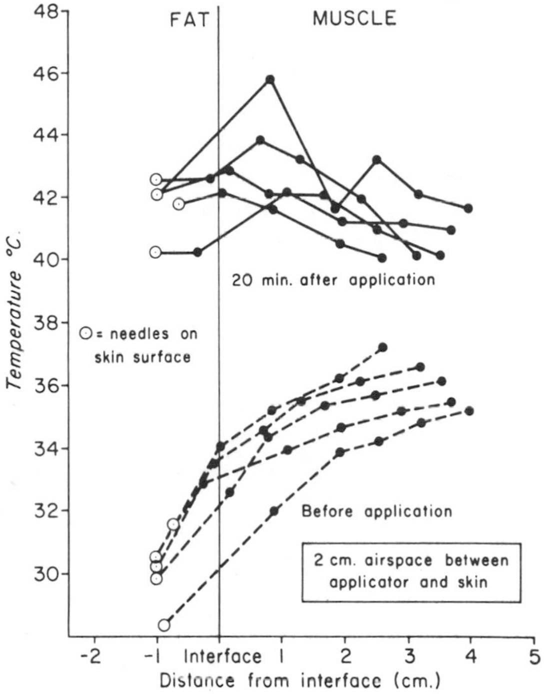

Fig. 10.44. Temperature distribution in the human thigh at the completion of 20 minutes of exposure to shortwave (27.12 MHz) applied with the monode with 2 cm air space between applicator and skin. From Lehmann et al. (239).

produced, but also the pain threshold may be reached. At the moment pain is experienced, the output of the equipment is reduced and adjusted to maintain a level just below the maximally tolerated output. The time of exposure is usually 20 to 30 minutes.

Common Indications

All therapeutic effects investigated so far are related to temperature elevations in the tissues. Thus, the location of the peak temperature in the distribution as produced by any technique of shortwave diathermy clearly relates to the selection of the modality for a given site of the pathology to be treated. All the common indications for heat therapy are also indications for shortwave diathermy. The modality is frequently used for musculo-skeletal diseases to relieve secondary muscle spasms, since it is able to heat down to the superficial musculature. It is frequently used in conditions which lead to secondary muscle spasms, including ankylosing spondylitis, and it is even used in deep seated joints with the presence of inflammatory processes. It does not heat the joint selectively, but alleviates the associated muscle spasm or stiffness (263).

However, in joints covered with little soft tissue, the joint may be selectively heated, high temperatures may be reached, and therefore, this application should be used only in chronic disease processes such as joint contractures. Shortwave diathermy application should only be applied vigorously in cases of rheumatic diseases where the arthritic process is essentially burned out. This treatment would be an adjunct to exercise for improved range of motion (159, 177). If the acute joint is selectively heated, potential damage could be done, since collagenase activity may be increased as was discussed under "enzymes." Also, vigorous heating would produce an inflammatory reaction which would be superimposed on the existing synovitis. In addition, Harris (159) showed that the radioactive sodium clearance in an active rheumatic joint was slowed after shortwave diathermy application to the knee, whereas it was accelerated in the normal.

Fibrositis or myofibrositis, a poorly defined syndrome, frequently responds to heat application, and shortwave diathermy has been found to be useful in combination with other types of therapy (50, 236, 360, 433). If mild heat application is indicated in epicondylitis (tennis elbow), which involves the myofascial interfaces, ligamentous structures, and tendons of the elbow, treatment is sometimes given in the form of shortwave diathermy, usually with an induction coil applicator (50, 360, 433). In traumatic arthritis, especially in joints with little soft tissue cover, shortwave diathermy is used in the later stages to increase blood flow and improve circulation to enhance the rate of resolution of edema and hemorrhage.

In peripheral arterial insufficiency, heat is sometimes applied as an adjunct to other therapy. Heating proximal to the vascular occlusion is safely done with shortwave diathermy application. The expectation is that reflex vasodilatation will occur in the distal area (1, 424). The question remaining is whether this leads only to the well-proven reflex vasodilatation of the skin vessels as part of the thermal regulatory mechanism of the body or whether collateral circulation to the deeper tissues can be developed this way. As discussed under "Technique of Application," the pelvic organs can be selectively heated using shortwave diathermy which is used only in chronic inflammatory pelvic diseases—this treatment seems to be effective because it produces a marked increase in the vascularity and blood flow to the point that even the cardiac output in the female may be significantly increased (39, 248). In addition, it is considered an adjunct to therapy with antibiotics since the vascularity may be increased to such a point that effective antibiotic levels can be increased in chronically inflamed tissues with previously poor vascularity.

Finally, Daily and Daily and Krusen (74, 209) described the application of shortwave diathermy to the eye in ocular disease. This application is controversial; its safety and effectiveness are unproven.

Specific Contraindications and Precautions

Heat therapy itself has well-established contraindications; these therefore, also represent contraindications to the application of shortwave diathermy. In addition, there are specific contraindications in which shortwave diathermy should not be used at all or should be used only with special precautions. In the presence of metal implants of any type, shortwave diathermy is contraindicated if it is felt that an appreciable amount of energy can reach the site of the implant (219). Even though it is theoretically possible to selectively reduce heating of a metal implant by proper orientation in the field, this is of no practical value since prediction of field orientation in tissues is too uncertain (361). The dangers involved are caused by shunting of currents through the metal implant or by increasing the current density surrounding the implant. In either case, locally high temperatures are produced. On the other hand, if metal implants are found at a site which is not reached by any appreciable amount of shortwave energy, application would be safe. When deep-seated implants like cup arthroplasties of the hip are present, the back, for instance, could be treated with shortwave diathermy since no appreciable amount of energy would reach the implant. Finally, until proven otherwise, intrauterine devices (IUD) containing copper or other metals should represent a contraindication to the use of internal electrodes. Too little is known about their conductivity to determine whether they represent a serious hazard when pelvic diathermy is used (350). Examples of metal implants where shortwave should not be used are metal plates attached to bones covered with little superficial tissue, metal wires used for fracture therapy, cardiac pacemakers, and electronic packets for controlling electrophysiological orthoses.

Contact lenses should be removed before diathermy application is applied in the vicinity of the eye. There may be a concentration of current, which may cause hot spots in the region of the ciliary body (359). It can also be assumed that the lenses may interfere with evaporative cooling of the cornea. In general, caution should be observed when irradiating areas around the eyes, even though no cataracts were produced in short-term exposure of monkeys (337).

If children are exposed to shortwave diathermy, the application should be done in such a way that a significant rise of temperature does not occur in the growth zones of their bones. Bone covered with minimal soft tissue may, under certain circumstances, be heated significantly. A built-in safeguard is provided by the fact that growth is disturbed only if intensities are applied which are painful. A few cases of burns have been reported in children after shortwave application (82). In animal experiments, on the other hand, stimulation of bone growth occurred if a significant but non-destructive temperature increase was achieved in the growing bone over a long period of time (85). Others have reported a slowdown in growth (192). The extent to which the results of these animal experiments can be applied to the conditions in human therapy is not yet known. In animal experiments, Hutchison observed that shortwave diathermy, applied repeatedly in clinical dosages, caused a delay in healing of fractures in rabbits and in the union of bone grafts in dogs. It must be noted that while the applied dose was similar to that used in humans in a clinical situation, the volume exposed was much less and therefore it can be assumed that this represents a very vigorous heating. Consistent with this assumption, the continued use of the diathermy produced edema of skin, subcutaneous and muscle tissue. Also, there was delay of the healing of the surgical wounds. These results are consistent with the findings of a detrimental effect on epiphyseal growth when ultrasonic diathermy is applied in high dosages (29).

Some clinicians have suggested that shortwave diathermy applied to the low back has resulted in an increased menstrual flow. It suffices to say that this does not necessarily represent a contraindication, but the patient should be made aware that this may happen (219).

Pregnant women should not be treated with pelvic diathermy using vaginal electrodes because of the possibility of thermal damage to the fetus. This is especially important during the first trimester when the conception may not yet be known to the patient (369). In addition, since pelvic shortwave diathermy may increase the blood flow significantly in the female, this form of treatment may, under certain circumstances, be contraindicated in cardiac patients in whom the work load of the heart could be seriously increased (205).

It is important to note that in some techniques of application, beads of perspiration may be formed and selectively heated. This is not a serious hazard since the use of terry cloth as a spacer prevents the accumulation of beads of perspiration. In addition, in several applications, adequate air spacing has been shown to allow surface cooling, in which case these beads rarely occur.

More recently, concern has been expressed about the potential hazards from stray radiation and inadvertent exposure of the therapist or of non-treated areas of the patient. Most of these concerns have been raised, however, with occupational hazards in mind, and therefore emphasize long-term exposure with relatively low energy levels (288, 296, 331). Much of the concern over hazards has been based on test tube and small-animal experiments (24–26). This makes extrapolation to man and specifically to the therapeutic situation difficult, particularly since quantification of absorbed power is difficult in humans. Most of these types of experiments and their results have been summarized by Michaelson (296).

In Sprague-Dawley rats irradiated at frequencies in the range of 3 to 30 MHz (104), no remarkable biological effects were found in their hemotological, metabolic, cardiovascular, or respiratory systems. There were no gross or microscopic pathological changes in the tissues, no change in the activity of the central nervous system, and no changes in gastric acidity, and only minor changes in gastrointestinal motility or cholinesterase activity. There was, however, increase of congenital abnormalities when pregnant albino mice were exposed. The authors concluded that further investigations would be necessary to determine the significance of the changes observed.

Bollinger (41) reported that short-term (1 hour) exposures of monkeys to 10.5, 19.3, and 26.6 MHz frequencies and 100 to 200 mW/cm^2 power densities did not produce discernible physiological effects. It was noted, however, that at 26.6 MHz with power densities of greater than 400 mW/cm^2, thermal stress in monkeys became evident. In another study, in monkeys (42), frequencies of 10.5, 19.3, and 26.6 MHz, with power densities ranging from 50 to 600 mW/cm^2 at a duty cycle of 17 percent were used. They also showed no gross changes and no significant biological damage or psychological effects which were attributable to rf radiation. Many eastern European countries have been investigating the possibility of industrial hazards produced by electromagnetic fields, especially in personnel working around radio, television, short-wave, and medium wave transmitters (201, 212, 213, 326). The results of these studies are rather inconclusive. They showed symptoms of vegetative dysfunction, red dermographism, and other hard-to-quantify observations. No organic lesions were found.

Michaelson (296) specifies the recommended safety standards for electromagnetic radiation of frequencies from 10 MHz to 100 GHz at a power density of 10 mW/cm^2; free space electric field strength 200 V/m rms; free space magnetic field strength 0.5 A/m rms (16). None of these values should be exceeded over an average 6-minute period. It is anticipated that the safety standard will be lower, especially at frequencies above 30 MHz, at which resonance may occur in total body exposure. One can conclude that there is foundation for concern about hazards of occupational exposure over long periods of time, especially when total body exposure may occur. However, most of the research supporting this concern is not directly applicable to the therapeutic situation of short-term exposure of both patient and therapist.

Non-Thermal Effects and Pulsed Application

One of the best-known nonthermal effects is the so-called pearl-chain formation of particles. Unicellular organisms, microorganisms, fat globules in milk, and red blood cells all are oriented parallel to the lines of force at frequencies in the lower megahertz range, and some lie at right angles to the lines of force at higher frequencies (353). Similarly, motile microorganisms travel only parallel to the lines of force at lower frequencies (8.5 MHz) and perpendicular to the lines of force at higher frequencies (389). Herrick (168, 169) showed that the effect can be produced by pulsed shortwave application as well as by continuous wave of the same average output. Possible nonthermal changes of macromolecules were reported by Bach (24, 25) and by Heller (163), who exposed gamma globulin in normal saline solution at 37.5°C to frequencies of 13.1, 13.2, 13.3, 13.5, 13.6, and 14.4 MHz, using a phosphate buffer of pH 7.6. They did find changes of the electrophoretic pattern and antigenic activity of these macromolecules which they did not relate to temperature rises. It must be noted, however, that these frequencies are not used in therapeutic pulsed shortwave diathermy machines. Thus, as far as is known, these nonthermal reactions neither have any therapeutic value nor do they suggest that specific effects can be produced by high peak intensities during the pulses which cannot be produced by the same average output applied with continuous wave (CW) application. Thus, it is difficult to use these observations as a basis for therapeutic indications specific to pulses shortwave diathermy. Using high field intensities at frequencies of 1 and 60 MHz, Takashima (381) studied the effect on alcohol dehydrogenase and DNA. The effects of heating were avoided and no alterations of alcohol dehydrogenase or of DNA were observed.

In addition, Cameron (53) applied shortwave diathermy to healing wounds in dogs. He found that transverse alignment of fibroblasts and collagen formation, white cell infiltration, phagocytosis, histiocytic activities, hematoma canalization, and metabolic activity all were speeded up by the application of pulsed shortwave. However, animals that did not receive any shortwave application served as controls. Thus, it is possible that CW application of the same average output as the pulsed diathermy could have produced some or all of these changes (134).

Constable *et al.* (64) compared the effects of pulsed shortwave with a control group of guinea pigs and found no difference in wound healing when the parameter of tensile strength was measured. In a preliminary study, Taylor (387) studied the influence of pulses shortwave application on oral wound healing in humans. In a small number of cases, he found that wound healing was accelerated by treatment with pulsed shortwave. No CW was used as control. Wong and Ehrlich (427) studied wound healing in rats; however, there were no controls with CW application. Experiments by Kaplan and Weinstock (202) on experimental healing after foot surgery found edema was decreased by pulsed application. Again, there was no comparision with the effectiveness of CW application of the same average output. Nadasdi (308) observed that experimental arthritis in rats was less pronounced when treated with pulsed shortwave; however, control animals were not treated and therefore, no conclusion as to the specific value of pulsed power in treating experimental arthritis can be drawn. No measurements of joint temperature were made; thus, it could not be concluded that this effect was not due to heating. Erdman (98) applied pulsed shortwave diathermy to the epigastric area and found an increase in skin temperature of 1.5°C in the area treated. He also found an increase in skin temperature of 2°C, due to blood flow changes, in the foot, but no change in rectal temperature. Again, it could not be concluded whether the same results might have been produced with continuous wave application of the same average output. The findings of Morrissey (304) are consistent with these data. At a low output of pulsed shortwave (40 W and 600 pulses per second), he found no increase in circulation and no change in blood flow. At a higher output of pulsed shortwave (80 W and 2000 pulses per second), he found a significant increase in both tissue temperature and blood flow. He concluded that an increase in blood flow in skeletal muscle could be obtained only when the temperature of the tissue was increased. Hedenius and others (162) studied the effects of pulsed shortwave application in cases of intermittent claudication. An average output of 38 W was applied over 80 cm^2 in the epigastric region, and in all cases skin temperature was increased after treatment for 20 minutes. Control subjects were not treated with CW power; thus, the findings are essentially the same as those of Erdman (98), and conclusions might be similarly cautious. Silverman and Pendleton (367) applied pulsed and CW shortwave diathermy of equal average power to the abdomen. He found no difference in the effects on circulation. D.H. Wilson (421) originally compared, in recent ankle sprains, the results of application of pulsed shortwave diathermy with a sham application and found better results with the pulsed application. The only study which compares pulsed with continuous shortwave application and apparently obtains better clinical results with the pulsed application has ambiguous results: Wilson (422) compared CW and pulsed shortwave diathermy in the treatment of soft tissue injury. Patients who had sustained an inversion injury of the ankle during the preceding 36 hours were graded by swelling, pain, and disability, and paired for age, weight, sex, and degree of trauma. One patient in each pair was treated each day for 3 days by CW shortwave diathermy. The other patient in each pair was given pulsed shortwave diathermy. In all of the measured categories there was less swelling, pain, and disability with the pulsed diathermy. Measurements of the total energy transmitted to the patient were made for each of the forms of treatment. Those given continuous shortwave diathermy received a total of approximately 22.5 W hours, and those treated with the diapulse machine received approximately 15 W hours. In contrast to the authors' conclusion that, "the results show a very clear preference for the pulse electromagnetic energy, as compared with (continuous wave) shortwave diathermy, in promoting the healing of recently injured soft tissue", the reverse may well have been the case. With an acute injury, diathermy was contraindicated. The fact that there was less swelling with the treatment with less power substantiates the contention that less vigorous heating in this situation promotes less swelling and other symptoms. The interpretation of these studies is, therefore, not necessarily that of the author. Pulsed shortwave diathermy of this dosage may have constituted a form of mild heating, which may have helped the symptoms. It was not compared to some other form of mild heating. It was, in fact, compared with CW application at high intensity, a form of vigorous heating. Vigorous heating in this clinical situation may aggravate both pain and edema.

Claims have been made that pulsed shortwave diathermy application has special effects on the body defense mechanism to bacterial infection and to other disease processes. The assertion that pulsed diathermy stimulates the body defense mechanism against bacterial infection could not be verified by Silverman (366) in an experimental situation where pulsed energy was compared with CW application of the same average power. In experiments conducted by Mackaness (283) mice with acute and chronic bacterial infections were irradiated with pulsed shortwave. No beneficial effect over a control group, either in acute or chronic infections, was observed. No control group irradiated with CW shortwave was used.

Fenn (103) studied resolution of hematomas in rabbit ears when treated with pulsed shortwave diathermy. Resolution of the hematomas was found to be accelerated in the treated group. The author states that no attempt was made to study the mechanism by which the increased rate of hematoma absorption occurred. No controls with CW were used. Wilson et al. (423) studied the effects of pulsed electromagnetic energy on peripheral nerve regeneration. They irradiated the median and ulnar nerves of rats with pulsed shortwave and found an increase in the rate of healing. Also, nerve conduction studies showed that after 45 days of treatment, the conduction tracings were identical to those of normals. No controls were irradiated with CW. Romero-Sierra and Tanner (344) studied the effect of electromagnetic radiation (27 MHz CW) on the exposed sciatic nerve and on wound healing in rats. Varying results were found in the nerve studies depending on the amount of energy absorbed in the tissue. They reported that wound healing was accelerated.

In addition, a large number of clinical claims have been made and published in the literature. Ginsberg (137) treated calcific bursitis and found improvement. Levy (274) treated sinusitis, lymphadenosis, recurrent otitis media and sinobronchitis. Trojel and Lebech (393) compared the effectiveness of pulsed shortwave as a treatment for pelvic inflammatory disease in 106 patients with a control group given simulated irradiation. They found no difference between the two groups and concluded that pulsed shortwave offers no advantage over the current methods used in the treatment of pelvic inflammatory disease. Too many other claims have been reported to list them all. However, in the absence of adequate clinical measurements to assess the efficacy of such applications, no conclusions can be built on these observations or on clinical impressions.

In summary, there is no evidence that the pulsed shortwave application can be readily used to discriminate between thermal and nonthermal effects. The assumption that peak powers during the pulses could exceed a threshold required for non-thermal effects could not be verified. The known proven thermal effects and non-thermal effects are produced equally with pulsed and continous wave application of the same average power.

Thus, at present, there is no specific therapeutic indication for the use of pulsed output.

Standards for Efficacy and Safety

While safety standards are being developed for the frequencies used in shortwave diathermy, equipment standards are not yet available. It would be desirable, for a given piece of equipment and its applicator, to have information regarding the temperature distribution, especially the location of the highest temperature that is produced. Research is in progress to develop substitute models for the human tissues to be used to obtain such information. Thus, it will be possible to measure the induced power absorption patterns thermographically (147). Further, it is necessary to assure the user that the equipment is powerful enough to raise the temperature into the therapeutic range. The approximate absorbed power which is required to do this is 170 W/kg. (142, 143, 198).

Further rise of temperature at these absorbed power densities is usually limited due to the cooling effect of increased blood flow. If compensation of blood flow cooling is considered desirable, then judged by the above considerations of power requirements, the equipment would have to have enough reserve power to increase the rate of power absorption by approximately 130 W/kg. Based on laboratory experiments, this is equivalent to a blood flow rate of 22 ml/100 g tissue/min (147). In addition, the diathermy equipment should have available various types of induction coil and capacitor pad or space pad applicators with a capacity for the use of internal rectal and vaginal electrodes. This allows it to locate the peak temperature in various types of tissues and thus permits a greater range of applications for vigorous heating.

The greatest present limitation of the equipment is the lack of power and, in many cases, its inability to produce peak temperatures any place except the subcutaneous fat. Thus, many of the commercially available pieces of equipment are safe but ineffective.

MICROWAVES

Microwaves are a form of electromagnetic radiation. FCC regulations allocate two frequencies for medical usage. These are the frequencies of 2,456 MHz and 915 MHz (109). In Europe, a frequency of 433.92 MHz (238) is available; however, other than slightly better capability of muscle heating, it does not have any major advantage over the application of microwaves at 915 MHz with modern, surface-cooled, direct-contact applicators.

Holmann (179, 180) writing in Germany in 1938 and 1939, introduced the idea of applying microwaves for the heating of deeply placed tissues. Hemingway and Stenstrom (164), writing about shortwaves (which at that time operated at frequencies up to 100 MHz), suggested the usage of higher frequency radiation for diathermy because of the ability to beam the energy to a selected tissue region, but equipment was not available to carry out the suggestion. Bell laboratories developed a magnetron tube in 1938. Although it was capable of generating microwave frequencies, the power output was low, only 2 to 3 W. Later, in 1938, RCA developed a magnetron with a 20-W output. Microwaves became unavailable for medical application during World War II, when they were used exclusively and secretly as radar. However, during that time, studies were conducted or sponsored by the armed forces (72, 108, 275) which demonstrated no ill effects of microwaves upon experimental animals. When, in 1946, Raytheon Company supplied an appropriate apparatus to the Mayo Clinic, Krusen et al. (211), Leden et al. (217), and Rae et al. (333) began work in dogs which became the first theoretical underpinnings of later therapeutic application. They found that, although temperature rises were higher in the skin and subcutaneous fat, the final temperature levels achieved in muscle were higher. Thus, deep heating was achieved without undue cutaneous and subcutaneous heating. However, these conclusions were based upon work in dogs, which have a much thinner layer of subcutaneous fat than humans.

Work done at the Massachusetts Institute of Technology during World War II showed that the absorption of microwaves at a frequency of 2,450 MHz in water at 100°F (37.8°C) was approximately 7,000 times greater than the absorption at the commonly used shortwave diathermy frequency of 27 MHz. Principally as a result of these data (and ignoring such important factors as electrical properties and geometry of tissue, as well as wavelength in tissue), the FCC in 1946 assigned the frequency of 2,456 MHz to physical medicine. Subsequently, Schwan (351, 354–357) carried out theoretical work which indicated that 2,456 MHz was not ideal for microwaves. He predicted that frequencies of 900 MHz or lower would be superior. Schwan's work has since been experimentally verified. Between 1960 and 1966, Lehmann et al. (238, 249, 257, 264) and Guy and Lehmann (146) demonstrated that frequencies of 900 MHz or lower could produce more therapeutically useful heating patterns.

Since 1966, Lehmann et al. (252), deLateur et al. (79), and Guy (142, 143) developed and tested, in normal human subjects, a direct-contact, 915-MHz microwave diathermy apparatus which gives very uniform muscle heating.

Biophysics: Propagation and Absorption in Tissues

The temperature distribution in the organism depends on the propagation and absorption characteristics of the tissues traversed by the microwaves (142, 143, 145, 174, 353). The attractiveness of microwave therapy has been that tissues with high water content predictably would absorb much more energy. Therefore, microwaves seem to be an ideal modality to selectively heat muscle for therapeutic purposes. In addition, it can be anticipated that fluid-filled organs such as the eye, joints with effusions, and external sweat beads, may be heated selectively to the point that undesirable high temperatures can be readily obtained.

As the microwaves travel through the layers, the relative amount of total energy which will be reflected at the interfaces is determined by the dielectric constants and the conductivity values. The type of reflection, plane wave, scattering or focusing will depend on the geometry of the tissue interfaces and their size. Tissue structures large as compared with the wavelength will represent reflecting obstacles. The wavelength λ in the range of the frequency used for therapeutic purposes in tissues is of the order of 1 cm. The absorption of the microwave energy also depends on the dielectric properties of the medium and its conductivity. The amount of energy converted at any given depth of the tissues resulting both from reflection and absorption has been calculated by Schwan (353) and confirmed by measurements by Lehmann and associates (249). From a therapeutic point of view, the limitation of the use of microwaves originally available only at the frequency of 2,456 MHz becomes obvious when the pattern of relative heating is studied. The interface value between subcutaneous fat and muscle is arbitrarily set as one, and the values elsewhere quantiatively compared with it, for the average subcutaneous fat thickness of 2 cm, too much energy is converted to heat in the subcutaneous tissues, too little in the musculature with the depth of penetration into the musculature which is limited due to rapid absorption.

As pointed out previously, lower frequencies would be more advantageous for therapeutic application (249, 353). The frequency of 915 MHz is available for medical purposes in this country (109).

Figure 10.45*b* shows for comparison the pattern of relative heating in the same specimen as in 10.45*a* at the lower frequency. For the average subcutaneous fat thickness of 2 cm, much less energy is converted into heat in the subcutaneous fat as compared with the musculature. Also, the depth of penetration into the musculature is much better, therefore if the purpose is to heat muscle selectively, this frequency should be preferred over the presently available equipment operating at 2,456 MHz (249).

The bone also represents a reflecting interface which potentially may produce a pattern of standing waves in front of the bone with hot spots (see Figure 10.46*a* and 10.46*b*).

This reflection may lead to increased energy absorption and a burn in thin layers overlying the bone as shown by Worden *et al.* (429) (see Figure 10.47) while the soft tissues without underlying bone exposed to the same beam are not adversely affected. Figure 10.47 also shows that because of the reflection at the bone there is very little energy available on the side of the bone distant from the applicator. Thus, in clinical practice, multiple field techniques have to be used exposing the soft tissue from either side of the bone without the need for the beam to travel through bone. The conclusions applicable to the clinical situations still hold at both 2,456 and 915 MHz. The experiments of Worden *et al.* also illustrate that, once a fluid-filled bleb

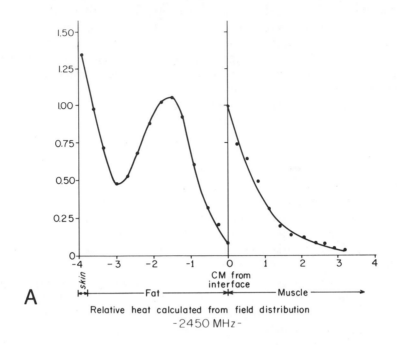

A
Relative heat calculated from field distribution
-2450 MHz-

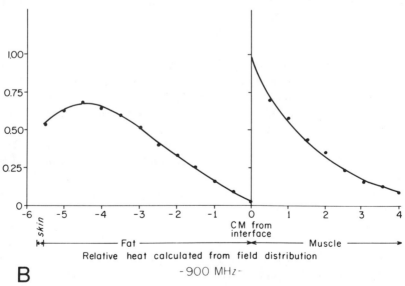

B
Relative heat calculated from field distribution
-900 MHz-

Fig. 10.45. *A*, Pattern of relative heating calculated from field distribution at a frequency of 2450 MHz. *B*, Pattern of relative heating calculated from field distribution at a frequency of 900 MHz. From Lehmann *et al.* (249).

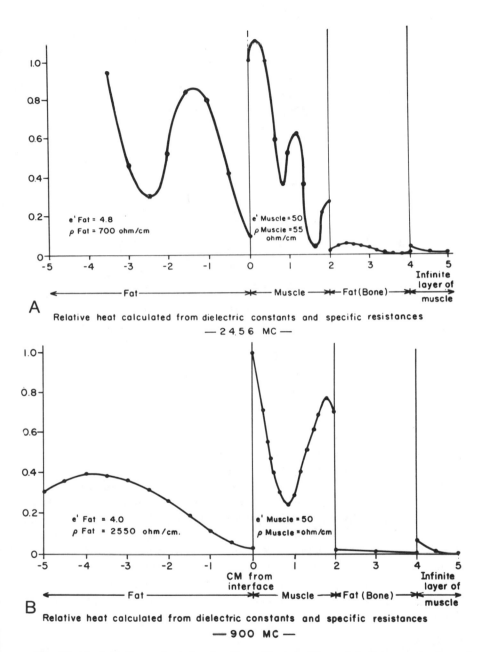

Fig. 10.46. *A*, Pattern of relative heating calculated from dielectric constants and specific resistances in a complex specimen at a frequency of 2450 MHz. *B*, Pattern of relative heating calculated from dielectric constants and specific resistances in a complex specimen at a frequency of 900 MHz. From Lehmann *et al.* (264).

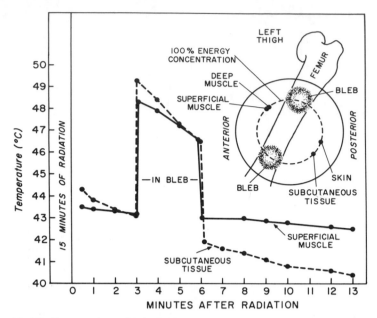

Fig. 10.47. Burns where high field intensity crosses over superficially located bone and selective rise of temperature in the bleb once formed. From Lehmann (219), modified from Worden et al. (429).

is raised, highly selective absorption in the blebs may occur with temperature rises to 49°C.

It should also be remembered that the temperature distribution produced by microwave absorption is superimposed upon the pre-existing temperature distribution with the high temperatures at the core and low temperatures in superficial tissues (203, 206, 217, 338, 339).

The blood flow also has an influence on the final temperature distribution. The blood flow in the heated tissues, especially the musculature, cannot only be increased by microwave application (338, 339) but the blood flow change in turn also greatly modifies the ultimate temperature distribution (234). After an initial temperature rise to a peak value in the 44°C range, the change in blood flow subsequently reduced the temperature by approximately 1 to 2°C (see Figure 10.48) (79, 234, 257), in spite of continuous microwave application. More recently, Sekins et al. (362), measured the blood flow change.

Equipment

Ideally, therapeutic equipment should have the following features. It should be able to selectively heat musculature with even temperature distribution from the subcutaneous fat-muscle interface to the bone. The

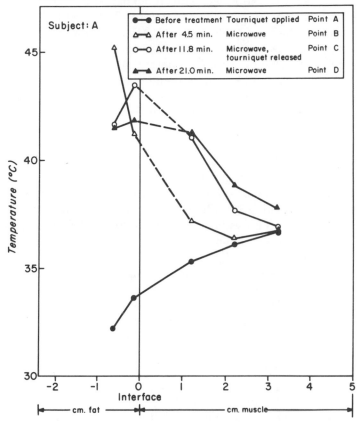

A Comparison of Temperature Distribution Produced in the
Human Thigh during Exposure to Microwave at 2456 MC.
Applied with Waveguide.

Subject: A

	Before treatment	Tourniquet applied	Point A
●——●	After 4.5 min.	Microwave	Point B
△——△	After 11.8 min.	Microwave, tourniquet released	Point C
▲——▲	After 21.0 min.	Microwave	Point D

Fig. 10.48. A comparison of temperature distribution produced at different times in the human thigh during exposure to microwave at 2,456 MHz applied with waveguide. From Lehmann *et al.* (234).

temperature throughout the field exposed from edge to edge should be as even as possible. The absorbed energy in W/kg should be adequate to raise the temperature in the tissues to tolerance levels. It is desirable to have enough reserve power to overcome the cooling effect due to the blood flow increase resulting from the temperature elevation. The equipment should be capable of producing a vigorous demonstrable physiological response. Stray radiation should be kept to a minimum to avoid exposure of sensitive organs of the patient and of the therapist. A meter should be available which quantitatively indicates the flow of power into the tissues. This type of measurement is commonly based on the measurement of the total output minus the reflected power. There should be an accurate timer to be set in order to limit the period of exposure. It should be possible to regulate the output within the available range. The frequency of the equipment should be limited to the frequency bands assigned by FCC regulations for therapeutic purposes, that is, 2,456 and 915 MHz. In order to fulfill these requirements, it has been shown that the lower frequency of 915 would be advantageous over 2,456 MHz. To get better coupling and less stray radiation, it is generally agreed that direct contact applicators whose aperture is in full contact with the skin of the patient would be preferred. The selection of the optimal frequency for these applicators was studied by Lehmann *et al.* (252).

Guy and Lehmann (146); Lehmann *et al.* (252); and Guy (143) analyzed the optimal frequency. The results show that the optimum frequency for therapeutic heating with a clinical size 12 × 16 applicator is 750 MHz, but that the results which can be obtained with the authorized frequency of 915 MHz are nearly as good (252). These studies indicated further that a 13 × 13 cm^2 aperture with a TE_{10} waveguide mode source distribution should give optimal results for the maximum muscle-to-fat heating ratio with the minimum size source at 915 MHz.

Applicators are also equipped with air cooling, the air being blown through the porous dielectric with which the cavity is loaded; a thin plastic radome with the proper distribution of grooves and holes assures even cooling of the skin and eliminates selective heating of the surface at the edges of the applicator (142, 143, 148, 250). These applicators have a fixed direction of the E field vector, they are linearly polarized. Experimental applicators, circularly polarized, with a rotating E field vector, are also available. Circularly polarized applicators operating at 2,456 and 915 MHz have been developed by Transco; the reduce stray radiation they have a circular quarter wavelength choke (see Figure 10.49).

Non-contact applicators operating at 2,456 MHz are still in clinical use. These include the A director, which consists of an antenna and a hemispheric reflector (diameter 9.3 cm) which produces a beam having a cross section field pattern in the shape of a ring (see Figure 10.50) (333). The intensity in the center of the field is half of the value of the intensity at the ring. However, if the applicator is applied directly to the skin, the highest intensity will be found in the center of the field in close proximity to the tip of the antenna rod.

The construction of the B director is similar to that of the A director, but the diameter of the reflector is approximately 15.3 cm and the field pattern is similar but larger than that of the A director. The C director consists of a half-wavelength (6.1 cm) dipole antenna with a corner reflector. It produces a beam with an oval cross section with the highest intensity found in the center of the field (see Figure 10.51). The E director consists of a full wave (12.2 cm dipole) antenna with corner reflector. The field pattern is

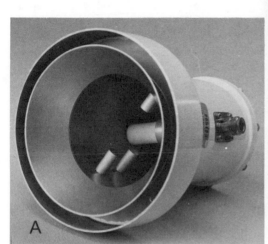
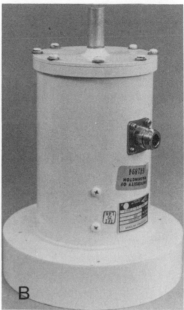

Fig. 10.49. 915 MHz Transco circularly polarized direct contact applicator with circular quarter wavelength choke around applicator edge.

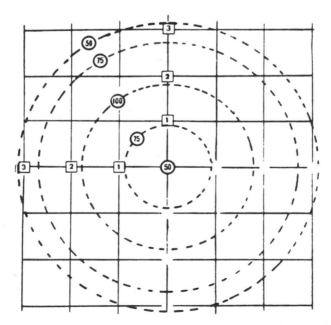

Fig. 10.50. Field pattern produced by ''A'' director at a distance of two inches in percent of maximal intensity (*circles*); distance from the center in inches (*squares*). From Lehmann (219).

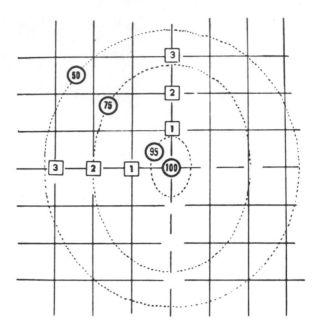

Fig. 10.51. Field pattern produced by "C" director at a distance of three inches in percent of maximal intensity (*circles*); distance from the center in inches (squares). From Lehmann (219).

similar to the C director; however, corresponding to the longer dipole it is more elongated. The beaming properties of these applicators are poor since the wavelength in air is 12.2 cm and, therefore, comparable in size to the antennae and reflectors. As a result the angle of divergence of the beams produced by these applicators will be significant (353). Consequently, the field intensity decreases rapidly with increasing distance from the applicator.

Technique of Application and Temperature Distribution

The temperature distribution of these commercially available noncontact applicators follows the radiation pattern (265). For instance, the A director, spaced 2 cm away from the skin, produces the typical ring pattern with highest temperature rises in the ring and lower temperatures in the center of the beam. However, when the A director has contact with the skin, the peak temperature is found directly under the antenna rod in the most superficial tissues; this defeats the deep-heating purpose. Direct contact should be avoided with any one of these applicators, which should be spaced about 2 cm above the skin to assure adequate heating. Spacing farther away markedly reduces the ability to heat vigorously.

Direct Contact Applicators. In order to test new applicator designs rapidly and effectively it was necessary to develop methods by which the pattern of relative heating, *i.e.*, the absorbed energy (W/kg) at any given tissue location could be evaluated. In order to do this, Guy (142) developed substances with dielectric constants identical to those of such human tissues as subcutaneous fat, muscle, and bone. These substances could also be used to develop geometric models of the anatomical structures (see Figure 10.52). Further, these substances had also thermal properties very close to the corresponding human tissues. These models were split, the two halves closely approximated and exposed to microwaves with the appropriate orientation of the E field vector across the split. After short-term exposure not allowing heat conduction to occur to any significant degree, the models were separated and immediately scanned with an infrared scanner (thermograph).

The thermograph output can be computerized and the direct plot of the temperature distribution obtained, also indicating the location of the peak temperatures (see Figure 10.53). From the original linear transient of the temperature rise, the absorbed power can be measured at any point in the model. If the same measurements are made in the human volunteer, with temperature probes in place, the absorbed power can be calculated where these measurements are taken and compared with the values obtained in the model (see Figure 10.54). Probes should be used which do not significantly interfere with the microwave field. There was good agreement in the

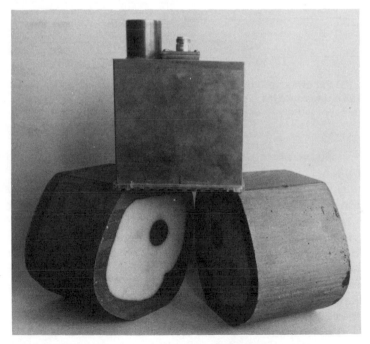

Fig. 10.52. Phantom thigh model with 13-cm square-contact microwave applicator with radome operating at 915 MHz. From Lehmann *et al.* (250).

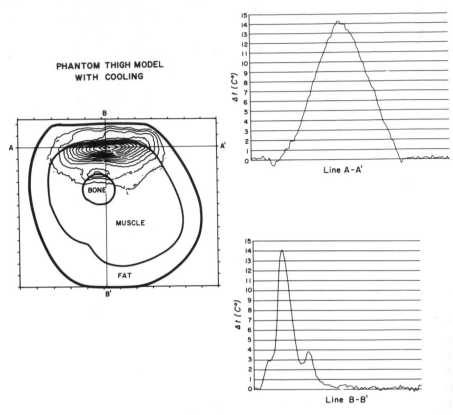

Fig. 10.53. Isotherms produced in phantom thigh model after exposure to a 13-cm square direct-contact microwave applicator operating at 915 MHz with radome and cooling. From Lehmann *et al.* (250).

calculated selective absorption rate in the human and in the model (see Figure 10.55).

More recently, methods have been developed to maintain direct electrical contact between the tissue layers of the split model so that rotating circularly polarized applicators can be assessed with the above described method without orientation of the electrical field vectors across the split (271).

In the human, the blood flow increase triggered by the temperature rise in the tissues produces a cooling effect which can be quantitively assessed (see Figure 10.56). Once the thermal properties of the tissues and blood are known, one can calculate the change in blood flow rate by measuring its cooling effect (Table 10.3). The calculated values of absorbed power in the human thigh at the point of pain are shown in Table 10.4. At these specific absorption rates, the calculated change in blood flow rate is shown in Table 10.5. In conclusion, at specific absorption rates of up to approximately 170

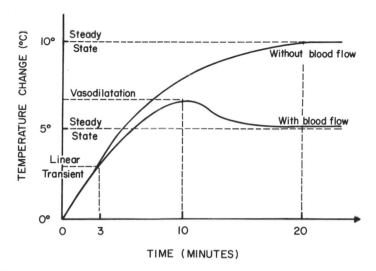

Fig. 10.54. Schematic representation of transient and steady-state temperatures for a typical tissue under diathermy exposure. From Lehmann *et al.* (250).

W/kg, blood flow increases up to approximately 30 ml/100 gm tissue/min are obtained. Thus, a vigorous physiological response is obtained, since blood flow increases under maximal exercise are of the order of 30 to 35 ml/100 gm tissue/min. The use of tissue substitute models allows quick determination of the maximum specific absorption rate in the muscle. In turn, the described human experiments allow one to predict whether the absorption rate is adequate to produce a significant vigorous biological response. Thus, applicators can be quickly tested and compared without human experimentation. Questions which can be answered include whether or not the heating pattern they will produce is therapeutically desirable, where the highest temperatures in the tissues can be expected, and whether the absorbed power in the tissues is adequate to produce desired biological responses (250).

The ultimate test of an applicator, *i.e.*, whether it is suitable for therapeutic purposes, rests with evaluation in the human. The described direct contact applicators with radome and surface cooling can produce, in an individual with less than 2 cm surface fat, a temperature distribution which shows the highest temperature in the musculature with an even temperature distribution from subcutaneous fat-muscle interface to periosteum (see Figure 10.57). In persons with more subcutaneous fat, slightly higher temperatures may still be found in the deep subcutaneous fat layers (79).

Dosimetry

Commercial equipment presently available with nondirect contact applicators does not allow accurate dosimetry. The meter on the control panel

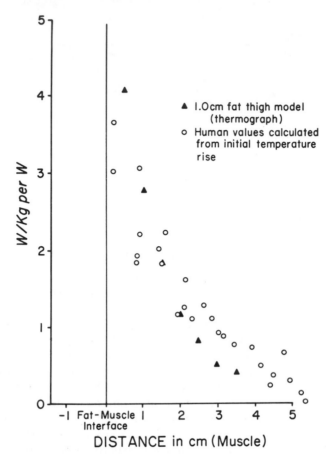

Fig. 10.55. Comparison of the calculations of the SAR in thighs of human beings and models. From Lehmann *et al.* (250).

does not read the energy entering the tissues. Therefore, as in shortwave diathermy, one has to rely on the sensation of pain as a warning that tolerance levels are exceeded. For vigorous heating, output should stay just below this threshold. For mild heating, a feeling of warmth is the best available guide. When direct contact applicators are used with equipment fulfilling the standards proposed by the FDA (109), a meter will indicate the forward power to the patient which is based on the measurement of total output minus the reflected power. For vigorous effect, the forward power would be of the order of 50 W (252) with an average intensity of the order of 500 mW/cm^2. Air-cooled applicators are useful to avoid undesirable temperature rise in skin and subcutaneous fat especially since optimum frequencies for muscle heating are below 915 MHz, the frequency allocated for medical purposes by the FCC (250, 269).

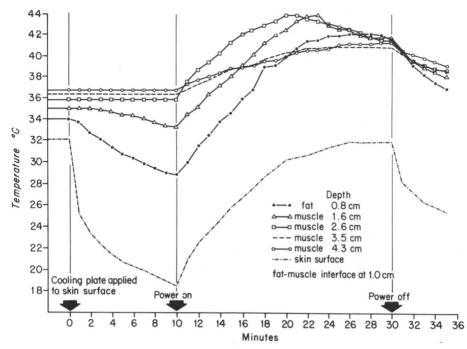

Fig. 10.56. Temperatures in a typical experiment at various depths of tissues resulting from application of microwave with a 915 MHz contact applicator. From de Lateur *et al.* (79).

TABLE 10.3. *Formula for Calculation of Blood Flow*[a]

Blood-Flow Rate in Muscle

$$m = \frac{W_b}{k_2 \cdot c \cdot \Delta T' \cdot \rho_b}$$

m = blood flow mm/100 gm/min
W_b = power dissipated by blood flow W/kg
ρ_b = gm/cm³
k_2 = Constant 0.698
c = specific heat of blood kcal/kg°C
$\Delta T = T - T_a$ = arterial temperature
T = tissue temperature

[a] From Lehmann *et al.* (250).

Common Indications

Microwave diathermy can be used for heating musculature selectively. It has been shown that treatment of fibrous muscular contractures may be successful when used in conjunction with stretch to utilize the effect on the extensibility of collagen tissues (see Figure 10.58) (80).

TABLE 10.4. *Calculated Values of Absorbed Power in Human Muscle*[a]

SAR in W/kg[1] in Musculature (1 to 2 cm)	
Run	Sar
1	121.60
2	78.17
3	118.70
4	75.27
5	167.93

1 at 555.55 mW/cm^2 maximum power density of incident radiation.

[a] From Lehmann *et al.* (250).

TABLE 10.5. *Calculated Values for Blood Flow in Human Muscle*[a]

Calculated Blood-Flow Rate in Muscle	
Run	ml/100 gm/minute
1	28.90
2	28.91
3	25.00
4	23.64
5	29.69

[a] From Lehmann *et al.* (250).

Microwave application may also be useful in treating secondary muscle spasm and in the treatment of the tender myofibrositic nodes as they are commonly found in the upper back (302).

Joints covered with heavy layers of soft tissues cannot be effectively treated with microwaves (263), whereas joints such as the interphalangeal and metacarpophalangeal joints and the wrist can be treated with microwaves since the soft tissue layer covering the joints is thin (334).

Specific Contraindications

Since microwave diathermy is a form of heat therapy the conditions listed under contraindications for heat therapy also apply to microwave application. In addition, as an electromagnetic radiation, microwaves should not be applied in the presence of surgical metal implants or such implants as cardiac pacemakers or electrophysiological braces; even though shielding has been improved, the high therapeutic intensities would likely either destroy the electronic equipment in the pacemaker and the electrophysiological braces or would produce selective overheating within or around the metallic surgical implants.

In addition, certain parts of the body are likely to be either selectively heated or to be more sensitive to temperature rise, and therefore, exposure

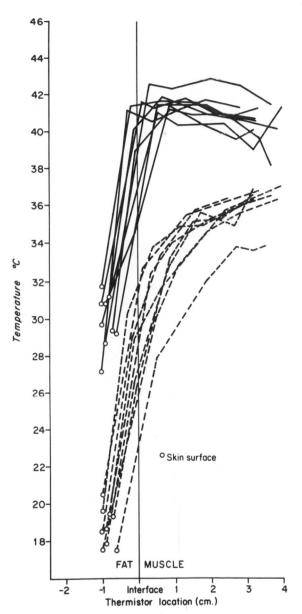

Fig. 10.57. Temperature distribution in all volunteers with, less than or equal to, 1 cm of subcutaneous fat before (- - - - - - - -) and 20 minutes after (————) microwave application. From de Lateur *et al.* (79).

of these organs should be prevented (401). These include the testicles because of their location external to the body within the scrotum. They are, therefore, easily exposed to stray radiation during therapeutic application. In contrast to the testicles, the ovaries are covered by such a thick layer of

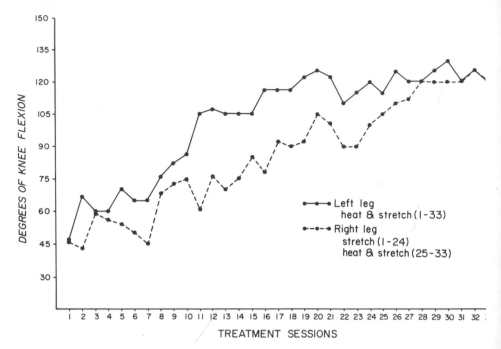

Fig. 10.58. The degrees of knee flexion due to residual elongation of the right and left rectus femoris muscles before each treatment session. From de Lateur *et al.* (80).

soft tissue that it is difficult to expose them to any significant amount of microwave radiation and heating (205).

Michaelson, in his preceding chapter of bioeffects of high frequency currents and electromagnetic radiation pointed out that exposure of the scrotal areas at high power densities of greater than 50 mW/cm^2 resulted in testicular damage such as edema, enlargement, atrophy, fibrosis, and necrosis of the seminiferous tubules in rats and rabbits. Intensities of 8 mW/cm^2 did not affect the mating of mice or rats. He related these responses to the heating of this organ. Pregnant small laboratory animals were exposed to radiation with resulting abnormalities in the offspring (see Chapter 7). Rubin and Erdman (346) reported on four women treated with microwave diathermy for chronic pelvic inflammatory disease who were or became pregnant during the course of therapy. The women were exposed to a frequency of 2,450 MHz and 100 W output of the at-that-time available therapeutic equipment. Three women delivered normal infants and one woman aborted on Day 67, but delivered a normal baby following a subsequent pregnancy during which she again received microwave therapy. Daels (70, 71) used microwaves to ease parturition without any evidence of injury in a 1-year follow-up of the children. While it is questionable that the fetus in the human can be reached with any significant microwave energy, that is not so in small laboratory animals. While it is also possible that the amniotic fluid selectively absorbs microwaves there is no evidence at this time that the uterine content in pregnancy would be selectively heated. However, in this absence of clear evidence to the contrary, and with the knowledge that temperatures of 38.9°C (160) are damaging to the human fetus, pregnancy should be considered a contraindication to microwave therapy applied in such a way that a significant amount of energy could reach the pregnant uterus.

In 1950 and 1951, Daily *et al.* and Richardson *et al.* (73, 75, 76, 340, 341) already demonstrated that cataracts can be formed in eyes of experimental animals exposed to microwaves. Williams *et al.* (418) studied the time and power density threshold for cataractogenesis in rabbits; with more accurate modern technology for the measurement of the power densities, these experiments were reported by Guy *et al.* (149) and Carpenter and van Ummerson (54, 55) and the results of these two studies were essentially the same and confirmed that very short-term exposures required very high densities to produce cataracts and that long-term exposure to power densities of approximately 150 mW/cm^2 and above were required to produce cataracts (see Figure 10.59).

Even very long-term exposures below this level would not produce the cataracts. By further temperature measurements and computer modeling of the temperature distribution the authors found that the minimum cataractogenic power density of 150 mW/cm^2 for 100 minutes corresponded to a maximum absorbed power density in the vitreous of 138 W/kg, and a possible threshold cataractogenic temperature around 41°C in the eye.

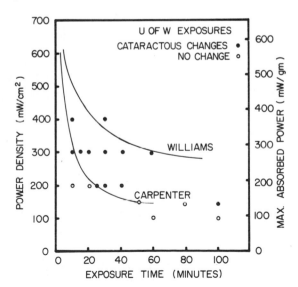

Fig. 10.59. Time and power-density threshold for cataractogenesis in rabbits exposed to near-zone 2450 MHz radiation. From Guy *et al.* (149).

Computer modeling showed the highest temperature at the posterior pole of the lenticular tissues (see Figure 10.60).

Guy *et al.* could demonstrate that this was indeed a temperature effect by hypothermia experiments where, by total body cooling the critical temperature rise in the eye was prevented in spite of microwave exposure above the cataractogenic level. It also should be noted that cataractogenic dosage is painful and anesthesia is required in the animals. This suggests that in man the cataractogenic doses cannot be applied without pain, which in turn would produce an immediate withdrawal from the exposure. From this discussion, it is quite obvious that the eye selectively absorbs microwaves and, therefore, is selectively heated. It is for that reason that exposure of the eye should be avoided at cataractogenic levels, in spite of the fact that there is no clear evidence that in man cataracts have been produced by microwave exposure.

Guy pointed out that concentration of the microwave energy and thus, spot heating may occur in the brain when the skull is exposed. He also demonstrated that processing of sensory input in the thalamus showed a decreased latency corresponding to the increase in temperature in the selectively heated area. These observations were reversible as the temperature returned to normal (198). Thus, these observed effects have to be dealt with as temperature effects when safety is considered. These effects were observed in cats at intensities as low as 5 mW/cm².

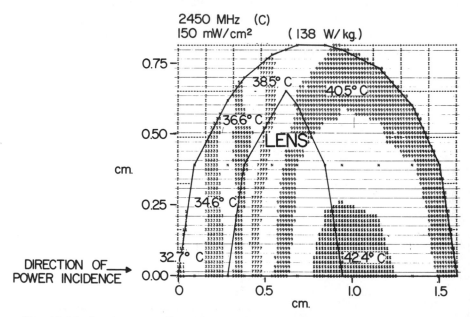

Fig. 10.60. Computer-predicted intraocular temperature in the rabbit exposed to 100 minutes of near-zone 2450 MHz at 150 W/cm². From Guy *et al.* (149).

However, because of the larger size of the human, one can expect such phenomena to occur at levels about 12 mW/cm^2. From these considerations, the exposure of the skull to high intensity levels should be avoided. In addition, many experiments observing for instance changes in EEG tracings can be related to the interference of the microwave fields producing enhanced absorption of energy because of the use of metallic electrodes in the electric field (144).

In addition, therapeutic application should take into consideration the possibility of enhanced absorption in thin layers of soft tissue covering reflecting bone. Such situations should be avoided to prevent burns. The unchecked accumulation of sweat beads on the skin exposed to microwaves may also lead to selective absorption and superficial burns which can be avoided by proper technique of application or by the use of air-cooled direct contact applicators.

Non-thermal Effects

Non-thermal effects have been definitely documented (207, 208). The so-called pearl chain formation is produced when particles such as fat globules in the milk or red blood cells in the serum arrange themselves in chain formation in the electromagnetic field. Saito and Schwan (348, 349) studied this effect and related it to the development of surface charges on these particles forming dipoles attracting each other. However, there is no evidence that non-thermal effects play any significant role in relation to the use of microwaves as a diathermy modality (219). None of these potential non-thermal effects has been related to a clearly identified therapeutic response.

Standards for Efficacy and Safety

Under the radiation control for health and safety act (332) and under the medical devices act, the FDA is in the process of developing standards for both efficacy and safety. In order to demonstrate that therapeutic microwave equipment is effective, it is necessary to demonstrate that it can heat adequately in order to produce physiological responses. The relationship between absorbed power, temperature rise, and biological reactions has been discussed in detail under "Dosimetry," as has the use of tissue substitute models for standardization.

In considering standards for safety, one must keep in mind that they should be developed for two purposes: to avoid inadvertent exposure of sensitive parts of the patient who is treated, and to avoid exposure of the therapist or the personnel to intensities which may produce detrimental effects. In the clinical application of any potent modality, there is always a potential trade-off between benefit and risk, whereas in the occupational exposure no hazards are acceptable. Two approaches to the development of the standard can be used. If a performance or emission standard for a piece of equipment is used, the output and stray radiation of the equipment is controlled in such a fashion that inadvertent exposure of the patient's sensitive organs or the therapist cannot occur. This type of approach has been used for the microwave oven. In a standard limiting use to certified personnel, safeguards have to be taken that neither the patient's sensitive organs nor the therapist are exposed to levels exceeding safety. This type of standard in the medical setting may rely heavily on the intelligent use of the equipment by trained personnel having adequate information about performance of the machine available. Control can be exerted to allow the use of such equipment only by physician or therapist. In either case, it is necessary to identify safe exposure levels.

The present safe exposure level of 10 mW/cm^2 over an average of 6 minutes was proposed by Schwan (353) and was based on the maximal thermal load that an adult could dissipate under usual environmental conditions without a rise in body temperature. This still allows for a safety factor of 10, since due to physiological thermal regulatory mechanisms the compensatory heat losses can be increased ten-fold. This standard assumes total body exposure, quite unlike the limited area which is usually exposed for therapeutic purposes. Michaelson (296) carried out intensive investigations in 1971 and found that none of them produced any evidence of a hazard at a proposed limit of 10 mW/cm^2. On the other hand, there is conclusive evidence that potentially hazardous thermal effects are produced at levels above 100 mW/cm^2. Presently, consideration has been given to lowering the level of safe exposure. From such extensive review of the literature Michaelson (296) came to the conclusion that most of the low intensity effects, if not all of them, could be explained on the basis of heat, often in the form of heat stress. Another extensive review of the literature by Justesen et al. (200) is essentially compatible with this conclusion. It is, therefore, doubtful that any useful purpose is served for the therapeutic application for the safety of patient and therapeutic personnel by lowering the safety level substantially, since such standards may significantly interfere with present and further therapeutic applications and the benefits derived from them (269, 270). Lehmann et al. (269) have shown that safety can be enforced by placing the equipment in the hands of knowledgable professionals. The use of strict performance standards of the equipment alone is not practical since no applicator readily available would fulfill the proposed performance standards of 5 or 10 mW/cm^2, 5 cm from the applicator edge in the patients (see Table 10.6). Even applicators designed to perfectly fit the large and small cylindrical and the plane layered tissue substitute models, as proposed by the FDA, would be unable to fulfill the same criteria in the human application to the corresponding parts of the anatomy, the arm, the leg, or the back. It has been demonstrated that leakage occurs primarily in the direction where direct contact is lost. In a linearly polarized applicator, leakage is always greater in the direction of the E field vector (see Figures 10.61 and 10.62, and Table 10.7).

Knowledgable use of such equipment would direct the stray radiation away from sensitive organs of the patient and from the therapist. Of course,

TABLE 10.6. *Data on a 2450-MHz Transco circularly polarized, direct-contact applicator with choke. The maximal distance is given between the 5 mW cm*$^{-2}$ *isopower-density level and the closest point of the external surface of the applicator. The input power was adjusted to 20 W net*[a]

Large cylinder 25 × 17.3 cm	Thigh model 21.6 cm long × 16.1 diameter flattened area 21.6 × 10 cm	Anterior human thigh 20 cm long × 16 cm diameter flattened area 29 cm × 14 cm in the center
+ × <5 cm	<5 cm	<5 cm
− × <5 cm	<5 cm	<5 cm
+y <5 cm	<5 cm	<5 cm
−y 6.7 cm	<5 cm	<5 cm
+z N.M.[b]	<5 cm	<5 cm
−z 10.8 cm	<5 cm	<5 cm

[a] From Lehmann *et al.* (269).
[b] Not measured.

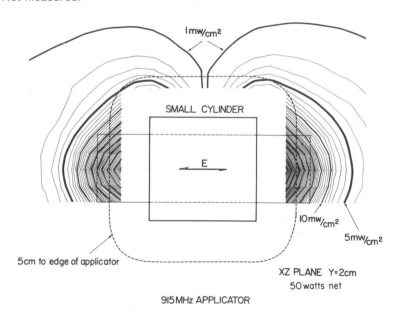

Fig. 10.61. Pattern of stray radiation around a tissue-substitute small cylinder with a 915 MHz direct-contact applicator on the model's surface. The E field is parallel to the cylinder axis. Graduated in 1 mW/cm^2 increments at 50 W net input power. From Lehmann *et al.* (269).

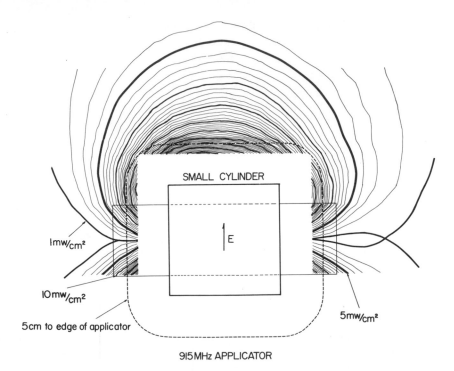

Fig. 10.62. Pattern of stray radiation around a tissue-substitute small cylinder with a 915 MHz direct contact applicator on the model's surface. The E field is perpendicular to the cylinder axis. Graduated in 1 mW/cm² increments at 50 W net input power. From Lehmann *et al.* (269).

such a standard based on the control as to who may apply such equipment will also require that the physician and therapist are equipped with enough information on the stray radiation pattern by the various applicators as applied to the proposed models that adequate judgment can be applied. This type of approach to the standard would be much more in keeping with the standards developed for ionizing radiation (298).

ULTRASOUND

Ultrasound is a form of diathermy often used to obtain specific therapeutic effects which cannot be achieved by other measures. It may be used alone or as a part of a treatment program which may include massage, exercise, and possibly other procedures. Although the three diathermy modalities have several features in common, there are some important differences in the individual characteristics and effects. In the following, the mechanisms determining indications and contraindications to this form of energy will be discussed in an attempt to establish the rationale for the therapeutic use of ultrasound. The parameters controlling proper dosage and technique of

TABLE 10.7 Stray Radiation Levels Produced at Sensitive Anatomic Sites[a]

Site Irradiated	Site Measured	915 MHz linearly polarized applicator		2450 MHz Transco applicator	2450 MHz E-director[b]		2450 MHz C-director	
		Parallel	Perpendicular		Parallel	Perpendicular	Parallel	Perpendicular
Thigh	Genitals	7	30	1	20	20	13	20
Anterior lateral aspect of shoulder	Eyes	20	2	1	20	13	NM[c]	NM
Posterior lateral aspect of shoulder	Eyes	12	2	3	10	8	NM	NM
Trapezius	Eyes	2	2	2	NM	NM	NM	NM
Posterior neck	Eyes	1	13	2	NM	6[d]	5	5

[a] From Lehmann et al. (270).
[b] Stray radiation levels in mW/cm^2 measured with E-field parallel and perpendicular to tissue axis. Input power normalized to 50 W net for 915 MHz, 20 W net for 2,450 MHz applicators.
[c] NM = not measured.
[d] On midline

application, as well as therapeutically desirable and potentially dangerous features, will be reviewed. Neither the diagnostic use of ultrasound nor the use of high intensity ultrasound to produce lesions will be discussed.

Definition and Physics

Ultrasound is defined as a form of acoustic vibration with frequencies so high that it cannot be perceived by the human ear (36). Thus, frequencies under 17,000 Hertz are usually called sound, while those above 17,000 Hz are defined as ultrasound. This is an arbitrary definition, however, since humans exhibit great variations in the upper limits of their acoustic perceptions. Younger individuals may hear frequencies as high as 18,000 Hz, while older persons may lack the ability to perceive frequencies above 12,000 Hz.

With exception of the difference in frequency, the physics of ultrasound is in no way different from that of audible sound waves. Sound waves within the audible and ultrasonic frequency range are longitudinal compression waves. The movement of the molecules or particles in the medium occurs parallel to the direction of wave propagation. In case of a cylindrical ultrasound beam, the propagation also occurs parallel to the axis of the beam. This propagation of ultrasound depends on the presence of a medium that can be compressed, since propagation does not occur in a vacuum.

The following relationship exists between the wavelength λ, the frequency n, and the velocity of the sound propagation in the medium c:

$$\lambda = c/n$$

Biophysics

Ultrasonic frequencies used for therapeutic purposes range between 0.8 and 1 MHz. The sound velocity in water and in tissues is approximately 1.5 $\times 10^5$ cm/second. The corresponding wavelength in water is approximately 0.15 cm. Thus, many tissue structures are large as compared with wavelength, although they are small as compared with the wavelength of audible sound. The result is that biological interfaces and tissue structures which are transparent to audible sound waves may reflect or scatter ultrasound, as will be explained later. Some tissue layers may have a thickness which does not allow transmission of ultrasound, whereas the same tissue structures may be considered as transparent for the long waves in the audible frequency range. The amount of the energy reflected at the biological interface depends on the mismatch of acoustic impedance. This acoustic impedance is the function of the specific acoustic impedance and the thickness of the membrane. The specific acoustic impedance is defined as a product of $\rho \cdot c$, where ρ is the density of the tissues and c is the sound velocity in the medium.

With perpendicular incidence of the sound waves on a plane layered tissue, maximal transmission occurs if the thickness of the tissue layer is an even multiple of the quarter wavelength in that medium, and maximal reflection at the interface occurs if the thickness is an uneven multiple of the quarter wavelength. If the layer is very thin as compared with the wavelength it is transparent.

At the therapeutic frequencies of 0.8 to 1 MHz, there is no technical difficulty in producing high ultrasonic intensities. Intensities of up to 40 W/cm^2 have been easily obtained without focusing.

The ultrasonic intensities used for therapy range up to 4 W/cm^2. These intensities are comparable to a noise level produced by ten thousand high output speakers in a room of one cubic centimeter (329).

The primary reactions occurring in the ultrasonic beam at therapeutic intensities can be graphically described as follows: the ultrasonic intensity I is in proportion to the square of the displacement amplitude A of the particles or molecules of the medium and in proportion to the square of the angular frequency ω, which equals $2\pi n$.

$$I = (\rho c/2)(\omega A)^2$$

The product $\omega \cdot A = U$

where U is the amplitude of the velocity of the medium particles. If P is the pressure amplitude, it follows that

$$P = \sqrt{2 \cdot I \cdot \rho \cdot c}$$

and

$$U = \sqrt{2 \cdot I / \rho \cdot c}$$

and

$$A = (U/2\pi n)$$

To find the acceleration, b, of the particles of the medium, the following formula is utilized:

$$b = 2\pi n U$$

Thus, it is possible to determine the amplitude of the displacement of the particles in the medium as rarefaction and compression occur alternatingly. It is also possible to calculate the pressure amplitude and the velocity of the particles. Additional information on the density of the medium is required. Let us assume that the therapeutically applied intensities are of the order of magnitude of 1 to 5 W/cm^2, that the ultrasonic frequencies are of the order of magnitude of 1 mHz, and that the density of the tissues is similar to water, that is, 1 gm/cm^3. Under those conditions, it can be calculated (329) that the pressure amplitude is approximately 1 to 5 atmospheres. It should be noted that the area of maximal pressure in the medium is separated by just a half wavelength that is, by approximately 0.75 mm from the area of maximal rarefraction. Thus, a great difference in pressure occurs over a relatively short distance. It is also noteworthy that the pressure in a given point changes one million times per second from the maximum to the minimum. The amplitude of the displacement of the particles of the medium is only of the order of 1×10^{-6} to 6×10^{-6} cm and the maximum velocity of the particles is approximately 10 to 26 cm/second. The accelerations which the particles are subjected to are about 5×10^7 to 16×10^7 cm/second^2. This represents an acceleration which is approximately 100,000 times that of gravity.

These mechanical forces can create secondary reactions in the tissues. Cavities can be produced in the fluid during the phase of rarefaction in the sound waves. During the following phase of compression, these cavities may again collapse creating a high-energy concentration in the form of shock waves. If the fluid does not contain any dissolved gas, this phenomenon is called true cavitation, in contrast to gaseous cavitation where degassing occurs during the phase of rarefaction, and gas bubbles are produced which may become larger or in turn may again collapse during the following phase of compression.

The growth of the gas bubbles can be explained as follows. During the phase of compression when the surface area of the gas bubble is relatively small, the gas moves out of the bubble into the surrounding fluid. Then, during the following phase of rarefaction, when the bubble is expanded and its surface is relatively large, the gas moves out of the fluid into the cavity. Since the amount of gas passing into or out of the bubble is in proportion to the bubble surface, there is a net gain of gas moving into the bubble (139).

Electrical and chemical phenomena have been described as resulting from cavitation. Cavitation also produces highly destructive mechanical forces. In biological material, since gases are always present, we deal only with gaseous cavitation. Even so, mechanical destruction can occur, since the gas bubble may collapse during compression or may expand to the extent that it tears tissues or may grow to such a size that it can vibrate in resonance with the sound waves (218). The occurrence of gaseous cavitation can be prevented by application of external pressure of a sufficient magnitude.

As sound is propagated through the tissues, it is gradually absorbed and converted into heat. The surface intensity is gradually attenuated, according to the following formula:

$$I = I_o \cdot e^{-\alpha x}$$

where I is the intensity in the tissues at the depth x, I_o is the surface intensity, α is the coefficient of absorption and e is the base of the natural logarithm. The coefficient of absorption α determines the depth, x_p, at which the incident sound intensity, I_o, is decreased to the value of $1/e$. This depth

$$x_p = (1/\alpha)$$

is called the depth of penetration. More commonly, the depth of penetration is defined as that depth of the tissues, x_L, where the surface intensity drops to one-half of its value.

$$x_L = \frac{ln\ 2}{\alpha} \quad \text{since} \quad I/I_o = 1/2$$

The sound intensity in a uniform medium decays (due to the absorption) exponentially. The end point of the curve cannot be determined where the sound intensity is totally absorbed and has dropped to zero.

Carstensen *et al.* (56) have demonstrated that ultrasonic absorption occurs primarily in the tissue proteins, although such structural elements as cellular membranes are responsible for a minor degree of absorption (352). Hueter and associate (182, 185) have shown that the attenuation of ultrasound in muscle tissue depends on whether or not the ultrasonic beam is parallel to the myofascial interfaces. Horvath and Hollander (181) demonstrated a selective rise of temperature at interfaces. The selective rise of temperature at interfaces of different tissues may be the result of relection, in the form of plane wave reflection at a smooth interface or resulting from scattering from an uneven surface or from focusing produced by a concave surface. Also, the longitudinal compression waves of ultrasound may be converted into transverse or shear waves which are rapidly attenuated. Finally, if the tissue presenting the interface is highly absorbing with rapid attenuation, the surface of this tissue will be heated selectively.

Chan *et al.* (59) demonstrated that that portion of ultrasonic heating resulting from shear waves at the tissue-bone interface depends on the angle of incidence (see Figure 10.63). The angle of incidence which produces maximal heating through shear waves is between 45 and 50°.

The reflection of the sound wave by a surface creates a radiation pressure. The radiation force produces a streaming in a viscous fluid medium because absorption of the sound in the fluid results in a spatial gradient of acoustic energy.

Pattern of Relative Heating. The pattern of relative heating of ultrasound in a three-layered system consisting of fat, muscle, and bone has been calculated by Schwan (353). Chan *et al.* (59) calculated this pattern for different angles of incidence (see Figure 10.64). This pattern clearly indicates that ultrasound is not a good heating modality for heating either subcutaneous fat or muscle. However, it produces a relatively high rise of temperature at the bone (21, 313). This indicates that in a uniform soft tissue not enough ultrasound is absorbed to make it a valuable diathermy modality for this purpose.

Chan *et al.* (58) used a numerical approach to obtaining the resultant temperature distribution in layered tissue, with thermal source and cooling inside the tissue. The calculation of the temperature distribution was based on a linear model of the tissue consisting of several layers of different kinds

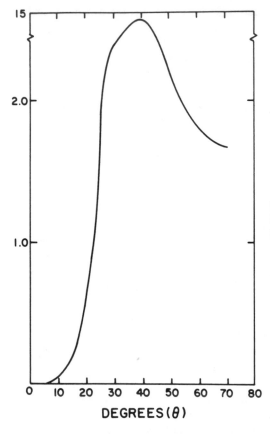

Fig. 10.63. Ratio of heating due to shear wave to heating due to longitudinal wave. From Chan *et al.* (59).

of tissue separated by parallel boundaries. The mathematical prediction, based on propagation and attenuation of acoustic ultrasound waves, as well as on microwaves and shortwave diathermy closely matched the experimental data.

For therapeutic application, it is important to recognize those areas which are selectively heated. One such area is the superficial bone, because bone attenuates ultrasound more than skeletal muscle and subcutaneous fat (see Table 10.8) (257). Also, the densities and sound velocities differ in these tissues (see Tables 10.9 and 10.10). As a result, a considerable amount of energy is reflected at the soft tissue-bone interface (see Table 10.11). Up to 30 percent may be reflected at this interface. As a result, it is possible to selectively raise the temperature in the capsule of a hip joint. This was done in an unanaesthetized, live pig, comparable in size to the human with temperatures in the upper therapeutic range. In contrast, microwaves and shortwaves applied to a dosage sufficient to produce a first-degree burn in the superficial tissue are ineffective at heating the hip (see Figures 10.65 and 10.66). Since a large amount of the incident ultrasonic energy is reflected at the bone surface, and whatever penetrates into the bone is rapidly

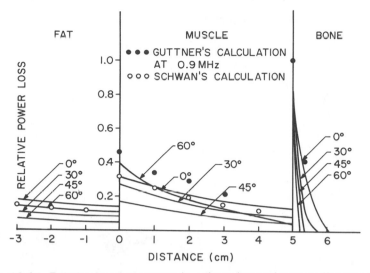

Fig. 10.64. Relative heating pattern in a three-layered system (fat-muscle-bone). Frequency: 1 MHz. Schwan's and Guttner's calculated values are superimposed, but these values are renormalized. From Chan *et al.* (59).

TABLE 10.8. *Ultrasonic Attenuation in Pig Tissues*[a]

Tissue	Number of Samples	Attenuation in Db/Cm	Standard Deviation
Whole bone	13	8.4	±1.2
Skeletal muscle	30	0.8	±0.1
Subcutaneous fat	28	1.8	±0.1

[a] From Lehmann *et al.* (256).

TABLE 10.9. *The Densities of Pig Fat, Muscle, and Bone*[a]

Tissue	Number of Samples	Density in gm/cc	Standard Deviation
Subcutaneous fat	8	0.937	±0.0046
Skeletal muscle	8	1.07	±0.008
Cortical bone	6	1.79	±0.008
Cancellous bone	5	1.25	±0.035
Bone marrow	1	0.93	

[a] From Lehmann *et al.* (256).

TABLE 10.10. *Ultrasonic Velocity in Pig Tissues*[a]

Tissues	Number of Samples	Velocity in m/second	Standard Deviation
Whole bone	1	2,814	
Cortical bone	3	2,941	+614
Cancellous bone	5	2,407	±554
Skeletal muscle	9	1,558	±30
Subcutaneous fat	12	1,454	±10

[a] From Lehmann *et al.* (256)

TABLE 10.11. *Experimental and Calculated Reflection of Ultrasonic Energy at Tissue Interfaces*[a]

Interface	Observed Reflection Percent of Incident Energy	Calculated Reflection Percent of Incident Energy
Water-fat (pig)	0	0.2
Water-muscle (pig)	0	0.3
Fat-muscle (pig)		1.1
Water-bone (pig)	30	30
Muscle-bone (pig)		26.8

[a] From Lehmann *et al.* (256).

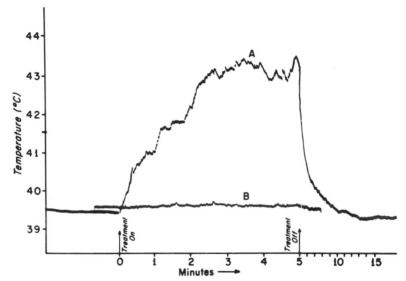

Fig. 10.65. Change in temperature inside hip joint during exposure to ultrasound (*A*) and microwave (*B*). From Lehmann *et al.* (263).

absorbed, the tissues behind the bone cannot be effectively heated (see Table 10.12).

A selective rise of temperature was also observed at myofascial interfaces by Pätzold and Born (322).

Carstensen *et al.* (56) measured absorption and velocity of sound in blood, plasma, and solutions of albumin and hemoglobin in the frequency range 800 to 3,000 MHz and temperature range 5 to 45°C. They found that absorption for the various solutions is in direct proportion to protein content (316). Goss and Dunn (138) found that absorption and velocity of ultrasound in collagen suspensions are much greater than in suspensions of globular proteins of equal unit concentration. This is consistent with the observation that scars, joint capsules, and tendons may be heated selectively.

Rosenberger (345) observed the selective temperature rise in the sciatic

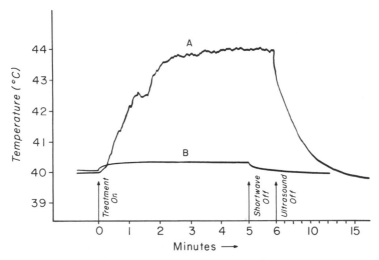

Fig. 10.66. Change in temperature inside hip joint during exposure to ultrasound (*A*) and shortwave (*B*). From Lehmann *et al.* (263).

nerve of experimental animals. Herrick *et al.* (167) demonstrated selective histological changes in the nerve after exposure to ultrasound without any detectable change in the musculature surrounding the nerve. These experimental findings suggested that ultrasound could be utilized specifically to treat larger nerve trunks imbedded in the myofascial interfaces; they also suggested that tendons and synovial tendon sheaths could be similarly treated because of their similar anatomical configuration and location. For the same reasons, scars within soft tissue can be selectively heated. Consistent with these findings, Lehmann and Nitsch (266) observed histological reactions at tissue interfaces when the tissues were exposed to ultrasound at a frequency of 0.175 and 1 MHz. The histological changes showed a frequency-dependent selective distribution different from that produced by heating through other means.

Acoustic properties of surgical metal implants have been investigated (261). It was found that the densities were considerably higher than those of bone (see Table 10.13). The measurement of the wavelength of 1 MHz showed a wavelength in titanium of 0.59 cm, and in stainless steel of 0.60 cm; correspondingly, the sound velocity in titanium is 5,723 m/second and in stainless steel 5,858 m/second. Therefore the acoustic impedance of implants of titanium is 2.575×10^6 gm/cm^2 second and for stainless steel 4.699×10^6 gm/cm^2 second. The acoustic impedance of soft tissue such as muscle is of the order of 1.667×10^5 gm/cm^2 second: that of bone is of the order of 4.459×10^5 gm/cm^2 second. It is apparent that the main problem with metal implants is that of reflection, since absorption in the implant is minimal. The area of maximal increase of intensity resulting from reflection

TABLE 10.12 Rise of Temperature (°C) in Hip Joint During Application of Diathermy[a]

Modality	Output	Duration of Treatment (Minutes)	Number of Exposures	Pre-Treatment Temperature (Mean)	Change of Temperature Inside Hip Joint[b]	
					Mean	Standard Deviation
Ultrasound[c]	1.5 to 2.0 W/cm²	5	6	39.79	1.43	0.479
	2.5 W/cm²	5	12	39.62	4.01	0.660
	3.0 W/cm²	10	7	39.34	0.48	0.060
					0.10	
Microwave	50 to 80 percent with C-director at 1 to 2 inch spacing	20	17	39.58	0.10	0.088
Shortwave	90 to 110 ma. with drum applicator at 1 to 2 inch spacing	20	11	40.05	0.30	0.136

[a] From Lehmann et al. (263).
[b] Thermistor located inside hip joint capsule on the opposite side from area treated.
[c] Radiating surface of applicator: 12.5 cm²

TABLE 10.13. *Densities of Metals Used as Metallic Implants*[a]

Stainless Steel (A.I.S.I. No. 304)	8.02 gm/cm³
Vitallium	8.29 gm/cm³
Titanium	4.5 gm/cm³

[a] From Lehmann *et al.* (261).

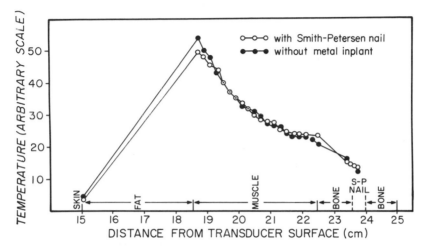

Fig. 10.67. Temperature distribution in a thigh specimen, with and without insertion of a Smith-Petersen nail. From Lehmann *et al.* (233).

was identified by the Schlieren method and found to be close to the metal implants. The factor by which the ultrasonic intensity was changed is shown in Table 10.14. When thigh specimens were exposed to ultrasound with and without a metal implant no selective rise of temperature occurred in the area of the implant (see Figure 10.67) (261). This was attributed to the fact that, in spite of the increased absorption resulting from reflection, the high thermal conductivity of the metal implant allowed rapid dissipation of the additional heat (see Table 10.15).

Ultrasound was applied in proper therapeutic dosage to both sides of unanaesthetized pigs, similar in size to the human. One side served as control; both control and treated side contained identical metal implants. It was found that the rise of temperature in the area of the implant could be well controlled. When therapeutic technique and dosage were used there was no histological evidence of damage or retarded healing on the side of the ultrasound treatment.

Equipment

The therapeutic ultrasound machine is a generator which produces a high-frequency alternating current of 0.8 to 1.0 MHz. This high frequency electric current is then converted by the transducer into mechanical, that is,

TABLE 10.14. *Change of Ultrasonic Intensity Resulting from the Presence of Metallic Implants*[a]

Type of Metal Implant	Mode of Application of Ultrasound and Location of Probe	Factor by Which Ultrasonic Intensity is Changed (Mean Value)	Standard Deviation of the Mean
Stainless steel disc	Probe in front of disc, ultrasound beam incident at angle of 90°	1.9	±.06
Stainless steel disc	Probe behind disc, ultrasound beam incident at angle of 90°	0.03	±.022
Vitallium hip cup (diameter 5 cm)	Ultrasound beam incident perpendicularly at opening of cup, probe in focal area	6.2	±.10
Vitallium hip cup (diameter 5 cm)	Ultrasound beam incident at convex side of cup, measurements within cup	0.086	±.007
Vitallium hip cup (diameter 5 cm)	Ultrsound beam incident at side of cup, measurements within cup	0.1	±.00
Vitallium hip cup (diameter 3.1 cm)	Ultrasound beam incident perpendicularly at opening of cup, probe in focal area	6.4	±.06
Smith–Petersen nail	Ultrasound beam incident between two flanges of the nail, probe in focal area	2.7	±.07
Smith–Petersen nail	One flange pointing toward ultrasound applicator, probe in focal area	1.1	±.001
Kuntscher nail	Ultrasound beam incident at groove of nail, probe in focal area	3.7	±.18

[a] From Lehmann *et al.* (261).

TABLE 10.15. *Physical Properties of Metallic Implants and Tissue*[a]

	Thermal Conductivity cal × cm / cm² × second × °C	Specific Heat at 20°C (cal/gm/°C)
Stainless Steel	0.039	0.12
Titanium	0.036	0.13
Muscle (pig)	0.0012	0.75
Bone (pig)	0.0035 (Whole bone)	0.323 (Cortical bone) 0.504 (Cancellous bone)

[a] From Lehmann *et al.* (233).

acoustic, vibration. The generator has a power supply with full wave rectification and filtering; this eliminates, within 1 percent, any modulation of the power output by the 60 Hz house current. Federal standard proposes that variations exceeding ± 20 percent for all emanations >10 percent of the maximum emission are not acceptable. The rf generator is tuned to the quartz crystal in the transducer to produce mechanical resonance in the crystal. The capacitance and inductance of the oscillating circuit are selected to produce an alternating current of the same frequency as the mechanical resonance frequency of the quartz crystal in the transducer. Adjustment of the frequency is made possible by tuning, usually by the insertion of a variable capacitor. In some apparatus, tuning is eliminated by a rigid control of the oscillating frequency, that is, through a quartz crystal or other frequency stabilizing device.

The 60 Hz alternating line current must be converted to high frequency oscillating current of 0.8 to 1.0 MHz and the voltage must be increased before application to the transducer crystal. For this reason, some machines have an amplifying circuit inserted between the oscillating and transducer circuits. The high-frequency alternating current is then transmitted to the transducer circuit, usually by inductive coupling.

The transducer or sound applicator is usually a crystal inserted between two electrodes. The crystal may be made from natural quartz, properly cut according to the electrical axis of the crystal lattice, or it may be a synthetic ceramic.

The conversion of the high-frequency alternating voltage into a mechanical vibration is accomplished by a reversal of the piezoelectric effect, which is illustrated in Figure 10.68. Figure 10.68 shows (in *a*) the natural state of the crystal, where the surface exhibits electrical neutrality, since the geometrical distribution of the charges is such that there is no measurable surface charge present. The charge of one sign is closer to the surface, and

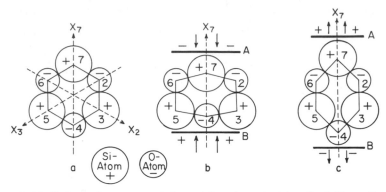

Fig. 10.68. Schematic representation of the piezoelectric effect. From Bergmann (36).

the two charges of the opposite sign are farther away from the surface, compensating for differences in the number of charges. In *b*, the schematic shows a compression of the crystal which results in alteration of the geometry to produce a positive surface charge on one side and a negative one on the other side. In *c*, the crystal is pulled apart and the surface charges are reversed. Conversely, if an alternating electrical charge is applied to the surfaces of the crystal, the crystal will be deformed, depending on the sign of the charges. Thus, an alternating increase and decrease of the thickness of the crystal will occur. The mechanical amplitude of this vibration will be maximal at the resonance frequency which depends on the thickness of the crystal. Thus, the higher the frequency, the thinner the crystal. The quartz crystal is enclosed in a metal housing. The "hot" electrode is applied to the opposite side of the crystal inside the housing. The metal plate in front of the crystal is thick, of the order of an even multiple of a quarter wavelength so as to permit maximal transmission of the sound waves.

Sound applicators produce an ultrasonic field in the vicinity of the applicator which shows a characteristic interference pattern. The intensity distribution produced by a therapeutic transducer was measured along the axis of the beam at various distances from the applicator surface (256). Figure 10.69 shows the maxima and minima in the near field and the last maximum at a distance of approximately 17 to 18 cm which marks the beginning of the far field.

The distance from the applicator at which the far field begins depends on frequency, that is, wavelength, and the diameter of the transducer's radiating surface (see Figure 10.70). From the last peak, the intensity curve shows a gradual decline.

Figure 10.71 shows the calculated intensity distribution along the axis of the beam in the far and near field for a different applicator operating at a different frequency.

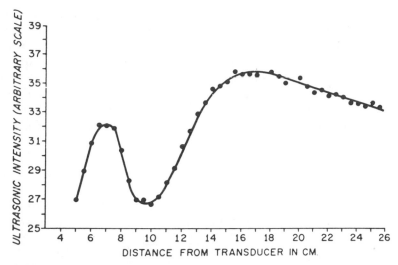

Fig. 10.69. Intensity distribution along the central axis of the ultrasonic beam. From Lehmann *et al.* (256).

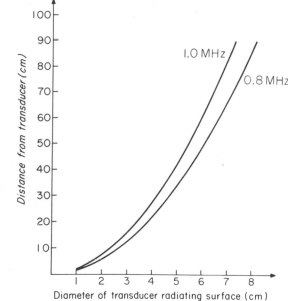

Fig. 10.70. Distance between transducer surface and last interference maximum dependent upon the diameter of the radiating surface of the applicator for the therapeutic frequencies of 0.8 and 1.0 MHz. Redrawn from Pohlman (329).

The intensity is especially non-uniform in the near field. This non-uniformity is inevitable and is the result of the development of an interference pattern of the sound wave in front of the transducer. Waves originating from A and B at the transducer travel to point P. Since the distance from A to P is shorter than the distance from B to P, the waves will arrive at P out of phase and interference may occur, leading to a decrease of the intensity; that is, the waves will cancel one another (see Figure 10.72). However, in Figure 10.73 the waves originating from A to B on the transducer meet at the point R in phase, thus causing an additive effect and a high intensity of ultrasound at this point. The intensity distribution across the far field of a therapeutic applicator was measured at a distance of 15 and 25 cm from the applicator (see Figure 10.74). It shows a bell-shaped distribution curve of the intensity. From these measurements it becomes apparent that we must define the radiating surface of the applicator accurately, since the intensity of the sound field drops gradually to zero at the edges.

A commonly used procedure to determine the radiating surface of the applicator is to insert baffles of decreasing diameter in front of the applicator to cut out the edge of the beam. The total output of the applicator is then measured behind the baffle. When the total output is decreased by 10

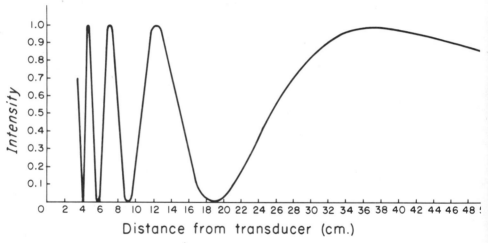

Fig. 10.71. Maxima and minima of intensity along the axis of the sound beam produced by a transducer of 8 cm diameter operating at a frequency of 0.35 MHz in water. Redrawn from Born (44).

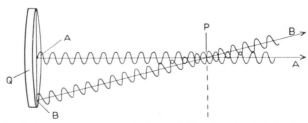

Fig. 10.72. Schematic representation of the development of an interference pattern in front of the ultrasound transducer. Waves cancel each other at P, since waves are out of phase. Redrawn from Pohlman (329).

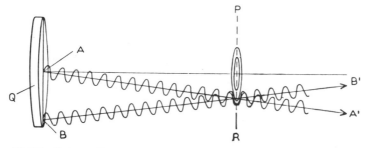

Fig. 10.73. Schematic representation of the development of an interference pattern in front of the ultrasound transducer. Waves enhance each other at *R*, since waves are in phase. Redrawn from Pohlman (329).

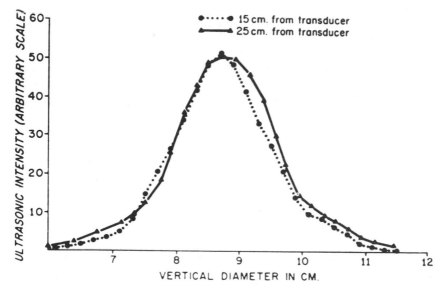

Fig. 10.74. Intensity distribution in the vertical diameter of the ultrasonic far field. From Lehmann *et al.* (256).

percent, the corresponding opening of the baffle is called the radiating surface area of the applicator. For therapeutic purposes, the applicator should have a radiating surface area which is only slightly smaller than the total applicator surface. This minimizes the problem of maintaining full contact between skin and applicator surface in areas of uneven body surface. For therapeutic application, the radiating surface area should be 7 to 13 cm^2. In order to be able to produce a vigorous therapeutic effect in the depths of the tissues, ultrasonic intensities of 3 to 4 W/cm^2 should be available. That is, the total output should be between 21 and 52 watts.

Figure 10.75 shows a schematic representation of the intensity distribution in ultrasound beams, at a frequency of 0.8 MHz, produced by applicators of

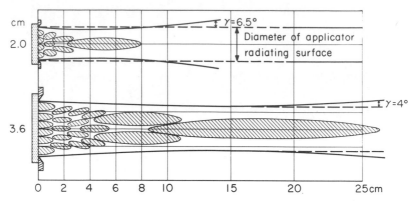

Fig. 10.75. Schematic representation of ultrasound beam; γ is the angle of divergence; *shaded areas* are zones of high ultrasound intensity. Redrawn from Pohlman (329).

different diameter. Both the non-uniformity of the near field and the single peak in the center of the beam in the far field are shown in Figure 10.75.

Figure 10.75 also shows that the longer the wavelength in relation to the diameter of the applicator, the greater the angle of divergence, that is, the more rapid the dispersion of ultrasonic energy. Therefore, it also holds that the smaller the diameter applicator, the greater is the angle of divergence.

$$\sin\gamma = 0.61 \ (\lambda/d/a)$$

here γ is the angle of divergence, λ the wavelength, and d the diameter of the applicator. One also notes that the last area of high intensity in a transducer of small diameter is closer to the transducer than in the case where the applicator has a large diameter.

A reasonable measure of the uniformity of the beam desirable for therapeutic purposes is a determination of the ratio of peak intensity (W/cm^2) in the far field to average intensity. This ratio should be 4:1 or less. Average intensity (W/cm^2) is measured by determining the total power (W) emanated from the radiating surface area and dividing by the radiating surface area.

The applicator should have a single synthetic or natural quartz crystal to produce a relatively uniform intensity distribution throughout the beam. Mosaic crystals usually produce high spatial peak intensities with a relatively low average intensity. This is undesirable, since peak intensities in these beams may exceed safe limits.

In addition, an applicator suitable for therapeutic application should have minimal internal losses to avoid excessive heating of the applicator surface during therapy. This may modify the therapeutic results that are dependent on temperature.

If the ultrasonic output is pulsed, duration of pulses and frequency, that is, the duty cycle, should be given. The shape of the pulses should be known as well as the average output to avoid excessive temporal intensity peaks which may produce undesirable side effects.

Finally, the machine should be equipped with a meter measuring accurately total power and average intensity emitted. A timer should also be available.

Measurement of Ultrasound

If ultrasound is incident at a right angle on a totally reflecting surface, a pressure, S, is exerted on the surface; I is the sound intensity and c is the sound velocity.

$$S = (2I/c)$$

Figure 10.76 shows a schematic arrangement of a so-called sound pressure balance. The sound pressure is measured in grams. Taking into consideration the angle of the reflecting surface to the beam, the ultrasonic output can be calculated, provided complete absorption of the reflected beam is assured. Another pressure measuring device is a reflecting inverted cone with a stem. The cone floats in a lightweight fluid medium with its stem partially immersed within a heavy-weight fluid. This arrangement centers itself in the sound beam. Sound pressure pushes the stem of the cone deeper into the heavier fluid beneath the light-weight fluid and the exerted pressure can again be calculated in grams.

Probes have been developed to determine sound intensities in a small area. One type of probe uses a crystal as a sound-sensing instrument. This basic operating principle is that the sound waves alternately deform the crystal, thus producing a piezoelectric effect, that is, an alternating surface

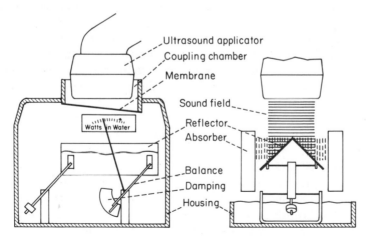

Fig. 10.76. Schematic arrangement of so-called sound pressure balance. Redrawn from Pohlman (329).

charge which can be demonstrated quantitatively by electrical means. Ceramic or synthetic crystals are most often used for small probes. Another type of probe consists of a temperature-recording device within a sound-absorbing material. The ultrasound is absorbed and converted into heat. Probes should be small as compared with the wavelength so as not to interfere with the propagation of the sound waves. The temperature change is recorded. In this type of probe, many factors modify the temperature rise in the absorbing material, for example, convection and conductivity of the surrounding material. Both types of probes must be calibrated for use (36, 152). Very accurate measurements have been developed by Fry and Fry (123) by inserting a small thermocouple junction into a sound-absorbing medium of known coefficient of absorption, for example, castor oil (265, 391). The initial rise of temperature can be utilized for calculation of the sound intensity when the absorption coefficient of the surrounding material is known.

Sound waves produce density changes in the material traversed which are in proportion to the ultrasonic intensity. This change of density can be made visible in transparent media such as glass or water by the so-called "Schlieren" method.

Thermal and Non-thermal Reactions to Ultrasound

In order to control dosage and technique of application of ultrasound, it is essential to know the biophysical mode of action which produces the desirable physiological changes. In the area of ultrasound therapy, a number of thermal and non-thermal reactions are known to occur as a result of the physical phenomena which occur in the sound wave as previously described. A large number of physiological effects have been investigated. In order to distinguish the responses resulting from temperature increase from those which are produced by other phenomena in the sound waves, several experimental designs have been repeatedly used. a) Once an ultrasound effect was produced, the associated temperature rise in the tissues was measured. In a subsequent experiment, the temperature in the tissues was raised to the same level but without ultrasound, *e.g.*, using a water bath. If the effect was thermal, it could be anticipated that the biological change could be reproduced quantitatively. In a variant of this experimental design, the tissues are exposed to different levels of ultrasonic intensities. The exposure occurs in water baths of different temperatures. The bath temperatures are selected such that the tissue temperature during sonation remains the same even though different ultrasonic intensities are used. In the experiments, the biological results would be the same at different ultrasonic intensities if the result is produced by heating (245). b) In a second set of experiments, tissues are exposed to ultrasound but the temperature rise to ultrasonic absorption is prevented by cooling. The physiological responses to ultrasound under these circumstances are prevented and the quantitative responses of biological phenomena under these circumstances arc the same as those of nontreated controls. On the other hand, if the temperature rise was allowed to occur during sonation, quantitative changes were observed. Any biological reaction which shows this type of behavior can be attributed to heating. c) The comparison of effects produced by continuous wave and pulsed ultrasound has been used to differentiate thermal and non-thermal mechanisms. The frequency of pulsing in these experiments was high enough that temperature changes averaged out and could not follow the pulses. The average ultrasonic intensity of the pulsed output was chosen to be equal to the continuous wave output. Thus, the heating effect of both would be the same, but if the high intensities during the pulses would exceed a minimal threshold required for producing a non-thermal phenomenon, the biological phenomena produced by the pulses could not be reproduced by the continuous wave output of the same intensity as the average of the pulsed ultrasound. It has been speculated (28, 220) that large molecular chains could be torn mechanically under such circumstances. While this type of experiment may distinguish between some non-thermal phenomena and the thermal effects, it must be recognized that also some non-thermal phenomena such as streaming are in proportion to the average output. Thus, even if the average intensity and the temperature are the same with pulsed and CW output, one may not conclude that the effects are necessarily thermal in origin. On the other hand, if the average intensity and temperature are kept the same, those effects which are seen only with the pulsed ultrasound may be assumed to be nonthermal in origin. d) If gaseous cavitation is to be ruled out as a cause of the observed biological effect, one must keep in mind that the occurrence of cavitation is frequency dependent. The higher the frequency, the less likely the occurrence of cavitation. Gaseous cavitation is also temperature dependent. The development of the gas bubbles does occur more readily at higher temperatures. Finally, the presence of cavitation can be demonstrated if the biological effect is prevented when irradiation occurs under increased pressure. The threshold of pressure which prevents the cavitation phenomena is higher the greater the ultrasonic intensity. The occurrence of gaseous cavitation can be prevented by application of external pressure of a sufficient magnitude. Cavitation is always suspect when producing a biologic phenomenon if macromolecules or cells are exposed in solution (303). The greater the viscosity of the solute, and the greater the volume percentage of cells in suspension, the less likely cavitation is the cause of the observed phenomena, but experiments with applied pressure are often needed to prove absence or presence of cavitation (221, 222).

Experimental evidence suggests that cavitation may occur more readily while pulsed ultrasonic energy is applied whereas the heating effect is minimized. This is true only if the ultrasonic intensity during the pulses exceeds threshold and provided the duration of the pulses is long enough to develop the cavitation.

The absence of experimental designs of this type, the difficulties in measuring acoustic intensities and the selectivity of the rise of temperature in some tissues, have resulted in a large number of observations of biological changes without clear explanation as to the mechanism by which they are produced.

In the following, only the physiological responses will be reviewed which are of therapeutic interest, and which have been observed under conditions similar to those in therapy.

Thermal Effects of Ultrasound. As discussed in the introduction, all the desirable therapeutic effects of heat can be produced by any modality, including ultrasound, provided that the modality elevates the temperature adequately in the area required for the specific response. The hallmark of the physiological responses produced by ultrasound is that ultrasound selectively raises the temperature in some well-circumscribed areas. The increase in extensibility of collagen tissues due to heating has been discussed previously. It also has been shown that ultrasound selectively raises the temperature in joint capsules and scar tissues containing large amounts of collagen. It has been shown experimentally that heating with ultrasound (133) raises the temperature in the collagen tissues of tendon and that the same temperature rises produced by other means result in a corresponding increase in the extensibility of this tissue. This is consistent with clinical studies which show that this effect can be used in the treatment of joint contractures and contracted scars (133).

The effect of ultrasonic energy on nerve tissues has also been studied extensively. Changes of chronaxie and rheobase after ultrasound application to live mice were found to be due to its heating effect. Greatly increased chronaxie values and elevation of the rheobase were confirmed by Hueter (182–184). Hueter and his associates (185, 186) and Lambert and his co-workers (216) studied the effect of ultrasound on the isolated bullfrog's nerve. They found a decrease in the amplitude of action potential and complete blocking of the nerve. These changes depend primarily on the thermal effect of ultrasound and have been duplicated by the use of direct heating alone. It was also found that fibers of different diameter showed differences in sensitivity to heating. Fully reversible blocking can be obtained with carefully graded doses (434). Currier *et al.* (69) measured the bilateral antidromic sensory conduction of the lateral cutaneous branch of the radial nerve in five men at intervals before and up to 15 minutes following ultrasound application. Ultrasound was applied at a frequency of 1 MHz for 5 minutes at an intensity of 1.5 W/cm^2. Amplitude and duration of the nerve action potential did not change. Latency decreased, indicating a corresponding increase in conduction velocity consistent with the observed temperature increases. Halle *et al.* (151) heated the tissues with infrared and ultrasound to the same temperature as measured by a thermistor and found the same reduction in nerve conduction latency. Therefore, they concluded that the effect of ultrasound on the nerve conduction is due to its thermal action rather than to its mechanical effects. Madsen and Gersten (284) found conduction velocity changes of borderline significance in the ulnar nerve. Anderson et al. (17) exposed the sciatic nerve of dogs to an ultrasonic frequency of 0.8 MHz with an applicator of a 10 cm^2 radiating surface area. They applied average intensities of 5 W/cm^2 for 10 minutes to six dogs. None of these animals showed any apparent evidence of impairment of function of the nerve 24 hours after the application. High intensity ultrasound produced a reduction and alternately a temporary abolishment of the nerve action potential (3.0 to 5.8 W/cm^2), a phenomenon which could be reproduced by direct heating to a maximum of 50°C.

When Anderson et al. (17) exposed the spinal cords of dogs to an average intensity of 5 W/cm^2 for 6 to 10 minutes with stationary technique, a paralysis of hind legs and tails was observed in 5 out of 7 dogs. None of the dogs recovered. Temperature recordings made during sonation showed temperatures up to 49°C. The cord was destroyed. It must be noted that all of these experiments were conducted by Anderson et al. at dosage and tissue temperature levels exceeding the therapeutic limits. On the other hand, reversible effects on the spinal reflexes were observed by Shealy and Henneman (365), who applied focused ultrasound with a frequency of 2.7 MHz to a cat's spinal cord. Spinal reflexes were elicited and recorded electrically as an indicator of the activity of the spinal cord. The initial effect of irradiation was usually an increase in the amplitude of spinal reflexes. After this there was sometimes a depression of reflex transmission. After a longer exposure, there was a complete disappearance of all reflex activity both monosynaptic and polysynaptic, but these effects were reversible. The mode of action of ultrasound was not studied in detail. Gersten (130) found both thermal and non-thermal effects of ultrasound on the spinal cord function. When the author exposed the cervical cord and the sciatic nerve, an increase in excitability occurred and was always followed by a rise of temperature in these areas. He found no evidence that this ultrasonic effect was independent of the temperature rise. On the other hand, when he exposed the lumbar cord, he found an increase in excitability which could be demonstrated before a significant increase in local temperature could be recorded. Taylor et al. (383, 386) exposed spinal cords of adult rats to pulsed ultrasound of intensities between 25 and 50 W/cm^2 during the pulses at 0.5 to 6.0 MHz with a 10 percent duty cycle. That is an average intensity of 2.5 to 5 W/cm^2. They observed paraplegia and hemorrhage. These results were discussed in terms of known effects of ultrasound. It is noted that these intensities should produce a significant increase in temperature. Since the effect decreased with increased frequency, the question of cavitation as a mechanism is raised. While Taylor et al. found that the vascular damage and its consequent hemorrhage were the most common lesions, Dunn and Fry (88) reported that the anterior horn cells were most sensitive.

Higashino (170) observed a striking increase in the frequency of the miniature motor endplate potentials when low ultrasonic intensities were applied. Higher intensities produced a decrease of these potentials. The associated temperature rise was 6.5°C.

The reduction of pain by heat application has been described in detail previously. In addition, it has been shown that ultrasound, when applied to the peripheral nerve or tissues with free nerve endings elevates the pain threshold in the tissues exposed directly to ultrasound or in the distribution of the peripheral nerve so exposed. The pain threshold was measured with the Hardy et al. (153) method. Ultrasound with an average intensity of 1.5 W/cm^2 and a total output of 15 W at 0.8 MHz was applied for 2 minutes. The nerve was exposed with the arm in a water bath of 35°C. The same results could be obtained with radiant heat provided the same temperatures that were obtained with ultrasound were produced in the tissues (235).

Schwartz (358) applied ultrasound paravertebrally to the autonomic nervous system. Patients with peripheral vascular disease as well as normal volunteers were treated. An increase in the skin temperature was found. Other investigators have applied ultrasound to the carotid sinus and stellate ganglion area with a total applicator output of 4 to 6 W. The only effects observed were cough (5 out of 29 patients), ventricular premature contractions (in 3 patients), and a burning sensation (in 5 patients). No major effect on heart rate or blood pressure was noted. The authors believe that the cough was provoked by the stimulation of the superior laryngeal nerve (408). Stuhlfauth (375) observed a number of vascular responses as well as an increase in the secretion of free acid by the gastric mucosa after applying ultrasound paravertebrally to nerve roots. These effects were produced reflexly; however, the mechanism remains obscure. The ultrasonic effect on muscle tissue has been studied by Gersten (133) who found that ultrasound applied to striated frog muscle with intensities of 0.5 W/cm^2 produced changes in the contractile protein and in isometric tension. These changes were reproducible by heating with infrared radiation or by heating in a water bath. If ultrasonic energy was increased to 3 W/cm^2, the observed changes could not be explained fully on the basis of temperature elevation. These experiments could neither rule out cavitation nor identify another mechanism. Zimny and Head (437) studied in vivo effects of ultrasound on ground squirrels and found that if ultrasound was applied at a frequency of 1 MHz at an intensity of 0.13 to 3 W/cm^2, ATP and phosphocreatine were decreased significantly with slight changes in inorganic phosphate and glycogen. Temperature measurements were not made in the tissues. Microscopically, there were no structural changes.

Furthermore, the changes in the metabolism of muscle were dependent on the temperature attained during exposure of ultrasound. When exposure took place at higher temperatures, the oxygen consumption was depressed (see Figure 10.77) (222), an effect which could be quantitatively reproduced by heating the tissue to the same temperature which was observed during sonation (255).

The same results were obtained when both oxygen consumption and carbon dioxide production were measured (see Figure 10.78). If the tissues were cooled during application of ultrasound so that no rise of temperature occurred, no difference was found between the oxygen consumption of the exposed tissues and that of the controls (see Figure 10.79).

In all these experiments, the average ultrasonic intensity used was 1.5 W/cm^2, with a total output of 15 W at 1 MHz. These findings were confirmed in part by Pauly and Hug (325).

The effect of ultrasound waves on biological membranes has been studied in detail. Frog skin was used as a prototype model. The work of a number of investigators (15, 114, 115, 176, 187–189, 278, 279, 377, 378, 382) indicates that three different potentials are found. The main potential is obtained when Ringer's solution is applied to both sides of the skin and is located in the epithelial layer of the skin. The second potential is characteristic of the isoelectric point of the proteins that form the physical and chemical structure of the epithelium. The third potential is a diffusion potential that is

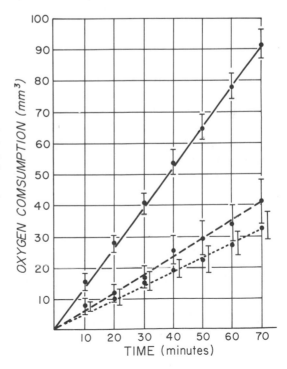

Fig. 10.77. Oxygen consumption of tissue after exposure to ultrasonic energy at 40.5°C (water bath): - - - - - - -; after heating tissue to 46.5°C: · · · · · · · · . Controls: ———. From Lehmann (222).

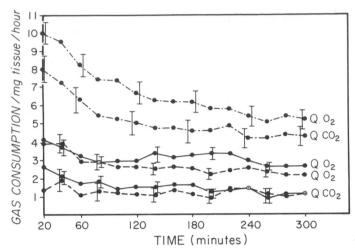

Fig. 10.78. Q_{O2} = oxygen consumption, mm^3 per hour per mg of tissue. Q_{CO2} = carbon dioxide formation, mm^3 per hour per mg. of tissue. Metabolism after exposure to ultrasonic energy. ●——●——●; after heating to the temperature measured during exposure ●- - -●- - -●. Controls; ●--●--●. From Lehmann (222).

encountered when a diluted solution is applied to the exterior surface of the skin. According to Höber (176), this third potential is located in the interior layers of the skin. It was found that the ultrasound application at 30°C depressed the main potential. This could be reproduced within the limits of the statistical error by heating to a temperature of 41°C. Heating to 36°C had no effect, and temperatures of 44°C produced a greater effect than ultrasound. Further experiments suggested that actual temperature in the epithelium during ultrasound treatment was 41°C. The ultrasonic effect on the isoelectric point of the proteins of the membrane could also be reproduced by heating at 41°C (see Figure 10.80).

Finally, a study was made of the ultrasonic effect on the so-called diffusion potential located in the interior layer of the skin (231). A marked increase in the permeability to ions was observed (see Table 10.16). The permeability increase after cessation of ultrasound application was reproducible by heating the membrane by other means to the same temperature as measured during ultrasound application. It was also recognized that a considerable temperature gradient could be produced across the comparatively thin membrane. The increase in ion permeability during the sonation could not be totally attributed to the temperature increase. It was found that this was due in part to an acceleration of the diffusion process by the streaming produced by the sound waves. The effect of pulsed and CW application of the same therapeutic intensites had essentially the same effect on active transport of ions through biological membranes, on permeability, and on

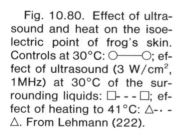

Fig. 10.79. Oxygen consumption of tissue after exposure to ultrasonic energy at 5°C: - - - - - - . Controls: ————. From Lehmann (222).

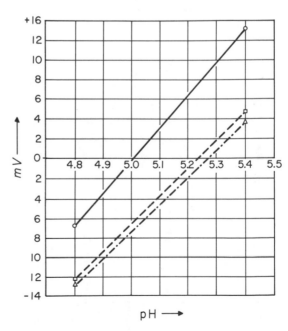

Fig. 10.80. Effect of ultrasound and heat on the isoelectric point of frog's skin. Controls at 30°C: O————O; effect of ultrasound (3 W/cm², 1MHz) at 30°C of the surrounding liquids: □- - -□; effect of heating to 41°C: △-·-△. From Lehmann (222).

TABLE 10.16. *Changes of the Permeability of the Frog's Skin after Irradiation with Ultrasonic Energy and after Heating*[a,b]

Experimental Conditions during the Period from 0 to 30 Minutes	Permeated Amount of NaCl, mol/cm² of the Skin	Experimental Conditions during the Period from 30 to 60 Minutes	Permeated Amount of NaCl, mol/cm² of the Skin
Control			
Temperature of the liquid 22°C	$1.5 \cdot 10^{-4}$		$1.4 \cdot 10^{-4}$
Temperature of the tissue 22°C	$M^c = \pm 0.3 \cdot 10^{-4}$		$M = \pm 0.3 \cdot 10^{-4}$
Irradiation			
Temperature of the liquid 22°C	$22.3 \cdot 10^{-4}$		
Temperature of the tissue 30°C	$M = \pm 0.8 \cdot 10^{-4}$	Temperature of the liquid 22°C	$19.8 \cdot 10^{-4}$
			$M = \pm 1.2 \cdot 10^{-4}$
Heating to 30°C			
Temperature of the liquid 30°C	$6.7 \cdot 10^{-4}$		
Temperature of the tissue 30°C	$M = 0.9 \cdot 10^{-4}$	Temperature of the tissue 22°C	$20.9 \cdot 10^{-4}$
			$M = \pm 0.2 \cdot 10^{-4}$
Heating to 37°C			
Temperature of the liquid 37°C	$22.0 \cdot 10^{-4}$		
Temperature of the tissue 37°C	$M = 0.6 \cdot 10^{-4}$		$33.6 \cdot 10^{-4}$
			$M = \pm 0.2 \cdot 10^{-4}$

[a] From Lehmann et al. (221).
[b] Velocity of the NaCl solution: 30 cm³/minutes cm²; velocity of the water: 10 cm³/minutes cm²; pressure of the NaCl solution: 30 cm H_2O; Ultrasound intensity: 3.7 W/cm².
[c] M is the standard error of the mean.

diffusion processes through membranes, provided the average intensity was the same (259).

Lota and Darling (277) measured the change in permeability of red blood cell membranes in suspension when ultrasound was applied. In an experiment with controlled temperatures, he found that the streaming or stirring effect of ultrasound was probably more important than the thermal effects.

Paul and Imig (324) and others found that the blood flow through the femoral artery as determined by an electromagnetic flow meter was increased more than 25 percent if ultrasound intensities between 2 and 3 W/cm^2 were applied. The authors also recorded a concomitant marked temperature increase in the tissues. They compared the effects of ultrasound with those produced by other diathermy modalities and found that the blood flow was related to the temperature increase regardless of the device which was used for heating. Abramson and co-workers (4) observed that pulsed ultrasound with a stationary sound applicator to a healthy subject produced a consistent increase in the blood flow through the forearm of the subjects as determined by the venous occlusion plethysmograph as well as an increase in the oxygen uptake of the tissues. The temperature rise occurring in the tissues was adequate to explain the change in blood flow. Imig *et al.* (193) also observed an increase in blood flow at ultrasonic intensities above 1 W/cm^2 applied for 15 minutes and found that blood flow increase related to the amount of tissue hyperthermia produced. Bickford and Duff (37) also found an increase in blood flow. Only Zankel (435) could not find any increase in blood flow due to ultrasound. Since the blood flow increase produced by ultrasound seems to be critically dependent on the introduction of enough energy (intensity and an adequate total output), this may explain the discrepancy.

It was also observed that reactions such as hyperemia and inflammatory responses in the tissues which are characterized by increase in vascularity, edema, and tissue necrosis, were all quantitatively explained on the basis of the heating effect of ultrasonic energy (225, 244, 245). It was possible to demonstrate that these reactions could be prevented by cooling. The reactions produced by ultrasound could be quantitatively reproduced by heating the tissues to the same temperature as had been measured in the tissues during exposure to ultrasound. It also was found that the dependence of these reactions on the particle amplitude of the medium was consistent with what could be expected in any reaction which would be produced by heat (225, 244, 245). Finally, it could be demonstrated that the dependence of these reactions on the ultrasonic frequency could be explained on the basis of the differences in the heating effect when ultrasound was applied with frequencies of 0.175 to 1.0 MHz (266).

The action of ultrasound on bone has been studied by Janes, Herrick, and their associates (21, 34, 167, 195, 196). Higher-than-therapeutic doses produced bone necrosis resulting in pathological fractures. This was attributed primarily to the temperature rise resulting from ultrasonic absorption. On the other hand, if a lower dose comparable to that in therapy was used, the authors found that the cell structure and distribution of inorganic phosphate in the femora of adult dogs apparently were unaffected. The ultrasonic output applied ranged from 6 to 20 W, the intensity varied from 0.6 to 2 W/cm^2. The animals were observed for periods of up to 2 years from the date of the last exposure to ultrasound. DeForrest $et\ al.$ applied ultrasound to immature epiphyses in animal experiments at doses higher than the therapeutic levels, with destructive effects on epiphyseal growth. Stationary technique was used (78).

These findings were consistent with early investigations of Barth and Bülow (29) who found that only high-intensity ultrasound applications, associated with severe pain, produced pathological fractures or retarded growth whereas lower intensities were tolerated without untoward effects. In these investigations, the epiphyseal lines of the bones in puppies were irradiated with ultrasound. The epiphyseal areas of growing bone of rabbits were treated with water coupling at 1 W/cm^2 with a sound head of 12 cm^2 radiating surface for 5 minutes daily from age 3 months until there was X-ray evidence of epiphyseal closure. The untreated leg served as control. Vaughen and Bender (402) found that there was no significant difference in bone length, microscopic space, rate or manner of epiphyseal closure between treated and the control leg. Maintz (285) examined the rate of callus formation after ultrasound treatment and found either no effect at all or destructive changes at higher intensities. It should be noted that the exposure times were comparatively short and that ultrasound was reapplied only a few times. Ardan $et\ al.$ (22) did not find that healing of fractures was accelerated when treated with ultrasound as had been suggested in certain clinical studies. More extensive investigations applying ultrasound under a greater variety of conditions would be of great interest.

$Non\text{-}thermal\ Effects\ of\ Ultrasound.$ As pointed out previously, most of the physiological responses important for therapy are produced by the thermal effects. However, in some of these instances, it has been shown that the entire reaction could not be explained on the basis of the heating effect. In part, the reaction was due to nonthermal effects. For instance, the effect on diffusion and other membrane potentials could be explained in part on the basis of streaming of fluids in the ultrasonic field, which increases in turn, the gradient of concentration of ions and other materials across a biological membrane, thus accelerating the rate of diffusion (218, 229). It also has been shown that this agitating effect of ultrasound could occur in single living cells. For example, eosinophilic leucocytes were studied and exhibited a marked increase of motion of the eosinophilic granules when exposed to ultrasound. The functional properties of the cell, however, such as ameboid mobility, were not impaired unless an excessive rise of temperature was associated with irradiation (230). Dyson $et\ al.$ (93) found in chick embryos that, if a pattern of standing waves was set up in the sound field, the red cell flow through blood vessels stopped and the cells accumulated in the wave nodes. They also pointed out that this phenomenon was observed when ultrasound was applied with stationary technique and can be prevented by moving the applicator.

Zarod and Williams (436) and Williams *et al.* (417) observed an *in vitro* platelet aggregation and an increase in re-calcification time of platelet-rich plasma. These authors suspected that shear stresses created by ultrasound might be part of the mechanism. However, no evidence that the same phenomena occur under therapeutic conditions *in vivo* is available.

Macintosh *et al.* (281, 282) found chromosome aberrations in white blood cells exposed to ultrasound at a frequency of 2 MHz applied for one hour. The leukocytes were exposed in culture. A threshold intensity of ultrasound of 8.2 mW/cm^2 was required. The mechanism of this effect is unknown. Other defects of chromosomes and mitoses have been related to the occurrence of cavitation (254). Developmental abnormalities of embryos have been observed resulting from temperature increases. Taylor and Dyson (384) insonated chick embryos at a peak intensity of 40 W/cm^2 with a 10 percent duty cycle and a frequency of 1 MHz. When pulse intensities were lowered to 10 W/cm^2 no abnormalities were produced. Even long exposure did not produce any defects. The average intensities of 4 W/cm^2 should produce enough temperature rise that the changes observed by the authors might be explained on that basis. The specific mechanism was not investigated.

Taylor and Dyson (385) further insonated chick embryos at a frequency of 1 MHz with 25 and 10 W/cm^2 with a 10 percent duty cycle for 5 minutes and found abnormalities. Again, the intensities applied to a small embryo would be enough to produce very significant temperature rises. Similarly, at 2.2 MHz and 100 mW/cm^2 CW output, abnormalities were observed.

Harvey *et al.* (161) exposed fibroblasts in cell culture to ultrasound and found that structural changes were induced in the suspended fibroblasts and the rate of protein synthesis was increased (see Figure 10.81). Cortisone pretreatment inhibited this effect. The mechanism by which these observations could be explained was not known. On the basis of the inhibition by corticosteroids and on the proposal by Szego (379, 380) that the lysozomes are the main method of hormone action, Harvey *et al.* speculated that the ultrasonic effect may be mediated through an effect on the lysozomes.

Dyson *et al.* (90, 91) found an enhancing effect on tissue regeneration by application of pulsed ultrasound at a frequency of 3.5 MHz. When 0.5 W/cm^2 peak intensities with a 20 percent duty cycle and 0.1 W/cm^2 continuous output were compared, it was shown that both had essentially the same enhancing effect. In both cases, the average intensity was 0.1 W/cm^2. In the third case, 8 W/cm^2 pulsed 1 msecond on and 79 mseconds off had a retarding effect. Possible mechanisms, such as streaming, were discussed. It

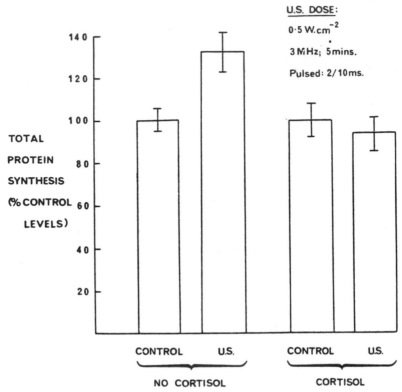

Fig. 10.81. Effect of ultrasound treatment on the stimulation of protein synthesis by ultrasound. From Harvey *et al.* (161).

should be pointed out that streaming as well as heating effects in the first two cases would be the same since the average intensity was 0.1 W/cm^2 in both. In the third experiment, one could also speculate that cavitation thresholds may have been exceeded in the pulses, with detrimental results. In this case, the average intensity was still the same as in the first two experiments, and therefore streaming, as well as the heating effect, should have been the same.

Mortimer *et al.* (305) found that ultrasound (1 MHz at an intensity of 2.4 W/cm^2 *in vitro*) appears to affect resting tension of the cardiac muscle without affecting the active tension. There were thermal and non-thermal effects. When the thermal effects were eliminated, the non-thermal component remained. It caused a decrease in resting tension without affecting developed tension.

There are numerous reactions to gaseous cavitation (220, 416). It is necessary to distinguish clearly between reactions which occur in the test tube and those which occur under therapeutic conditions. The following examples may serve to illustrate this point. Typically, destructive reactions such as hemolysis and the dissolution of bacteria and cancer cells in suspension (218, 258) occur only if there is a low concentration of cells in the suspension and the viscosity of the suspending medium is low as compared with the therapeutic conditions under which ultrasound is applied to a live organism. In these examples, it could be clearly demonstrated that the cells were destroyed mainly by the mechanical and other effects of cavitation. The occurrence of cavitation and its destructive effects can be prevented by application of external pressure, by increasing the viscosity of the suspension fluid, or by increasing the volume percentage of cells in suspension. It was found that even in normal blood which has a 40 percent volume of red cells and a high viscosity of the serum, cavitation did not occur under conditions similar to those in therapy. Cavitation then was studied (254) in uniform tissue without blood vessels (onion root tips). The histological appearance of cavitation reactions was rather characteristic. The destruction of cells was spotty (see Figure 10.82).

This appearance could be explained by the spotty occurrence of gas bubbles in the tissues. It could be demonstrated that the conditions under which the reactions occurred clearly indicated that they were produced by cavitation. Intensity thresholds of 1 to 2 W/cm^2 were required to produce these lesions. The reactions could be prevented by the application of external pressure. Histologically the lesions were quite different from the more diffuse reactions due to the heating effect of ultrasonic energy. The reactions to cavitation also consisted of damaging effects on chromosomes, mitotic figures, and nuclei (see Figure 10.83).

Finally, experiments were performed to discover whether or not gaseous

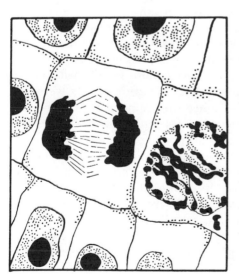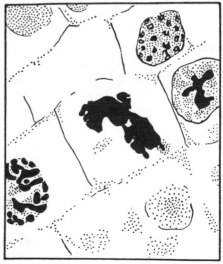

Fig. 10.82. Spotty reaction to cavitation with most severe destruction in center (iron hematoxylin, Heidenhain). Magnification of 125. From Lehmann *et al.* (254).

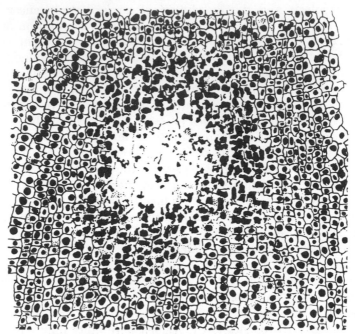

Fig. 10.83. Mitotic figure. At *left*, normal figure; at *right*, destructive effect of cavitation on mitotic figure at a similar stage. From Lehmann *et al.* (254).

cavitation would occur under therapeutic conditions in live animals. Live mice developed petechial hemorrhages as a result of cavitation (253). It was shown that the biological reaction was due to cavitation since it was suppressed by the application of high pressure during irradiation. The threshold of pressure required to prevent the reaction increased with the ultrasonic intensity. The reactions were also dependent on frequency as is the case with cavitation. Lesions were produced more readily with lower ultrasonic frequencies. It was also shown that cavitation effects were dependent upon temperature. The dependence on temperature can be explained by the fact that the solubility of gases is diminished when the temperature is elevated; more reactions were observed at higher temperatures. Biologically these reactions had the characteristic appearance of focal lesions where the destructive effect rapidly decreased with greater distance from the central zone (see Figure 10.84). It was noted that at intensities of 1 W/cm^2 or below, applied with stationary technique, the destructive cavitation did not occur. When the stroking technique of therapeutic application was simulated and intensities of up to 4 W/cm^2 average were applied with an applicator having a radiating surface of 10 cm^2, no destructive effects were produced. It also could be demonstrated that the potential danger of producing cavitation under therapeutic conditions is increased if

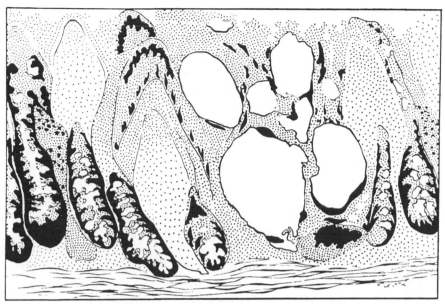

Fig. 10.84. Histological evidence of cavitation in intestinal tract mucosa of a mouse. The empty space in the center of the lesion presumably had been occupied by gas bubbles. From Lehmann *et al.* (253).

unsuitable equipment is used. Animals were irradiated with a stationary applicator at an intensity of 1.5 W/cm^2 and a total applicator output of 15 W. The machine had a power supply with full wave rectification. In one series of irradiations, filters were used to produce a steady ultrasound output. In another series the filters were removed, producing a greatly modulated ultrasound output. In the animals treated with steady ultrasound output, cavitation reactions were observed in only 5 percent. On the other hand, if the ultrasound was applied with the same machine with the same output but the filters removed, cavitation effects were observed in 55 percent of the animals. These experiments point out that peak ultrasonic intensities occurring from lack of filtering of the rectified line voltage may be potentially dangerous. The same detrimental effect can be expected, if, instead of full-wave rectification, half-wave rectification is used.

The mechanism of high-intensity ultrasound was studied by Fry and co-workers and by Lehmann and associates (87, 118–122, 124–127, 227, 228); some of the high-intensity effects on brain tissue were reversible. The destructive effects on nerve and on plant tissues could not be explained on the basis of cavitation nor on the basis of heat development. The exact mechanism is still unknown. It must be recognized that these effects are produced by intensities of magnitude different from those used for therapeutic purposes. The intensities discussed here are of the order of 100 to

1,000 W/cm^2 in contrast with about 1 to 4 W/cm^2 used in treatment. The high intensities are usually produced by focusing or by the multiple beam method.

This brief review of biological reactions to ultrasound, with special emphasis on those reactions of potential therapeutic significance, clearly indicates that most of the effects produced by ultrasound are due to the temperature elevation resulting from the absorption and conversion of ultrasonic energy (62). In addition, a few effects have been demonstrated such as the acceleration of the diffusion process across biological membranes, which may be therapeutically useful and are non-thermal in nature. It must be recognized that these effects are also dependent on temperature elevation. There are other effects where the mechanism by which they are produced is not clear, but experimental evidence suggests a non-thermal component. These include the effects on protein synthesis and wound healing (90, 91). Beyond this, destructive effects due to cavitation have been observed which fortunately do not occur under therapeutic conditions. A more detailed investigation of the nonthermal effects could lead to new, specific indications for ultrasonic therapy.

These investigations have also shown that there are differences between thermal reactions produced by ultrasound and those produced by other heating modalities (266). The reactions which are produced by various ultrasonic frequencies can also be different. Such differences have been attributed mainly to the variations in temperature distribution throughout the live organisms as they are produced by ultrasound of different frequencies.

Technique of Application

More than in any other modality, the proper technique of application is required to obtain the desirable therapeutic effect. Therefore, it is essential to consider in detail the technique of application and its modification for specific purposes.

Stroking Technique. Ultrasound is usually applied with a stroking technique, that is, the applicator is moved over the area to be treated. The applicator is moved slowly with one stroke overlapping the next. The field to be treated at a given time is usually limited to an area of approximately 3 to 4 in^2. The strokes may be circular or longitudinal. This technique allows adequate and uniform heating of the area treated with only slight ripples of the tissue temperature produced by the overlapping strokes. This technique also averages out the interference pattern in the near field, as well as the high intensity center portion of the beam in the far field avoiding development of hot spots. If a larger area is to be covered or if a joint is treated with bone intervening between the surface of the joint close to the applicator and the part of the joint distant to the applicator, multiple field applications, with the exposure of one field after the other, are necessary. Specifically, in the shoulder joint, three fields of application are necessary, one anteriorly, one laterally, and the third posteriorly. In this application, one must avoid aiming the beam so that it transverses the acromion and acromio-clavicular joint. Similarly, the hip joint should be treated with ultrasound applied to an anterior, a lateral, and a posterior aspect, again aiming the beam at the joint above the greater trochanter. This is necessary because it has been shown (263) that ultrasound cannot be effectively transmitted through bone. If the objective is to heat a contracted joint capsule vigorously, it is essential to treat each field over a period of at least 5 minutes. Ten minutes would be better. With very brief exposure, the highest rise of temperature occurs in the most superficial bone (241). The temperature in the joint capsule is just below that of the bone. This selective rise in the bone is produced quickly and therefore, time has to be allowed for heat conduction to occur from the superficial bone to the area of the contracted tissues in front of the bone in order to get temperatures in this area high enough to produce the desired effect. This was demonstrated by experimentation with human volunteers to whom ultrasound was applied with two intensity levels, 1.0 W/cm^2 and 1.5 W/cm^2. One group of volunteers had a large amount of soft tissue cover (soft tissue thickness overlying the bone greater than 8 cm). The other group had soft tissue in that region less than 8 cm in thickness. The ultrasound was turned off at the first occurrence of pain and at this time the temperature in front of the bone was recorded. Results are shown in Figure 10.85 which indicates that the same ultrasonic intensity of 1.5 W/cm^2 produced a higher temperature rise in front of the bone in the thigh with a thick absorbing soft tissue layer than in the thigh with a thin soft tissue layer superficial to the bone. If the time was recorded until pain occurred under these two conditions, it was shown that it took considerably longer to pain with a thick soft tissue cover than with a thin one. Interpretation of the results was based on the fact that the most superficial bone is heated

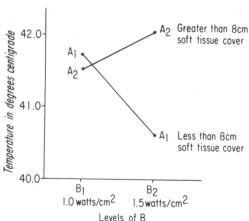

Fig. 10.85. Temperatures in front of bone at pain. From Lehmann et al. (240).

most and that a significantly longer period of time is required to allow heat conduction from bone to soft tissue in front in order to significantly elevate the temperature in this location. Therefore, the temperature as measured in front of the bone was higher than in the thin people where the temperature in the superficial bone rapidly reached pain threshold without elevating the temperature in front of the bone by heat conduction.

Multiple Field Application. In case of multiple field applications, techniques of exercise and stretching in combination with ultrasound have been developed. To maximize the ultrasonic effect after each field of application, the increased extensibility of the contracted tissues in that particular area is used by a corresponding stretch and exercise. Thus stretch immediately follows each field of application (292). The anterior portion of the hip joint can be readily stretched while ultrasound is applied. The patient is stretched by strapping him in the "Thomas Test" position. Intensities of up to 4 W/cm^2 average with a total output up to 40 W have been used with this type of application. The output selected will depend on whether or not vigorous or mild heating is required and also will depend on the thickness of the absorbing soft tissue layer superficial to the tight joint or other structure to be treated. For instance, the maximal output may have to be utilized in an obese person with a hip joint contracture. In order to ascertain whether vigorous treatment is achieved, it is necessary to increase the output just to the maximally tolerated level. Clinically that is done by increasing the ultrasonic output or reducing the area of application until the patient feels the first dull aching pain. Then the output is slightly decreased or the area of application increased so that the condition of treatment stays just below the pain threshold.

Stationary Technique. Ultrasound application with a stationary sound head is rarely, if ever, used. The reason is that heating is very non-uniform because of the hot spots in the interference pattern and in the center of the beam in the far field. In addition, the temperature control in the tissue is extremely difficult because of a very rapid rise of temperature at moderate ultrasonic outputs (166). Without continuously controlling the output, it is impossible to predict where the temperature in the tissue will level off. Because of the limited size of the applicator only a small area can be treated. And finally, the accumulation of the red cells in the wave nodes with disruption of blood flow may occur with this technique of application, whereas it can be avoided when the applicator is moved (384). The use of large applicators with a mosaic of crystals producing the ultrasound has been advocated for ultrasound application with stationary technique. These applicators are unacceptable by FDA standards because of the non-uniformity of the beam. The high pack intensities may render these applicators potentially hazardous. They are safe only if the maximal average output is too low to produce vigorous therapeutic results.

Pulsed Application. Application of pulsed ultrasound has also been advocated. Acceptable equipment produces well-defined square pulses with a specified intensity during the pulse and with a controlled rate of pulsing and duty cycle (110). If pulsed ultrasound is applied the temperature rise would be equal to that produced by a CW application of the same average output, provided that the rate of pulsing is fast enough to prevent major temperature fluctuations between pauses and pulses. Therefore, all thermal reactions can be equally and less expensively produced by CW application; also, many non-thermal reactions such as streaming are in proportion to the average output and therefore, can be produced equally well by CW application (222, 259). In other physiological responses where non-thermal mechanisms may be involved, there is no evidence that these reactions could not be produced by a corresponding CW output (89–92). Therefore, at this time, there seems to be very little evidence for the need of pulsed output for therapeutic purposes.

Coupling Medium. Unlike microwave application, a coupling medium must be inserted between the sound applicator and the skin of the patient in order to obtain adequate transmission of ultrasound into the tissues. The coupling medium, in addition, should have lubricating qualities so that gliding of the applicator against the skin surface can be easily achieved when stroking technique is used. Since the amount of ultrasound reflected at an interface between two media depends on the mismatch of acoustic impedance, it is necessary that the coupling medium matches the impedance of the tissues. An air layer between applicator and skin must be avoided since the acoustic impedance of the air is so different that almost 100 percent reflection would occur. Even microscopic gas bubbles may produce significant losses in transmission. Because a thin layer of coupling medium is used, the coefficient of absorption of the coupling medium is of secondary importance. Degassed water can be used as a standard for transmission. It has been shown that commercial gels such as Soni-gel, Aqua-sonic, Medco, and mineral oil are adequate coupling media (see Figure 10.86). However, the ultrasound transmission of any coupling medium deteriorates markedly

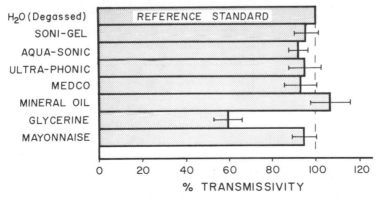

Fig. 10.86. Percent transmissivities of several coupling agents using ultrasound generator without transducer voltage control circuit. From Warren *et al.* (409).

when air is mixed in the medium (see Figure 10.87). If water is used as a coupling medium, the part to be treated has to be submerged and the applicator has to be moved over the skin surface without touching, since water is a poor lubricant. Also, special care should be taken that the water is not saturated with gas and that bubbles do not collect at applicator or skin surfaces. Ideally, degassed water should be used; however, the procedures of degassing are too cumbersome to be practical.

The main purpose of ultrasound application is to selectively raise the temperature in certain areas in the depth of the tissues where treatable pathology is found. Whether such a selective rise of temperature can be achieved will depend on the temperature of applicator and coupling medium (237). In human experimentation, it has been demonstrated that a selective rise of temperature, for instance, in front of the bone where contracted joint structures may be found, can be produced provided that the mineral oil coupling medium is kept at a temperature of 18°C or less. At a temperature of 24°C, skin surface temperature will exceed the deep temperatures and therefore limit vigorous heating (see Figures 10.88 and 10.89). If the coupling medium is water, temperatures as high as 24°C have been shown to be suitable without defeating the deep heating purpose. This is probably due to the high specific heat of water and therefore, its better cooling capability of the surface area. To minimize surface heating it is also important that adequate applicators are used which do not have large internal losses heating the applicator surface unduly during application. It is also recommended that between each field of application the applicator is cooled down to room temperature which can be readily achieved by dipping it briefly in tap water. Units were available which thermostatically controlled the temperature of the applicator. On the other hand, it has been demonstrated that hot pack application preceding ultrasound application does not defeat the deep heating purpose of the ultrasound application primarily because

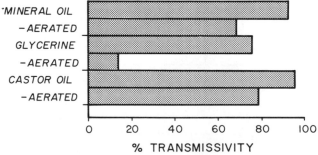

Fig. 10.87. Percent transmissivities for several common coupling media in aerated and non-aerated forms using ultrasound generator without voltage control circuit. From Warren *et al.* (409).

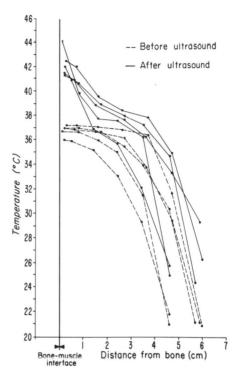

Fig. 10.88. Comparison of temperature distributions in five human thighs before and after exposure to ultrasound using a mineral oil coupling medium at 18°C. From Lehmann *et al.* (237).

the large increase in blood flow to the skin triggered by the hot pack application cools the superficial tissues enough that subsequent ultrasound application is still effective in heating deep structures (268).

Cavitation. To avoid the occurrence of gaseous cavitation and its destructive effects during therapeutic application, it has been demonstrated that the application of ultrasonic average intensities up to 4 W/cm^2 with a total output of 4 W at an ultrasonic frequency of 1 MHz are tolerated without producing cavitation effects. However, with stationary technique of application, the cavitation threshold for small animals is between 1 and 2 W/cm^2. It must also be remembered that cavitation is inhibited during most therapeutic applications by the high viscosity of serum and the high volume concentration of cells in blood tissues (222), but this inhibition does not occur when ultrasound is applied, for instance, to the fluid media of the eye, the amniotic fluid of the pregnant uterus, and fluid-filled joints. These organs or conditions, therefore, represent contraindications because cavitation is likely to occur at therapeutic intensities and frequencies.

From these experiments, it is also concluded that applicators which produce a less uniform intensity distribution in the beam than the federal standard requires are potentially dangerous in that the peak intensities in the beam may exceed cavitation thresholds. The cavitation thresholds may

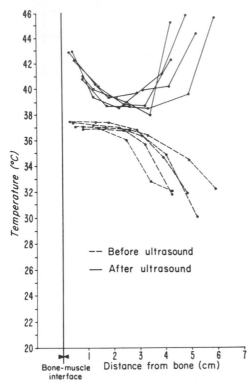

Fig. 10.89. Comparison of temperature distributions in human thighs before and after exposure to ultrasound using mineral oil coupling medium at 24°C. From Lehmann *et al.* (237).

also be exceeded with equipment without rectification and filtering. Uncontrolled temporal peaks of intensity may produce cavitation, as does pulsed application with high peak intensities during the pulses.

Metallic Implants. Ultrasound also can be utilized in the presence of surgical metallic implants. Marked reflection with a resulting pattern of standing waves or focusing occurs at the interface of the tissue and the metal implant. This leads to a large increase in ultrasound intensity near the metal. Lehmann *et al.* (233) studied the temperature distribution throughout specimens exposed to ultrasound with and without metal implants. A selective rise of temperature in the presence of the metal implant did not occur (see Figure 10.90) and the temperature in the specimen close to the metal frequently was lower than the temperatures measured without the metal present. Since the metal has a very high thermal conductivity as compared with tissue (see Table 10.15), the increase amount of energy absorbed close to the metal implant is more than compensated for by the rapid conduction of heat through the metal to cooler, unexposed areas.

The experimental findings obtained in specimens were confirmed in live pigs (232) with surgical metal implants where foci or standing waves would be produced during the period of ultrasonic treatment (see Figure 10.91). Nevertheless, the temperatures obtained in these areas were within the therapeutic range and could be well-controlled.

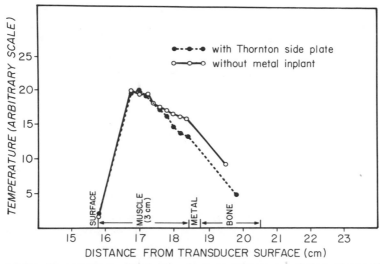

Fig. 10.90. Temperature distribution in a specimen consisting of muscle and bone with and without a Thornton side plate inserted in front of the bone. From Lehmann *et al.* (233).

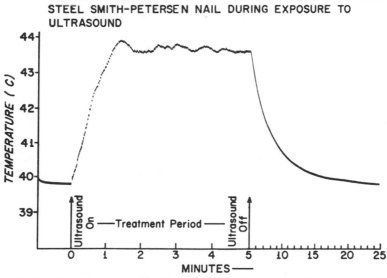

Fig. 10.91. Change in temperature between flanges of stainless steel Smith-Petersen nail during exposure of a live pig to ultrasound. From Lehmann (232).

In a second series of experiments, identical metal implants were inserted bilaterally into live pigs. One side served as control; the other one was exposed to ultrasound. After the pigs were sacrificed, histological examination did not show any signs of untoward nonthermal effects.

Ultrasound energy appears to be the only type of diathermy which can be used safely and effectively with metallic implants in the treatment field, a finding consistent with previous observations of Gersten (131). The modern joint replacements using plastics such as high-density polyethylene or methyl methacrylate should at this point in time not be treated with ultrasound. The coefficient of absorption of these materials is high, and no data are available as to whether or not under the conditions of therapy this material would be heated to the point of destruction or to the point of damage to the surrounding tissues. Further experimentation is necessary before therapeutic application of ultrasound under these conditions (226).

Dosimetry

Dosimetry in itself is easy with ultrasound application, since the therapeutic machine is equipped with a meter which reads the ultrasonic average intensity and total output going into the tissues, provided proper coupling is used. A timer will accurately measure the duration of the application. However, since the main purpose of the application is to produce a specific temperature in the depth of the tissues, these measurements are not adequate to predict the effectiveness of the treatment. The tissue temperature will depend not only upon the wattage but also upon the technique of application as discussed above, and the propagation and absorption characteristics of the tissues exposed. For vigorous effects, temperatures have to be brought to the maximal tolerated level which can be done by staying just below the pain threshold. For mild therapeutic effects, one has to stay significantly below that level. However, accurate dosimetry is not available in this area and a physiological guide of sensation of temperature is absent since in most of the deep structures which ultrasound heats, temperature receptors are not present.

In combination with the proper technique of application, for deep-seated structures, intensities up to 4 W/cm^2 with a total output of 40 W may be needed when vigorous results are to be obtained. For most joints covered with a significant amount of soft tissue (*e.g.*, shoulder, hip), outputs for mild heating are of the order of 1 to 2 W/cm^2 with a total output of 10 to 20 W. For smaller beams, allowances have to be made. For very mild treatment, average outputs of 0.1 to 1 W/cm^2 are used with a total output of 1 to 10 W. For structures with little soft tissue cover such as small joints the above outputs may be adequate for mild heating. However, it must be emphasized that these are rough guidelines which are greatly modified by the technique of application.

Common Indications

The indications for ultrasound therapy are primarily based on the physiological effects which can be produced by raising the temperature (223, 224,

247). The location of the selective rise of temperature in the tissue matches very well the empirically developed indications. In some of these, the efficacy of ultrasound has been tested in controlled studies. According to the results of these studies, the indications to ultrasound therapy may be assigned to one of three groups: a) where effectiveness superior to other modalities has been proven, b) indications where ultrasound is of suggested value; and c) indications where ultrasound has been used purely on an empirical basis. In the first group, controlled studies are available. In the second group, clinical observations are available consistent with the selective temperature distribution ultrasound produces. In the third group, the use of ultrasound is suggested on the basis of case studies only. A full diagnostic evaluation of the patient's problems is required to intelligently select ultrasound over any other modality and to adapt the technique of application appropriately. Evaluation must include detailed information as to the type of pathology, as to acuteness or chronicity of the processes, and its location in the tissues. On the basis of this evaluation and the knowledge of the selective temperature distribution ultrasound produces, together with the knowledge of the physiological responses to heating, the clinical indications have been developed.

Indications Where Ultrasound is of Proven Effectiveness. Conditions in which ultrasound is of established value include joint contractures resulting from tightness of periarticular structures or scarring of capsular tissues, irrespective of the cause, whether immobilization, rheumatic processes, degenerative joint disease, or trauma. The rationale for this treatment is that these structures can be heated adequately and perhaps selectively by ultrasound. This results in an increase in extensibility of the tight structures limiting joint motion, which greatly augments the effects of physical therapy, such as range of motion exercises given with or without stretching. Other effects of ultrasound, such as the relief of pain, may contribute to the favorable results.

Many reports in the literature have indicated that ultrasound can be useful in periarthritis of the shoulder, if given in conjunction with other forms of physical therapy (13, 14, 33, 65, 141, 199, 301, 433). A statistical comparison has been made between the results obtained after exposure to ultrasound and those obtained with microwaves. Ultrasound selectively raises the temperature of the tight capsular structures whereas microwaves at the frequency of 2,450 MHz may selectively heat muscle and/or subcutaneous fat. Ultrasound and microwaves were given in conjunction with a standard physical therapy program consisting of massage and exercise (243, 260). The two groups of patients with periarthritis were comparable for statistical purposes, in terms of age distribution and duration of symptoms prior to therapy (Figures 10.92 and 10.93) and available range of motion prior to treatment (Figure 10.94). Thus a valid comparison could be made

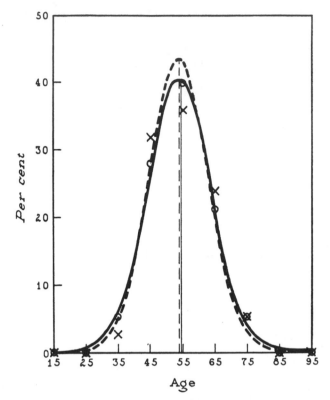

Fig. 10.92. Calculated distribution of age within the group of patients treated with ultrasound (*solid line*) and with microwave (*broken line*). Data from ultrasound observations indicated by *circles*; data from microwave observations shown by *crosses*. From Lehmann *et al.* (243).

between the effects produced by ultrasound and microwaves. Evaluation after treatment showed that the gain in the range of motion was significantly greater when the patients were treated with ultrasound than when they were treated with microwave diathermy (see Table 10.17).

In conclusion, ultrasound is of value for this condition when given in conjunction with a standard exercise program.

Mueller *et al.* (306) treated 14 cases of periarthritis. Eight were treated with ultrasound, six received a sham exposure without output of the applicator. All patients had to forego all supplemental treatment or medications during the experimental period. The patients were evaluated semi-objectively before and after the experimental period. The evaluation included goniometric measurements of the active range of motion. There was no statistically significant improvement in either group. Subsequent laboratory studies have explained this result (262). It could be demonstrated that when

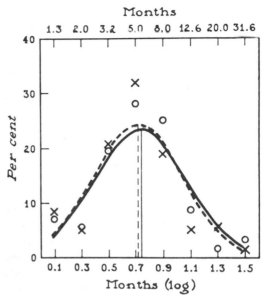

Fig. 10.93. Calculated distribution of the duration of symptoms prior to first visit in patients treated with ultrasound (*solid line*) and with microwave (*broken line*). Data observed in ultrasound group indicated by *circles*, data from microwave group indicated by *crosses*. From Lehmann *et al.* (243).

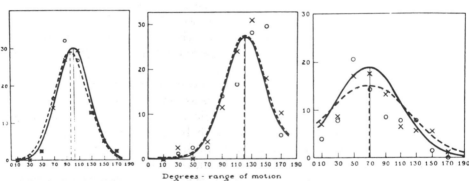

Fig. 10.94. Calculated distribution of range of motion before treatment in group of patients later treated with ultrasound (*solid lines*) and with microwave (*broken lines*). Data observed after ultrasound indicated by *circles*; after microwave by *crosses*. *Left*—range of abduction; *center*—range of forward flexion; *right*—range of rotation. From Lehmann *et al.* (243).

collagen tissue was heated but not stretched, there was no residual elongation, and the measured length was equal to the control. Residual increase in length could be obtained only after heating and stretching, which was not done in Mueller's study, whereas all studies reporting good results in ultrasound treatment of periarthritis used range-of-motion exercises and stretch in addition to the ultrasound.

The results obtained in the previously described studies on periarthritis

TABLE 10.17. *Gain in Range of Motion after Ultrasonic and Microwave Treatment*[a]

Gain In	After Treatment with:	
	Ultrasound	Microwaves
Forward flexion	$27.4° \pm 2.3°$[b]	$16.1° \pm 1.5°$
Abduction	$32.6° \pm 2.5°$	$21.2° \pm 2.1°$
Rotation	$45.4° \pm 2.8°$	$17.3° \pm 4.0°$

[a] From Lehmann et al. (243).
[b] Standard error of the mean.

of the shoulder are also in agreement with clinical observations by Friedland (117), DePreux (81), and Reese et al. (336), who treated conditions such as rheumatoid arthritis and degenerative joint disease with ultrasound. A thorough evaluation including X-rays as to the cause of contractures is essential in the degenerative joint disease of the hip. Ultrasound is useless if bony spurs interfere with the range of motion. It is useful only if one deals with the soft tissue contracture of joint capsule and ligaments. A side benefit is that ultrasound often temporarily relieves pain. It is most important that treatment is used in conjunction with range of motion exercise and stretch, which preferably is given as a long-term stretch extending over 0.5 to 2 hours which is statically applied by weight with a pulley while at the same time ultrasound is given for the normal period of time (5 to 10 minutes per field).

Another clinical study was designed to evaluate statistically the efficacy of the ultrasonic treatment of contractures associated with internal fixation of hip fractures (246). In this study, geriatric patients who had sustained hip fractures which were fixed internally with Richard's screws were treated either with ultrasound or with infrared. Both groups received, in addition, standard range of motion exercises. Geriatric patients of this type were selected because hip contractures almost invariably develop which becomes a problem in treatment, since any physical therapy procedures involving vigorous stretch cannot be applied without endangering the surgical results. It was found in this study that all patients treated with ultrasound gained in range of motion, whereas the majority of the patients who were treated with infrared developed further limitations of the range of motion (see Table 10.18). The results were statistically significant.

In summary, there is good clinical and statistical evidence that ultrasound is an efficient modality, when used for the treatment of all types of joint contractures resulting from the development of capsular tightness and scarring. This form of energy can be used safely in the presence of surgical metallic implants. Ultrasound is the modality of choice if the joint is covered by a thick layer of soft tissues, since neither microwave nor shortwave diathermy is able to heat such structures to a therapeutic level and produce

TABLE 10.18. *Comparison of Amount of Change in Range of Motion after 1 Week of Treatment*[a, b]

	With Ultrasound			With Infrared			t	p
	N	Mean	S.D.	N	Mean	S.D.		
Hip								
Flexion	15	21.67	9.7	15	5.40	11.4	4.057	.01
Extension	15	10.40	8.2	15	−3.20[c]	7.7	4.503	.01
Abduction	15	06.33	7.4	15	−1.67[c]	5.6	3.225	.01
Adduction	15	09.67	6.6	15	−1.20[c]	6.0	4.567	.01
External Rotation	14	12.86	7.9	15	0.20	7.9	4.178	.01
Internal Rotation	14	10.93	7.6	15	−1.60[c]	8.8	3.965	.01
Knee								
Flexion	15	18.33	14.9	15	10.33	13.3	1.498	.20
Extension	15	03.60	3.9	15	−3.47[c]	4.8	4.259	.01

[a] From Lehmann *et al.* (246)
[b] US and IR groups compared using independent samples method.
[c] When the mean is expressed as a negative value, range of motion has been lost during treatment.

results comparable to ultrasound treatment. Ultrasound is certainly preferred to superficial heating modalities such as infrared. Whether ultrasound can be used in the presence of plastics such as high-density polyethylene and methyl methacrylate needs to be investigated further.

Indications Where Ultrasound is of Suggested Value. Listed in this category are conditions in which it is the clinical impression of many authors that ultrasound is of therapeutic value. However, evaluations by statistical or other objective means of the efficacy of ultrasound in these conditions are not available.

During the First International Congress of Ultrasound in Medicine held in 1949, a statistical study was presented on the successful treatment of ankylosing spondylitis with ultrasound (291). Evaluation was done on an entirely subjective basis and no controls were mentioned. Hintzelmann (171, 172) on the other hand, substantiated this clinical impression to a certain extent by measuring the change in vital capacity and chest expansion before and after treatment with ultrasound (see Figure 10.95). He observed an appreciable and consistent increase in both values. No control subjects were presented in this study. Thus, even if the evidence suggests that ultrasound may be used in this condition, the final value of the treatment remains to be established. The ultrasound therapy was applied in such a fashion that the costovertebral joints were treated in combination with deep breathing, stretch, and exercise. Therefore, the same rationale for the use of ultrasound applies in this case as to the other joint contractures. Pain relief is an associated benefit.

Ultrasonic treatment of joint contractures secondary to the scarring

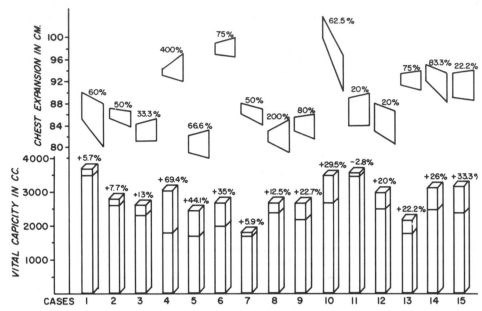

Fig. 10.95. Chest expansion and vital capacity before and after ultrasound treatment of patient with ankylosing spondylitis. From Hintzelmann (171).

associated with rheumatoid arthritis has been proposed by several investigators (117, 315, 317, 336). It seems to be justified to conclude that ultrasound treatment in rheumatoid arthritis should be reserved for the chronic burned out processes with residual contractures lest an aggravation of the symptoms occur.

Limitation of the range of motion of a joint can develop not only as a result of shortening of capsule and ligaments, but also as a result of scarring and fibrosis of musculature, skin, and subcutaneous tissues. In most of these cases, with the exception of diffuse muscular fibrosis, these contracted collagen tissues are likely to be selectively heated by ultrasound. The temperature in these tissues may be elevated enough to produce an increase in extensibility. This effect can be utilized by use of physical therapy designed to increase the range of motion. Therefore, it seems reasonable that such fibrosis and scarring, irrespective of their cause, should represent an indication for ultrasound treatment. Scarring of the skin may be due to trauma, burns, or diseases such as scleroderma (398). Bierman (38) showed that contractures of the hand resulting from scars due to electrical burns, due to laceration of the palm or due to Dupuytren's contracture, and secondary to X-ray burns were treated successfully (see Figure 10.96). Calcific bursitis and tendinitis of the shoulder have been treated successfully with ultrasound by various authors (14, 33, 433). It can be assumed that the

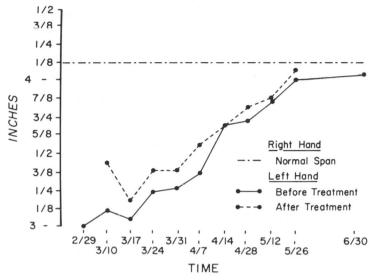

Fig. 10.96. Influence of ultrasound on scar of left hand indicating span before and directly after each treatment. From Bierman (38).

rationale for this type of treatment is the selective heating of areas where calcific deposits occur, that is, in the bursae or tendons. The calcium deposit probably has a high coefficient of absorption and the resulting hyperemia and mild inflammatory reaction may be comparable in their therapeutic effects to needling or other accepted procedures. Even though several studies suggest that calcific deposits may disappear after the sound treatment, there is no statistical evidence that this occurrence is more frequent than would be anticipated by the natural course of the disease. Flax (106) specifically investigated whether ultrasound could resolve the calcium deposits. He found that calcium deposits were resolved as frequently in the control group as in the treated group. Thus, ultrasound therapy does not assist in the resolution of calcium deposits. However, from the previously described data, it can be used to treat the associated joint contractures if present. Ultrasound used in combination with hydrocortisone injection seems to be more effective than either procedure applied alone (314). Experimentally it could be demonstrated that the cortisone is more evenly distributed when ultrasound is applied following the injection (13).

In acute subacromial bursitis with an associated acute inflammatory reaction, ultrasound should not be used, since it probably produces a selective rise of temperature at the bursa which in turn promotes further inflammatory reaction with hyperemia and exudate, acutely aggravating the pain. It has been demonstrated that the pain is largely due to pressure in the bursa. It can be relieved by removing the bursal content with the syringe and can be reproduced by replacing the volume withdrawn. This may help to explain the acute exacerbations which are found with vigorous ultrasound treatment in this condition. Ice would be the modality of choice with other local procedures such as withdrawal of the pasty bursal content, hydrocortisone and/or lidocaine injection, and mild physical therapy such as Codman's (63) pendulum exercises. At a later stage, the condition would be best treated with either ice or mild heat.

Another clinical application that has been described is the treatment of pain as it occurs in postamputation neurofibromas, especially where they are imbedded in scar tissues. Frequently, phantom pain is associated with this syndrome. Chateau (60), Tepperberg and Marjey (388), Rubin and Kuitert (347), and their associates agreed in their clinical observations that marked and sometimes even dramatic improvement could be observed after ultrasound application. This was true even in cases which had been resistant to most other forms of therapy over a long period of time. Experimental evidence seems to support the clinical observations since nerve and scar tissues can both be heated selectively with apparent alteration in the nerve function by ultrasound application (166, 345). Ultrasound treatment requires a small field of application with relatively high dosage. It is essential though that the symptom of pain is not of psychological origin, but pain produced at the neuroma site by local conditions.

Chronic skin ulcerations resulting from various causes, such as peripheral venous insufficiency (varicose ulcers), decubital ulcers, and x-ray burns, have been treated (36, 320, 323). Some of these conditions often heal under general management such as bed rest or relief of pressure, and since no controlled studies are available, it remains open to question whether they represent indication for ultrasound therapy.

However, there is one study on stimulation of healing of varicose ulcers by ultrasound where Dyson *et al.* (89, 92) showed in a controlled study that ultrasound was effective in accelerating the healing of varicose ulcers. Actual insonation was alternated with mock insonation. They found a significantly more rapid decrease of the ulcerated area with the ultrasonic treatment than without it (see Figure 10.97). The ultrasonic average intensity was 1 W/cm^2, the frequency of 3 MHz, which was applied pulsed with a 20 percent duty cycle and pulse duration of 2 msecond. Treatment was given three times weekly for a minimum of four weeks.

Conditions Where Ultrasound is Used Purely on an Empirical Basis. Among the conditions where ultrasound may be helpful on the basis of clinical experience is the tennis elbow or epicondylitis. The treatment should be primarily that of rest, splinting, as combined with other forms of heat, superficial heat or shortwave diathermy combined with injection of lidocaine and hydrocortisone. Ultrasound is likely to selectively raise the temperature of the common tendon of origin and fascia of the extensors at the lateral

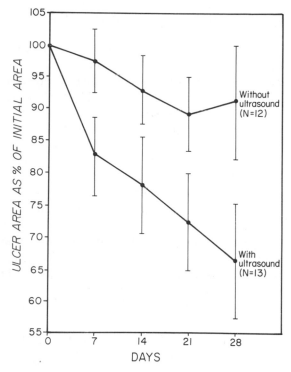

Fig. 10.97. Effect of treatment with ultrasound on varicose ulcer area. From Dyson *et al.* (89).

epicondyle. Ultrasound usually is contraindicated in the acute stage, but may be helpful in the presence of prolonged pain, especially when the patient does not follow the prescribed regimen of immobilization. It should then be given in low dosage (0.5 w/cm^2) (11, 52, 397).

Pain which sometimes persists following sprains can be relieved by ultrasound in a comparatively short period of time (66, 232, 241, 246, 306). It is also possible that the healing of the injury and the absorption of hemorrhages may be speeded up by the thermal component of the ultrasound effect. The pain relief is perhaps the reason why athletes often go back to competitive sports events immediately after the occurrence of the injury and its treatment with ultrasound. However, the very acute injury should be treated with ice and not heat. In scleroderma associated with Raynaud's phenomenon, ultrasound has been used in order to improve the joint range and vascularity (10, 396). Friction massage to mobilize the scarred skin against the underlying structures may also be used in addition to stretch and range of motion exercises (49, 157, 397).

The treatment of arterial insufficiency in the extremities has been suggested (36). This proposal is based on the result of biological research showing that an increase in blood flow can be obtained in the extremities when either the sympathetic nerves or ganglia are treated. However, ultrasound, as other types of heat, should never be applied to the ischemic area itself.

Treatment of the nerve roots or the sympathetic ganglia and nerves has been advocated for a large variety of conditions. So-called segmental treatment has been advocated by Tschannen (394, 395), Sonnen (370), Thiele (390), and Sonnenschein (371). This type of treatment technique has been recommended for treatment of rheumatic diseases and peripheral vascular disorders. The rationale for this treatment is doubtful with the exception of the fact that perhaps pain relief can be obtained and the vascularity of the area increased (276). The effectiveness of such treatment in clinical practice has not been clearly established.

Ultrasonic therapy of sympathetic reflex dystrophies related to the shoulder-hand syndrome, Sudeck's atrophy and causalgia, has been advocated by several authors (38, 214, 314, 405, 426) who favor treatment both of the sympathetics and the involved joints. Stuhlfauth (375) and Woeber (426) claimed that ultrasound exposure of the sympathetics gave results similar to those obtained with stellate ganglion block, but this has not been substantiated.

Buchtala (49) treated Raynaud's phenomena and found an increase in the cutaneous temperature of 2.5°C if ultrasound was used locally or applied to the appropriate sympathetic ganglia. These findings were confirmed by Stuhlfauth (375). Woeber (426) published a statistical study on treatment of reflex dystrophies. His results were similar to those obtained elsewhere by stellate ganglion blocks, the major difference being that it took longer to achieve the same results when ultrasound was applied to either the peripheral sympathetic fibers or sympathetic ganglia. More clinical investigations and experimental evidence will be necessary in order to confirm these clinical impressions.

Bonica (43) developed the rationale for the management of the so-called myofascial pain syndrome. Ultrasound has also been used to treat the focal irritation or to interrupt the reflexes perpetuating the pain syndrome (392). Again, even though the clinical impression is that ultrasound is useful for the treatment of this condition, final proof is not available. Because of the non-uniformity of the etiology and the clinical symptomatology, statistical studies which assess the final value of the ultrasound treatment of this condition are difficult to obtain.

The combined use of ultrasound and electrical stimulation has been advocated, using the sound applicator as a stimulating electrode. It is imperative in this case to use an aqueous gel as coupling agent, because mineral oil is a poor conductor of electricity and other media are poor coupling agents for ultrasound. In the literature, there is no clearly established physiological basis nor any clinical evidence demonstrating that this type of treatment is superior to either electrical stimulation or ultrasound treatment alone or used consecutively.

Kuitert (214) has advocated ultrasound treatment for referred pain and radiculitis. In addition, it has been advocated for the post-herpetic pain after herpes zoster has been treated (280). The potential basis for this type of treatment is that nerves themselves as a result of their coefficient of absorption and their location at myofascial interfaces may be selectively heated and their function altered (12).

Several authors advocated the treatment of plantar warts with ultrasound because they selectively absorb ultrasound (203). Bender and associates (35) found supportive evidence which suggested that this treatment is of value. Since this is sometimes a therapeutically difficult problem, and since ultrasound has no significant side effects in this application, a trial of ultrasound therapy may be worthwhile.

Specific Contraindications to Ultrasound Therapy

In addition to the general contraindications to heating, ultrasound should not be applied to fluid media in the body because cavitation can be readily produced at therapeutic dosages and may potentially damage the tissues. This applies to the exposure of the eye and the pregnant uterus to therapeutic ultrasonic intensities. In the latter situation, of course, heating of the fetus would also be detrimental. However, it should be recognized that because of the excellent beaming properties of ultrasound, it is quite possible to treat other parts of the body without affecting the two organs mentioned. Specifically, treatment of contractures or degenerative joint disease of the temporomandibular joint can be done without affecting the eye. Unless a deliberate attempt is made to expose the pregnant uterus, it is virtually impossible to reach the uterus with significant ultrasonic energy if ultrasound is applied in the described common indications such as joint pathology. Special precautions in adjusting the dosage should be taken when the area of the spinal cord is treated after laminectomy since the absorbing soft tissues and intervening bone have been removed in part. Therefore, under these circumstances, intensities at the level of the spinal cord may be high enough to produce cavitation in the cerebrospinal fluid and may also affect the cord function by heating. Again, because of the excellent beaming properties of the ultrasound, the facet joints can be treated even in these cases without exposing the spinal cord. Finally, the controversy about the safety of exposing growing bone has been resolved in that at therapeutic dosage, without exceeding pain threshold, growth disturbances have not been observed in animals or in men.

Standards for Efficacy and Safety

Desirable equipment characteristics for therapeutic ultrasound include the following items.

The appropriate frequency for therapeutic ultrasound is about 0.8 to 1 MHz because this frequency range produces the desired selective rise in the described areas of the tissue. It has a good depth of penetration in soft tissues. The short wavelength together with the size of the applicator produces an ultrasonic beam with little divergence. To assure optimal uniformity of the ultrasonic field, a single synthetic or natural crystal should be used.

The ratio of the peak intensity in the beam in the far field to the average intensity should be 4 to 1 or less.

The diameter of the applicator should be close to the diameter of the radiating surface area to allow optimal contact of the applicator and skin in the area of uneven body surfaces. The radiating surface area of the applicator ideally should be 7 to 13 cm^2.

Full wave rectification with filtering assures avoidance of temporal potentially dangerous peaks of ultrasound intensity. The fluctuation from the 60 Hz house current should be less than 1 percent even though the federal standard allows the fluctuation of 20 percent for all emissions greater than 10 percent of the maximum emission. The meter on the panel should accurately indicate both the average intensity (W/cm^2) and the total output (W) irradiating into the tissues provided the coupling is adequate. There should be a timer which shuts off the output after a pre-set period of time. Unfortunately a minimum output for therapeutic effectiveness has not been stated in the FDA standard (110). At present it is possible to manufacture a piece of equipment which meets all the criteria for FDA approval without having enough output to be therapeutically effective. Based on animal experiments, it will be necessary to have available a total output of 40 W with an average intensity of 4 W/cm^2 to be able to vigorously heat the deep-seated structures such as the hip joint in an obese person. It has been also demonstrated that these intensities are safe with regard to the occurrence of cavitation provided proper technique of application and adequate equipment are used. It is desirable to have applicators which have an output of this magnitude so that vigorous effects could be obtained. The FDA standard so far has controlled only the design of equipment. Efforts are on the way to assure safety and efficacy by limiting the use of therapeutic equipment to physicians and therapists. This restriction seems reasonable because selection of patients and the use of proper technique is complex. Desirable results can be achieved only with proper training. Without it, severe burns have been observed as a result of incorrect application.

Summary

This review of the literature basic to the therapeutic application of the superficial and deep-heating modalities forces the conclusions that most of the therapeutic effects are produced by heating the tissues. One might then infer that all the modalities are interchangeable. However, the reason for having so many modalities is that in most cases the temperature distribution produced by each modality is significantly different. It also has been demonstrated that in order to get a vigorous therapeutic effect the temperature should be brought to the maximally tolerated level. Therefore, nowhere else could this temperature level be exceeded without damage. Thus, for a given pathology at a given site, one must select the modality which produces a selective rise in this area with the peak temperature nowhere else to be exceeded. The selection therefore depends on the specific temperature distribution of the modality more than upon any other factor discussed. The areas selectively treated by the given modalities are as follows:

Skin and subcutaneous tissues are selectively heated by infrared, visible light, hot packs, paraffin baths, fluidotherapy, hydrotherapy, and moist air cabinets.

The deeper subcutaneous tissues and superficial musculature can be selectively heated by the application of shortwave diathermy with capacitor plates or using microwave radiation at a frequency of 2,456 MHz. The superficial musculature is selectively heated by shortwave application at 27 MHz using an induction coil applicator.

Muscle throughout is selectively heated by microwave direct contact applicators at 915 MHz using air cooling of the skin surface.

Joints, ligaments, fibrous scars, myofascial interfaces, nerve trunks, tendon and tendon sheaths are selectively heated by ultrasound at 0.8 to 1.0 MHz.

The pelvic organs can be selectively heated with shortwave diathermy application at 27 MHz using internal electrodes.

REFERENCES

1. ABRAMSON, D. I. Physiologic basis for the use of physical agents in peripheral vascular disorders. *Arch. Phys. Med. Rehabil.*, 46: 216–244, 1965.
2. ABRAMSON, D. I., BELL, Y., REJAL, H., TUCK, S. JR., BURNETT C. AND FLEISCHER C. J. Changes in blood flow, oxygen uptake and tissue temperatures produced by therapeutic physical agents; II. Effect of short-wave diathermy. *Am. J. Phys. Med.*, 39: 87–95, 1960.
3. ABRAMSON, D. I., BELL, Y., TUCK, S. JR., MITCHELL, R. AND CHANDRASEKHARAPPA G. Changes in blood flow, oxygen uptake and tissue temperatures produced by therapeutic physical agents: III. Effect of indirect or reflex vaodilatation. *Am. J. Phys. Med.*, 40: 5–13, 1961.
4. ABRAMSON, D. I., BURNETT, C., BELL, Y., TUCK, S. JR., REJAL, H. AND FLEISCHER, C. J. Changes in blood flow, oxygen uptake and tissue temperatures produced by therapeutic physical agents; I. Effect of ultrasound. *Am. J. Phys. Med.*, 39: 51–62, 1960.
5. ABRAMSON, D. I., FLACHS, K., FREIBERG, J. AND MIRSKY, I. A. Blood flow in extremities affected by anterior poliomyelitis. *Arch. Intern. Med.*, 71: 391–396, 1943.
6. ABRAMSON, D. I., HARRIS, A. J., BEACONSFIELD, P. AND SCHROEDER, J. M. Changes in

peripheral blood flow produced by shortwave diathermy. *Arch. Phys. Med. Rehabil., 38:* 369–376, 1957.

7. ABRAMSON, D. I., KAHN, A., TUCK, S. JR., TURMAN, G. A., REJAL H. AND FLEISCHER, C. J. Relationship between a range of tissue temperature and local oxygen uptake in the human forearm. I. Changes observed under resting conditions. *J. Clin. Invest., 37:* 1031–1038, 1958.

8. ABRAMSON, D. I., MITCHELL, R. E., TUCK, S. JR., BELL, Y. AND ZAYAS, A. M. Changes in blood flow, oxygen uptake and tissue temperatures produced by the topical application of wet heat. *Arch. Phys. Med. Rehabil., 42:* 305–318, 1961.

9. ABRAMSON, D. I., TUCK, S. JR., CHU, L. S. W. AND AGUSTIN, C. Effect of paraffin bath and hot fomentations on local tissue temperatures. *Arch. Phys. Med. Rehabil., 45:* 87–94, 1964.

10. ALARCON-SEGOVIA, D. AND OSMUNDSON, P. J. Peripheral vascular syndromes associated with systemic lupus erythematosus. *Ann. Intern. Med., 62:* 907, 1965.

11. ALDES, J. H. Ultrasonic radiation in the treatment of epicondylitis. *Gen. Pract., 13:* 89, 1956.

12. ALDES, J., EDMUNDSON, E., AGRESTI, M. AND RHODEN, R. The use of ultrasonic radiation for the treatment of herpes zoster. American Institute of Ultrasonics in Medicine Proc. 4th Ann. Conf on Ultrasonic Therapy, Detroit, pp. 115–123, 1955.

13. ALDES, J. H., JADESON, W. J. AND GRABINSKI, S. A. A new approach to the treatment of subdeltoid bursitis. *Am. J. Phys. Med., 33:* 79–88, 1954.

14. ALDES, J. H. AND KLARAS, T. Use of ultrasonic radiation in the treatment of subdeltoid bursitis with and without calcareous deposits. *West J. Surg., 62:* 369, 1954.

15. AMBERSON, W. R. AND KLEIN, H. The influence of pH upon the concentration potentials across the skin of the frog. *J. Gen. Physiol., 11:* 823, 1928.

16. AMERICAN NATIONAL STANDARDS INSTITUTE: AN AMERICAN NATIONAL STANDARD. Safety level of electromagnetic radiation with respect to personnel. Approved November 15, 1974 (ANSI C95.1–1974), Institute of Electrical and Electronics Engineers, 345 East 47th Street, New York, NY 10017, 1974.

17. ANDERSON, T. P., WAKIM, K. G., HERRICK, J. E., BENNETT, W. A. AND KRUSEN, F. H. An experimental study of the effects of ultrasonic energy on the lower part of the spinal cord and peripheral nerves. *Arch. Phys. Med., 32:* 71–83, 1951.

18. ANNE, A. Scattering and absorption of microwaves by dissipative dielectric objects: the biological significance and hazard to mankind. PhD dissertation, University of Pennsylvania, Philadelphia, 106p, cont NONR 551505, ASTIA Doc 408 997, 1963.

19. ANNE, A., SAITO, M., SALATI, O. M. AND SCHWAN, H. P. Penetration and thermal dissipation of microwaves in tissues. University of Pennsylvania, Philadelphia, Tech. Rept. RADC-TDR-62-244. Cont AF 3-(602)-2344, ASTIA Doc. 281 981, 1962.

20. ANNE, A., SAITO, M., SALATI, O. M. AND SCHWAN, H. P. Relative microwave absorption cross sections of biological radiation. *In: Biological Effects of Microwave Radiation.* Plenum Press, New York, pp. 153–176. 1960.

21. ARDAN, N. I., JANES, M. J. AND HERRICK, J. F. Changes in bone after exposure to ultrasonic energy. *Minn. Med., 37:* 415, 1954.

22. ARDAN, N. I., JANES, J. M. AND HERRICK, J. F. Ultrasonic energy and surgically produced defects in bone. *J.B.J.S., 39A:* 394–402, 1957.

23. ARON, H. C. S., CRAIG, R. M., FARMER, C. J., KENDELL, H. W. AND SCHWEMLEIN, G. X. Effect of elevated body temperature on plasma vitamin A and carotene. *Proc. Soc. Exp. Biol. Med., 61:* 271–276, 1946.

24. BACH, S. A. Biological sensitivity to radio-frequency and microwave energy. *Fed. Proc., 24:* suppl 14:S-22–S-26, 1965.

25. BACH, S. A., LUZZIO, A. J. AND BROWNELL, A. S. Effects of radio-frequency energy on human gamma globulin. *Proc. Fourth Ann. Tri-Serv. Conf. Biol. Effects Microwave Radiation, 1:* 117–133, 1960.

26. BACH, S. A., LUZZIO, A. J. AND BROWNELL, A. S. *J. Med. Electronics, 1:* 9, 1961.
27. BÄCKLUND, L. AND TISELIUS, P. Objective measurement of joint stiffness in rheumatoid arthritis. *Acta. Rheum. Scand., 13:* 275-288, 1967.
28. BALDES, E. J., HERRICK, J. F. AND STROEBEL, C. F. Biologic effects of ultrasound. *Am. J. Phys. Med., 37:* 111, 1958.
29. BARTH, G. AND BÜLOW, H. A. Zur Frage der Ultraschallschädigung jugendlicher Knochen. *Strahlentherapie, 79:* 271-280, 1949.
30. BARTH, G. AND KELLNER, K. Über den Wirkungsmechanismus biologischer Ultraschall-reaktionen; IV. Mitteilung; Versuche an Kaninchenextremitaten bei normaler und unterbundener Blutzirkulation. *Strahlentherapie, 81:* 654-658, 1950.
31. BASS, A. L. Treatment of muscle, tendon and minor joint injuries in sport. *Proc. Roy. Soc. Med., 62:* 925-928, 1969.
32. BAUWENS, P. AND SCOTT, B. O. The value of measurements in diathermy. *Ann. Phys. Med., 1:* 191-197, 1953.
33. BEARZY, H. J. Clinical applications of ultrasonic energy in the treatment of acute and chronic subacromial bursitis. *Arch. Phys. Med. Rehab., 34:* 228, 1953.
34. BENDER, L. F., JANES, J. M. AND HERRICK, J. F. Histologic studies following exposure of bone to ultrasound. *Arch. Phys. Med. Rehab., 35:* 555, 1954.
35. BENDER, L. F. AND NICK, C. Treatment of plantar warts with ultrasound: Report given at the American Congress of Physical Medicine and Rehabilitation. 40th Ann Session. *Arch. Phys. Med., 43:* 371, 1962.
36. BERGMANN, L. *Der Ultraschall und seine Anwendung in Wissenschaft und Technik.* S. Hirzel Verlag, 1949.
37. BICKFORD, R. H. AND DUFF, R. S. Influences of ultrasonic radiation on temperature and blood flow in the human skeletal muscle. *Circ. Res., 1:* 134, 1953.
38. BIERMAN, W. Ultrasound in the treatment of scars. *Arch. Phys. Med. Rehab., 35:* 209, 1954.
39. BIERMAN, W. AND HOROWITZ, E. A. A new vaginal diathermy electrode. *Arch. Phys. Ther., 17:* 15-16, 1956.
40. BISGARD, J. D. AND NYE, D. The influence of hot and cold application upon gastric and intestinal motor activity. *Surg. Gynecol. Obstet., 71:* 172-180, 1940.
41. BOLLINGER, J. N. Detection and evaluation of radiofrequency electromagnetic radiation-induced biological damage in Macaca mulatta. Southwest Research Inst., San Antonio, Texas, Final Report under contract F41609-70-C-0025, SWRI 05-2808-01, February 1971.
42. BOLLINGER, J. N. Induced biological damage in Macaca mulatta. Final report on detection and evaluation of radiofrequency electromagnetic radiation. USAF School of Aerospace Medicine (AFSC). Contract No. F41609-70-C0025. SWRI No. 05-2808-01, February, 1971.
43. BONICA, J. J. Management of myofascial pain syndromes in general practice. *J.A.M.A., 164:* 732, 1957.
44. BORN, H. Zur Frage der Absorptionsmessungen im Ultraschallgebiet. *Zeitschrift Phys., 120:* 383, 1943.
45. BORRELL, R. M., HENLEY, E. J., HO, P. AND HUBBELL, M. K. Fluidotherapy: evaluation of a new heat modality. *Arch. Phys. Med. Rehabil., 58:* 69-71, 1977.
46. BORRELL, R. M., PARKER, R., HENLEY, E. J., MASLEY, D. AND REPINECZ, M. Comparison of *in vivo* temperatures produced by hydrotherapy, paraffin wax treatment, and fluidotherapy. *Phys. Ther., 60:* 1273-1276, 1980.
47. BROWN, A. M. Physical medicine in athletic rehabilitation. *Maryland Med. J., 19:* 61-64, 1970.
48. BUCHTALA, V. Die Ultraschallwirkung auf den wachsenden Knochen. *Strahlentherapie, 78:* 127-142, 1948.
49. BUCHTALA, V. The present state of ultrasonic therapy. *Br. J. Phys. Med., 15:* 3, 1952.
50. BURDICK CORPORATION. *Burdick Syllabus.* Seventh edition. The Burdick Corporation, 1969.

51. BURRY, H. C. Late effects of neglected soft tissue injury. *Proc. Roy. Soc. Med.*, *62:* 930–932, 1969.
52. BURT, H. A. Heat in chronic rheumatic diseases. *In: Therapeutic Heat and Cold.* Licht, S. (ed). Second edition. Chapter 14. Waverly Press, Inc., Baltimore, pp. 387–397, 1965.
53. CAMERON, B. M. Experimental acceleration of wound healing. *Am. J. Orthoped.*, *3:* 336–343, 1961.
54. CARPENTER, R. L. AND VAN UMMERSON, C. A. The action of microwave power on the eye. *J. Microwave Power*, *3:* 3–19, 1968.
55. CARPENTER, R. L. Experimental microwave cataract: a review. *Proc Public Health Service Symp Biological Effects and Health Implications Microwave Radiation*, Bur Radiolog Health Dept., BRH/DBE 70-2, 1970.
56. CARSTENSEN, E. L., LI, K. AND SCHWAN, H. P. Determination of the acoustic properties of blood and its components. *J. Acoust. Soc. Am.*, *25:* 286–289, 1953.
57. CASTOR, C. W. AND YARON, M. Connective tissue activation: VIII. The effects of temperature studied *in vitro*. *Arch. Phys. Med. Rehabil.*, *57:* 5–9, 1976.
58. CHAN, A. K. SIGELMANN, R. A., GUY, A. W. AND LEHMANN, J. F. Calculation by the method of finite differences of the temperature distribution in layered tissues. *IEEE Trans. Biomed. Eng.*, *BME-20:* 86–90, 1973.
59. CHAN, A. K., SIGELMANN, R. A. AND GUY, A. W. Calculations of therapeutic heat generated by ultrasound in fat-muscle-bone layers. *IEEE Trans. Biomed. Eng.*, *BME-21:* 280–284, 1973.
60. CHATEAU, A. Quelques applications récentes en ultrasonthérapie. Les algies des amputés. *J. Radiol. Electrol.*, *32:* 513, 1951.
61. CLAFF, C. L. AND CRANE, C. Self-heating insulated sleeve to replace the conventional hot pack poultice. *Am. J. Surg.*, *81:* 695–697, 1951.
62. COAKLEY, W. T. Biophysical effects of ultrasound at therapeutic intensities. *Physiother.*, *64:* 166–169, 1978.
63. CODMAN, E. A. *The Shoulder.* T. Todd Co. Boston, 1934.
64. CONSTABLE, J. D., SCAPICCHIO, A. P. AND OPITZ, B. Studies of the effects of diapulse treatment of various aspects of wound healing in experimental animals. *J. Surg. Res.*, *11:* 254–257, 1971.
65. CORRADI, C. AND DEL MORO, V. M. Risultati di un biennio di ultrasuonoterapia nel campo ortopedico. *Arch. Orto.*, *66:* 52, 1953.
66. COVENTRY, M. B. Problem of painful shoulder. *J.A.M.A.*, *151:* 177, 1953.
67. CROCKFORD, G. W. AND HELLON, R. F. Vascular responses of human skin to infrared radiation. *J. Physiol.*, *149:* 424–432, 1959.
68. CROCKFORD, G. W., HELLON, R. F. AND PARKHOUSE, J. Thermal vasomotor responses in human skin mediated by local mechanisms. *J. Physiol.*, *161:* 10–20, 1962.
69. CURRIER, D. P., GREATHOUSE, D. AND SWIFT, T. Sensory nerve conduction: effect of ultrasound. *Arch. Phys. Med. Rehabil.*, *59:* 181–185, 1978.
70. DAELS, J. Microwave heating of the uterine wall during parturition. *Obstet. Gynecol.*, *42:* 76–79, 1973.
71. DAELS, J. Microwave heating of the uterine wall during parturition. *J. Microwave Power*, *11:* 166–168, 1976.
72. DAILY, L. E. A clinical study of the results of exposure of laboratory personnel to radar and high frequency radio. *U.S. Navy Med. Bull.*, *41:* 1052–1056, 1943.
73. DAILY, L. JR. AND BENEDICT, W. L. The effects of microwave diathermy on the eye of the rabbit. *Am. J. Ophthalmol.*, *35:* 1001, 1952.
74. DAILY, L. AND DAILY, R. K. Heat in diseases of the eye. *In: Therapeutic Heat and Cold.* Licht, S. (Ed) Second edition. Chapter 19. Waverly Press, Inc., Baltimore, pp. 491–501, 1965.
75. DAILY, L. JR., WAKIM, K. G., HERRICK, J. F., PARKHILL, E. M. AND BENEDICT, W. L. The effects of microwave diathermy on the eye. *Am. J. Ophthal.*, *33:* 1241–1254, 1950.

76. DAILY, L. JR., ZELLER, E. A., WAKIM, K. G., HERRICK, J. F. AND BENEDICT, W. L. Influence of microwaves on certain enzyme systems in the lens of the eye. *Am. J. Ophthal.*, *34:* 1301–1306, 1951.

77. DALICHO, W. A. Die Praxis der Kurzwellentherapie. *Handbuch Medizinischer Elektronik.* Frucht, A. H., Matauschek, J., and Kahl, W. (Eds). Berlin, Germany, pp. 521–591, Ch. 5, 1960.

78. DE FOREST, R. E., HERRICK, J. F., JANES, J. M. AND KRUSEN, F. H. Effects of ultrasound on growing bone: an experimental study. *Arch. Phys. Med.*, *34:* 21, 1953.

79. DE LATEUR, B. J., LEHMANN, J. F., STONEBRIDGE, J. B., WARREN, C. G., AND GUY, A. W. Muscle heating in human subjects with 915 MHz microwave contact applicator. *Arch. Phys. Med. Rehabil.*, *51:* 147–151, 1970.

80. DE LATEUR, B. J., STONEBRIDGE, J. B. AND LEHMANN, J. F. Fibrous muscular contractures: treatment with a new direct contact microwave applicator operating at 915 MHz. *Arch. Phys. Med. Rehabil.*, *59:* 488–490, 1978.

81. DEPREUX, T. Ultrasonic wave therapy of osteoarthritis of the hip joint. *Br. J. Phys. Med.*, *15:* 14, 1952.

82. DIETZEL, F. AND KERN, W. Kann hohes mütterliches Fieber beim Kind auslösen. Originalmitteilungen ist ausschliesslich der Verfasser verantwortlich. *Die Naturwissenschaften*, *2:* 24–26, 1971.

83. DIETZEL, F. AND KERN, W. Kann hohes mütterliches Fieber Missbildungen beim Kind auslösen? *Gerburtshilfe und Frauenheilkund*, *31:* 1074–1079, 1971.

84. DIETZEL, F., KERN, W. AND STECKENMESSER, R. Missbildungen und intrauterines Absterben nach Kurzwellenbehandlung in der Frühschwangerschaft. *Munch. Med. Wochenschr.*, *114:* 228–230, 1972.

85. DOYLE, J. R. AND SMART, B. W. Stimulation of bone growth by shortwave diathermy. *J.B.J.S.*, *45-A:* 15–24, 1963.

86. DUBOIS, E. L. Management of systemic lupus erythematosus. *Mod. Treatment, 3:* 1245–1279, 1966.

87. DUNN, F. Physical mechanisms of action of intense ultrasound on tissue. *Am. J. Phys. Med.*, *37:* 148, 1958.

88. DUNN, F. AND FRY, F. J. Ultrasonic threshold dosages for the mammalian central nervous system. *IEEE Trans. Biomed. Eng.*, *BME-18:* 253–256, 1971.

89. DYSON, M., FRANKS, C. AND SUCKLING, J. Stimulation of healing of varicose ulcers by ultrasound. *Ultrasonics*, *14:* 232–236, 1976.

90. DYSON, M. AND POND, J. B. The effect of pulsed ultrasound on tissue regeneration. *Physiother.*, *56:* 136–142, 1970.

91. DYSON, M., POND, J. B., JOSEPH J. AND WARWICK, R. The stimulation of tissue regeneration by means of ultrasound. *Clin. Sci.*, *35:* 273–285, 1968.

92. DYSON, M. AND SUCKLING, J. Stimulation of tissue repair by ultrasound: a survey of the mechanisms involved. *Physiother.*, *64:* 105–108, 1978.

93. DYSON, M. WOODWARD, B. AND POND, J. B. Flow of red blood cells stopped by ultrasound. *Nature*, *232:* 572–573, 1971.

94. EDHOLM, O. G., FOX, R. H. AND MACPHERSON, R. K. The effect of cutaneous anaesthesia on skin blood flow. *J. Physiol.*, *132:* 15P–16P, 1956.

95. EDWARDS, M. J. Congenital defects in guinea pigs. *Arch. Pathol.*, *84:* 42–48, 1967.

96. EDWARDS, M. J. Influenza, hyperthermia, and congenital malformation. *Lancet, 1:* 320–321, 1972.

97. EDWARDS, M. J., MULLEY, R., RING, S. AND WANNER, R. A. Mitotic cell death and delay of mitotic activity in guinea-pig embryos following brief maternal hyperthermia. *J. Embryol. Exp. Morph.*, *32:* 593–602, 1974.

98. ERDMAN, W. J. II. Peripheral blood flow measurements during application of pulsed high-frequency currents. *Am. J. Orth.*, *2:* 196–197, 1960.

99. ERDMAN, W. J. II AND STONER, E. K. Comparative heating effects of Moistaire and

Hydrocollator hot packs. *Arch. Phys. Med. Rehabil.*, *37:* 71–74, 1956.

100. EVANS, D. S. AND MENDELSSOHN, K. The physical basis of radiant heat therapy. *Proc. Roy. Soc. Med.*, *28:* 578–586, 1945.

101. FEDERAL COMMUNICATIONS COMMISSION. *Rules and Regulations.* Vol. 2, Sub-part A, Section 18.13, 1964.

102. FELLMANN, N. Behandlungsergebnisse mit einer kombinierten physikalischbalneologischen und sportlichen Behandlung bei der Spondylitis ankylopoetica. *Arch. Phys. Ther.*, *17:* 319–322, 1965.

103. FENN, J. E. Effect of pulsed electromagnetic energy (Diapulse) on experimental hematomas. *Canad. Med. Assoc. J.*, *100:* 251–254, 1969.

104. FINAL TECHNICAL REPORT ON RESEARCH PROJECT TO STUDY RADIATION HAZARDS CAUSED BY HIGH POWER, HIGH FREQUENCY FIELDS (Volume I, August 1969 to June 1971). Submitted by Ark Electronics Corporation, Willow Grove, Pennsylvania, to United States Information Agency, Washington D.C., Contract No. 1A–14121.

105. FISCHER, E. AND SOLOMON, S. Physiological responses to heat and cold. *In: Therapeutic Heat and Cold.* Licht, S. (Ed). Chapter 4, Second edition, Waverly Press, Baltimore, pp. 126–169, 1965.

106. FLAX, H. J. Ultrasound treatment of peritendinitis calcarea of the shoulder. *Am. J. Phys. Med.*, *43:* 117–124, 1964.

107. FLORY, P. J. AND GARRETT, R. R. Phase transitions in collagen and gelatin systems. *J. Am. Chem. Soc.*, *80:* 4836–4845, 1958.

108. FOLLIS, R. H. JR. Studies on the biological effect of high frequency radio waves (radar). *Am. J. Physiol.*, *147:* 281–283, 1946.

109. FOOD AND DRUG ADMINISTRATION, U.S. DHEW: Performance standard for microwave diathermy products. *Fed. Reg.*, *40:* 23877–23878, 1975.

110. FOOD AND DRUG ADMINISTRATION, U.S. DHEW Performance standards for sonic infrasonic, and ultrasonic radiation-emitting products. *Fed. Reg.*, *43:* 7166, 1978.

111. FORSYTHE, W. E. AND CHRISTIAN, F. Ultraviolet radiation from sun and heated tungsten. *J. Opt. Soc. Am.*, *20:* 396, 1930.

112. FOUNTAIN, F. P. GERSTEN, J. W. AND SENGIR, O. Decrease in muscle spasm produced by ultrasound, hot packs, and infrared radiation. *Arch. Phys. Med. Rehabil.*, *41:* 293–298, 1960.

113. FOX, R. H. AND HILTON, S. M. Bradykinin formation in human skin as a factor in heat vasodilatation. *J. Physiol.*, *142:* 219–232, 1958.

114. FRANCIS, W. L. The electrical properties of isolated frog skin. Part II. The relation of the skin potential to oxygen consumption and to the oxygen concentration of the medium. *J. Exp. Biol.*, *11:* 35–47, 1934.

115. FRANCIS, W. L. AND HUMPHREY, R. J. The electrical properties of isolated frog skin. Part I. Introductory. *J. Exp. Biol.*, *10:* 379–385, 1933.

116. FREEMAN, N. E. Influence of temperature on the development of gangrene in peripheral vascular disease. *Arch. Surg.*, *40:* 326–333, 1940.

117. FRIEDLAND, F. Ultrasonic therapy in rheumatic diseases. *J.A.M.A.*, *163:* 799, 1957.

118. FRY, W. J. Action of ultrasound on nerve tissue. A review. *J. Acoust. Soc. Am.*, *25:* 1, 1953.

119. FRY, W. J. Comments on a recent paper on cerebral ultrasonics. *Ultraschall. Med. Grenzgeb.*, *9:* 1, 1956.

120. FRY, W. J. Intensiver Ultraschall, ein Werkzeug der Neurologie. *Internat. Rundschau. Physikal. Med.*, *11:* 4, 1958.

121. FRY, W. J. Mechanism of acoustic absorption in tissue. *J. Acoust. Soc. Am.*, *24:* 412, 1952.

122. FRY, W. J. AND DUNN, F. Ultrasonic irradiation of the central nervous system at high sound levels. *J. Acoust. Soc. Am.*, *28:* 129, 1956.

123. FRY, W. J. AND FRY, R. B. Determination of absolute sound levels and acoustic absorption coefficients by thermocouple probes—experiment. *J. Acoust. Soc. Am.*, *26:* 311, 1954.

124. FRY, W. J., FRY, R. B. AND KELLY, P. Effects of high intensity ultrasound on the mechanical response of excised biceps muscle of the frog. *Physiologist, 2:* 3, 1959.
125. FRY, W. J., MEYERS, R. AND EGGLETON, R. C. The use of ultrasound in neurosurgery. *Proc. Third Internat. Conf. Med. Electronics.* London, 1960.
126. FRY, W. J., TUCKER, D., FRY, F. J. AND WULFF, V. J. Physical factors involved in ultrasonically induced changes in living systems. II. Amplitude duration relations and the effect of hydrostatic pressure for nerve tissue. *J. Acoust. Soc. Am., 23:* 364, 1951.
127. FRY, W. J., WULFF, V. J., TUCKER, D. AND FRY, F. J. Physical factors involved in ultrasonically induced changes in living systems. I. Identification of nontemperature effects. *J. Acoust. Soc. Am., 22:* 867, 1950.
128. GAMMON, G. D. AND STARR, I. Studies on the relief of pain by counterirritation. *J. Clin. Invest., 20:* 13–20, 1941.
129. GANONG, W. F. *The Nervous System.* Second edition. Lange, 1979.
130. GERSTEN, J. W. Changes in spinal cord thresholds following the application of ultrasound. Paper given at Fourth Annual Conference Amer. Instit. Ultrasonics in Med., Detroit, 1955.
131. GERSTEN, J. W. Effect of metallic objects on temperature rises produced in tissues by ultrasound. *Am. J. Phys. Med., 37:* 75, 1958.
132. GERSTEN, J. W. Effect of ultrasound on tendon extensibility. *Am. J. Phys. Med., 34:* 362–369, 1955.
133. GERSTEN, J. W. Ultrasonics and muscle disease. *Am. J. Phys. Med., 33:* 68, 1954.
134. GERSTEN, J. W., WAKIM, K. G., HERRICK, J. F. AND KRUSEN, F. H. The effect of microwave diathermy on the peripheral circulation and on tissue temperature in man. *Arch. Phys. Med., 30:* 7–25, 1949.
135. GHIETTI, A. Embriopatia da onde corte. *Minerva Nipiologica, 5:* 7–12, 1955.
136. GIBBON, J. H. JR. AND LANDIS, E. M. Vasodilatation in the lower extremities in response to immersing the forearms in warm water. *J. Clin. Invest., 11:* 1019–1036, 1932.
137. GINSBERG, A. J. Pulsed shortwave in the treatment of bursitis with calcification. *Internat. Rec. Med., 174:* 71–75, 1961.
138. GOSS, S. A. AND DUNN, F. Ultrasonic propagation properties of collagen. *Phys. Med. Biol., 25:* 827–837, 1980.
139. GOULD, R. K. Rectified diffusion in the presence of, and absence of acoustic streaming. *J. Acoust. Soc. Am., 56:* 1740–1746, 1974.
140. GRANT, R. T. AND HOLLING, H. E. Further observations on the vascular responses of the human limb to body warming; evidence for sympathetic vasodilator nerves in the normal subject. *Clin. Sci., 3:* 273–285, 1938.
141. GRYNBAUM, B. B. An evaluation of the clinical use of ultrasonics. *Am. J. Phys. Med., 33:* 75, 1954.
142. GUY, A. W. Analyses of electromagnetic fields induced in biological tissues by thermographic studies on equivalent phantom models. *IEEE, MTT-19:* 205–214, 1971.
143. GUY, A. W. Electromagnetic fields and relative heating patterns due to a rectangular aperture source in direct contact with bilayered biological tissue. *IEEE, MTT-19:* 214–223, 1971.
144. GUY, A. W. Quantitation of induced electromagnetic field patterns in tissue and associated biologic effects. Biologic Effects and Health Hazards of Microwave Radiation, Proceedings of an International Symposium, Warsaw, 15–18 October 1973; Polish Medical Publishers, Warsaw, pp. 203–216. 1974.
145. GUY, A. W. AND LEHMANN, J. F. Comparative evaluation of electromagnetic diathermy modalities in 433 MHz to 2450 MHz. 21st ACEMB - Shamrock Hilton Hotel, Houston, TX, Nov. 18–21, 1968.
146. GUY, A. W. AND LEHMANN, J. F. On the determination of an optimum microwave diathermy frequency for a direct contact applicator. *IEEE, BME-13:* 76–87, 1966.
147. GUY, A. W., LEHMANN, J. F. AND STONEBRIDGE, J. B. Therapeutic applications of

electromagnetic power. *Proc. IEEE, 62:* 55–75, 1974.

148. GUY, A. W., LEHMANN, J. F., STONEBRIDGE, J. B. AND SORENSEN, C. C. Development of a 915-MHz direct-contact applicator for therapeutic heating of tissues. *IEEE Trans. Microwave Theory Tech., MTT-26:* 550–556, 1978.

149. GUY, A. W., LIN, J. C., KRAMAR, P. O. AND EMERY, A. F. Effect of 2450-MHz radiation on the rabbit eye. *IEEE Trans. Microwave Theory Tech., MTT-23:* 492–498, 1975.

150. HALES, J. R. S. AND IRIKI, M. Differential thermal influences on skin blood flow through capillaries and arteriovenous anastomoses, and on sympathetic activity. *Bibl. Anat. (16 Pt 2):* 189–191, 1977.

151. HALLE, J. S., SCOVILLE, C. R. AND GREATHOUSE, D. G. Ultrasound's effect on the conduction latency of the superficial radial nerve in man. *Phys. Therapy, 61:* 345–350, 1981.

152. HANEL, R. Ein neues Messverfahren mit thermoelektrischer Sone für modulierten Ultraschall. *Ultraschall, 9:* 53, 1956.

153. HARDY, J. D., WOLFF, H. G. AND GOODELL, H. Studies on pain. A new method for measuring pain threshold: observations on spatial summation of pain. *J. Clin. Invest., 19:* 649–657, 1940.

154. HARELL, A., MUELLER, E. E. AND MEAD, S. Electrically heated hot packs. *Arch. Phys. Med., 32:* 211–218, 1951.

155. HARRIS, E. JR. AND KRANE, S. M. Cartilage collagen: substrate in soluble and fibrillar form for rheumatoid collagenase. *Trans. Assoc. Am. Phy., 86:* 82–94, 1973.

156. HARRIS, E. JR. AND McCROSKERY, P. A. The influence of temperature and fibril stability on degradation of cartilage collagen by rheumatoid synovial collagenase. *N. Engl. J. Med., 290:* 1–6, 1974.

157. HARRIS, R. Heat in vascular disorders. *In: Therapeutic Heat and Cold.* Licht, S. (Ed). Second Edition, Chapter 16. Waverly Press, Inc., Baltimore, pp. 407–432. 1965.

158. HARRIS, R. Physical methods in the management of rheumatoid arthritis. *Med. Clin. North. Am., 52:* 707–716, 1968.

159. HARRIS, R. The effect of various forms of physical therapy on radiosodium clearance from the normal and arthritic knee joint. *Ann. Phys. Med., 3:* 1–10, 1963.

160. HARVEY, M. A. S., McRORIE, M. M. AND SMITH, D. W. Suggested limits of exposure in the hot tub and sauna for the pregnant woman. *J. Canad. Med. Assoc., 125:* 50–53, 1981.

161. HARVEY, W., DYSON, M., POND, J. B. AND GRAHAME, R. The 'in vitro' stimulation of protein synthesis in human fibroblasts by therapeutic levels of ultrasound. Proc. Second Europ Cong on Ultrasound in Med. *Excerpta Med. Int. Cong. Series, 363:* 10–21, 1975.

162. HEDENIUS, P., ODEBLAD, E. AND WAHLSTRÖM, L. Some preliminary investigations on the therapeutic effect of pulsed shortwaves in intermittent claudication. *Curr. Ther. Res., 8:* 317–321, 1966.

163. HELLER, J. H. *Reticuloendothelial Structure and Function.* Chapt. 12. New York, The Roland Press Co., 1960.

164. HEMINGWAY, A. AND STENSTROM, K. W. Physical characteristics of shortwave diathermy. *Handbook of Phys Therap.* AMA Press, pp. 214–229, 1939.

165. HENDRICKX, A. G., STONE, G. W., HENRICKSON, R. V. AND MATAYOSHI, K. Teratogenic effects of hyperthermia in the bonnet monkey (*Macaca radiata*). *Tetratology, 19:* 177–182, 1979.

166. HERRICK, J. F. Temperatures produced in tissues by ultrasound: experimental study using various technics. *J. Acoust. Soc. Am., 25:* 12–16, 1953.

167. HERRICK, J. F., JANES, J. M. AND ARDAN, N. I. Experimental studies relative to the therapeutic use of ultrasound. *J. Am. Vet. Med. Assoc., 128:* 571, 1956.

168. HERRICK, J. F., JELATIS, D. G. AND LEE, G. M. Dielectric properties of tissues important in microwave diathermy. *Fed. Proc., 9:* 60, 1950.

169. HERRICK, J. F. AND KRUSEN, F. H. Certain physiologic and pathologic effects of microwaves. *Elec. Eng., 72:* 239–244, 1953.

170 HIGASHINO, S. The action of ultrasound on the neuromuscular junctions. *J. Cell. Comp. Physiol.*, 54: 251, 1959.

171. HINTZELMANN, U. Ultraschalltherapie rheumatischer Erkrankungen. *Deutsche Med. Wschr.*, 72: 350, 1947.

172. HINTZELMANN, U. Ultraschalltherapie rheumatischer Erkrankungen. *Deutsche Med. Wschr.*, 74: 869, 1949.

173. HO, H. S., GUY, A. W., SIGELMANN, R. A. AND LEHMANN, J. F. Electromagnetic heating patterns in circular cylindrical models of human tissue. Proc 8th Int Conf on Med and Biol Eng, Chicago, IL, Sess 27.4, 1969.

174. HO, H. S., GUY, A. W., SIGELMANN, R. A. AND LEHMANN, J. F. Microwave heating of simulated human limbs by aperture sources. *IEEE, MTT-19*: 224–231, 1971.

175. HO, H. S., SIGELMANN, R. A., GUY, A. W. AND LEHMANN, J. F. Electromagnetic heating of simulated human limbs by aperture sources. *Proc. 23rd Ann Conf on Eng in Med and Biol*, Washington D.C., pp. 159, 1970.

176. HÖBER, R. *Physikalische Chemie der Zellen und Gewebe.* Stämpfli & Cie, 1947.

177. HOLLANDER, J. L. AND HORVATH, S. M. The influence of physical therapy procedures on the intra-articular temperature of normal and arthritic subjects. *Am. J. Med. Sci.*, 218: 543–548, 1949.

178. HOLLANDER, J. L., STONER, E. K., BROWN, E. M. JR. AND deMOOR, P. Joint temperature measurement in the evaluation of anti-arthritic agents. *J. Clin. Invest.*, 30: 701–706, 1951.

179. HOLMANN, H. E. Das Problem der Behandlung biologischer Körper in ultrakurz-Wellen-Strahlungsfeld. Ultrakurz-wellen in ihren medizinische-biologischen Anwendungen. Leipzig, Germany, Thieme, Sec. 4, pp. 232–249, 1938.

180. HOLMAN, H. E. Zum Problem der ultrakurz Wellen Behandlung durch Austrahlung. *Strahlentherapie*, 64: 691–702, 1939.

181. HORVATH, S. M. AND HOLLANDER, J. L. Intra-articular temperature as a measure of joint reaction. *J. Clin. Invest.*, 28: 469–473, 1949.

182. HUETER, T. Messung der ultraschallabsorption in tierischen Geweben und ihre Abhängigkeit von der Frequenz. *Naturwissenschaften*, 35: 285, 1948.

183. HUETER, T. On the mechansim of biological effects produced by ultrasound. *Chem. Engin. Prog. Symp.*, 47: 57, 1951.

184. HUETER, T. Ultraschallwellen als neue therapeutische Energieform. *Ärztl Praxis, 1*: 2, 1949.

185. HUETER, T. AND BOLT, F. H. An ultrasonic method for outlining the cerebral ventricles. *J. Acoust. Soc. Am.*, 23: 160, 1951.

186. HUETER, T., DYER, J., LUDWIG, G. D. AND KYRAZIA, D. Thresholds of damage in nervous tissues. MIT Quart Prog Rept, October 1950.

187. HUF, E. Versuche über den Zusammenhang zwischen Stoffwechsel, potential Bildung und Funktion der Froschhaut. *Arch. ges. Physiol. (Pflügers)*, 235: 655, 1935.

188. HUF, E. Über aktiven Wasser- und Salztransport durch die Froschhaut. *Arch. ges. Physiol. (Pflügers)*, 237: 143, 1936.

189. HUF, E. Über den Anteil vitaler Kräfte bei der Resorption von Flüssigkeit durch die Froschhaut. *Arch. ges. Physiol., (Pflügers)* 236: 1–19, 1935.

190. HUNTER, J., KERR, E. H. AND WHILLANS, M. G. The relation between joint stiffness upon exposure to cold and the characteristics of synovial fluid. *Canad. J. Med. Sci.*, 30: 367–377, 1952.

191. HUSTLER, J. E., ZAROD, A. P. AND WILLIAMS, A. R. Ultrasonic modification of experimental bruising in the guinea-pig pinna. *Ultrasonics, 16*: 223–228, 1978.

192. HUTCHISON, W. J. AND BURDEAUX, B. D. The effects of shortwave diathermy on bone repair. *J.B.J.S., 33-A*: 155–165, 1951.

193. IMIG, C. J., RANDALL, B. F. AND HINES, H. M. Effect of ultrasonic energy on blood flow. *Am. J. Phys. Med.*, 53: 100–102, 1954.

194. JACKSON, D. W. AND FEAGIN, J. A. Quadriceps contusions in young athletes. *J.B.J.S., 55-*

A: 95–105, 1973.

195. JANES, J. M., DAHLEN, D. C., HERRICK, J. F. AND HIGGINS, G. M. The effect of ultrasonic energy on osteogenic sarcoma: an experimental study. *Arch. Phys. Med. Rehabil.*, *38:* 148–156, 1957.

196. JANES, J. M., HERRICK, J. F., KELLY, P. J. AND PETERSON, L. F. A. Long-term effect of ultrasonic energy on femora of the dog. *Proc. Staff. Meet. Mayo Clin.*, *35:* 663–671, 1960.

197. JOHNS, R. J. AND WRIGHT, V. Relative importance of various tissues in joint stiffness. *J. Appl. Physiol.*, *17:* 824–828, 1962.

198. JOHNSON, C. C. AND GUY, A. W. Nonionizing electromagnetic wave effects in biological materials and systems. *Proc. IEEE*, *66:* 692–718, 1972.

199. JONES, A. C. Clinical observations in the use of ultrasound. *Am. J. Phys. Med.*, *33:* 46, 1954.

200. JUSTESEN, D. R., RAGAN, H. A., ROGERS, L. E., GUY, A. W. HJERESEN, D. L. AND HINDS, W. T. Compilation and assessment of microwave bioeffects, AO–02–01/EA81028; final report: a selective review of the literature on biological effects of microwaves in relation to the satellite power system. For Division of Solar Energy, Department of Energy, contract no. EY-76-C-06-1830, May 1978.

201. KALAYADA, T. V. Biologic effects of radiation in 30–300 MHz range. *Proc. IEEE*, *60:* 389–421, 1972.

202. KAPLAN, E. G., AND WEINSTOCK, R. E. Clinical evaluation of diapulse as adjunctive therapy following foot surgery. *J. Am. Pod. Assoc.*, *58:* 218–221, 1968.

203. KENT, H. Plantar warts—treatment with ultrasound. *Arch. Phys. Med. Rehabil.*, *40:* 15–18, 1959.

204. KERSLAKE, D. McK. AND COOPER, K. E. Vasodilatation in the hand in response to heating the skin elsewhere. *Clin. Sci.*, *9:* 31–47, 1950.

205. KOTTKE, F. J. Heat in pelvic diseases. *In: Therapeutic Heat and Cold.* Licht, S. (Ed). Second edition, Chapter 18, Waverly Press, Baltimore, pp. 474–490. 1965.

206. KOTTKE, F. J., KOZA, D. W., KUBICEK, W. G. AND OLSON, M. Studies of deep circulatory response to short wave diathermy and microwave diathermy in man. *Arch. Phys. Med.*, *30:* 431–437, 1949.

207. KRASNY-ERGEN, W. *Hochfreq. techn. Elektroak.*, *49:* 195, 1937.

208. KRASNY-ERGEN, W. Nicht-thermische Wirkungen elektrischer Schwingungen auf Kolloide. *Hochfreq. Tech. Elektroak.*, *48:* 126–133, 1936.

209 KRUSEN, F. H. *Physical Medicine.* WB Saunders, Philadelphia, 1942.

210. KRUSEN, F. H. AND ELKINS, E. C. Investigations in fever therapy. *Arch. Phys. Ther.*, *20:* 77–84, *passim,* 1939.

211. KRUSEN, F. H., HERRICK, J. F., LEDEN, U. AND WAKIM, K. G. Microkymatotherapy: preliminary report of experimental studies of the heating effect of microwaves ("radar") in living tissues. *Proc. Staff. Meet. Mayo Clin.*, *22:* 209–224, 1947.

212. KUCIA, H. R. Accuracy limitation in measurements of HF field intensities for protection against radiation hazards. *IEEE Trans. Inst. Measurement*, *1M21(4):* 412–415, Nov. 1972.

213. KUCIA, H. R. Electromagnetic radiation safety in Poland. XVII th General Assembly of URS, Warsaw, Poland, *1:* 21–29, Aug. 1972.

214. KUHLER, E. Der Einfluss des Ultraschalls auf das Sudeck'sche Syndrom. *Strahlentherap.*, 87: 575, 1952.

215. KUITERT, J. H. Ultrasonic energy as an adjunct in the management of radiculitis and similar referred pain. *Am. J. Phys. Med.*, *33:* 61–65, 1954.

216. LAMBERT, E. H., TREANOR, W. J., HERRICK, J. F. AND KRUSEN, F. H. Comparative study of the effects of heat and ultrasound on nerve conduction. *Fed. Proc.*, *10:* 78, 1951.

217. LEDEN, U. M., HERRICK, J. F., WAKIM, G. K. AND KRUSEN, F. H. Preliminary studies on the heating and circulatory effects of micro-waves—"radar." *Br. J. Phys. Med.*, *10:* 177–184, 1947.

218. LEHMANN, J. Beitrag zur Ultraschallhämolyse. *Strahlentherapie*, 70: 533–542, 1950.

219. LEHMANN, J. F. Diathermy: *In: Handbook of Phys Med and Rehabil.* Krusen, F. H., Kottke, F. J. and Ellwood, P. M. Jr. (Eds). Second edition Chapter 11. WB Saunders, Philadelphia, pp. 273-345, 1971.

220. LEHMANN, J. F. Die Therapie mit Ultraschall und ihre Grundlagen. *In: Ergebnisse physikalischdiätetischen Therapie.* Verlag Steinkopff. Dresden, 1951.

221. LEHMANN, J. F. The biophysical basis of biologic ultrasonic reactions with special reference to ultrasonic therapy. *Arch. Phys. Med. Rehabil., 34:* 139-152, 1953.

222. LEHMANN, J. F. The biophysical mode of action of biologic and therapeutic ultrasonic reactions. *J. Acoust. Soc. Am., 25:* 17-25, 1953.

223. LEHMANN, J. F. The present status of ultrasonic therapy. *Arch. Phys. Med. Rehabil., 34:* 741-749, 1953.

224. LEHMANN, J. F. AND KRUSEN, F. H. Therapeutic application of ultrasound in physical medicine. *Am. J. Phys. Med., 37:* 173-183, 1958.

225. LEHMANN, J. F. Über die Temperaturabhängigkeit therapeutsicher Ultraschallreaktionen und der besonderer Berücksichtigung der Wirkung auf Nerven. *Strahlentherap, 79:* 543, 1950.

226. LEHMANN, J. F. Unpublished data.

227. LEHMANN, J. F., BALDES, E. AND KRUSEN, F. H. Destructive effects of high intensity on plant tissues. *In: Ultrasound in Biology and Medicine.* Kelly, E. (Ed). American Institute of Biological Sciences, Washington, 1957.

228. LEHMANN, J. F., BALDES, E. J. AND KRUSEN, F. H. Effects of ultrasound of high intensity on cellular structures. *Arch. Phys. Med. Rehabil., 37:* 90-95, 1956.

229. LEHMANN, J. F., BECKER, G. AND JAENICKE, W. Über die Wirkung von Ultraschallwellen auf den Ionendurchtritt durch biologische Membranen als Beitrag zur Theorie des therapeutischen Wirkungmechanismus. *Strahlentherap, 83:* 311, 1950.

230. LEHMANN, J. F., BECKER, G. AND OTTO, J. Thermische und mechanische Wirkungen des Ultraschalles auf einzelne Zellen. Untersucht am Beispiel der eosinophilen Leucocyten. *Strahlentherap., 87:* 411, 1954.

231. LEHMAN, J. F. AND BIEGLER, R. Changes of potentials and temperature gradients in membranes caused by ultrasound. *Arch. Phys. Med. Rehabil., 35:* 287-295, 1954.

232. LEHMANN, J. F., BRUNNER, G. D., MARTINIS, A. J. AND McMILLAN, J. A. Ultrasonic effects as demonstrated in live pigs with surgical metallic implants. *Arch. Phys. Med. Rehabil., 40:* 483-488, 1959.

233. LEHMANN, J. F., BRUNNER, G. D. AND McMILLAN, J. A. The influence of surgical implants on the temperature distribution in thigh specimens exposed to ultrasound. *Arch. Phys. Med. Rehab., 39:* 692, 1958.

234. LEHMANN, J. F., BRUNNER, G. D., McMILLAN, J. A., SILVERMAN, D. R. AND JOHNSON V. C. Modification of heating patterns produced by microwaves at the frequencies of 2456 and 900 mc. by physiologic factors in the human. *Arch. Phys. Med. Rehabil., 45:* 555-563, 1964.

235. LEHMANN, J. F., BRUNNER, G. D. AND STOW, R. W. Pain threshold measurements after therapeutic application of ultrasound, microwaves, and infrared. *Arch. Phys. Med. Rehabil., 39:* 560-565, 1958.

236. LEHMANN, J. F. AND DELATEUR, B. J. Heat and cold in the treatment of arthritis. *In: Arthritis and Physical Medicine,* Licht, S. (Ed). Chapter 14. Waverly Press, Baltimore, pp. 315-378, 1969.

237. LEHMANN, J. F., DELATEUR, B. J. AND SILVERMAN, D. R. Selective heating effects of ultrasound in human beings. *Arch. Phys. Med. Rehabil. 47:* 331-339, 1966.

238. LEHMANN, J. F., DELATEUR, B. J. AND STONEBRIDGE, J. B. Heating patterns produced in humans by 433.92 MHz round field applicator and 915 MHz contact applicator. *Arch. Phys. Med. Rehabil., 56:* 442-448, 1975.

239. LEHMANN, J. F., DELATEUR, B. J. AND STONEBRIDGE, J. B. Selective muscle heating by shortwave diathermy with a helical coil. *Arch. Phys. Med. Rehabil., 50:* 117-123, 1969.

240. LEHMANN, J. F., DELATEUR, B. J., STONEBRIDGE, J. B. AND WARREN, C. G. Therapeutic temperature distribution produced by ultrasound as modified by dosage and volume of tissue exposed. *Arch. Phys. Med. Rehabil.*, 48: 662–666, 1967.

241. LEHMANN, J. F., DELATEUR, B. J., WARREN, C. G. AND STONEBRIDGE, J. B. Heating of joint structures by ultrasound. *Arch. Phys. Med. Rehabil.*, 49: 28–30, 1968.

242. LEHMANN, J. F., DUNDORE, D. AND ESSELMAN, P. Unpublished data.

243. LEHMANN, J. F., ERICKSON, D. J., MARTIN, G. M. AND KRUSEN, F. H. Comparison of ultrasonic and microwave diathermy in the physical treatment of peri-arthritis of the shoulder. *Arch. Phys. Med. Rehabil.*, 35: 627–634, 1954.

244. LEHMANN, J. F. AND FEISSEL, H. J. Inwieweit lässt sich die Ultraschall-Leistung durch Zufuhr von Wärmeenergie in ihrer biologischen Wirkung ersetzen? *Strahlentherap.*, 85: 615, 1951.

245. LEHMANN, J. F. AND FEISSEL, H. J. Über die Abhangigkeit biologischer Ultraschallreaktionen von der Teilchenamplitude als Beitrag zum therapeutischen Wirkungsmechanismus. *Strahlentherap.*, 82: 293, 1950.

246. LEHMANN, J. F., FORDYCE, W. E., RATHBUN, L. A., LARSON, R. E. AND WOOD, D. H. Clinical evaluation of a new approach in the treatment of contracture associated with hip fracture after internal fixation. *Arch. Phys. Med. Rehabil.*, 42: 95, 1961.

247. LEHMANN, J. F. AND GUY, A. W. Ultrasound therapy. *In: Interaction of Ultrasound and Biological Tissues.* Reid, J. M. and Sikov, M. R. (Eds). Proceedings of a workshop held at Battelle Seattle Research Center 11/8/71 to 11/11/71, DHEW Pub (FDA) 73–8008, Session 3:8, pp. 141–152, 1971.

248 LEHMANN, J. F., GUY, A. W., DELATEUR, B. J., STONEBRIDGE, J. B. AND WARREN, C. G. Heating patterns produced by short-wave diathermy using helical induction coil applicators. *Arch. Phys. Med. Rehabil.*, 49: 193–198, 1968.

249. LEHMANN, J. F., GUY, A. W., JOHNSTON, V. C., BRUNNER, G. D. AND BELL, J. W. Comparison of relative heating patterns produced in tissues by exposure to microwave energy at frequencies of 2,450 and 900 megacycles. *Arch. Phys. Med. Rehabil.*, 43: 69–76, 1962.

250. LEHMANN, J. F., GUY, A. W., STONEBRIDGE, J. B. AND DELATEUR, B. J. Evaluation of a therapeutic direct-contact 915-MHz microwave applicator for effective deep-tissue heating in humans. *IEEE Trans. Microwave Theory Tech.*, MTT-26: 556–563, 1978.

251. LEHMANN, J. F., GUY, A. W., STONEBRIDGE, J. B. AND WARREN, C. G. Review of evidence for indications, techniques of application, contraindications, hazards, and clinical effectiveness of shortwave diathermy. Report No. FDA/HFK-75-1, to Office of DHEW/Public Health Service, Food and Drug Administration, 1/1/74 to 12/31/74, Contract No. FDA 74–32.

252. LEHMANN, J. F., GUY, A. W., WARREN, C. G., DELATEUR, B. J. AND STONEBRIDGE, J. B. Evaluation of microwave contact applicator. *Arch. Phys. Med. Rehabil.*, 51: 143–147, 1970.

253. LEHMANN, J. F. AND HERRICK, J. F. Biologic reactions to cavitation, a consideration for ultrasonic therapy. *Arch. Phys. Med. Rehabil.*, 34: 86–98, 1953.

254. LEHMANN, J. F., HERRICK, J. F. AND KRUSEN, F. H. The effects of ultrasound on chromosomes, nuclei and other structures of the cells in plant tissue. *Arch. Phys. Med. Rehabil.*, 35: 141–148, 1954.

255. LEHMANN, J. AND HOHLFELD, R. Der Gewebestoffwechsel nach Ultraschall und Wärmeeinwirkung. *Strahlentherapie*, 87: 544–549, 1952.

256. LEHMANN, J. F. AND JOHNSON, E. W. Some factors influencing the temperature distribution in thighs exposed to ultrasound. *Arch. Phys. Med. Rehabil.*, 39: 347–356, 1958.

257. LEHMANN, J. F., JOHNSTON, V. C., MCMILLAN, J. A., SILVERMAN, D. R., BRUNNER, G. D. AND RATHBUN, L. A. Comparison of deep heating by microwaves at frequencies 2456 and 900 megacycles. *Arch. Phys. Med. Rehabil.*, 46: 307–314, 1965.

258. LEHMANN, J. F. AND KRUSEN, F. H. Biophysical effects of ultrasonic energy on carcinoma

and their possible significance. *Arch. Phys. Med. Rehabil.*, *36*: 452–459, 1955.

259. LEHMANN, J. F. AND KRUSEN, F. H. Effect of pulsed and continuous application of ultrasound on transport of ions through biologic membranes. *Arch. Phys. Med. Rehabil.*, *35*: 20–23, 1954.

260. LEHMANN, J. F., KRUSEN, F. H., ERICKSON, D. AND MARTIN, G. The present value of ultrasonic diathermy. *J.A.M.A.*, *157*: 996, 1955.

261. LEHMANN, J. F., LANE, C. E., BELL, J. W. AND BRUNNER, G. D. Influence of surgical metal implants on the distribution of the intensity in the ultrasonic field. *Arch. Phys. Med. Rehabil.*, *39*: 756–760, 1958.

262. LEHMANN, J. F., MASOCK, A. J., WARREN, C. G. AND KOBLANSKI, J. N. Effect of therapeutic temperatures on tendon extensibility. *Arch. Phys. Med. Rehabil.*, *51*: 481–487, 1970.

263. LEHMANN, J. F., McMILLAN, J. A., BRUNNER, G. D. AND BLUMBERG, J. B. Comparative study of the efficiency of shortwave, microwave and ultrasonic diathermy in heating the hip joint. *Arch. Phys. Med. Rehabil.*, *40*: 510–512, 1959.

264. LEHMANN, J. F., McMILLAN, J. A., BRUNNER, G. D. AND GUY, A. W. A comparative evaluation of temperature distributions produced by microwaves at 2,456 and 900 megacycles in geometrically complex specimens. *Arch. Phys. Med. Rehabil.*, *43*: 502–507, 1962.

265. LEHMANN, J. F., McMILLAN, J. A., BRUNNER, G. D. AND JOHNSTON, V. C. Heating patterns produced in specimens by microwaves of the frequency of 2,456 megacycles when applied with the "A", "B" and "C" directors. *Arch. Phys. Med. Rehabil.*, *43*: 538–546, 1962.

266. LEHMANN, J. F. AND NITSCH, W. Über die Frequenzabhängigkeit biologischer Ultraschallreaktionen mit besonderer Berücksichtigung der spezifischen Temperaturverteilung im Organismus. *Strahlentherap.*, *85*: 606, 1951.

267. LEHMANN, J. F., SILVERMAN, D. R., BAUM, B. A., KIRK, N. L. AND JOHNSTON, V. C. Temperature distributions in the human thigh, produced by infrared, hot pack and microwave applications. *Arch. Phys. Med. Rehabil.*, *47*: 291–299, 1966.

268. LEHMANN, J. F., STONEBRIDGE, J. B., DELATEUR, B. J., WARREN, C. G. AND HALAR, E. Temperatures in human thighs after hot pack treatment followed by ultrasound. *Arch. Phys. Med. Rehabil.*, *59*: 472–476, 1978.

269. LEHMANN, J. F., STONEBRIDGE, J. B. AND GUY, A. W. A comparison of patterns of stray radiation from therapeutic microwave applicators measured near tissue substitute models and human subjects. *Radio Sci.*, *14*: 271–283, 1979.

270. LEHMANN, J. F., STONEBRIDGE, J. B., WALLACE, J. E., WARREN, C. G. AND GUY, A. W. Microwave therapy: stray radiation, safety and effectiveness. *Arch. Phys. Med. Rehabil.*, *60*: 578–584, 1979.

271. LEHMANN, J. F. AND WALLACE, J. Development of new phantom material for testing diathermy applicators. Progress Report, National Institute of Handicapped Research Grant, 16-P56818–18, Rehabilitation Research and Training Center, University of Washington, School of Medicine, Seattle, WA 4/1/79 to 3/31/80: project number R-135, pp. 175–180, 1980.

272. LEHMANN, J. F., WARREN, C. G. AND GUY, A. W. Therapy with continuous wave ultrasound. *In: Ultrasound: Its Applications in Medicine and Biology*. Fry, F. J. (Ed). Vol. 3 of Methods and Phenomena: Their applications in science and technology, part II. Elsevier, Chapter 10, pp. 561–587, 1978.

273. LEHMANN, J. F., WARREN, C. G. AND SCHAM, S. M. Therapeutic heat and cold. *Clin. Orthop.*, *(99)*: 207–245, 1974.

274. LEVY, H. Pulsed shortwaves in sinus and allied conditions in childhood. *Western Med.*, 2: 246, 1961.

275. LIDMAN, B. I. AND COHN, C. Effect of radar emanations on the hematopoietic system. *Air Surg. Bull.*, 2: 448–449, 1945.

276. LOTA, M. J. Electronic plethysmographic and tissue temperature studies of effect of

ultrasound on blood flow. *Arch. Phys. Med. Rehabil.*, *46:* 315–322, 1965.

277. LOTA, M. J. AND DARLING, R. C. Change in permeability of the red blood cell membrane in a homogeneous ultrasonic field. *Arch. Phys. Med. Rehabil.*, *36:* 282–287, 1955.

278. LUND, E. J. Relation between continuous bio-electric currents and cell respiration II. *J. Exp. Zool.*, *51:* 265–290, 1928.

279. LUND, E. J. Relation between continuous bio-electric currents and cell respiration III. *J. Exp. Zool.*, *51:* 291–307, 1928.

280. LUZES, F. Contribution au traitement de l'herpes zoster par les ultrasons. *Acta Physiother. Rheum. Belg.*, *7:* 354–356, 1952.

281. MacINTOSH, I. J. C., AND DAVEY, D. A. Chromosome aberrations induced by an ultrasonic fetal pulse detector. *Br. Med. J.*, *4:* 92–93, 1970.

282. MacINTOSH, I. J. C. AND DAVEY, D. A. Relationship between intensity of ultrasound and induction of chromosome aberrations. *Br. J. Radiol.*, *45:* 320–327, 1972.

283. MACKANESS, S. B. The effect of diapulse treatment on acute and chronic bacterial infections in mice. Final report and addendum submitted to the Food and Drug Administration, Jan 23, 1967.

284. MADSEN, P. W. AND GERSTEN, J. W. The effect of ultrasound on conduction velocity of peripheral nerve. *Arch. Phys. Med. Rehabil.*, *42:* 645–649, 1961.

285. MAINTZ, G. Tierexperimentelle Untersuchungen über die Wirkung der Ultraschallwellen auf die Knochenregeneration. *Strahlentherapie*, *82:* 631–638, 1950.

286. MAREK, J., JEZDINSKÝ, J. AND OCHONSKÝ, P. Effects of local cold and heat therapy on traumatic oedema of the rat hind paw; II. Effects of various kinds of compresses on the course of traumatic oedema. *Acta. Univ. Olomuc. Fac. Med.*, *66:* 203–228, 1973.

287. MAREK, J., JEZDINSKÝ, J. AND OCHONSKÝ, P. Effects of local cold and heat therapy on traumatic oedema of the rat hind paw: III. The effect of heat radiation on the course of traumatic oedema. *Acta Univ. Olomuc. Fac. Med.*, *70:* 149–160, 1974.

288. MARHA, K. MUSIL, J. AND TUHA, H. *Electromagnetic Fields Life Environment.* San Francisco Press, Inc., San Francisco, 1971.

289. MARTIN, G. M., ROTH, G. M., ELKINS, E. C. AND KRUSEN, F. H. Cutaneous temperature of the extremities of normal subjects and of patients with rheumatoid arthritis. *Arch. Phys. Med.*, *27:* 665, 1946.

290. MASON, P. AND RIGBY, B. J. Thermal transitions in collagen. *Biochim. Biophys. Acta.*, *66:* 448–450, 1963.

291. MATTHES, K. AND RECH, W. *Der Ultraschall in der Medizin.* S. Hirzel Verlag, Zürich, 1949.

292. McGEE, M. AND FRESHMAN, S. Ultrasound and stretch: a treatment for decreased range of motion. A slide-tape presentation, Health Sciences Learning Resources Center, University of Washington, 1978.

293. MELZACK, R. AND WALL, P. D. Pain mechanisms: a new theory: *Science, 150:* 971–979, 1965.

294. MENSE, S. Effects of temperature on the discharges of muscle spindles and tendon organs. *Plfügers Arch.*, *374:* 159–166, 1978.

295. MENSER, M. Does hyperthermia affect the human fetus? *Med. J. Austral.*, *2:* 550, 1978.

296. MICHAELSON, S. M. Human exposure to nonionizing radiant energy—potential hazards and safety standards. *Proc. IEEE, 60:* 389–421, 1972.

297. MICHAËLSSON, G. AND ROS, A. M. Familial localized heat urticaria of delayed type. *Acta Dermatovener, 51:* 279–283, 1971.

298. MICROWAVE NEWS. Comments on the proposed BRH/FDA standard for diathermy products. *Microwave News, February* 4, 1981.

299. MOAYER, M. die morphologischen Veränderungen der Plazenta unter dem Einfluss der Kurzwellendurchflutung. Tierexperimentelle Untersuchungen. *Strahlentherapie, 142:* 609–614, 1971.

300. MOLANDER, C. O. Physiologic basis of heat. *Arch. Phys. Ther.*, *22:* 335–340 *passim,* 1941.

301. MONCUR, J. A. Ultrasonic therapy in rehabilitation. A supplement to active exercise. *Br. J. Phys. Med., 20:* 25, 1957.

302. MOOR, F. B. Microwave diathermy. *In: Therapeutic Heat and Cold.* Licht, S. (Ed). Second edition, Chapter 12. Waverly Press, Baltimore, pp. 310–320, 1965.

303. MOORE, J. L. AND COAKLEY, W. T. Ultrasonic treatment of Chinese hamster cells at high intensities and long exposure times. *Br. J. Radiol., 50:* 46–50, 1977.

304. MORRISSEY, L. J. Effect of pulsed short-wave diathermy upon volume blood flow through the calf of the leg. Plethysmographic studies. *J. Am. Phys. Ther. Assoc., 46:* 946–952, 1966.

305. MORTIMER, A. J., ROY, O. Z., TAICHMAN, G. C., KEON, W. J. AND TROLLOPE, B. J. The effects of ultrasound on the mechanical properties of rat cardiac muscle. *Ultrasonics, 16:* 179–182, 1978.

306. MUELLER, E. E., MEAD, S., SCHULZ, B. F. AND VADEN, M. R. A placebo-controlled study of ultrasound treatment for periarthritis. *Am. J. Phys. Med., 33:* 31–35, 1954.

307. MUSSA, B. Embriopatie da cause fisiche. *Minerva Nipiologica, 5:* 69–72, 1955.

308. NADASDI, M. Inhibition of experimental arthritis by athermic pulsing shortwave in rats. *Am. J. Orthop., 2:* 105–107, 1960.

309. NAGELSCHMIDT, F. A new method of applying heat by diathermy. *Proc. Second. Internat. Cong. Light Heat.* London, 1928.

310. NAGELSCHMIDT, F. *Lehrbuch der Diathermie.* Berlin, 1913.

311. NARENDRANATH, R. AND KIRACOFE, G. H. Effects of heat-stress in rats. I. Critical period and reduced survival of post-implantation heat-stress inducted in early gestation. *Indian J. Physiol. Pharmac., 19:* 135–139, 1975.

312. NARENDRANATH, R. AND KIRACOFE, G. H. Effects of heat-stress in rats. II. Factor(s) responsible for reduced embryonic and/or foetal survival percentage. *Indian J. Physiol. Pharmac., 19:* 140–145, 1975.

313. NELSON, P. A., HERRICK, J. F. AND KRUSEN, F. H. Temperatures produced in bone marrow, bone and adjacent tissues by ultrasonic diathermy. *Arch. Phys. Med., 31:* 687–695, 1950.

314. NEWMAN, M. K., KILL, M. AND FRAMPTON, G. Effects of ultrasound alone and combined with hydrocortisone injections by needle or hypospray. *Am. J. Phys. Med., 37:* 206, 1958.

315. NEWMAN, M. K., AND MURPHY, A. Application of ultrasonics in chronic rheumatic diseases. *J. Mich. St. Med. Soc., 51:* 1211, 1952.

316. O'BRIEN, W. D. JR. AND DUNN, F. Ultrasonic absorption by biomacromolecules. Session 1.1. *In: Interaction of Ultrasound and Biological Tissues.* Reid, J. M., Sikov, M. R. (Eds). Proceedings of a workshop held at Battelle Seattle Research Center 11/8/71 to 11/11/71, DHEW Pub (FDA) 73-8008. pp. 13–19, 1971.

317. ODERMANN, E. Die Ultraschallbehandlung rheumatischer Krankheiten am Landesbad Aachen. *Med. Klin., 46:* 329, 1951.

318. O'DONOGHUE, D. H. General principles involved in the treatment of injuries to athletes. *Med. Times, 87:* 1246–1260, 1959.

319. O'DONOGHUE, D. H. Principles in the management of specific injuries. *In: Treatment of Injuries to Athletes.* Third edition. WB Saunders, Philadelphia, pp. 47–50, 1976.

320. PARONI, F. Die Ultraschall-Therapie beim Tropengeschwür. *Arch. Radiol. (Rome), 270:* 14, 1955.

321. PASILA, M., VISURI, T. AND SUNDHOLM, A. Pulsating shortwave diathermy: valuable in treatment of recent ankle and foot sprains. *Arch. Phys. Med. Rehabil., 59:* 383–386, 1978.

322. PÄTZOLD, J. AND BORN, H. Behandlung biologischer Gewebe mit gebündeltem Ultraschall. *Strahlentherap., 76:* 486, 1947.

323. PAUL, B. J., LAFRATTA, C. W., DAWSON, A. R., BAAB, E. AND BULLOCK, F. Use of ultrasound in the treatment of pressure sores in patients with spinal cord injury. *Arch. Phys. Med. Rehabil., 41:* 438–440, 1960.

324. PAUL, W. D. AND IMIG, C. J. Temperature and blood flow studies after ultrasonic

irradiation. *Am. J. Phys. Med., 34:* 370–375, 1955.

325. PAULY, H. AND HUG, O. Untersuchungen über den Einfluss von Ultraschallwellen und von Wärme auf den Stoffwechsel überlebender Gewebe. *Strahlentherap., 95:* 116, 1954.

326. PAZDEROVA, J. Blood proteins in personnel of T.V. and radio transmitting stations. Biologic effects and health hazards of microwave radiation. Proc. of an International Symposium, Warsaw, Polish Medical Publishers, pp. 281–287, Oct. 15–18, 1973.

327. PETAJAN, J. H. AND EAGAN, C. J. Effect of temperature, exercise, and physical fitness on the triceps surae reflex. *J. Appl. Physiol., 25:* 16–20, 1968.

328. PICKERING, G. W. The vasomotor regulation of heat loss from the human skin in relation to external temperature. *Heart, 16:* 115–135, 1932.

329. POHLMAN, R. *Die Ultraschalltherapie.* Georg Thieme Verlag, Stuttgart, 1951.

330. POLLEY, H. F. Physical treatment of arthritis. In: *Medicine and Rehabilitation for the Clinician,* Krusen, F. H. (Ed). WB Saunders, Philadelphia, 1951.

331. PRESSMAN, A. S. *Electromagnetic Fields Life.* Plenum Press, New York, 1970.

332. RADIATION CONTROL FOR HEALTH AND SAFETY ACT. Public Law 90–602.

333. RAE, J. W. JR., HERRICK, J. F., WAKIM, K. G. AND KRUSEN, F. H. A comparative study of the temperatures produced by microwave and shortwave diathermy. *Arch. Phys. Med., 30:* 199–211, 1949.

334. RAE, J. W., MARTIN, G. M., TREANOR, W. J. AND KRUSEN, F. H. Clinical experience with microwave diathermy. *Proc. Staff Meet. Mayo Clin., 24:* 441, 1950.

335. RANDALL, L. M. AND KRUSEN, F. H. A consideration of the Elliott treatment of pelvic inflammatory disease of women. *Arch. Phys. Ther., 18:* 283–287, 1937.

336. REESE, E. P., KINNISON, D. M. AND JACOBUS, H. J. Observations and evaluation of ultrasonic therapy in treatment of arthritis. Paper read at Third Annual Conference, Amer. Instit. Ultrasonics in Medicine, Washington, 1954.

337. REIDER, D. R., EPSTEIN, D. L. AND KRIK, J. H. Possible cataractogenic effects of radiofrequency radiation. *Aeromed. Rev.* ADH 730922, 1971.

338. RICHARDSON, A. W. Effect of microwave-induced heating on the blood flow through peripheral skeletal muscles. *Am. J. Phys. Med., 33:* 103–107, 1954.

339. RICHARDSON, A. W. The effectiveness of microwave diathermy therapy as a hyperthermic agent upon vascularized and avascular tissue. *Br. J. Phys. Med. 18:* 143–149, 1955.

340. RICHARDSON, A. W., DUANE, T. D. AND HINES, H. M. Experimental lenticular opacities produced by microwave irradiation. *Arch. Phys. Med., 29:* 765–769, 1948.

341. RICHARDSON, A. W., LOMAX, D. H., NICHOLS, J. AND GREEN, H. D. The role of energy, pupillary diameter, and alloxan diabetes in the production of ocular damage by microwave irradiations. *Am. J. Ophthal., 35:* 993–1000, 1952.

342. ROBBINS, S. L. *Pathology.* Vol 1. Third edition. WB Saunders, Philadelphia, 1967.

343. RODDIE, I. C., SHEPHERD, J. T. AND WHELAN, R. F. Evidence from venous oxygen saturation measurements that the increase in forearm blood flow during body heating is confined to the skin. *J. Physiol., 134:* 444–450, 1956.

344. ROMERO-SIERRA, C. AND TANNER, J. A. Biological effects of nonionizing radiation: An outline of fundamental laws. *Ann. N.Y. Acad. Sci., 238:* 263–272, 1974.

345. ROSENBERGER, H. Über den Wirkungsmechanismus der Ultraschallbehandlung, insbesondere bei Ischias und Neuralgien. *Der Chirurg., 21:* 404, 1950.

346. RUBIN, A. AND ERDMAN, W. J. Microwave exposure of the human female pelvis during early pregnancy and prior to conception. *Am. J. Phys. Med., 38:* 219–220, 1959.

347. RUBIN, D. AND KUITERT, J. Use of ultrasonic vibration in the treatment of pain arising from phantom limbs, scars and neuromas. *Arch. Phys. Med. Rehab., 35:* 445, 1955.

348. SAITO, M. AND SCHWAN, H. P. Cited by Schwan (353).

349. SAITO, M. AND SCHWAN, H. P. The time constants of pearl-chain formation. Biological Effects of Microwave Radiation. *Proc. Fourth Ann. Triservice Conf. Biol. Effects of Microwave Radiation, 1:* 85–97, Plenum Press, New York, 1961.

350. SANDLER, B. Heat and the I.U.C.D. *Br. Med. J.*, *25:* 458, 1973.

351. SCHWAN, H. P Alternating current spectroscopy of biological substances. *Proc. IRE, 47:* 1841–1855, 1959.

352. SCHWAN, H. P. Absorption and energy transfer of microwaves and ultra sound in tissues: characteristics *In: Medical Physics.* Vol. III. Glaser O. (Ed). The Year Book Publishers, Inc., Chicago, pp. 1–7, 1960.

353. SCHWAN, H. P. Biophysics of diathermy. *In: Therapeutic Heat and Cold.* Licht, S. (Ed). Second edition, Chapter 3, Waverly Press, Baltimore, pp. 63–125, 1965.

354. SCHWAN, H. P. Electrical properties of tissues and cells. *Advan. Biol. Med. Phys., 5:* 147–209, 1957.

355. SCHWAN, H. P. Survey of microwave absorption characteristics of body tissues. *Proc. Second Tri-Serv. Conf. Biol. Effects of Microwave Energy,* 126–145, 1958.

356. SCHWAN, H. P. AND PIERSOL, G. M. The absorption of electromagnetic energy in body tissues. Part 1, Biophysical aspects. *Am. J. Phys. Med. 33:* 371–404, 1954.

357. SCHWAN, H. P. AND PIERSOL, G. M. The absorption of electromagnetic energy in body tissues. Part II, Physiological and clinical aspects. *Am. J. Phys. Med., 34:* 425–448, 1955.

358. SCHWARTZ, F. The value of ultrasonics in physical medicine. *Am. J. Phys. . Med., 33:* 38, 1954.

359. SCOTT, B. O. Effect of contact lenses on shortwave field distribution. *Br. J. Ophthal., 40:* 696–697, 1956.

360. SCOTT, B. O. Short wave diathermy. *In: Therapeutic Heat and Cold.* Licht, S. (Ed). Second edition, Chapter 11. Waverly Press, Baltimore, pp. 279–309, 1965.

361. SCOTT, B. O. The effects of metal on short-wave field distribution. *Ann. Phys. Med., 1:* 238–244, 1953.

362. SEKINS, K. M., DUNDORE, D. EMERY A. F., LEHMANN, J. F., MCGRATH, P. W. AND NELP, W. B. Muscle blood flow changes in response to 915 MHz diathermy with surface cooling as measured by Xe^{133} clearance. *Arch. Phys. Med. Rehabil., 61:* 105–113, 1980.

363. SEVRINGHAUS, E. L. A constant temperature foot cradle. *Am. J. Med. Sci., 187:* 509–511, 1934.

364. SHAPIRO, A. R., LUTOMIRSKI, R. F. AND YURA, H. T. Induced fields and heating within a cranial structure irradiated by an electromagnetic plane wave. *IEEE Tran. Microwave Theory Tech.* (special issue on biological effects of microwaves), *MTT-19:* 187–196, 1971.

365. SHEALY, C. N. AND HENNEMAN, E. Reversible effects of ultrasound on spinal reflexes. *Arch. Neurol., 6:* 374–386, 1962.

366. SILVERMAN, D. R. A comparison of the continuous and pulsed shortwave diathermy resistance to bacterial infection of mice. *Arch. Phys. Med., 45:* 491–499, 1964.

367. SILVERMAN, D. R. AND PENDLETON, L. A comparison of the effects of continuous and pulsed short-wave diathermy on peripheral circulation. *Arch. Phys. Med. Rehabil., 49:* 429–436, 1968.

368. SIMON, H. B. Gram-positive cocci. *In: Scientific American Medicine.* Rubenstein, E. and Federman, D. D. (Eds). Vol. 2, Section 7, pp. I2–I23, Scientific American, 1980.

369. SMITH, D. W., CLARREN, S. K. AND HARVEY, M. A. S. Hyperthermia as a possible teratogenic agent. *J. Pediatr., 92:* 878–883, 1978.

370. SONNEN, V. G. Pathophysiologic bases of ultrasonic treatment of rheumatoid disease. Paper read at Third Annual Conference, *Amer Instit. Ultrasonics in Medicine,* Washington, 1954.

371. SONNENSCHEIN, V. Die pathophysiologischen Grundlagen der Ultraschalltherapie rheumatischer Erkrankungen. *Schweiz. med. Wschr., 82:* 1137, 1952.

372. STARR, I. JR. A thermoregulated foot cradle for the treatment of peripheral vascular disease. *Proc. Soc. Exp. Biol. Med., 29:* 166–167, 1931.

373. STEIN, R. B. Peripheral control of movement. Physiol. Rev., 54: 215–243, 1974.

374. STILLWELL, G. K. General principles of thermotherapy *In: Therapeutic Heat and Cold.*

Licht, S. (Ed). Chapter 7, Second edition, Waverly Press, Baltimore, pp. 232–239, 1965.

375. STUHLFAUTH, K. Neurological effects of ultrasonic waves. *Br. J. Phys. Med.*, *15:* 10, 1952.

376. SULZBERGER, M. B., WOLF, J., WITTEN, V. H. AND KOPF, A. W. *Dermatology, Diagnosis Treatment.* Year Book Publishers, Chicago, 1961.

377. SUMWALT, M. Ion effects upon ion permeability of the Fundulus chorion. *Biol. Bull.*, *64:* 114, 1933.

378. SUMWALT, M., AMBERSON, W. R., MICHAELIS, E.: Factors concerned in the origin of concentration potentials across the skin of the frog. *J. Cellular Comp. Physiol.*, *4:* 49–59, 1933.

379. SZEGO, C. M. The lysosomal membrane complex as a proximate target for steroid hormone action. *In: The Sex Steroids.* McKerns, K. W. (Ed). First edition, Chapter 1, pp. 1–51, 1971.

380. SZEGO, C. M. The lysosome as a mediator of hormone action. *Rec. Prog. Hormone Res.*, *30:* 171–233, 1974.

381. TAKASHIMA, S. Studies on the effect of radio-frequency waves on biological macromolecules. *IEEE Trans. Biomed. Eng.*, *BME-13:* 28–31, 1966.

382. TAYLOR, A. B. Studies of the electromotive force in biological systems. IV. The effect of various nitrogen-oxygen and carbon monoxide-oxygen mixtures on the E.M.F. and oxygen consumption of frog skin. *J. Cell. Comp. Phys.*, *7:* 1, 1935.

383. TAYLOR, K. J. W. Ultrasonic damage to spinal cord and the synergistic effect of hypoxia. *J. Pathol.*, *102:* 41–47, 1970.

384. TAYLOR, K. J. W. AND DYSON, M. Possible hazards of diagnostic ultrasound. *Br. J. Hosp. Med.*, *8:* 571–579, 1972.

385. TAYLOR, K. J. W. AND DYSON, M. Toxicity studies on the interaction of ultrasound on embryonic and adult tissues. *Proc. Second World Cong. on Ultrasonics in Med.* Excerpta Medica, Rotterdam, pp. 353–359, 1973.

386. TAYLOR, K. J. W. AND POND, J. B. A study of the production of haemorrhagic injury and paraplegia in rat spinal cord by pulsed ultrasound of low mega-Hertz frequencies in the context of the safety for clinical usage. *Br. J. Radiol.*, *45:* 343–353, 1972.

387. TAYLOR, R. G. The effect of diapulse (pulsed high frequency energy) on wound healing in humans. Cited by Lehmann *et al.* (251).

388. TEPPERBERG, I. AND MARJEY, E. Ultrasound therapy of painful post-operative neurofibromas. *Am. J. Phys. Med.*, *32:* 27, 1953.

389. TEXEIRA-PINTO, A. A., NEJELSKI, L. L., CUTLER, J. L. AND HELLER, J. H. The behavior of unicellular organisms in an electromagnetic field. *Exp. Cell. Res.*, *20:* 548–564, 1960.

390. THIELE, W. Die Ultraschallbehandlung bei rheumatischen Erkrankungen. *Arztl. Wschr.*, *7:* 193, 1952.

391. TORR, G. R. AND WATMOUGH, D. J. A constant-flow calorimeter for the measurement of acoustic power at megahertz frequencies. *Phys. Med. Biol.*, *22:* 444–450, 1977.

392. TRAVELL, J. AND RINZLER, S. H. The myofascial genesis of pain. *Postgrad. Med.*, *11:* 425, 1952.

393. TROJEL, H. AND LEBECH, P. E. Intermitterende kortbølge (Diapulse) i behandlingen af inflammatoriske underlivslidelser. *Nordisk Medicin*, *81:* 307–310, 1969.

394. TSCHANNEN, F. Effects of ultrasonic therapy on rheumatic diseases and circulatory disorders. *Br. J. Phys. Med.*, *15:* 7, 1952.

395. TSCHANNEN, F. Ultraschallwirkung bei rheumatischen Erkrankungen und Durchblutungsstörungen. *Schweiz. med. Wschr.*, *82:* 301, 1952.

396. TUCHMAN, L. S. Role of ultrasound in scleroderma. *Am. J. Phys. Med.*, *35:* 118, 1956.

397. TUREK, L. S. *Orthopaedics, Principles and Their Application.* JP Lippincott, Philadelphia, 1959.

398. UCHMAN, L. S. Role of ultrasound in scleroderma. A preliminary report of two cases. *Am. J. Phys. Med.*, *35:* 118, 1956.

399. UNITED STATES CONSUMER PRODUCT SAFETY COMMISSION. CPSC warns of hot tub temperatures. News from CPSC, December 31, 1979.
400. UPRUS, V., GAYLOR, J. B., AND CARMICHAEL, E. A. Vasodilatation and vasoconstriction in response to warming and cooling the body. A criticism of methods. *Clin. Sci., 2:* 301–316, 1936.
401. VANDEMARK, W. R. AND FREE, J. R. Temperature effects. *In: The Testis.* Johnson, A. D. *et al.* (Eds). Vol. 3. Academic Press, New York, pp. 233–312, 1973.
402. VAUGHEN, J. L. AND BENDER, L. F. Effects of ultrasound on growing bone. *Arch. Phys. Med. Rehabil., 40:* 158–160, 1959.
403. VERRIER, M., ASHBY, P. AND CRAWFORD, J. S. Effects of thermotherapy on the electrical and mechanical properties of human skeletal muscle. *Physiother. Canada, 30:* 117–120, 1978.
404. VERZÁR, F. Liberation of mechanical tension by heating of collagen fibres. *Experientia, 18:* 310–311, 1962.
405. WACHSMUTH, W. Ultraschall bei Sudeckscher Krankheit. *Der Ultraschall in der Medizin.* Zurich, 1949.
406. WAKIM, K. G. AND KRUSEN, F. H. Influence of physical agents and of certain drugs on intra-articular temperature. *Arch. Phys. Med., 32:* 714–721, 1951.
407. WAKIM, K. G., GERSTEN, J. W., HERRICK, J. F., ELKINS, E. C. AND KRUSEN, F. H. The effects of diathermy on the flow of blood in the extremities. *Arch. Phys. Med., 29:* 583–593, 1948.
408. WALLACE, L. AND ZACH, F. Ultrasound, its effect on the cardiovascular system when applied over the carotid sinus and stellate ganglion. *Calif. Med., 91:* 21, 1959.
409. WARREN, C. G., KOBLANSKI, J. N. AND SIGELMANN, R. A. Ultrasound Coupling Media: Their Relative Transmissivity. *Arch. Phys. Med. Rehabil., 57:* 218–222, 1976.
410. WARREN, C. G., LEHMANN, J. F. AND KOBLANSKI, J. N. Elongation of rat tail tendon: effect of load and temperature. *Arch. Phys. Med. Rehabil., 52:* 465–475, 1971.
411. WARREN, C. G., LEHMANN, J. F. AND KOBLANSKI, J. N. Heat and stretch procedures: an evaluation using rat tail tendon. *Arch. Phys. Med. Rehabil. 57:* 122–126, 1976.
412. WEBER, R. L., WHITE, M. W. AND MANNING, K. V. *College Physics.* Second edition, McGraw-Hill, p. 275, 1952.
413. WEIDENBACKER, R. A. AND SMITH, C. Does heat cause relaxation? *Phys. Ther. Rev., 40:* 261–265, 1960.
414. WEISS, N. S., DODELL, P. AND BROWN, H. E. Thermal urticaria: an unusual case. *Ann. Allergy, 37:* 55–57, 1976.
415. WHYTE, H. M. AND READER, S. P. Effectiveness of different forms of heating. *Ann. Rheum. Dis., 10:* 449–452, 1951.
416. WILLIAMS, A. R., CHATER, B. V., ALLEN, K. A., SHERWOOD, M. R. AND SANDERSON, J. H. Release of β-thromboglobulin from human platelets by therapeutic intensities of ultrasound. *Br. J. Haematol., 40:* 133–142, 1978.
417. WILLIAMS, A. R., O'BRIEN, W. D. AND COLLER, B. S. Exposure to ultrasound decreases the recalcification time of platelet rich plasma. *Ultrasound Med. Biol., 2:* 113–118, 1976.
418. WILLIAMS, D. B., MONAHAN, J. P., NICHOLSON, W. J. AND ALDRICH, J. J. Biologic effects of microwave radiation. U.S.A.F. School of Aviation Medicine Report No. 55–94. Washington, 1955.
419. WILLIAMS, J. G. P. AND SPERRYN, P. N. *Sports Medicine.* Arnold, E. (Ed). pp. 292–309, 1976.
420. WILLIS, I. AND EPSTEIN, J. H. Solar- vs. heat-induced urticaria. *Arch. Dermatol., 110:* 389–392, 1974.
421. WILSON, D. H. *Br. Med. J., 2:* 269–270, 1972.
422. WILSON, D. H. Comparison of short wave diathermy and pulsed electromagnetic energy in treatment of soft tissue injuries. *Physiother., 60:* 309–310, 1974.

423. WILSON, D. H., JAGADEESH, P., NEWMAN, P. P. AND HARRIMAN, D. G. F. The effects of pulsed electromagnetic energy on peripheral nerve regeneration. *Ann. N.Y. Acad. Sci.,* *238:* 575–585, 1974.

424. WISE, C. S. The effect of diathermy on blood flow. *Arch. Phys. Med., 29:* 17–21, 1948.

425. WISE, D. D. Physiotherapeutic treatment of athletic injuries to the muscle-tendon complex of the leg. *CMA. J. 117:* 635–639, 1977.

426. WOEBER, K. Biological basis and application of ultrasound in medicine. *Ultrasonics Biol. Med., 1:* 9, 1956.

427. WONG, C. AND EHRLICH, H. P. A preliminary report on pulsed high frequency energy (diapulse therapy) in wound healing. Cited by Lehmann *et al.* (251).

428. WOODMANSEY, A., COLLINS, D. H. AND ERNST, M. M. Vascular reactions to the contrast bath in health and in rheumatoid arthritis. *Lancet 2:* 1350–1353, 1938.

429. WORDEN, R. E., HERRICK, J. F., WAKIM, K. G. AND KRUSEN, F. H. The heating effects of microwaves with and without ischemia. *Arch. Phys. Med., 29:* 751–758, 1948.

430. WRIGHT, S. *Applied Physiology.* Oxford University, pp. 316–317, 1952.

431. WRIGHT, V. AND JOHNS, R. J. Physical factors concerned with the stiffness of normal and diseased joints. *Bull. Johns Hopkins Hosp., 106:* 215–231, 1960.

432. WRIGHT, V. AND JOHNS, R. J. Quantitative and qualitative analysis of joint stiffness in normal subjects and in patients with connective tissue diseases. *Ann. Rheum. Dis., 20:* 36–46, 1961.

433. WULFF, D. Behandlungsergebnisse mit Ultraschall. *Der Ultraschall in der Medizin, 7:* 111, 1954.

434. YOUNG, R. R. AND HENNEMAN, D. Functional effects of focused ultrasound in mammalian nerves. *Science, 134:* 1521, 1961.

435. ZANKEL, H. T. Effect of ultrasound on leg blood flow. *In Scientific Proc. Seventh Ann. Conf. Am. Inst. Ultrasonics in Med.* pp. 7–17, August 25, 1962.

436. ZAROD, A. P. AND WILLIAMS, A. R. Platelet aggregation *in vivo* by therapeutic ultrasound. *Lancet, 1:* 1266, 1977.

437. ZIMNY, M. AND HEAD, L. H. Effects of ultrasound on skeletal and carotid muscle in the ground squirrel. *Am. J. Phys., 200:* 672, 1961.

11

Cryotherapy[1]

JUSTUS F. LEHMANN
BARBARA J. DE LATEUR

Introduction

The following is a discussion of the therapeutic use of local cold applications, *i.e.*, cryotherapy. The clinical selection of cold therapy for certain conditions is based on the knowledge of physiological responses to cold which seem to be desirable for therapeutic purposes. It is also based on clinical evaluation of the effectiveness of this type of therapeutic modality. In this chapter, information on physiological responses will be closely related to the established clinical use of cryotherapy. Informational gaps will also be pointed out, as well as the need for further basic and clinical research.

The application of cold has been found useful to reduce muscle tone in cases of muscle spasms secondary to underlying skeletal and joint pathology or resulting from nerve root irritation as in low back syndromes. In these cases, the primary objective is usually to break a vicious cycle of secondary muscle spasm with ischemia and pain and more muscle spasms. Cold application is also used in the spasticity of upper motor neuron lesions. In these cases, cooling is used to reduce or abolish clonus spasticity so that other physical therapy and training programs can be initiated for appropriate motor skill learning. There is no evidence that cold at temperatures within the therapeutic range permanently changes muscle tone. It is, however, important that the effect last long enough that appropriate therapies can be given to the patient while the interfering spasticity is eliminated. Superficial cold application has also been used for re-education purposes to facilitate muscle contraction.

Cold is applied in mechanical trauma primarily to reduce bleeding and edema formation by vasoconstriction. This therapy is commonly combined

---

[1] This chapter is in part based on research supported by Research Grant # G008003029 from the National Institute of Handicapped Research, Department of Education, Washington, D.C. 20202.

with compression. There is also evidence that thermal burns can be alleviated by immediate cold application.

Pain is relieved by elevating the pain threshold as a direct effect of temperature reduction on nerve fibers and receptors. Pain is also alleviated indirectly by relieving painful conditions such as muscle spasms, spasticity, and swelling. Arthritic joints are treated with cold to reduce the inflammatory reaction and activity of destructive enzymes, as well as to reduce pain.

Physiological Effects as a Basis for Therapy

EFFECTS ON THE SPINDLE MECHANISM AS A BASIS FOR THE TREATMENT OF SPASTICITY, MUSCLE SPASM, AND FACILITATION

The physiological effects on the spindle mechanism will be discussed as a basis for the treatment of spasticity, muscle spasms, and as a physiological basis for neuromuscular facilitation. Ottoson (72) has shown that the responsiveness of the spindle to stretching increases linearly with temperature in the range from 3°C to about 32°C. At 32°C, maximal responsiveness to stretch is obtained. The sensitivity of the spindle drops off as the temperature is elevated further (Figure 11.1).

Eldred and associates (27) varied the temperature of the total muscle and recorded from the afferents arising from flower-spray and annulospiral endings. They found that the rate of discharge paralleled the change in temperature; the cooler the muscle, the lower the rate of firing. In addition,

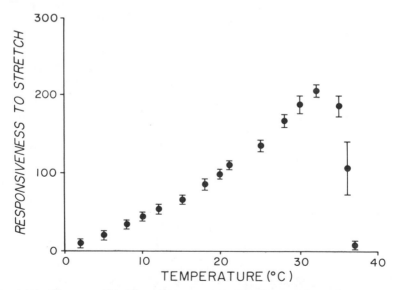

Fig. 11.1. Change of impulse response with temperature. Mean values of eleven experiments. *Ordinate:* number of spikes elicited by test stretch as a percentage of value at 20°C. *Vertical lines* indicate ± 1 S.E. of the mean (72).

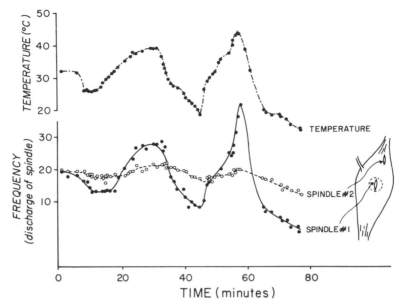

Fig. 11.2. Effect of local change in temperature on discharge of spindle (27).

they selectively cooled single spindles and found that the responsiveness to the temperature change was at least as great and followed the temperature curves precisely, while other spindles in the muscle were not much affected (Figure 11.2).

Whereas the relationship between muscle stretch and frequency of spindle discharge was maintained, the entire curves were shifted as the temperature increased from 28.8°C to 39.3°C. Finally, the rate of spontaneous spindle discharge in a "precollicular" decerebrate animal with intact dorsal roots decreased with decreasing temperature. Also, the rate of discharge from the Golgi tendon organs was temperature-dependent.

Theoretically, the change in discharge of the muscle spindle may result from the effect of cold on the extrafusal muscle, the intrafusal fibers or the sensory endings. Eldred and associates concluded from their experiments and observations that the cooling primarily affects the sensory wrappings in the spindles. They believed that under the conditions of the experiments, the length-tension relationships of the gross muscle were not changed enough to affect spindle firing. They suggested that the visco-elastic properties of intrafusal fibers were not significantly affected. Since the tendon organs, which do not have any intrafusal fibers, were also influenced by temperature changes, the effect of cold on the spindle could not be explained through changes in the intrafusal fibers. Moreover, the changes in the excitability of the large medullated axons by cooling were, in their opinion, not responsible. Local cooling of a single spindle could at best have affected the non-myelinated portion of the nerve. Ischemia was probably not involved, since gradual cooling of the muscle did not produce blanching; and local cooling, which presumably is less likely to cause vasoconstriction, produced the greatest effect on the rate of spindle firing.

Eldred and associates concluded that the site of the thermal effect is the sensory terminal itself and is likely the result of changes in membrane stability similar to those induced in axons by lowering of the temperature.

Lippold *et al.* (58) measured the minimal stretch which produced a single action potential as spindle response. When they lowered the temperature, the sensitivity of the spindle initially increased with a minimum of stretch required for a response at 30°C. As temperatures were lowered further, the stretch required to produce a response was markedly increased (Figure 11.3).

Thus, their findings are in good agreement with those of Ottoson (Figure 11.1). In addition, Lippold *et al.* found that increase of the potassium concentration or direct current polarization accelerated spindle discharge. Conversely, hyperpolarization of the membrane or low potassium concentration reduced or abolished the activity, suggesting that the effect of cold application is related to the rate of change in membrane polarization.

Michalski and Seguin (66) studied the discharge of single afferents from 162 de-efferented muscle spindles in the gastrocnemius of the anesthetized cat during cooling of the muscle from 37 to 24°C. On the basis of conduction velocity, the endings were classified as primary or secondary endings. The dividing line was set at 70 M/s. A response to cooling was obtained only in

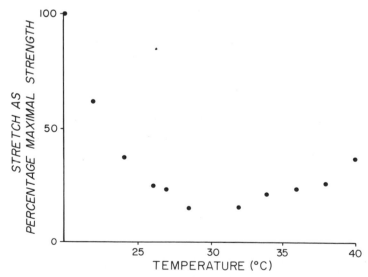

Fig. 11.3. Minimal stretch required to produce a single action potential as a spindle response from 0 to 40°C (58).

endings with conduction velocities of 20 to 70 M/s, that is, in 65 percent of the secondary endings studied. This "cold response" was described as follows: there was no activity from these spindle endings at 37°C, but when the muscle was gradually cooled, an afferent discharge began at 33.2°C, reached a maximum near 31°C and decreased during further cooling to 25°C. The remainder of the secondary endings and the primary endings showed no activity during cooling. During maintained stretches, the responsiveness of these endings was reduced by cooling.

Knutsson and Mattsson (49) studied the effects of local cooling on both the H response and the Achilles tendon jerk in man. In both cases, the amplitude of the electrical activity of the muscle was recorded. The tendon jerk was mechanically induced. The H reflex was evoked by submaximal electrical stimulation of the tibial nerve. The common pathway in both responses is the α motor neuron. Stimulation of the peripheral nerve elicits an orthodromic impulse in the IA afferents, which in turn monosynaptically facilitates α motor neuron discharge, resulting in a muscle contraction. Thus, the H reflex largely bypasses the spindle and the γ bias on the intrafusal fibers.

The γ efferents produce a contraction of the intrafusal fibers, taking up the slack in the spindle resulting from contraction of the extrafusal muscle fibers in parallel with the spindle; the γ efferents thus increase the sensitivity of the spindle to stretch. The mechanical stimulation of the Achilles tendon leads to a stretch of the muscle spindles with a corresponding IA afferent discharge, monosynaptically stimulating the α motor neurons. The amplitude of the stretch reflex thus is dependent upon the pre-existing γ bias.

Knutsson and Mattsson observed that ice application produced an increase in the amplitude of the H response, suggesting an increase in α motor neuron excitability at a time when a significant temperature decrease had occurred only in the skin. As the temperature of the muscle dropped, there was a decrease of the Achilles tendon jerk; thus, stimulation of the exteroceptors of the skin produced a reflex facilitation of the α motor neuron, whereas the direct effect on the spindle, and perhaps also on the γ efferents, produced a reduction of the spindle sensitivity and a consequent reduction of the tendon reflex. Specifically, the latter mechanism may form the basis for reduction of muscle tone through a reduction of spindle sensitivity. On the other hand, the skin stimulation with the resulting facilitation of the α motor neuron discharge may be the basis for ice massage used in neuromuscular facilitation techniques as part of muscle re-education (Figure 11.4).

Urbscheit and Bishop (90) also studied the facilitation, by hand grip, of the electrically recorded amplitude of both the H response and the Achilles tendon reflex. In the non-cooled state, they found a facilitation of both the H response and the Achilles tendon reflex at 20 percent of maximal grip strength. This facilitation was maintained (90) or even increased (11) at 80

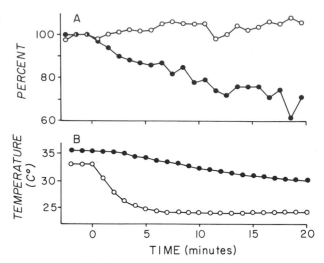

Fig. 11.4. Mean reflex (EMG) and temperature changes in normal triceps surae during local cooling. (A) Amplitude of H response (*open circle*) and amplitude of tendon jerk (*solid circle*). (B) Subcutaneous (*open circle*) and intramuscular (*solid circle*) temperatures (49).

percent of grip strength for the Achilles tendon reflex (ATR), but dropped in the case of the H response. The increase of the ATR can only be explained by an effect on the spindle sensitivity which may be reflexly produced by γ efferent excitation.

At the same time, the drop of the H response may be explained by simultaneous inhibition of the α motor neuron. On cooling, there was a marked increase of the H response and a slight but statistically insignificant decrease of the ATR. The drop of facilitation at 80 percent hand grip for the H response was not observable. These latter two findings again indicate a differential effect of cold on the α and γ systems, reflexly increasing the α excitability and suppressing the excitability of the spindle mechanism.

Figures 11.5 and 11.6 show that the increase in the H response was significant when cooling was applied; the decrease of the ATR was not statistically significant. The authors' interpretation of these findings was that the amplitude of the ATR showed only a small change, suggesting a decrease in the excitability of the γ motor neurons, whereas the H response and the extent of hand grip facilitation were markedly increased, suggesting an increased excitability of the α motor neuron. The authors assumed that the observed changes were produced reflexly via exteroceptors in the skin. However, the duration of cold application in the experiments was sufficient that cooling of the muscle itself may have occurred, directly affecting the spindles and γ efferents. From the measurements of other authors, it was concluded that a significant temperature drop occurs in the muscle after 10 minutes of ice application.

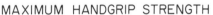

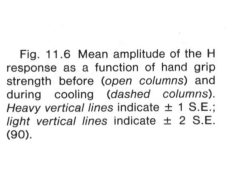

Fig. 11.5. Mean amplitude of the ATR as a function of hand grip strength before (*open columns*) and during cooling (*dashed columns*). *Heavy vertical lines* indicate ± 1 S.E.; *light vertical lines* indicate ± 2 S.E. (90).

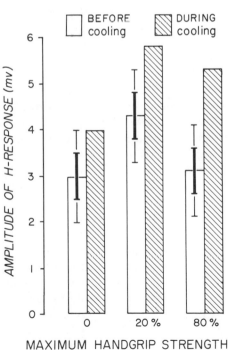

Fig. 11.6 Mean amplitude of the H response as a function of hand grip strength before (*open columns*) and during cooling (*dashed columns*). *Heavy vertical lines* indicate ± 1 S.E.; *light vertical lines* indicate ± 2 S.E. (90).

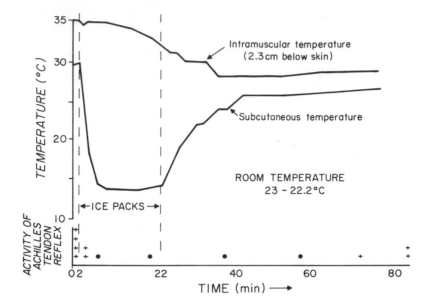

Fig. 11.7. Subcutaneous and intramuscular temperatures produced in the gastrocnemius by application of ice packs (40).

Hartviksen (40) (see Figure 11.7) applied ice packs to the gastrocnemius muscles of patients with upper motor neuron lesions and spasticity, and found that while the subcutaneous temperature dropped sharply, there was an initial increase in spasticity. The muscle temperature at 2.3 cm below the skin dropped on continuing application of ice packs, and the clonus and spasticity disappeared. It is important to note that spasticity and muscle temperature had not yet returned to normal at the end of the experiment, 58 minutes after ice packing. The long duration of the effect is essential, since therapeutically an adequate period of time is needed during which range of motion exercises and training in motor tasks can be done without interference of spasticity. All ten patients studied had clonus with an increase in spasticity when the skin was cooled, and with a decrease of the spasticity later.

Hartviksen additionally stipulated that spasticity had already disappeared while the intramuscular temperature was still normal. He found that skin temperature had to drop to 20°C before spasticity is affected. However, he made no temperature measurements in the superficial musculature. Therefore, it is possible that the spindles or the γ efferents were cooled and directly affected. He tried to explain the effect on the basis of experiments by Granit (35) who demonstrated that skin receptors may have an influence on the γ efferent cell activity in the spinal cord. However, Granit never demonstrated such an influence from cold applications.

In clinical investigation, Miglietta (67) observed that clonus and spasticity were not abolished unless the muscle temperature dropped significantly. Finally, Miglietta mentioned the possibility that sympathetic fibers reflexly may reduce spindle sensitivity. He based this possibility on the fact that sympathetic fibers do enter the spindle, and that Hunt (44) showed a change in spindle response with electrical stimulation of the sympathetic trunk. With mild, short-duration stimulation, the spindle sensitivity was increased; with more vigorous and continued stimulation it was decreased. While it is possible that by superficial cold application, reflex sympathetic stimulation not only produces vasoconstriction but also decreases spindle sensitivity, the experiments of Hunt have not demonstrated this (Figure 11.8).

EFFECTS OF THE NEUROMUSCULAR JUNCTION

When muscle is cooled, there is an effect on the neuromuscular junction. Li (56) demonstrated that at a temperature of 5°C, blockage of the neuromuscular junction occurred and did so prior to the failure of nerve conduction. Li and Gouras (57) observed that as temperature decreased, the amplitude and duration of the miniature endplate potentials increased, and their frequency decreased.

EFFECTS ON PERIPHERAL NERVES AS A BASIS FOR TREATMENT OF SPASTICITY AND PAIN

The effects of cooling on peripheral nerves were also assessed. These effects may in part explain the changes in muscle tone and the occurrence of pain relief. The sensitivity of nerve fibers to cold seems to depend largely upon myelination and upon fiber diameter (Table 11.1).

The largest myelinated fibers are the A α fibers which includes both the sensory fibers for proprioception and the alpha motor neurons. The γ

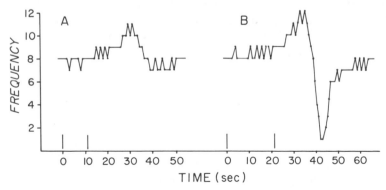

Fig. 11.8. Changes in the rate of discharge of afferents from a muscle spindle in the soleus. Sympathetic stimulation (100/second) for 11 seconds in *A* and 21 seconds in *B*. Period of stimulation noted by vertical lines above the abscissa (44).

TABLE 11.1. *Nerve Fiber Type, Function, Diameter and Conduction Velocity (31)*

Fiber Type	Function	Fiber Diameter (μm)	Conduction Velocity (msecond)
Aα	Proprioception, somatic motor	12–20	70–120
β	Touch, pressure	5–12	30–70
γ	Motor to muscle spindles	3–6	15–30
δ	Pain, temperature, touch	2–5	12–30
B	Preganglionic autonomic	<3	3–15
C Dorsal root	Pain, reflex responses	0.4–1.2	0.5–2
Sympathetic	Postganglionic sympathetics	0.3–1.3	0.7–2.3

efferents to the muscle spindles are all significantly smaller in diameter, even smaller are the myelinated pain fibers. Of interest also is the C group of fibers which includes the non-myelinated pain fibers and the post-ganglionic sympathetics, both fibers of small diameter. In general, all of the fibers are affected by cooling. Douglas and Malcolm (26), in experiments with cats, studied the differential effect of cold on fibers of various diameters. Small medullated fibers were affected first, then the large medullated fibers, and finally the unmedullated fibers. Specifically, they found that the smaller γ efferent fibers were more sensitive to cold than the larger α efferents. Unfortunately, data like these are somewhat species-dependent; therefore, generalization can only be tentative. It has been shown, for instance, that there is a difference in thresholds for blockage of nerve conduction by cold between hibernating and nonhibernating animals (18, 85). The motor nerve conduction velocity in man decreases linearly at the rate of 1.84 M/s/°C between 36°C and 23°C (24). Goodgold and Eberstein (33) quoted a decrease of 2 to 2.4 M/s for each drop in temperature of 1°C. Below 20°C the current threshold for successful electrical stimulation rises rapidly and the conduction velocity falls sharply, according to de Jong *et al.* (24). Li and Gouras (57) found that the strength of an electrical stimulus to produce a propagated spike potential of the peripheral nerve showed a marked increase at temperatures below 10°C. Li (56) found that nerve fibers ceased conduction at 4°C, that is, at a temperature below the blocking of the neuromuscular junction. However, muscle contraction could be produced by direct stimulation at temperatures as low as 1°C. Other changes in nerve function as a result of cooling have been described by Douglas and Malcolm (26). They found that the duration of the recovery cycle after excitation was increased with cooling. In addition, Schoepfle and Erlanger (82) observed an increase in the absolute refractory period after stimulation. According to Li (56) and Li and Gouras (57) the duration of the spike action potentials rapidly increased as the temperature was lowered from 30°C to 0°C. On the other hand, they found that the resting membrane potentials were not changed by cooling. The touch receptors in the skin, as tested with the two-edge threshold, changed significantly only at temperatures below 6°C (77). This is consistent with findings of Douglas and Malcolm that the sensory fibers important for motor learning, such as those which carry proprioception, are relatively insensitive to cold, since they are myelinated, large-diameter fibers (see Table 11.1).

EFFECTS ON MUSCLE STRENGTH AND ENDURANCE

Since it is a therapeutic objective to eliminate muscle spasticity and clonus to allow training for motor tasks, it is important that cooling not simultaneously abolish or significantly reduce the muscle strength and the endurance to continue with the performance of a given task. Therefore, physiological studies of the effect of cold upon strength and endurance are important. Walker (92) studied the changes in the characteristics of a twitch contraction after electrical nerve stimulation at temperatures ranging from 37°C to 24.5°C. He found an increase in tension, an increase in the duration of the rise of contraction, and an increase in the one-half relaxation time with decreasing temperature. These changes were associated with an increase of the height and duration of the action potentials. The height of the action potentials showed a peak value around 28°C. Maclagan and Zaimis (60) and Miglietta (67) found a similar slowing of the twitch contraction, but with a decrease in tension. Walker compared the effect of cooling and change in potassium concentration. He concluded that the duration of the membrane breakdown produced by the passage of excitation along the muscle fiber is slowed by cooling. More important for clinical application, perhaps, is the fact that the rate of stimulation required to obtain a fusion of the twitches to a complete tetanus drops as the temperature is lowered. Chatfield (17) found that cooling the muscle increased tension at lower frequencies of stimulation. At lower temperatures there was a greater fusion of contraction. At all frequencies of stimulation, tension was greater at 26.5°C than at 37°C. At no frequency was the normal physiological temperature the optimum for the function of the muscle. On the other hand, Maclagan and Zaimis (60) found that maximal tetanic tension was slightly decreased at lower temperatures. The effects of indirect stimulation observed by Walker were duplicated by Chatfield by direct stimulation of the muscle after the animals were curarized. This implied that hypothermia produces the observed effects by directly affecting the contractile mechanism itself. Boes (12) studied the mechanically elicited patellar tendon reflex in stroke patients. She found that during cooling the electrical activity in the muscle, used as a measure of the ankle jerk, was markedly reduced during and after ice application (Figure 11.9).

Petajan and Watts (76) observed that the half-relaxation of the ankle jerk was increased during and after cooling in the iced extremity, but not in the contralateral limb. This effect lasted more than 210 minutes. Neither the half-relaxation time nor the muscle temperature had returned to normal after the ice application had been discontinued for 30 minutes, an important

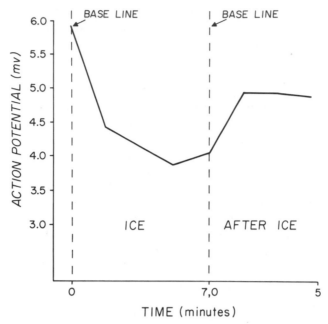

Fig. 11.9. ATR as measured by electrical output from muscle during and after ice application (12).

finding supporting the suggestion that the effect on spasticity lasts long after the ice application. This allows therapeutic intervention with training for skilled motor tasks (Figure 11.10).

Coppin *et al.* (22) submersed the right arm in cold water and found that the grip strength was decreased as compared with the contralateral extremity, which was not cooled. The difference was statistically significant.

The effect of cooling upon endurance has also been studied. Clarke *et al.* (19) investigated the ability to sustain a contraction over a period of time at different muscle temperatures. They found a maximal duration of sustained contraction could be achieved at 27°C (Figure 11.11). At temperatures below 27°C, the duration of the contraction was shortened. Below 20°C, the contractions could be sustained only over a significantly shorter period of time than at normal temperatures. When Clarke *et al.* predicted the duration of the contraction on the basis of muscle temperature, the predicted values agreed very well with the observed duration. There was no relationship between the actual values and those predicted on the basis of the subcutaneous temperatures. There also was no relationship between forearm blood flow and ability to sustain a contraction. Clarke *et al.* considered it likely that when the muscle temperature increased above 27°C, the rate of metabolism increased with the resulting early accumulation of metabolites, and therefore, the earlier onset of fatigue. At temperatures below 27°C, they

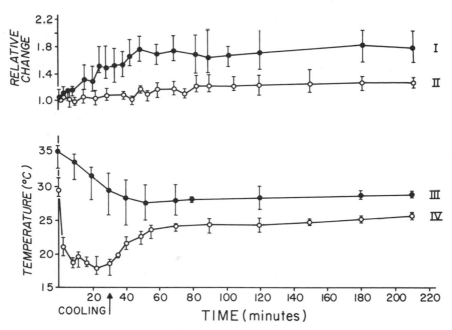

Fig. 11.10. Mean changes of the ATR as dependent on temperature. Line *I* shows the relative change in half-relaxation time in the cooled limb. Line *II* shows the relative change in half-relaxation time in the uncooled limb. Line *III* shows the change in muscle temperature, and Line *IV*, the change in skin temperature of the cooled limb. The range is indicated by *vertical lines* (76).

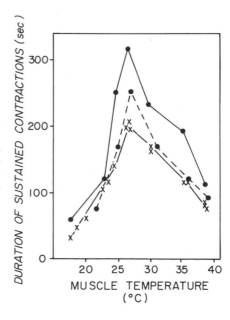

Fig. 11.11. Average duration of five sustained contractions at various muscle temperatures. The *upper curve* represents the first contraction; the *intermediate curve*, the second contraction; while the third, fourth and fifth contractions are all represented by the *lower curve* (19).

assumed that the more superficial muscle may not contract properly as a result of interference with the neuromuscular control. From the previously discussed experiments, it is also possible that the contractile mechanism of the muscle fiber itself is disturbed. The initial maximal tension that could be developed after immersion in water of 18°C was about the same as at normal tissue temperatures. This bath temperature corresponds to approximately 27°C intramuscular temperature. Below the water temperature of 18°C, the tension which could be exerted fell sharply with decreasing muscle temperature to a value of 40 percent of the maximum in water temperatures of 2°C. Integrated muscle action potentials showed that at the termination of the contraction there was no difference in electrical activity over the muscle when its temperature was 27°C or 35°C, but when it was reduced to 20°C there was considerably less electrical activity at the end of the contraction. On reviewing the data discussed previously, it seems feasible to reduce spasticity by cooling without grossly interfering with muscle function. The experiments therefore support clinical experience that the reduction of abnormal muscle tone can be utilized to allow training of motor tasks with sufficient muscular function, strength and endurance.

EFFECTS ON SKILLED MOTOR TASKS

If the clinical objective is to allow motor learning after spasticity has been reduced or eliminated by ice application, it is important to review the information available on the effect of cooling on skilled performance.

In well-controlled experiments, Gaydos and Dusek (32) found that if the extremity was cooled either by total body or local cooling, the performance scores in block stringing and knot tying dropped sharply as compared with the control at normal temperature. Similarly, Teichner (86) found that for a given task the performance time increased as the mean skin and digital temperatures dropped. He exposed volunteers to low temperatures under various conditions. Under cold exposure, the performance time increased when the Minnesota Rate of Manipulation Test was used. Fox (29) measured typing speeds with a standardized test. After both hands and forearms had been immersed for half an hour in water of temperatures ranging from 10°C to 42°C, he found that the time for completion of the task increased from the pretest mean as hand temperatures dropped. This drop occurred before grip strength decreased. At lower temperatures, grip strength decreased while the performance time rapidly increased (Figure 11.12).

EFFECTS ON BLOOD VESSELS AS A BASIS FOR TREATMENT OF TRAUMA AND INFLAMMATION

The vasoconstriction produced by cold application is considered the principal mechanism by which swelling and bleeding are reduced after trauma or edema is reduced in inflammatory reactions. Pain may also be reduced, either directly or indirectly. Indirectly, pain can be reduced by

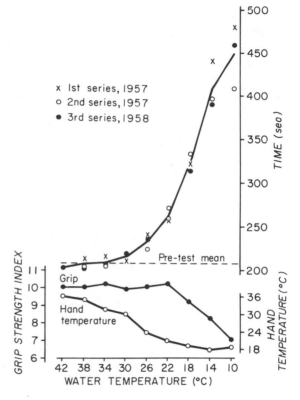

x 1st series, 1957
o 2nd series, 1957
● 3rd series, 1958

Fig. 11.12. Effect on copy-typing speed, grip strength, and hand temperature of immersing both hands and forearms for a half-hour in water at temperatures ranging from 10 to 42°C (29).

TABLE 11.2. *Blood Vessel Responses of Effector Organs to Autonomic Nerve Impulses and Circulating Catecholamines (34)*

Effector Organs	Cholinergic Impulses	Adrenergic Impulses	
	Response	Receptor Type	Response
Blood vessels, skin, and mucosa	...	α	Constriction
Skeletal muscle	Dilatation	α	Constriction
		β	Dilatation

reducing painful swelling and muscle spasms. There is a direct effect on the sensory endings and the pain fibers.

The innervation of the blood vessels of the skin, mucosa and skeletal muscles is shown in Table 11.2.

It is well-documented that cold application produces a reflex vasoconstriction via the sympathetic fibers. In addition, Perkins *et al.* (75) showed that vasoconstriction can be produced by a direct effect of cooling on the blood vessels. They demonstrated that the blood flow drop, determined by skin temperature measurements, was much less pronounced in the sympathectomized leg than in the remaining three extremities of a dog. If the room temperature was lowered from 15°C to 10°C, the authors found that after some delay, the sympathectomized leg also showed the signs of full vasoconstriction. These findings suggest that cooling to low temperatures may produce vasoconstriction through a direct effect on the blood vessels. Clarke *et al.* (20) found a decrease in blood flow as temperatures decreased to 18°C, with a marked increase in blood flow at 2°C. The latter increase is probably consistent with the Hunting reaction described by Clarke *et al.* (20), Lewis (54, 55), and Nelms and Soper (70) which explains blood flow increase as an effort of the organism to maintain temperatures at the level adequate to prevent tissue damage. This opening of the blood vessels, in spite of cooling, occurs on and off as necessary to maintain a minimum safe temperature level. Clarke *et al.* believed that the dilatation of the blood vessels which produced the blood flow increase at lower temperatures occurred largely in the muscle. It was independent of blood pressure changes and hormonal factors. Since the reaction was still present in a subject who had undergone cervical sympathectomy, but not in the patient who had a denervated arm, they concluded that the dilatation of the vessels is mediated by somatic nerves and possibly through an axon reflex. Adrenergic fibers with β receptors and cholinergic fibers are also available for such vasodilatation of the musculature.

Clarke *et al.* (19) found that the post-exercise hyperemia in the arm was decreased when the temperature was dropped from 39°C to 27°C. The finding was probably due to the changed metabolic rate at different temperatures.

Coles and Cooper (21) showed a similar decrease of reactive hyperemia after arrest of the limb circulation by a tourniquet. In agreement with Clarke *et al.* they found a decrease in the post-exercise hyperemia produced by immersion in water of 12°C for 20 minutes. The corresponding muscle temperature was between 19°C and 20°C.

The effect of local cooling in rabbits, post-femoral fracture, has been investigated by Matsen *et al.* (63). Contrary to expectation, it was found that the lower the applied temperature, the greater the swellings; however, the differences were not statistically significant (Figure 11.13). The observation extended over a period of 72 hours post-fracture. This observation is in agreement with the findings of Marek *et al.* (61), who treated posttraumatic edema by mild cooling with water at 12°C. Jezdinský *et al.* (45) found that cold applied immediately after injury for 2, 5, 7, and 10 hours, respectively, did not exert an inhibitory effect on the development of edema, and in fact, revealed a tendency to increase it. After discontinuation of application, a significant increase in edema volume always appeared. However, Schmidt *et al.* (81) produced reduction of edema by application of ice and frozen gel packs. According to Schmidt *et al.*, the development of inflammatory edema depends on the agent that produces the inflammation

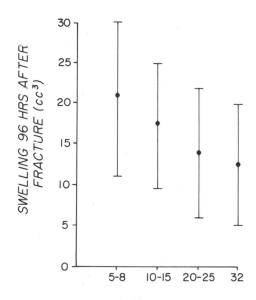

Fig. 11.13. Swelling of limbs 96 hours after fracture as a function of the temperature with which they were treated. Values shown are the means ± 1 S.D. All treatment periods were 24 hours. The 32°C value is the mean of all control limbs (63).

and on the time when the edema is measured and compared with the control. These authors produced experimental inflammatory reactions in the paws of the rat by injection of dextran and carrageenan, and then applied cold. They found an initial reduction and later increase of the edema as compared with the controls. With local kaolin injection, cold application aggravated edema at all times, while formol injection showed a late reduction (24 hours) of edema. When an adjuvant arthritis was produced in rats by injecting the paws, the edema was greater in the cold treated animals than in the controls. No difference was observed in the developing edema of the non-injected paws of the same rats. These experiments suggest that more studies are necessary on the mode of application, and on the condition in which cold is applied, before one can safely predict how and when edema will be influenced by cold therapy. It is interesting to note that the experiments described by Schmidt et al. showed that in all the cases heat application produced different effects, mostly in the opposite direction of that produced by cold application.

EFFECTS ON SMOOTH MUSCULATURE, INTESTINAL BLOOD FLOW, AND GASTRIC ACIDITY

Bisgard and Nye (10) studied the effect of cold packs applied to the abdomen and found an increase in the peristalsis in the stomach, the small bowel, and the colon. They found the opposite effect when heat was applied in the form of hot packs to the abdominal wall. A marked decrease or disappearance of the peristaltic waves occurred. Cold application also has been found to increase the blood flow through the mucous membrane of the alimentary canal and to increase acid secretion in the stomach (28). These findings explain the aggravation of stomach cramps and gastrointestinal upset with cold application and the relaxation of cramping with external abdominal heat application. Increased gastric acidity is undesirable in the presence of pathology, particularly peptic ulcers.

Clinical Studies

Cold application is commonly used to reduce muscle spasm and spasticity. It is used both in mechanical and thermal trauma. It is frequently used to relieve pain through its direct effect on nerve fibers and receptors and by improving painful conditions such as muscle spasm, spasticity, and swelling and edema. It is used to reduce the symptoms of inflammation, including those that occur in rheumatoid joints.

THE TREATMENT OF MUSCLE SPASM AND SPASTICITY

There is ample documentation that spasticity and muscle clonus can be reduced when ice is applied (76) (Figures 11.14 and 11.15).

Knutsson (48) found that passive resistance to stretch of the chilled muscle was reduced in 10 of 15 cases. Clonus was abolished or diminished in eight. The strength of the chilled muscles did not increase, but the power of the antagonist was enhanced by more than 50 percent in 11 of 29 cases. The antagonist could function better because it was unopposed by the spastic muscle.

Miglietta (67) studied 40 spastic patients with a diagnosis of hemiplegia in 30 patients, and paraplegia and multiple sclerosis in five each. The half-relaxation time was markedly increased after 30 minutes of cold application (Figure 11.16). When cooling started, 100 percent of his patients had ankle clonus. At the end of the cooling period, this number was reduced to 13 percent. Clonus had reappeared in 100 percent of the patients 90 minutes

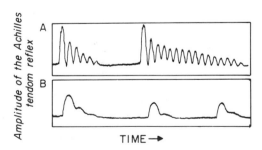

Fig. 11.14. Effect of cooling on amplitude of ankle clonus recorded by photo-motograph, (A) before and (B) after 20 minutes of cold application with water at 13°C in a spinal-cord-injured patient (76).

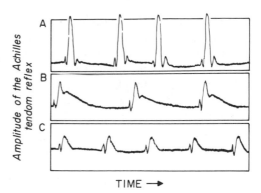

Fig. 11.15. Effect of cooling on the amplitude of the ATR in a patient with spinal-cord injury, (A) before cooling, (B) after 10 minutes of immersion in water at 15.6°C, and (C) 20 minutes after immersion (76).

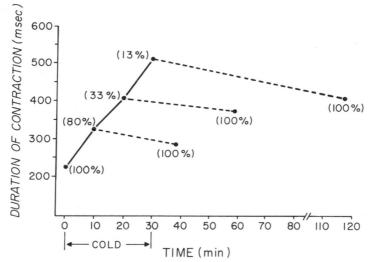

Fig. 11.16. Change of half-relaxation time of contraction of triceps surae resulting from single supramaximal indirect stimuli to the posterior tibial nerve after immersion of leg in water of 7°C for 30 minutes. Recordings at 10, 20, and 30 minutes. Figures in parentheses give the percentage of patients who exhibited a clonus at a given time (67).

after cold treatment was stopped. Thus, the effect on clonus was retained in part over a period as long as 90 minutes after ice application ended. Most important was Miglietta's finding that clonus started to decrease and disappeared only if the intramuscular temperature of the triceps surae started to drop. This observation suggests that techniques of ice application which solely or primarily lower the temperature in the skin may not be effective in reducing muscle tone. It has been shown that cooling of the skin alone stimulates exteroceptors and facilitates the H reflex, that is the α motor neuron discharge. It has been speculated that skin cooling may reflexly set up a sympathetic discharge to the spindle, decreasing its sensitivity, but this, according to Miglietta's observation, does not occur.

In addition, Knutsson (48) found that 12 patients with upper motor neuron lesions and spasticity had a restricted range of motion as a result of the spasticity. In eight of these cases, the voluntary range of motion increased from 15° to 70° with a mean of 35°. In neither Knutsson's nor Miglietta's experiments did all the patients respond.

Knutsson observed that in some cases there was even an increased passive resistance to motion that may have been the result of α motor neuron facilitation. In kinematic studies of a paraparetic patient, he found that after 20 minutes of cold application to the triceps surae muscle, the gait pattern changed.

Urbscheit et al. (91) investigated the changes in the H response and the Achilles tendon jerk in both involved and uninvolved limbs of hemiplegic patients. They found that the uninvolved limbs in four of the patients failed to respond in the same manner as the limbs of normal volunteers, implying that the apparently uninvolved limb of the hemiplegic may not be neurologically normal. Five of the six hemiplegic limbs responded differently from either the normal person or the uninvolved limb of the patient. Each patient's response to cooling was unique, or at least unpredictable, indicating the complexity of the neural mechanism underlying his spasticity. This may explain why, in some cases of spasticity, patients did not respond in terms of reduced clonus and muscle tone during ice application. The authors suggested that local cooling might decrease, increase, or exert no effect on the spastic state of hemiplegic patients.

Based on the preceding review of the literature, it appears that in order to give an optimal trial of cold therapy, it is essential to reduce the muscle temperature. This is necessary because the effects from skin exteroceptors and sympathetic stimulation are less well-documented, and in clinical practice seem to play less of a role.

THE TREATMENT OF MECHANICAL TRAUMA

The clinical application of cold in mechanical trauma is primarily based on vasoconstriction which leads to reduction of swelling and bleeding. There are numerous clinical observations suggesting the effectiveness of cold, of which only a few will be discussed in detail. Basur et al. (5) treated ankle sprains in 60 patients without radiological evidence of cartilagenous or bone trauma. They treated two groups of patients with compression bandages, one with additional ice therapy and the other without. They found that recovery occurred earlier in the group treated with ice (Figure 11.17).

More serious injuries were studied by Moore and Cardea (69). These authors studied 15 patients with closed fractures of the distal tibia and fibula, and measured the pressures in the anterior, lateral, superficial posterior, and deep posterior compartments. Five patients were treated con-

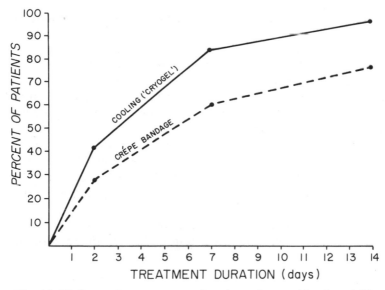

Fig. 11.17. Percentage recovery at various stages of treatment (5).

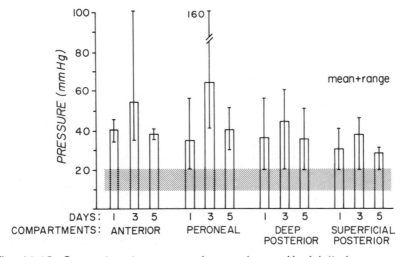

Fig. 11.18. Compartment pressure changes in mm Hg (plotted as mean and range) after distal tibial fracture in 10 patients treated conventionally. *Horizontal axis* represents days after fracture. *Shaded area* represents range of normal values obtained from uninjured legs (69).

ventionally, and five patients were placed in a prototype water-jacketed boot which provided cooling and intermittent compression. They found that the compartment pressures in the conventionally-treated group were significantly elevated over the norm (Figure 11.18), even at 5 days after injury.

In the second group, the pressures returned to normal without 24 hours (Figure 11.19).

It must be recognized that two factors in the treatment are different. The patients treated with cooling were also subjected to intermittent compression of the injured limb.

Schaubel (80) applied cold to a large number of patients with different types of operations which required casting. Procedures included knee surgery, wrist fusions, foot surgery, hip surgery, fractures, tendon surgery, shoulder surgery, bone grafts, tumor excisions, osteotomies, manipulations, nerve surgery, fusions, and amputations. The group treated with cast applications and cooling with ice totaled 207 cases. The group which was casted without ice represented 312 cases. With ice application, the necessity of splitting the cast on account of swelling was reduced from 42.3 percent to 5.3 percent. Unfortunately, while these figures are very impressive, they are not necessarily conclusive due to the non-uniformity of the surgical proce-

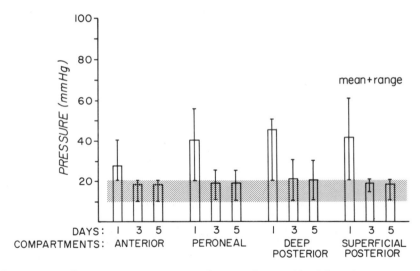

Fig. 11.19. Compartment pressure changes in mm Hg (plotted as range and mean) during prototype boot application in five patients. *Horizontal axis* represents days after fracture. *Shaded area* represents range of normal values obtained from uninjured legs (69).

TABLE 11.3. *Average of Total Amount of Narcotics Required during the First 72 Hours after Operation, with and without Ice Treatment (80)*

Average Dosage mg/Case	Cases with ice			Cases without ice		
	Codeine	Morphine	Demerol	Codeine	Morphine	Demerol
	89.2	11.8	3.8	268.5	25.1	12.0

dures in this group and the fact that the author did not control the severity of the conditions. The author also found that the requirement for narcotics was markedly reduced when ice was applied (Table 11.3).

Hayden (41) in a military practice setting, treated a thousand patients with minor injuries with ice. Her clinical impression was that the patients responded well, since 850 of them returned to duty within 1 hour after reporting for treatment, and 970 returned to duty the same day they reported. All except three patients returned to duty within 2 days.

THE TREATMENT OF BURNS

Zitowitz and Hardy (99) demonstrated, in animal experiments, that cold application inhibited the development of experimental burns. Severity was reduced and healing time shortened. They found that the milder, more superficial burns responded best, but that delaying the cold exposure by 2 days caused an increase in burn severity and healing time. These findings were essentially confirmed by Shulman (84) in patients with burns of all degrees involving less than 20 percent of the body surface. He treated 150 patients as promptly as possible after the burn by immersion of the burned areas in baths of ice water with hexachlorophene or by application of ice cold compresses. He found that pain was immediately relieved and the extent of redness and blistering visibly reduced. Local cooling was continued for several hours and was reapplied if pain recurred when the cold application was discontinued. He stated that timing is essential and that cold should be applied as soon as possible. Consistent with these findings, Demling et al. (25) found that immediate application of cold by immersion in 15°C saline reached the edema of a deep second-degree burn and did not impair the resorption rate compared with the control limbs. Fluid content returned to baseline after 1 week. Cold treatment beginning 2 minutes after the burn did not decrease edema formation and did impair resorption.

THE TREATMENT OF PAIN

As mentioned previously, the pain threshold can be elevated by a direct effect of cooling on the pain receptors and fibers. Also, pain can be relieved indirectly by reducing painful spasms and spasticity or by reducing painful swelling resulting from trauma or from inflammatory reaction. Parsons and Goetzl (73), in addition, showed that cold could be used as a counter-irritant to relieve pain. This finding can also be explained by the gate theory of Melzack and Wall (65). For this specific effect, Parsons and Goetzl used evaporative cooling by spraying ethyl chloride on the skin of the leg to the point of pain. Under these circumstances, they obtained a much more marked effect on the pain threshold than by just producing a sensation of cold. The pain threshold was tested by electrical stimulation of a tooth filling (Figure 11.20).

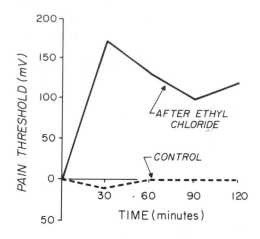

Fig. 11.20. Effect of a pain induced by ethyl chloride spray on the pain threshold of normal human subjects (73).

THE TREATMENT OF INFLAMMATION—ARTHRITIDES AND BURSITIS

The inflammatory reaction is influenced by cold application through the vasoconstriction with reduction of edema. The pain is frequently relieved. It has been documented that bacterial inflammatory reactions show retardation of toxicity and spread when cold is applied (2, 3, 8, 9).

The application of ice to acutely or subacutely involved rheumatoid joints has become more popular since Harris and McCroskery (38) found that destructive enzymes are more active at higher temperatures. Synovial collagenase, which is found in rheumatoid joints and destroys collagen fibers in cartilage, is one of these enzymes. They studied the temperature range between 30°C and 35°C. These findings support the clinical concern that heat applied directly to the joint might actually worsen the inflammatory reaction; cold application may not only reduce the inflammatory reactions, but also retard the destruction resulting from these enzymes. It must be recognized that the evaluation of any type of therapy in rheumatoid arthritis is extremely difficult. Evaluation of effectiveness is virtually impossible without objective measurements in a controlled series in a disease which shows a natural history of exacerbations followed by improvements. Such controlled studies are not available at this time; however, studies are available in the literature which give the clinical impression, on a mostly subjective basis, that ice application may alleviate rheumatoid symptomatology. Pegg *et al.* (74) studied 35 joints and found a reduction of the complaint of stiffness with an immediate improvement between 91 and 100 percent, with a residual benefit of 100 percent over a series of 11 treatments. The authors found a similar reduction of joint pain between 62 and 93 percent and a residual benefit ranging between 53 and 93 percent. They also measured the range of motion and found an improvement. Kirk and Kersley (47) examined the pain and stiffness in 20 rheumatoid knees and found an improvement of pain with cold application in seven cases, and with heat application in six cases. There was a lessening of stiffness with cold in six cases, and in two by heat applications.

Landen (51) treated 117 patients with low back pain. She divided the patients into eight groups: those with minimal, with moderate, or with marked increase in low back pain; those with minimal, with moderate, or with marked decrease in low back pain; those with no change; and those who were asymptomatic. When she compared the percentage of patients falling within any one of those categories before treatment with ice and after treatment, she found the major shift toward the group with marked decrease in low back pain. However, if she treated with heat, she found the same change. She also compared the duration of the hospital stay in patients treated with ice and those treated with heat. The group of patients with acute pain stayed for a shorter period in the hospital when treated with heat as compared with cold treatment. Patients with chronic back pain, on the other hand, stayed in the hospital for a shorter period of time when treated with cold as compared with those treated with heat. The author did not find any difference in hospital stay when ice and heat treatment were compared in the total population (Figure 11.21).

While these clinical impressions suggest that ice is a useful modality in these conditions, there is still not enough information available on the basis of objective experiments to explain some of the discrepancies in the findings of various authors. Bäcklund and Tiselius (4) and Wright and Johns (98)

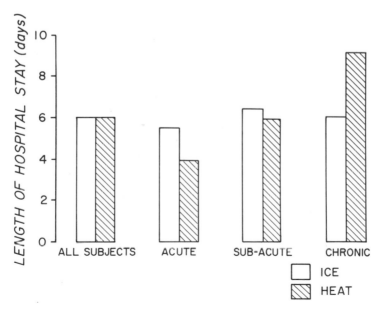

Fig. 11.21. Average days of hospitalization after heat and ice treatment of back pain syndromes (51).

developed a crank which moved the relaxed finger through the full range of extension and flexion at the second metacarpophalangeal joint. They measured the resistance to motion by attaching a strain gauge to the lever arm of the crank and found that the resistance was different in the upstroke than in the downstroke. A hysteresis loop was observed. Detailed analysis of this loop allows both quantitative assessment of the elastic and viscous properties of the tissues, and estimation of the friction in the joint (Figure 11.22). By and large, the steepness of the hysteresis loop indicated the degree of stiffness. Bäcklund and Tiselius found in a series of normal females and males that the joints of females were slightly less stiff than those of males (Figure 11.23). By comparison, they found in rheumatoid patients that the stiffness, that is, the steepness of the loop, was markedly increased (Figure 11.24).

They also observed that there was a strong correlation between the subjective feeling of stiffness and the steepness of the hysteresis loop. When they heated the joints of rheumatoid patients, they found a decrease in the stiffness, whereas cooling increased the stiffness. Wright and Johns also found increased stiffness with cold (Figure 11.25).

The previously described clinical observations, indicating a decrease in stiffness, and these objective measurements of Bäcklund and Tiselius do

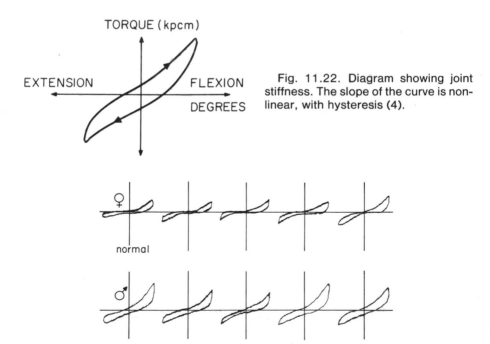

Fig. 11.22. Diagram showing joint stiffness. The slope of the curve is nonlinear, with hysteresis (4).

Fig. 11.23. Resistance to passive flexion and extension of the second metacarpophalangeal joint in healthy young females and males (4).

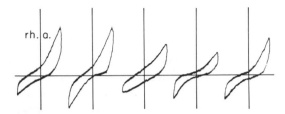

Fig. 11.24. Resistance to passive flexion and extension of the second metacarpophalangeal joint in five patients with rheumatoid arthritis (4).

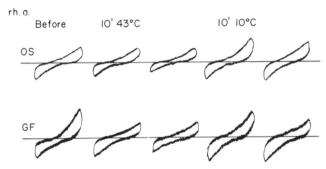

Fig. 11.25. Effect of temperature on joint stiffness in two patients with rheumatoid arthritis (4).

not necessarily have to be contradictory, but further information is needed. Conceivably, the subjective reduction of stiffness by ice application to the joint may depend on the vigor with which ice is applied. If the temperature is lowered enough, sensation may be impaired to the point that the patient does not perceive stiffness any more, even though objectively the joint becomes appreciably stiffer.

In acute subacromial or subdeltoid bursitis, cold is usually preferred to heat since it reduces swelling and, therefore, reduces pain. It has been documented that if one aspirates the content of the bursa, thereby reducing the pressure, the pain is relieved; when one reinjects a volume of fluid equal to that which had been withdrawn, the pain recurs. Although in other acute conditions, such as acute peri-arthritis of the shoulder, cold is used, heat may be used at a later stage. Heat applied to such inflammatory reactions as bursitis may acutely aggravate the pain of the patient (37).

Cold, in the form of ethyl chloride spray, has also been used extensively by Kraus (50), Travell (89), Bonica (13, 14), Grant (36), and others for treating so-called trigger points, myofascial pain and myofibrositis. However, since these conditions are still poorly understood and not well-defined, it is difficult to assess the effectiveness of this type of therapy beyond the possibility that it may act as a counter-irritant.

Cold, alternating with heat, is used in contrast baths (15, 30, 39, 42, 62, 97). A contrast bath produces a marked increase in blood flow to the hands and feet. It relieves stiffness and pain in such conditions as Heberden's nodes and chronic arthritides of the small joints of hands and feet.

In cases with excessive vasodilatation during the early phase of Sudeck's atrophy, cold application may reduce vasodilatation and metabolic demand resulting from alleviation of the tissue temperature, and thus, decrease destruction of tissue. However, as soon as the period of reactive hyperemia has disappeared, cold should be discontinued, since in a later stage of this disease, vasospasm is predominantly present.

Techniques of Cold Application

The vast majority of cold applications use melting ice together with water; this produces a steady temperature of 0°C. The part may be treated by immersion in ice water, by application of compresses containing melting ice with water or by application of a terry cloth, dipped in water with ice shavings, wrung out, and then applied repeatedly. Also, ice massage has been used, moving a block of ice over the surface to be cooled. In any one of these applications, the result is an almost instantaneous drop in the skin temperature with a drop, almost as rapid, of the superficial subcutaneous

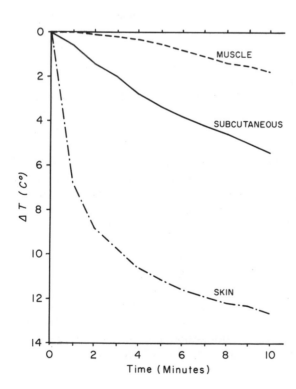

Fig. 11.26. Change of skin, subcutaneous, and muscle temperatures during topical (thigh) ice application in a person with less than 1 cm of subcutaneous fat.

temperature, and a much slower reduction of the muscle temperature. The slowness of the drop of the muscle temperature depends largely upon the thickness of the subcutaneous fat.

It has been demonstrated (Figure 11.26) that in patients with less than 1 cm of subcutaneous fat, there is a significant reduction of muscle temperature after 10 minutes of cold application. If the temperature distribution is plotted at this time, cooling can be seen to occur to a maximal depth of 2 cm into the muscle (Figure 11.27).

If the patient has more than 2 cm of fat, the muscle temperature hardly drops after 10 minutes of ice application (Figure 11.28). The depth of the temperature change in the muscle is about 1 cm (Figure 11.29).

It takes a long time to rewarm the muscle after ice application is discontinued, as shown by Hartviksen (40) and Bierman and Friedlander (7). When ice is applied to the skin, vasoconstriction occurs; cooling then has to occur through the subcutaneous fat layer, which is an excellent thermal insulator. Therefore, the thicker the fat layer, the more time it takes to cool the muscle. Once the muscle is cooled, the blood flow to the muscle is reduced, and therefore, warming via an increase in blood flow does not occur rapidly. At the same time, the muscle is shielded against rewarming from ambient higher temperatures through the insulating subcutaneous fat. This

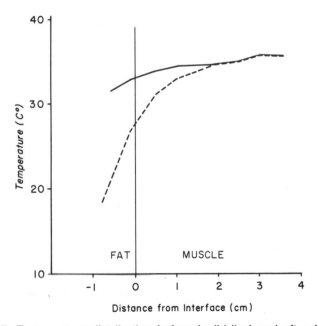

Fig. 11.27. Temperature distribution before (*solid line*) and after (*dashed line*) topical (thigh) ice application for 10 minutes in a person with less than 1 cm of subcutaneous fat.

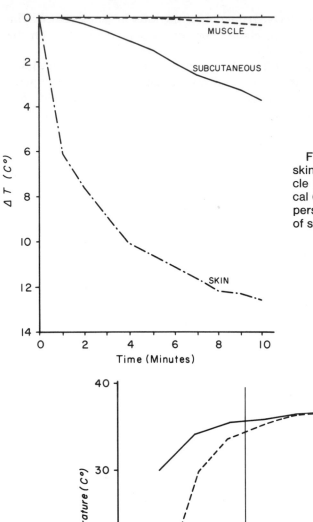

Fig. 11.28. Change of skin, subcutaneous, and muscle temperatures during topical (thigh) ice application in a person with greater than 2 cm of subcutaneous fat.

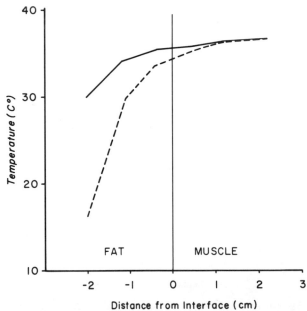

Fig. 11.29. Temperature distribution before (*solid line*) and after (*dashed line*) topical (thigh) ice application for 10 minutes in a person with greater than 2 cm of subcutaneous fat.

is the most important known reason why there is a long period after ice application when spasticity is reduced. This enables the therapist to increase the range of motion in joints, to stretch tight muscle groups, and to train the patient in order to improve motor skills. It is not known whether reduction of spasticity lasts longer than the cooling of the muscle. There is no evidence that spasticity is permanently relieved. However, in secondary muscle spasms a permanent resolution can be obtained. It is likely that once a vicious cycle of secondary muscle spasm, ischemia, pain, with resulting stimulation of more spasms, can be broken, the spasms may not return.

Cooling to relieve muscle spasm or spasticity should extend over a sufficiently long time. For a slender individual, cooling should last longer than 10 minutes; for an obese individual, it should last longer than one-half hour. The same methods of cooling can also be used in minor injuries to prevent the development of swelling and hemorrhage. The therapeutic effect in part is the result of vasoconstriction. Therefore, simultaneous compression of the injured part is often helpful. Cooling of this type is usually done for 4 to 6 hours (79). It may be extended over a period of 24 to 48 hours; however, it should be remembered that once swelling has been prevented, once hemostasis has been produced, further cooling serves no purpose, since pain is rarely a problem at that time. Lundgren *et al.* (59) produced experimental wounds in rabbits and assessed wound healing by measuring the tensile strength. They found that healing was decreased when they cooled the wounds to 12°C as compared with a temperature of 20°C. Tensile strength was reduced 20 percent (Figure 11.30). They also found that this retardation in wound healing was due to vasoconstriction. Slowing of wound healing did not occur in the presence of sympathectomy. However, one should remember that, with more intense cooling, vasoconstriction can be produced in the presence of sympathectomies by a direct action on the blood vessels.

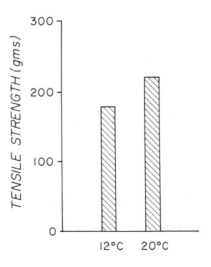

Fig. 11.30. Mean values of tensile strength of healing wounds at 12 and 20°C (59).

Evaporative cooling with ethyl chloride spray is usually done by spraying the skin from a distance of one meter with a stroking motion. Bierman (6) suggested a movement of the spray 4 in/second and suggested that each area should be sprayed only for a few seconds, followed by a pause. With this type of spray, frosting of the skin should be avoided. More recently, chlorofluoromethanes have been suggested (88) to replace ethyl chloride because of the high flammability of ethyl chloride.

McMaster *et al.* (64) compared various newer modalities for cold application: a frozen gel, a chemical ice envelope (a chemical which can be broken within the package and the package applied when the endothermal reaction cools the pack), refrigerant-inflated bladders, and chipped ice. They found that the standardized application with melting ice water cooled better than any one of the other more recently available methods. Refrigeration units based on thermoelectric or evaporative principles (93, 94) may produce temperatures significantly below the freezing point and, unless they have special features, frostbite is a possibility.

Contrast bathing is a method of combined heat and cold application, with resulting increase in blood flow and decrease in joint stiffness. Alternate immersion of the limb in hot and cold water at approximately 40°C (104°F) and approximately 15°C (59°F) is used. An initial period of 10 minutes in hot water is followed by a 1-minute exposure to cold water. This, in turn, is followed by 4 minutes immersion in hot water and 1 minute in cold water, to be repeated until a total treatment of 30 minutes has been completed (68).

Adverse effects

Fortunately, severe adverse effects of cold application are rare. The major group is due to hypersensitivity to cold. Juhlin and Shelley (46) divided cold hypersensitivity syndromes into three categories. The first group of cold hypersensitivity syndromes is the result of release of histamine or histamine-like substances. It presents itself frequently as the classical cold urticaria. The effects are primarily those of histamine on capillary vessels and smooth musculature throughout the body. Skin manifestations in addition to the urticaria include erythema, itching, and sweating. A facial flush may also be observed. There is puffiness of the eyelids and laryngeal edema; respiratory embarrassment may be present. In more severe cases, there is shock or so-called cold anaphylaxis with syncope, hypotension, tachycardia, and extrasystoles. Gastrointestinal symptoms are associated with gastric hyperacidity and include dysphagia, abdominal pain, diarrhea, and vomiting. A passive transfer is possible only in the idiopathic type of cold sensitivity. Tennenbaum and Lowney (87) repeated the occurrence of localized heat and cold urticaria in the same individual.

Horton *et al.* (43) found that this type of sensitivity is amenable to treatment. They observed patients who collapsed and were unconscious for a limited period of time after a short swim in a cold lake. In a series of 22 subjects, they found that 14 had systemic reactions. Eleven of the 14 developed syncope. Horton *et al.* found that the syndrome was treatable by desensitization to cold. They had the patients immerse the hand in water at 10°C for 1 to 2 minutes twice a day for 3 to 4 weeks (Figure 11.31). An alternate method was daily immersion of the hand in cool water starting at 65°F (18°C) and decreasing the temperature to 45°F (7°C) for increasing periods of time. Of the 22 patients Horton *et al.* studied, 16 became completely well and 5 were improved. They also suggested that patients can be desensitized to cold by subcutaneous administration of 0.1 mg. or less of histamine twice daily for 2 to 3 weeks.

The second group of hypersensitivity syndromes described by Juhlin and Shelley is the result of the presence of cold hemolysins and agglutinins. They primarily produce general symptoms such as malaise, chills and fever, with a significant anemia. The presence of cold hemolysins and agglutinins can be demonstrated in the blood. Renal symptomatology includes paroxysmal cold hemoglobinuria. The skin manifestations are cold urticaria, ulcers, Raynaud's phenomenon, and acrocyanosis.

The third group of hypersensitivity syndromes are the result of the

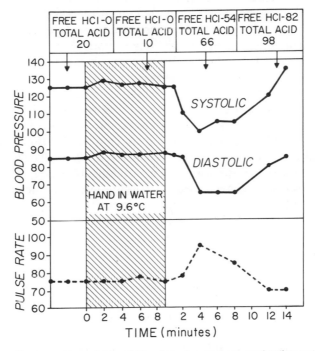

Fig. 11.31. Changes in gastric acidity, blood pressure, and pulse rate in a patient with hypersensitivity to cold after immersion of a hand in water at 9.6°C for 9 minutes (43).

presence of cryoglobulins, which in turn produce chills and fever and seriously affect both vision and hearing to the point of blindness and deafness. Also, conjunctival hemorrhages and epistaxis may be present. An anemia with fibrinogenopenia, elevated sedimentation rate, cryoglobulin inclusion cells, and cryoglobulins are observed. There is no passive transfer possible except with cryoprotein. The skin manifestations include erythema, itching, purpura, cold urticaria, Raynaud's phenomenon, and ulceration and necrosis. Dyspnea may be present, gastrointestinal symptoms may include stomatitis, melena, and gingival bleeding.

Some of the syndromes occur in the presence of associated disease, such as lupus erythematosus, atypical pneumonia, leucocytoclastic vasculitis, rheumatoid disease, progressive systemic sclerosis, or multiple myeloma. From this description, it is obvious that some of these side effects may be serious. Necrosis after injudicious immersion in ice water for diagnostic purposes was observed in all fingers of both hands of one patient. Prevention of such occurrences is possible only by a thorough medical evaluation including history and physical examination, which should include appropriate lab tests. A high degree of suspicion should be entertained in the presence of predisposing diseases.

It is also interesting to note that Nielsen *et al.* (71) found that patients with Raynaud's disease showed a pathological increase in arterial tone at 23.5°C with closure of the digital arteries at a mean temperature of 18.5°C. The temperature eliciting these reactions in patients with thromboangiitis obliterans was about 7°C lower; the increase in arterial tone occurred at 16.5°C and the closure of the arteries at 11°C. That implies that even moderately cool temperatures such as 18.5°C can create problems in some of these conditions. A marked cold pressor response, as in a patient with submersion of limbs in ice water, is also a contraindication to such cold application. In addition, pain produced by cold application seems to be a major stimulus for the vasopressor response (16, 53, 83, 95, 96).

In peripheral vascular diseases with arterial insufficiency, cold is contraindicated because of its potent vasoconstricting effect, reducing the already compromised blood flow through the extremity (1).

The rare observation by Raifman *et al.* (78) indicated that rhabdomyolysis may occasionally be the result of cold exposure.

Tissue damage resulting from frostbite is possible, though rare, with the use of modalities capable of dropping the temperature below the freezing point, and perhaps with the use of supercooled ice blocks for massage. Frostbite can be readily produced by excessive evaporative cooling using ethyl chloride and chlorofluoromethanes. Frostbite resulting from improper technique is usually not severe.

The overexposure to cold leads to a marked increase in capillary permeability that produces a rapid loss of plasma with stranding of the red cells in the capillaries. The red cells stick together and form occlusive masses which finally undergo hyalinization (52). Dawson and Hardenbergh (23) found that the severity of the frostbite depends to a lesser degree on the time the tissues are frozen than on the duration of the thawing period. Immediate immersion in warm water improves survival of the tissues. A water temperature of 43°C has been suggested. In summary, at least three independent factors apparently contribute to the final injury of frozen tissues: the length of time frozen, the temperature during the frozen state, and the duration of thawing. However, Lange *et al.* (52) showed that rewarming to a relatively high temperature of 44°C for 24 hours after exposure increases severity of the lesion.

Cold Versus Heat Therapy

On the basis of various authors' findings, there are conditions where apparently both heat and cold application may be used successfully. In addition, there are specific indications for cold or heat application where these two modalities cannot be used interchangeably. It, therefore, is worthwhile to briefly review the similarities and differences of these two types of therapy.

There are similarities between the two extremes of the temperature spectrum in the following conditions: heat and cold both decrease muscle spasms resulting from underlying skeletal and joint pathology and from nerve root irritation as it is encountered in low back syndromes. Cold is a very effective treatment of spasticity in cases of upper motor neuron lesions. Heat, on the other hand, may also reduce spasticity, but only on a short-term basis, so that the decrease of spasticity cannot be used for other therapeutic purposes such as training in motor skills. Because of the thermodynamics of the heat exchange in tissues, once a muscle is cooled, it takes a long time for the tissue to return to normal temperatures. With heat application, because of the great increase in blood flow, the return to normal temperature occurs within minutes. It is assumed that the effectiveness of heat application in relieving secondary muscle spasm is due to the fact that it breaks up a vicious cycle where spasm leads to ischemia and pain, and triggers, in turn, more muscle spasm. Even a short-term interruption of this cycle may permanently relieve the symptom. The pain sensation is directly and indirectly reduced by heat and by cold application.

In other areas, heat and cold produce the opposite physiological phenomena. A sustained contraction can be maintained only for a short period of time if the tissues are heated. Moderate cooling to approximately 27°C increases the capability to sustain the contraction. The strength of contraction according to some authors is increased by slightly lowering the tissue temperature, but decreased with further cooling, whereas there seems to be slight increase with heating. The tissue metabolism is clearly reduced due to cold application and increased when the tissue temperature is elevated. The blood flow is decreased with cold application and increased with heating. Therefore, the tendency to bleed is decreased with cold application and increased with heating. It is generally assumed that edema is produced more readily with heating and is reduced with cooling. However, there is evidence in experimentally produced inflammatory reactions that cold may not always alleviate edema and that what happened may be specific for a given type of inflammation. In some cases, heat application may be more effective in reducing the edema. Also, in trauma, effectiveness in reducing edema may depend on the type of cold application (Matsen *et al.* (63)). Capillary permeability may be increased in both cases, depending on the degree of cooling or heating. Burns can be alleviated by immediate cooling, while the effects of frostbite can be reduced by quick warming. Joint stiffness is increased with cold application and is decreased with heat application. Skilled movements are impaired by cold. Orthostatic hypotension is readily produced by heat application to larger parts of the body or total exposure. It is decreased due to vasoconstriction during cold application (61, 63, 81).

Cold can be used acutely in injuries or in acute inflammatory responses, and heat can be used late to assist in their resolution. Thus, each modality, cold or heat, has its indications, its contraindications, and, in some cases, both modalities can be used interchangeably. More understanding, specifically in the management of joint diseases with these two modalities, is necessary to clearly delineate when cold and when heat should be applied.

REFERENCES

1. ABRAMSON, D. I. Physiologic basis for the use of physical agents in peripheral vascular disorders. *Arch. Phys. Med. Rehabil.*, *46:* 216–244, 1965.
2. ALLEN, F. M. Experiments concerning ligation and refrigeration in relation to local intoxication and infection. *Surg. Gynecol. Obstet.*, *68:* 1047–1051, 1937.
3. ALLEN, F. M. Reduced temperatures in surgery. I. Surgery of limbs. *Am. J. Surg.*, *52:* 225–237, 1941.
4. BÄCKLUND, L. AND TISELIUS, P. Objective measurement of joint stiffness in rheumatoid arthritis. *Acta Rheum. Scand.*, *13:* 275–288, 1967.
5. BASUR, R. L., SHEPHARD, E. AND MOUZAS, G. L. A cooling method in the treatment of ankle sprains. *Practitioner, 216:* 708–711, 1976.
6. BIERMAN, W. Therapeutic use of cold. *J.A.M.A.*, *157:* 1189–1192, 1955.
7. BIERMAN, W. AND FRIEDLANDER, M. The penetrative effect of cold. *Arch. Phys. Ther., 21:* 585–591, 1940.
8. BINGHAM, R. The therapeutic effect of cold in bone and joint infection, part I. *Am. J. Orthop. Surg., 10:* 158–165, 1968.
9. BINGHAM, R. The therapeutic effect of cold in bone and joint infection, conclusion. *Am. J. Orthop. Surg., 10:* 186–189, 1968.
10. BISGARD, J. D. AND NYE, D. The influence of hot and cold application upon gastric and intestinal motor activity. *Surg. Gynecol. Obstet., 71:* 172–180, 1940.
11. BISHOP, B., MACHOVER, S., JOHNSTON, R., ANDERSON, M. A quantitative assessment of gamma motoneuron contribution to the Achilles tendon reflex in normal subjects. *Arch. Phys. Med. Rehabil., 49:* 145–154, 1968.
12. BOES, M. C. Reduction of spasticity by cold. *J. Am. Phys. Ther. Assoc., 42:* 29–32, 1962.
13. BONICA, J. J. Management of myofascial pain syndromes in general practice. *J.A.M.A., 164:* 732–738, 1957.

14. BONICA, J. J. The management of myofascial pain syndromes. *Phys. Ther. Rev., 39:* 389–396, 1959.

15. BOWIE, M. A. Physical therapy in arthritis. *In: Arthritis and Allied Conditions.* Hollander, J. L. (Ed). Seventh edition. Lea and Febiger, Chapter 28, pp. 481–527, 1966.

16. BOYER, J. T., FRASER, J. R. E. AND DOYLE, A. E. The haemodynamic effects of cold immersion. *Clin. Sci., 19:* 539–550, 1960.

17. CHATFIELD, P. O. Hypothermia and its effects on the sensory and peripheral motor systems. *Ann. N.Y. Acad. Sci., 80:* 445–448, 1959.

18. CHATFIELD, P. O., BATTISTA, A. F., LYMAN, C. P., *et al.* Effects of cooling on nerve conduction in a hibernator (golden hamster) and non-hibernator (albino rat). *Am. J. Physiol., 155:* 179–185, 1948.

19. CLARKE, R. S. J., HELLON, R. F. AND LIND, A. R. The duration of sustained contractions of the human forearm at different muscle temperatures. *J. Physiol., 143:* 454–473, 1958.

20. CLARKE, R. S. J., HELLON, R. F. AND LIND, A. R. Vascular reactions of the human forearm to cold. *Clin. Sci., 17:* 165–179, 1958.

21. COLES, D. R. AND COOPER, K. E. Hyperaemia following arterial occlusion or exercise in the warm and cold human forearm. *J. Physiol., 145:* 241–250, 1959.

22. COPPIN, E. G., LIVINGSTONE, S. D. AND KUEHN, L. A. Effects on handgrip strength due to arm immersion in a 10° water bath. *Aviat. Space Environ. Med., 49:* 1322–1326, 1978.

23. DAWSON, D. AND HARDENBERGH, E. Effect of rapid rewarming on tissue survival of frozen rabbits' feet. *J. Appl. Physiol., 12:* 155–163, 1958.

24. DE JONG, P. H., HERSHEY, W. N. AND WAGMAN, I. H. Nerve conduction velocity during hypothermia in man. *Anesthesiology, 27:* 805–810, 1966.

25. DEMLING, R. H., MAZESS, R. B. AND WOLBERG, W. The effect of immediate and delayed cold immersion on burn edema formation and resorption. *J. Trauma, 17:* 56–60, 1979.

26. DOUGLAS, W. W. AND MALCOLM, J. L. The effect of localized cooling on conduction in cat nerves. *J. Physiol., 130:* 53–71, 1955.

27. ELDRED, E., LINDSLEY, D. F. AND BUCHWALD, J. S. The effect of cooling on mammalian muscle spindles. *Exp. Neurol., 2:* 144–157, 1960.

28. FISCHER, E. AND SOLOMON, S. Physiological responses to heat and cold. *In: Therapeutic Heat and Cold.* Licht, S. (Ed). Second edition, Chapter 4, Waverly Press, Baltimore, pp. 126–169, 1965.

29. FOX, R. H. Local cooling in man. *Br. Med. Bull., 17:* 14–18, 1961.

30. FRICKE, E. J. AND GERSTEN, J. W. Effect of contrast baths on the vasomotor response of rheumatoid arthritis patients. *Arch. Phys. Med., 33:* 210–216, 1952.

31. GANONG, W. F. *The Nervous System.* Second edition. Lange Medical Publications, 1979.

32. GAYDOS, H. F. AND DUSEK, E. R. Effects of localized hand cooling versus total body cooling on manual performance. *J. Appl. Physiol., 12:* 377–380, 1958.

33. GOODGOLD, J. AND EBERSTEIN, A. *Electrodiagnosis of Neuromuscular Diseases.* Second edition. The Williams and Wilkins Company, Baltimore, 1977.

34. GOODMAN, L. S. AND GILMAN, A. *The Pharmacological Basis of Therapeutics.* Fifth edition. Macmillan, 1975.

35. GRANIT, R. *Receptors and Sensory Perception.* Yale University Press, New Haven, 1955.

36. GRANT, A. E. Massage with ice (cryokinetics) in the treatment of painful conditions of the musculoskeletal system. *Arch. Phys. Med. Rehabil., 45:* 233–238, 1964.

37. GUCKER, T. III. The use of heat and cold in orthopedics. *In: Therapeutic Heat and Cold.* Licht, S. (ed). Second edition, Chapter 15. Waverly Press, Baltimore, pp. 398–406, 1965.

38. HARRIS, E. D. AND McCROSKERY, P. A. The influence of temperature and fibril stability on degradation of cartilage collagen by rheumatoid synovial collagenase. *N. Engl. J. Med., 290:* 1–6, 1974.

39. HARRIS, R. Heat in vascular disorders. *In: Therapeutic Heat and Cold.* Licht, S. (ed). Second edition, Chapter 16. Waverly Press, Baltimore, pp. 407–432, 1965.

40. HARTVIKSEN, K. Ice therapy in spasticity. *Acta Neurol. Scand. 38 [suppl 3]:* 79–84, 1962.

41. HAYDEN, C. A. Cryokinetics in an early treatment program. *J. Am. Phys. Ther. Assoc., 44:* 990–993, 1964.
42. HOLMES, G. Hydrotherapy as a means of rehabilitation. *Br. J. Phys. Med., 5:* 93–95, 1942.
43. HORTON, B. T., BROWNE, G. E. AND ROTH, G. M. Hypersensitiveness to cold. *J.A.M.A., 107:* 1263–1268, 1936.
44. HUNT, C. C. The effect of sympathetic stimulation on mammalian muscle spindles. *J. Physiol., 151:* 332–341, 1960.
45. JEZDINSKÝ, J., MAREK, J. AND OCHONSKÝ, P. Effects of local cold and heat therapy on traumatic oedema of the rat hind paw. I. Effects of cooling on the course of traumatic oedema. *Acta Univ. Olomuc. Fac. Med., 66:* 185–201, 1973.
46. JUHLIN, L. AND SHELLEY, W. B. Role of mast cell and basophil in cold urticaria with associated systemic reactions. *J.A.M.A., 117:* 371–377, 1961.
47. KIRK, J. A. AND KERSLEY, G. D. Heat and cold in the physical treatment of rheumatoid arthritis of the knee. *Ann. Phys. Med., 9:* 270–274, 1968.
48. KNUTSSON, E. Topical cryotherapy in spasticity. *Scand. J. Rehabil. Med., 2:* 159–163, 1970.
49. KNUTSSON, E. AND MATTSSON, E. Effects of local cooling on monosynaptic reflexes in man. *Scand. J. Rehabil. Med., 1:* 126–132, 1969.
50. KRAUS, H. *Therapeutic Exercise.* Charles C Thomas, Springfield, IL, 1949.
51. LANDEN, B. R. Heat or cold for the relief of low back pain? *Phys. Ther., 47:* 1126–1128, 1967.
52. LANGE, K., WEINER, D. AND BOYD, L. J. Frostbite. Physiology, pathology and therapy. *N. Engl. J. Med., 237:* 383–389, 1947.
53. LARSON, D. L. *Systemic Lupus Erythematosus.* Little, Brown, 1961.
54. LEWIS, T. Observation on some normal and injurious effects of cold upon the skin and underlying tissues. I. Reactions to cold, and injury of normal skin. *Br. Med. J., 2:* 795–797, 1941.
55. LEWIS, T. Observations upon the reactions of the vessels of the human skin to cold. *Heart, 15:* 177–208, 1930.
56. LI, C.-L. Effect of cooling on neuromuscular transmission in the rat. *Am. J. Physiol., 194:* 200–206, 1958.
57. LI, C.-L. AND GOURAS, P. Effect of cooling on neuromuscular transmission in the frog. *Am. J. Physiol., 192:* 464–470, 1958.
58. LIPPOLD, O. C. J., NICHOLLS, J. G. AND REDFEARN, J. W. T. A study of the afferent discharge produced by cooling a mammalian muscle spindle. *J. Physiol., 153:* 218–231, 1960.
59. LUNDGREN, C., MUREN, A. AND ZEDERFELDT, B. Effect of cold vasoconstriction on wound healing in the rabbit. *Acta Chir. Scand., 118:* 1–4, 1959.
60. MACLAGAN, J. AND ZAIMIS, E. The effect of muscle temperature on twitch and tetanus in the cat. *J. Physiol., 137:* 89P–90P, 1957.
61. MAREK, J., JEZDINSKÝ, J. AND OCHONSKÝ, P. Effects of local cold and heat therapy on traumatic oedema of the rat hind paw. III. Effects of various kinds of compresses on the course of traumatic oedema. *Acta Univ. Olomuc. Fac., 66:* 203–228, 1973.
62. MARTIN, G. M., ROTH, G. M., ELKINS, E. C., *et al.* Cutaneous temperature of the extremities of normal subjects and of patients with rheumatoid arthritis. *Arch. Phys. Med., 27:* 665–682, 1946.
63. MATSEN, F. A. III, QUESTAD, K. AND MATSEN, A. L. The effect of local cooling on post fracture swelling. *Clin. Orthop., 109:* 201–206, 1975.
64. MCMASTER, W. C., LIDDLE, S. AND WAUGH, T. R. Laboratory evaluation of various cold therapy modalities. *Am. J. Sports Med., 6:* 291–294, 1978.
65. MELZACK, R. AND WALL, P. D. Pain mechanisms: a new theory. *Science, 150:* 971–979, 1965.
66. MICHALSKI, W. J. AND SEGUIN, J. J. The effect of muscle cooling and stretch on muscle spindle secondary endings in the cat. *J. Physiol., 253:* 341–356, 1975.

67. MIGLIETTA, O. Action of cold on spasticity. *Am. J. Phys. Med.*, *52:* 198–205, 1973.
68. MILLARD, J. B. Conductive heating. *In: Therapeutic Heat and Cold.* Licht, S. (Ed). Second edition, Chapter 8. Waverly Press, Baltimore, pp. 240–251, 1965.
69. MOORE, C. D. AND CARDEA, J. A. Vascular changes in leg trauma. *South Med. J.*, *70:* 1285–1286 *passim*, 1977.
70. NELMS, J. D. AND SOPER, D. J. G. Cold vasodilatation and cold acclimatization in the hands of British fish filleters. *J. Appl. Physiol.*, *17:* 444–448, 1962.
71. NIELSEN, S. L., NOBIN, B. A., HIRAI, M., *et al.* Raynaud's phenomenon in arterial obstructive disease of the hand demonstrated by locally provoked cooling. *Scand. J. Thorac. Cardiovasc. Surg.*, *12:* 105–109, 1978.
72. OTTOSON, D. The effects of temperature on the isolated muscle spindle. *J. Physiol.*, *180:* 636–648, 1965.
73. PARSONS, C. M. AND GOETZL, F. R. Effect of induced pain on pain threshold. *Proc. Soc. Exp. Biol. Med.*, *60:* 327–329, 1945.
74. PEGG, S. M. H., LITTLER, T. R. AND LITTLER, E. N. A Trial of ice therapy and exercise in chronic arthritis. *Physiotherapy*, *55:* 51–56, 1969.
75. PERKINS, J. F., LI, M.-C., HOFFMAN, F., *et al.* Sudden vasoconstriction in denervated or sympathectomized paws exposed to cold. *Am. J. Physiol.*, *155:* 165–178, 1948.
76. PETAJAN, R. H. AND WATTS, N. Effects of cooling on the triceps surae reflex. *Am. J. Phys. Med.*, *41:* 240–251, 1962.
77. PROVINS, K. A. AND MORTON, R. Tactile discrimination and skin temperature. *J. Appl. Physiol.*, *15:* 155–160, 1960.
78. RAIFMAN, M. A., BERANT, M. AND LENARSKY, C. Cold weather and rhabdomyolysis. *J. Pediatr.*, *93:* 970–971, 1978.
79. RYAN, A. J. Traumatic injuries: office treatment of strain. *Postgrad. Med.*, *61:* 215–218, 1977.
80. SCHAUBEL, H. J. The local use of ice after orthopedic procedures. *Am. J. Surg.*, *72:* 711–714, 1946.
81. SCHMIDT, K. L., OTT, V. R., RÖCHER, G., *et al.* Heat, cold and inflammation. *Rheumatol.*, *38:* 391–404, 1979.
82. SCHOEPFLE, G. M. AND ERLANGER, J. The action of temperature on the excitability, spike height and configuration, and the refractory period observed in the responses of single medullated nerve fibers. *Am. J. Physiol.*, *134:* 694–704, 1941.
83. SHELLEY, W. B. AND CARO, W. A. Cold erythema. *J.A.M.A.*, *180:* 639–642, 1962.
84. SHULMAN, A. G. Ice water as primary treatment of burns. *J.A.M.A.*, *173:* 1916–1919, 1960.
85. TAIT, J. The heart of hibernating animals. *Am. J. Physiol.*, *59:* 467, 1922.
86. TEICHNER, W. H. Manual dexterity in the cold. *J. Appl. Physiol.*, *11:* 333–338, 1957.
87. TENNENBAUM, J. I. AND LOWNEY, E. Localized heat and cold urticaria. *J. Allergy Clin. Immunol.*, *51:* 57–59, 1973.
88. TRAHERNE, J. B. Evaluation of the cold spray technique in the treatment of muscle pain in general practice. *Practitioner*, *189:* 210–212, 1962.
89. TRAVELL, J. Ethyl chloride spray for painful muscle spasm. *Arch. Phys. Med.*, *33:* 291–298, 1952.
90. URBSCHEIT, N. AND BISHOP, B. Effects of cooling on the ankle jerk and H-response. *Phys. Ther.*, *50:* 1041–1049, 1970.
91. URBSCHEIT, N., JOHNSTON, R. AND BISHOP, B. Effects of cooling on the ankle jerk and H-response in hemiplegic patients. *Phys. Ther.*, *51:* 983–988, 1971.
92. WALKER, S. M. Potentiation of twitch tension and prolongation of action potential induced by reduction of temperature in rat and frog muscle. *Am. J. Physiol.*, *157:* 429–435, 1949.
93. WOLF, S. L. AND BASMAJIAN, J. V. A rapid cooling device for controlled cutaneous stimulation. *Phys. Ther.*, *53:* 25–27, 1973.
94. WOLF, S. L. AND BASMAJIAN, J. V. Intramuscular temperature changes deep to localized cutaneous cold stimulation. *Phys. Ther.*, *53:* 1284–1288, 1973.

95. WOLF, S. AND HARDY, J. D. Studies on pain. Observations on pain due to local cooling and on factors involved in the "cold pressor" effect. *J. Clin. Invest., 20:* 521–533, 1941.

96. WOLFF, H. H. The mechanism and significance of the cold pressor response. *Q. J. Med., 20:* 261–273, 1951.

97. WOODMANSEY, A., COLLINS, D. H. AND ERNST, M. M. Vascular reactions to contrast both in health and in rheumatoid arthritis. *Lancet, 2:* 1350–1353, 1938.

98. WRIGHT, V. AND JOHNS, R. J. Physical factors concerned with the stiffness of normal and diseased joints. *Bull. Johns Hopkins Hosp., 106:* 215–231, 1960.

99. ZITOWITZ, L. AND HARDY, J. D. Influence of cold exposure on thermal burns in the rat. *J. Appl. Physiol., 12:* 147–154, 1958.

12

Hyperthermia in the Treatment of Malignancies

JAMES R. OLESON
EUGENE W. GERNER[1]

Introduction

BIOLOGICAL RATIONALE

While the historical development of hyperthermia dates from the nineteenth century and before (1), the past decade has witnessed an explosion in research results showing the potential, and more recently, the clinical utility of hyperthermia in human cancer therapy. Until 1971, reports on the potential applicability of heat in clinical oncology appeared sporadically and were often lacking controls and quantification of results so that significance could be assessed. Up to this time, a variety of investigators had suggested that heat was selectively lethal to cancer cells (2, 3, 4), and there were anecdotal clinical reports that heat was effective in treating human malignancies (5–8) either as a single agent or in combination with radiation therapy. In 1963, Belli and Bonte (9) published a significant paper, quantifying the radiosensitizing effects of hyperthermia. Unfortunately, this work attracted little attention, and the field was generally dormant during the next few years.

In 1971, a paper appeared which has had a dramatic influence on the

[1] The authors wish to recognize and thank their co-workers who have participated in this work over the past 7 years in the Hyperthermia Program at the University of Arizona. These include Drs. M.R. Manning, T.C. Cetas, S. Aristizabal, E. Surwit, T.S. Herman, R.C. Miller, M.L.M. Boone, W.G. Connor, J.M. Landig-Hevezi, M.J. Schneider, R.S. Heusinkveld, J.T. Leith, A.E. Cress, D.J.M. Fuller, B.E. Magun, D.S. Alberts, R.C. Jones, T. Bowen, R. Nassoni, M. Dewhirst, E. Ozimek, and Mr. P. Stauffer. This work was supported by a Program Project Grant from the U.S. National Cancer Institute, CA 17343.

modern field of hyperthermic biology in that it provided the first new rationale in nearly four decades for the use of heat in cancer therapy. In this publication, Westra and Dewey (10) demonstrated that the cell cycle specific response of mammalian cells to heat was nearly the mirror image of that for ionizing radiation. Thus, heat seemed to be selectively lethal to radioresistant cells. In addition, this paper quantified thermodynamic parameters for heat cell killing and for the interaction of heat and radiation. It also provided insight on the mechanism of action for heat alone and heat radiosensitization. This paper was followed closely by the work of Ben-Hur et al. (11, 12) on heat radiosensitization in cultured cells, by Robinson and co-workers (13–15), and Gillette and co-workers (16, 17) on thermal enhancement ratios for the radioresponse of normal and tumor tissues in rodents, and by Mondovi and co-workers (18–21), the Overgaards (22), and Hahn (23) on mechanisms of hyperthermia action.

These workers confirmed and extended understandings from previous work on the synergistic interaction of heat with radiation. More importantly, their work demonstrated that heat was selectively lethal to radioresistant cells for a number of reasons, in addition to the cell cycle considerations of Westra and Dewey. These early workers laid the foundation for subsequent work that, along with the original observations, would show that environmental factors of tumors which tend to make them radioresistant, such as hypoxia, nutritional deprivation, and low pH, are parameters that make cells sensitive to heat induced cell killing and heat radiosensitization. A large volume of additional data has subsequently been generated on the interaction of heat and radiation in cells in culture and in normal tissues and tumor in vivo. These studies have shown that the sequence of application of these two agents greatly affects their synergistic interaction and that specific sequencing may be required to optimize the therapeutic gain factor when heat is combined with radiation. This topic has been recently reviewed in depth by Dewey and co-workers (24).

Laboratory studies on the effects of heat on radioresponsiveness have also been important in laying the foundation for clinical studies for reasons in addition to those previously cited. Normal tissue studies have addressed the effects of heat on both acute and chronic radiation responses. Miller et al. (25) and Goffinet et al. (26) have shown the need for caution, as they demonstrated that hyperthermia enhances late effects of radiation, such as injury to the spinal cord of rats and mice in terms of induced myelitis. The thermal enhancement of radio-response in these tissues, however, seems to be less than that for tumors (24). Perhaps the most convincing studies during the past 10 years about the potential clinical efficacy of hyperthermia are those which have used heat and radiation to treat spontaneously occurring tumors in large animals, such as dogs and cats. Groups at New Mexico, Stanford, and Arizona (see 27 for review) have observed significant clinical results in canine and feline tumors that resemble human tumors in terms of tumor volume, histologies, and growth kinetics. Of great importance, these studies all reported rather innocuous normal tissue reactions using heat and radiation doses resembling those which would be used in human therapy. Thus, these studies provided important Phase I preclinical toxicity information. The results in these large animal trials demonstrated that heat (43 to 45°C) combined with radiation was both safe and effective. These findings have been borne out in the Phase I/II human studies which have been recently reported and will be discussed later in this chapter.

During this past decade, hyperthermia has been shown to sensitize cells to the cytotoxic effects of a number of chemotherapeutic drugs (see 28 for review). George Hahn from Stanford has been a leader in this area. Results from his lab, and from other investigators, have shown that heat potentiates drug responses for a variety of reasons. Heat can increase drug uptake, inhibit repair mechanisms, inhibit efflux systems, affect interaction of drugs with target molecules, and affect intracellular metabolism of drugs. A major rationale which has evolved from these studies is that heat may be quite effective at overcoming drug resistance, which is known to limit the effectiveness of certain forms of chemotherapy. It is clear that beneficial interactions of heat will *not* occur with all chemotherapy agents. An example is actinomycin D, which interacts less than additively with hyperthermia (29). However, heat has been shown to interact at least additively and in some cases synergistically with a rather large number of drugs (see 28 for review), implying that this combination may also be of benefit in the treatment of human cancers.

Work over the past decade has firmly established the rationale for hyperthermia in human cancer therapy. Hyperthermia clearly enhances radioresponses, and results strongly suggest that tumors can be selectively sensitized with combinations of heat and radiation. Heat also enhances the action of certain chemotherapeutic drugs; and the use of novel approaches, such as those described by Yatvin and co-workers (30, 31) may be of significant benefit clinically. This group has described techniques employing encapsulation of drugs in liposomes that melt at hyperthermic temperatures. Then, by employing local heating of tumor volumes, selective release of the drug could be accomplished to give targeted tumoricidal effects. Additionally, Alberts et al. (32) have reported that heat may selectively potentiate the killing effect of a specific drug, cis-platinum, on tumor cells compared to normal cells. This may be due to differential effects on drug uptake.

Recent work has cast doubt on the original rationale for the use of heat in cancer therapy, that of selective heat sensitivity of tumor cells. The current status of this concept seems to be that some transformed and tumor cells may be more heat sensitive than their normal tissue counterparts, but this is probably not a general phenomenon. Work by Giovanella and co-workers (33), and Kase and Hahn (34) certainly shows that this selective lethal effect on tumor cells occurs in some instances. However, others have observed the opposite effects (35, 36). The mode of transformation seems to have a considerable effect on this differential heat response, with DNA tumor virus and certain chemically transformed cells being more heat sensitive than normal cells, while RNA tumor virus transformed cells are more heat resistant than normal cells. What may be more important than the innate cellular heat sensitivity to the clinical response of human tumors are the physiological characteristics of tumors. Environmental factors such as low pH, poor nutritional supply, and hypoxia may act to override quantitative differences in cellular sensitivities and lead to selective tumoricidal effects, even in instances where the tumor cells may be more resistant than normal tissues under similar *in vitro* conditions. Thus, recent work has tended to support the earlier concept of selective thermal sensitivity, but for reasons based on differences in the physiology of tumors compared to normal tissues rather than on presumed differences in innate cellular sensitivities.

MECHANISMS OF CYTOTOXICITY

Heat Alone

Scientific understanding of the mechanism(s) by which heat exerts its effects on normal and tumor cells has greatly increased over the past 10 years. Many investigators have contributed significantly in this area; details of each of their contributions are too numerous to discuss here. Rather, three recent models which incorporate many of these findings will be discussed.

Based on the work of his post-doctoral fellow Arthur Westra (10) and substantial subsequent work in his and other laboratories, William Dewey presented a model for the mechanism of heat cell killing of S phase mammalian cells and for heat radio-sensitization (37). His model speculates that killing occurs as a result of a defect in rejoining of DNA strand breaks. Hyperthermia-induced accumulation of nuclear proteins acts to restrict this rejoining. Chromosome aberrations result and correlate with cell death. This model implies that the mechanism of heat cell killing may be different for cells in various cell cycle phases and for heat resistant and heat sensitive cells.

The authors' group has presented a second model to explain the cytotoxic effects of heat on mammalian cells (38). This model is general for cells in all growth phases and relates heat sensitivity to resistance. The model suggests that damage to the plasma membrane is an integral and possibly limiting event in heat-induced cell killing. Changes in membrane permeability are speculated to be especially important, with heat sensitivity associated with a state of increased membrane permeability, and heat resistance associated with a decrease in membrane permeability. Membrane components affecting permeability are thus thought to be quite important, particularly cholesterol and protein levels (36, 38). A further aspect of this model involves the ubiquitously occurring organic cations, the polyamines (38, 39). It is thought that these polycations act to affect molecular interactions within the membrane, thus affecting permeability.

This model was constructed to be general for both normal and thermotolerant cells. Thermotolerance is the phenomenon of heat-induced heat resistance (40–44). It is a transient, non-heritable form of heat resistance. The authors' model speculates that killing of these cells is similar to that for non-tolerant cells, and involves damage to plasma membrane function. Genetic heat resistance has been reported by others, especially Harris (45). However, Reeves (46) has reported that heat-induced cell death in these genetic variants also involves alterations in cell membrane permeability. Thus, while membrane changes may be linked to genetic expression, the authors believe plasma membrane damage is an integral and general aspect of the mechanism by which heat kills cells.

A third model for heat-induced cytotoxicity and heat radiosensitization has been formulated by Roti Roti and co-workers (47). This model attempts to encompass the two previous models and be comprehensive for heat effects on cells and tissues. It takes account of known thermodynamic parameters of heat cell killing and temperature range dependencies of heat effects. The model speculates that the cytotoxic effects of heat in the 43 to 49°C temperature range result from a series of coupled events. It incorporates aspects of the authors' membrane damage model and postulates that this damage is translated to nuclear damage similar to that described in Dewey's model. The important advance here is that Roti Roti's model addresses the fact that heat causes rather immediate alterations in the plasma membrane, yet a significant percent of cells die a proliferative type of death in this temperature range. If membrane damage were the only type of significant damage, one would predict that mammalian cells would die an interphase type death in response to hyperthermia doses. This model also includes effects of environmental factors, since these can be easily translated into nuclear damage because of resulting damage to the plasma membrane. This concept of a series of interacting reactions being involved in heat damage was first documented by Landry and Marceau (48).

While these models have been useful to summarize current results and point out directions for future studies, they are by no means complete descriptions of heat effects on cells and tissues. Many investigators have focused on thermal effects on lysosomes. Overgaard (49) and Hume et al. (50) have presented evidence suggesting that heat-induced increases in lysosome number and lysosomal enzyme activity correlate with cell killing. These workers speculate that hyperthermia may lead to an increase in lysosomal activity followed by rupture due to lysosomal membrane damage. Further, they propose that the released degradating enzymes then damage other cellular structures and cell death ensues. This view has been criticized by Hofer *et al.* (51) and Magun and Fennie (52). The latter authors argue that increased lysosomal enzyme activity may be an artifact of the assay procedure, which is an *in vitro* technique using fixed tissue as the source. In contrast to the results of Hume *et al.* (50) Magun reported a decrease in a specific lysosomal degradative enzyme activity in treated whole cells. The role of lysosomes in heat-induced cell death remains controversial.

A relatively recent concept of the mechanism(s) of heat damage in mammalian cells involves heat-shock proteins. Heat-shock proteins have been extensively studied in Drosophila melanogaster (53). They have also been identified in a variety of mammalian cell types (54, 55). One recent study shows a close correlation between a specific heat-shock protein and resistance to heat-induced cell killing in yeast (56). Unfortunately, several other factors, cholesterol for example, also show a high degree of correlation with heat-induced cell killing (36). How these various parameters interact remains to be fully understood.

The cellular mechanism(s) by which heat exerts its action on cells is most certainly only one component of the mechanism(s) by which heat affects organized tissues and tumor *in vivo*. Physiological characteristics of tumor and normal tissues have been shown to have effects on responses to hyperthermia. Several groups have demonstrated that hyperthermia acts to shut down tissue microcirculation (57–60), and that this may occur at lower temperatures in tumors, compared to normal tissues. Heat effects on tissue microcirculation could lead to a number of states which might influence responses. One is that tumors in which circulation is reduced might preferentially heat to higher temperatures than surrounding tissues that have greater heat loss via vascular flow. Increased sensitivity then could result because of higher temperatures in cells within the tumor. A second effect of heat on tumors, resulting from a shutdown of blood flow, could be expressed due to a now deficient delivery system. Since the vascular network delivers factors such as oxygen and nutrients to tissues, a block of this network could lead to hypoxia and nutrient deprivation, both factors known to sensitize cells to thermal effects. A third effect is that of a blocked disposal system which could result in lowered tissue pH or accumulation of cytotoxic molecules. These latter two effects are clearly extracellular and could change tumor responses, even in the situation where temperature may not be selectively *raised* above surrounding normal tissue temperatures. All three effects, however, are related, and it will await further work to clarify the relative importance of innate cellular sensitivity and physiological changes in determining the overall responses of tumors and tissues *in vivo* to hyperthermia.

A final physiological parameter of possible significance in thermal responses of tumors *in vivo* is that of immunological effects. Dickson and Calderwood (61) have recently reviewed this very controversial area. Studies in rodent and rabbit models bearing immunogenic tumors have shown that stimulated immunity may contribute to the overall response of the tumor to *localized* heat. The preliminary human clinical trials which have been carried out have not significantly contributed to understanding of this area. It is generally agreed that systemic hyperthermia leads to a reduction in immune competence of the host. That local or regional heating leads to a stimulation of immune competence is thought to occur by some, but the evidence is conflicting. This issue remains unclear at the present time.

Heat with Radiation

As discussed in the papers by Dewey *et al.* (24, 37) and Roti Roti (47), heat is known to interact synergistically with ionizing radiation. In part, it does so by inhibiting radiation repair mechanisms. One aspect of this inhibition involves restricted access of repair enzymes to substrate (DNA). Heat may directly affect DNA repair mechanisms as well, since certain DNA repair enzymes are heat sensitive (see 24, 37, and 47 for reviews). Current understanding of the mechanism of heat radiosensitization is that repair is inhibited, some new damage may be fixed, and death then occurs due to increased frequencies of chromosome aberration production (24, 37, 47).

Heat with Chemotherapeutic Drugs

Hyperthermia interacts with drugs in a variety of ways. Bronk *et al.* (62) have shown that heat interacts with certain alkylating agents by increasing the rate of alkylation and that this increase correlates with increased cell kill. Hahn (28) has shown that heat enhances adriamycin cytotoxicity by increasing drug uptake, but that uptake does not correlate with enhanced killing when bleomycin and heat are combined. In the case of some drugs, repair mechanisms are inhibited. Heat can also affect the metabolism of drugs *in vitro* and *in vivo*. David Alberts (personal communication) has shown that melphalan is quite heat labile and that thermal lability *in vitro* correlates with decreased effectiveness when used to treat cells in culture in combination with 42°C compared to 37°C. There are also physiological considerations to the mechanism(s) of heat-drug interactions, as drugs require a delivery system. The finding that this delivery system is quite heat sensitive and that differentials may exist between normal tissues and tumor have already been discussed. This heat effect on drug distribution could be deleterious to therapy in the event heat reduced tumor blood flow prior to the drug reaching the tumor. It would be advantageous if heat were used to trap the active drug in the tumor by preventing it from being carried away by the vascular system. This would act to increase the effective biological half-life of the drug; and it is known that for most drugs cytotoxic effects are both concentration and time dependent.

Techniques for Producing Hyperthermia in Treatment of Human Cancers

The long history of the therapeutic use of heat is punctuated by numerous observations that malignant tumors may regress after exposure to elevated temperatures. In 1891, for instance, Coley noted regression of a sarcoma in the neck of a patient having fever associated with erysipelas. He then deliberately attempted to induce erysipelas in a series of patients having malignancy as a means of producing fever (63). Many subsequent investigators have also employed heat in treatment of malignancy, but techniques have progressed and multiplied since Coley's time. For the most part, heating techniques have been borrowed from those commonly used in physical medicine: water baths, paraffin application, ultrasound waves, and electromagnetic fields. The latter include inductively or capacitively coupled radiofrequency fields and radiated microwave fields. Other techniques have been developed more specifically for use in cancer therapy. Stehlin, for instance, has isolated the vessels to a limb and perfused heated blood through the limb for treatment of sarcomas and melanomas (64–68). Parks et al. have used an extracorporeal heat exchanger apparatus together with an arteriovenous access to heat blood as a means of achieving systemic hyperthermia (69). Manning et al. have implanted accessible tumors with metallic needles that are used as electrodes for radiofrequency currents (70, 71). Recent developments have also been made in using electromagnetic techniques for regional heating. In this section, the various techniques currently being used in oncologic practice will be summarized, and will be organized in terms of the body volume to be heated: local, regional, or systemic approaches. In reviewing these techniques, it may be noted that in one sense, trials using hyperthermia are as much tests of techniques as they are of the efficacy of hyperthermia. Temperature distributions in tumors and normal tissues with all techniques are non-uniform and inadequately characterized. A falsely negative clinical trial may thus result because portions of a tumor were inadequately treated with the technique used. The investigator must constantly bear in mind the limitations of his technique.

LOCAL TECHNIQUES FOR TREATMENT

Capacitively and inductively coupled radiofrequency and microwave applicators have all been used intermittently over the last 50 years to locally heat tumors (72, 73). Most recent studies, however, have used 915 MHz and 2,450 MHz microwave applicators, inductive "pancake" coils at 27.12 MHz and 13.56 MHz, capacitively coupled radiofrequency at 13.45 MHz and 500 KHz, and ultrasound (70, 71, 74, 75). The biophysics of these devices is discussed in previous chapters. Here these devices will be considered in their clinical contexts.

Inductive pancake coils (27.12 MHz and 13.56 MHz): Kim et al. (74–76) have used an inductive unit of approximately 5 cm radius made by International Medical Electronics, Limited, that operates at 27.12 MHz. Patients with multiple superficial cutaneous lesions were selected for their study designed to treat individual lesions with hyperthermia alone, radiation alone, or radiation followed immediately by hyperthermia. The very localized heating resulting from the inductive coil was thus appropriate for their study. Thermocouple probes were placed into normal tissue and tumor at similar depths (1.0 to 1.5 cm) and at sites expected to receive maximum power deposition. In 17 of 24 lesions, temperatures greater than or equal to 42°C were noted, and these were greater than temperatures in normal tissue in 20 of 24 cases (77, 78). These results are consistent with the hypothesis that the thermoregulatory system of normal tissues is absent from tumors, so that heat loss from the tumor via the circulatory system is reduced relative to normal tissue. The absorbed power from an inductive coil decays nearly linearly with depth, so that one could expect temperature gradients within a tumor for this reason alone. Also, there will be a zone on the periphery of many tumors characterized by normal tissue having a variable degree of tumor infiltration. Unless temperatures at these peripheries as well as at the deep extension of the tumor are known, sub-optimal temperatures may be obtained.

Microwave (915 MHz and 2,450 MHz): Many groups are utilizing microwave applicators for treatment of relatively superficial tumors (71, 74–77, 79–84). U and collaborators reported their experience (81) in which patients with multiple subcutaneous or cutaneous metastases were selected for treatment to individual lesions with radiation alone, hyperthermia alone, or radiation followed within 10 minutes by heating. Thermistor probes were placed in the tumor center and in adjacent normal skin. Tumor core temperatures were 42 to 44°C, and were 1.0 to 8.5°C higher than the surrounding normal tissue temperatures. Again, relatively poorer perfusion of tumor than normal tissue is thought to explain the preferential tumor heating.

Capacitively coupled radiofrequency (500 MHz to 13.56 MHz): Because of the limited depth of penetration of the electromagnetic fields with the above techniques, plate electrodes on the body surface have been used to direct RF currents through larger and deeper volumes containing tumor. LeVeen et al. (85, 86) used multiple surface electrodes with electronic switching to achieve multiple current paths which intersected the tumor and lessened heating in surrounding normal tissue, especially the high resistance subcutaneous fat layer which was in series with the currents. These authors have not reported details of tumor versus normal tissue temperatures but indicate that tumor temperatures greater than 45°C can be achieved. In the experience of the authors at the University of Arizona (87), the clinical situations suitable for heating with capacitive coupling (not including electronically switched electrodes) have been infrequent. Generally, the large tumors that the authors have attempted to heat required substantial applied power in the range of 100 Watts to several kilowatts. Preferential heating of the high resistance subcutaneous fat layer occurred. Heating of the tumor at depth was often diminished because of spreading of the currents. Channeling of the currents around poorly conductive bone led to hot spots as well. A phantom model illustrating capacitive coupling is shown in Figure 12.1.

Interstitial radiofrequency (500 KHz): Direct placement of radiofrequency coaxial probes into tissue has been reported (80, 88). In Phase I trials at the University of Arizona (70, 71, 84, 89), placement under general anesthesia of 17 gauge stainless steel needle guides into accessible cutaneous, subcutaneous, and pelvic tumors was used. The needles themselves were electrically connected to form two planes, each of which was an electrode for the 500 KHz current. Tumor temperatures were measured with thermistors at multiple sites and were between 42.5°C and 45°C within 3 to 10 minutes. They were maintained for 30 to 40 minutes. This technique has a number of advantages over previously mentioned techniques: the heating is localized to the tumor; temperatures may be measured at multiple sites using implanted catheters as guides for flexible thermistors; electrode configurations

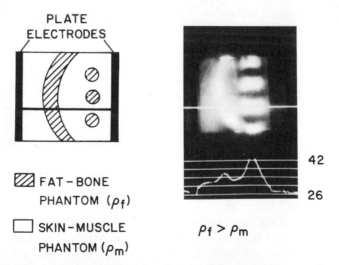

Fig. 12.1. A phantom model of heating by RF capacitive coupling is shown. Resistivities ρ_f, and ρ_m of fat and muscle, respectively, lead to greater ohmic heating not only in the fat layer, but also in muscle when currents are channeled around poorly conductive bone. On the thermographic camera photograph, *white* areas are hot, *black* areas are cold. Temperatures are sampled along the indicated line passing through the phantom, and plotted as a function of position in the lower half of the photograph.

may be easily modified to alter the heating pattern; and the needle guides may serve as holders for radioactive sources giving low dose rate radiation to the tumor. The disadvantages of this technique are that the needle implantation and heating usually require general anesthesia, that because both the hyperthermia and radiation are highly localized, great care must be given to ensure that all tumor margins are within the implanted volume, and that not all sites or tumors can be appropriately implanted in this manner.

Ultrasound (0.2 to 3 MHz): Ultrasound is being also used for tumor heating (78, 90). Lele (91) has developed a prototype computer-controlled focused ultrasound device specifically for investigation of tumor heating. Clinical Phase I experience with a single piezoelectric crystal transducer is reported by Marmor and Hahn (90). Twenty-five patients with metastatic or locally recurrent superficial tumors no greater than 4 cm in diameter and 3 cm deep were selected. Temperatures at multiple sites in the tumor and at the periphery were measured in the first treatment in each case; thereafter, only central tumor temperatures were measured with thermocouples. With incident power of 0.5 to 1.2 W/cm^2, tumor temperatures of 44 to 45°C were observed. Non-uniform heating of tumors was noted, generally with variations of 1 to 2°C and with the highest temperature centrally. Ultrasound does have relatively better depth dose distribution characteristics with single or multiple arrays than electromagnetic arrangements and has little interaction with metallic thermometers, compared to the electromagnetic techniques discussed. On the other hand, attenuation of ultrasound through air-filled spaces precludes treatment in the thoracic area. Preferential absorption in bone or reflections from bone-soft tissue interfaces may lead to undesirable excessive heating (92).

Several points may be made with respect to all these techniques for local heating: a) The volume over which power *deposition* is uniform is a function not only of the electromagnetic or ultrasonic field distribution, but also of the tumor and tissue properties characterizing the field and matter interaction. b) Resulting *temperature* distributions depend, in addition, upon thermal conductivities, thermal transport via the circulation, specific heats, and local metabolic heat production. It is not surprising that non-uniform heating of tumors results. c) The thermal *responsiveness* of a tumor may be spatially and time variable depending upon local conditions of oxygenation, nutrition, pH, and preceeding or following second modality treatment such as chemotherapy or radiation. State-of-the-art heating techniques are thus intimately associated with intense research into parameters entering the bioheat equation as well as the biological aspects of tumor response. It is premature to identify one technique as better than another. All have areas of appropriate application, and the modern hyperthermia clinic needs to have several techniques available for specific situations.

REGIONAL TECHNIQUES FOR TREATMENT

Regional hyperthermia denotes temperature elevation throughout the thorax, abdomen, pelvis, or an extremity. In general, the potential morbidity associated with elevation of regional temperatures to 43 to 44°C is greater than that with local hyperthermia, and the specialization of techniques to cancer therapy is greater. Again various methods are considered in their clinical context.

Heated perfusates: Stehlin *et al.* have a long experience with isolated perfusion of extremities (64–68). They added heat to existing practice of chemotherapeutic perfusion in 1967 in treatment of extremity malignant melanoma. Stehlin's technique involved exposing the axillary vein and artery surgically in the case of upper extremity perfusion and popliteal or iliac vessels in the case of lower extremity perfusion. Blood from the arteriovenous access was heated by a closed water circulator-heat exchanger unit to 43 to 46°C; blankets perfused with heated water were also wrapped around the extremity to elevate skin temperature. Perfusion was continued for 2 hours. Temperatures were monitored in skin and muscle and maintained at 38.8 to 40.0°C. Tumor temperatures were measured when possible, but tumor temperatures *per se* have not been reported. It should also be noted that melphalan was used consistently in the perfusate in Stehlin's series.

Heated water bath: For certain superficial lesions on an extremity, a heated water bath is an appealing approach. Kim *et al.* (74) have reported on this technique in their series of patients with malignant cutaneous lesions in which extremities were immersed immediately post irradiation in a water bath temperature controlled to within 0.05°C. Intradermal needle probes were placed to monitor temperatures; and it was found that with the skin surface held at 43.5°C, the temperature at 5 mm depth slowly increased from 40°C to about 41°C after a more rapid initial transient. The corresponding temperatures at 10 mm depth increased from 38.5 to 39.5°C. In hyperthermia for cancer therapy, tumor temperatures of at least 42°C are generally required so that the disadvantageous depth dose distribution with water bath immersion is apparent.

Magnetic induction: Storm *et al.* (93) have reported on a new hyperthermic device (the Magnetrode, Henry Electronics, Inc.) for cancer therapy, consisting of a 1kw, 13.56 MHz generator that drives a cylindrical resonant coil electrode circumferentially surrounding the patient. The magnetic field produced within the coil induces eddy currents in the selected body region that in turn produce ohmic heating in tissue. The power deposition in tissue resulting from eddy currents is very non-uniform (94), being greatest in muscle and other relatively highly conductive tissue deep to the subcutaneous fat layer, and then diminishing rapidly with increasing depth. On the other hand, heat transport by the circulatory system appears to produce a temperature distribution more uniform than expected. In a number of animal experiments, temperatures were observed to vary from 43 to 44°C in normal subcutaneous tissues (muscle) to 41 to 42°C in core tissues. Storm et al. (95) have reported tumor temperatures obtained in a series of 46 patients, 27 of whom had tumors deeper than 1 cm below the skin surface and were treated with the Magnetrode. The other 19 patients were treated with capacitively-coupled RF fields. The tumor temperatures obtained were not separately analyzed by heating technique. Storm et al. found that 44 percent of tumors were heated to greater than or equal to 45°C, 37 percent to 42.0 to 44.9°C, and 19 percent to less than 42°C. Thus, temperatures exceeding 42°C were reached in 81 percent of tumors. The biophysics of this inductive heating technique is incompletely characterized at this time. On the basis of the initial work, the authors believe that tumors at moderate depth (1 to 8 cm) may receive significant direct power deposition. If the perfusion of the tumor is impaired relative to normal tissue, as Storm et al. postulate, then the tumor temperature may significantly exceed that of surrounding normal tissue. A tumor on the longitudinal body axis will receive little direct power deposition. It may heat, however, by virtue of thermal conduction from peripheral tissues. This implies that tumor temperatures achieved on the longitudinal body axis may be limited to less than 41 to 42°C. Much remains to be done to better understand the biophysics and bioeffects of this technique.

Microwave phased array: P. F. Turner, with the BSD Corporation, Salt Lake City, Utah, has developed another original approach to regional heating consisting of synchronously phased microwave apertures radiating toward a selected deep volume of tissue (96). The electric field amplitudes E from n asynchronous applicators will add as the sum of E^2 from each field. The central power deposition is proportional to nE^2. Synchronous fields result in addition of the E vectors, so that if polarities of the E vectors are similar, the central power deposition is proportional to n^2E^2. The factor of n increase in power deposition in the latter case can offset the effect of beam attenuation to result in relatively uniform volume heating. Multiple unphased applicators produce minimal power deposition centrally with maximum power deposited superficially. In a number of animal experiments, Turner has shown initial heating rates in the esophagus of a living pig to be 70 percent that of superficial tissues; central temperatures in the sacrificed pig may exceed those in the subcutaneous tissue. Clinical investigation of this device is being done by Dr. F. A. Gibbs, Jr. at the University of Utah Medical Center.

The latter two approaches represent state-of-the-art electromagnetic methods of heating large volumes of the body. All the remarks made regarding local heating techniques apply here as well: non-uniform temperature distributions can be expected. In addition, the problem of measuring temperatures in deep normal tissues and tumors is much more difficult than in the case of superficial tumors. More invasive thermometry is required. Characterizing temperature variations in a larger volume requires measurement at a greater number of points. Regional heating combined with radiation or chemotherapy, or both, exposes larger volumes of normal tissue to as yet undetermined toxicity. Use of regional electromagnetic heating techniques must thus be developed cautiously, with thorough evaluation of the heating method alone, and with other therapeutic modalities.

SYSTEMIC TECHNIQUES FOR TREATMENT

Coley's use of toxins to produce systemic hyperthermia has been mentioned; and the history of pyrogen therapy of cancer has been reviewed by Nauts (1). Only approaches to total body heating that do not involve use of pyrogens will be considered here.

Pettigrew *et al.* (97–100) selected patients with advanced malignancy for their trial. Patients were prepared with narcotics, curare, epidural block, and intubation. Ventilation with heated gases, skin insulation with a sealed polyethylene bag followed by immersion in heated wax, and continued metabolic heat production accounted for heating rates of 500, 1,500, and 1,250 calories per minute, respectively, leading to a 4°C/hour core temperature rise. Concern regarding toxicity to the liver at temperatures exceeding 42°C led Pettigrew *et al.* to use a maximum body temperature of 41.8°C.

Larkin *et al.* also selected patients with advanced malignancy (101, 102). General anesthesia and endotracheal intubation were given. Heated ventilation gases were used to minimize respiratory heat loss and polyethylene wrappings were placed around the patient to lessen evaporative heat loss. A wrapping of water blankets completed the preparation. Core temperature (indicated on esophageal and rectal probes) was brought to 42°C and maintained for 2 hours. A heating time of 90 to 120 minutes was required to achieve 42°C at a rate of about 2 to 3°C/hour.

Bull and colleagues used a high-flow, heated-water perfusion suit covered with insulating material in patients given intravenous sedation and analgesia (103). Maximum inlet water temperatures were limited to 44.5°C and were feedback regulated to bring the esophageal temperature to 41.8°C. A heatup period of about 2 hours (2 to 3°C/hour) was required.

Parks and colleagues investigated systemic heating in patients with advanced bronchogenic cancer (69). A Dacron shunt was surgically anastomosed to the common femoral artery and vein, serving as access during heating for arterial to venous flow through connections to an extracoporeal heat exchanger device regulated initially to 49.0°C. Outflowing blood reached 45°C. Blood temperatures were reduced as systemic temperature (measured in the bladder) reached 41.5°C. This temperature was typically maintained for 5 to 6 hours. Regulation of systemic temperature to ± 0.1°C was possible with the feedback controlled heat exchanger. Heating rates were in the range of 5 to 6°C/hour. Patients in this series were given general anesthesia, endotracheal intubation, and positive end-expiratory pressure ventilation.

The principal advantages and disadvantages of the systemic heating methods discussed relate to time and personnel requirements, toxicity, rate of temperature elevation, degree of precision in regulation of temperature, and probably less importantly to temperature distribution, although no extensive investigation of the latter has been done. The arteriovenous shunt with an extracoporeal pump and heat exchanger presently appears advantageous in most respects.

Thermal Dosimetry

The goal of heat delivery systems in cancer therapy is to elevate malignant tumors to known or knowable temperatures greater than or equal to 42°C, and to limit the heating of normal tissues to temperatures consistent with acceptable toxicity. At the present time, measurement of a temperature deeper than the skin surface requires invasive placement of a thermometer into tissue. Interaction between the heating field, especially if it is electromagnetic, and the thermometer may lead to erroneous measurements. Cetas has discussed this problem in Chapter 2. Even if time-temperature profiles are measured at several points in normal tissue and tumor, can the time-temperature distribution at intermediate points be interpolated or inferred? In practice, this would require numerical solution of the bioheat equation with known parameters describing power deposition, heat dissipation and boundary conditions. Although such solution is a long-term goal, current clinical thermometry yields more limited information. Summarized here is the approach to thermometry taken at the University of Arizona in the hyperthermia clinic.

Cetas has discussed thermometric instrumentation in Chapter 2. Patients who are candidates for local heating in many cases have been simulated by constructing tissue and bone-equivalent phantoms based upon the methods of Guy et al. (104–107). Various arrangements of surface electrodes for capacitively coupled RF fields may be tested, as well as the 915 MHz applicator designed by Guy et al. (106, 107) or the 2,450 MHz applicator designed by Kantor et al. (108) Interstitial needle electrode heating has similarly been studied (84, 109). Thermistor probes can be inserted into the phantom through Teflon catheters (oriented perpendicularly to the electric field vector) to obtain point measurements. Split phantoms may be opened along different planes to expose surfaces to the thermographic camera and thereby reveal selected temperature distributions. It is realized that this approach at best simulates only temperature profiles resulting from direct power deposition and does not model the perfused tissue. Nevertheless, the phantom approach has been very useful to select the best heating techniques for deposition of power in the tumor region and avoiding delivery of excessive power to normal tissue volumes. A clinical example of this approach may clarify the methodology:

Case Report: A patient with bulky neck metastases from a squamous cell carcinoma of the tonsil was considered for combined hyperthermia and radiation. The left neck mass measured 6 cm × 7 cm × 9 cm, and the right neck mass was 5 cm × 10 cm × 11 cm. Both masses were in the anterior neck superior to a tracheostomy; little subcutaneous fat was present beneath the intact skin surfaces. A phantom trial was performed to evaluate power deposition with capacitively coupled radiofrequency currents. Large parallel plate electrodes extended from the prevertebral plane to the anterior skin surface, enclosing the hyoid bone (Figure 12.2 *A*). Thermograms are shown in 12.2 *B*, 12.2 *C*, and 12.2 *D*. Scans along lines *A*, *B*, and *C* yielded temperatures shown on the corresponding graphs. Relatively uniform heating of the region representing tumor anterior to the hyoid was seen. Currents

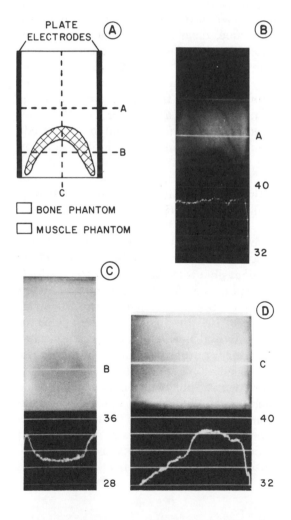

Fig. 12.2. Phantom study of power deposition patterns using capacitively coupled RF at 3 MHz. *Panel A*: Schematic of phantom showing plate electrodes, anterior neck mass, and hyoid bone. *Dashed lines* correspond to white scan lines on thermograms. *Panels B, C, D*: Thermograms of surface temperatures. *White* is warm, *dark* is cool. The temperatures are scanned along the white lines and plotted below the thermogram in degrees Celsius.

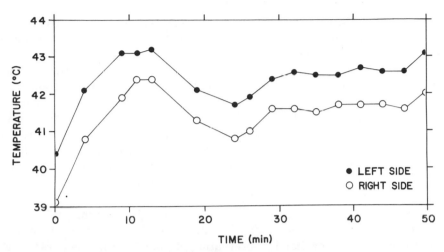

Fig. 12.3. Thermistor probes at 2 cm depth from each lateral neck surface into the anterior tumor recorded these temperatures during the actual patient treatment corresponding to the phantom model in Figure 12.2.

passed around the hyoid bone and enclosed tracheal air column, but no area of excessive heating was noted. For the actual patient treatment, capacitively coupled radiofrequency at 3 MHz was used. The plate electrodes were maintained at 40°C with circulating water. Hyperthermia was given twice weekly for 40 to 45 minutes, and radiation treatments were given within ten minutes of completion of heating. Ten daily radiation fractions of 200 rad were given. Thermistors for temperature measurement included two placed at 2 cm depth beneath the skin on each side into the central parts of the tumors. Temperatures measured at these sites during one treatment are shown in Figure 12.3. Within 2 weeks after completion of therapy, there was central necrosis and ulceration of each mass with a 70 percent reduction in overall volume. The patient died 1 month after completion, however, because of uncontrolled disease in other areas.

In heating patients, three to eight thermistor probes are placed through Teflon catheters into tumor and normal tissue sites under local anesthesia. Care is taken to measure temperatures at the center, periphery, and deepest extension of tumor. Temperatures are recorded and displayed in real time using a microprocessor instrumentation computer. Surface temperatures are also observed and recorded with the thermographic camera. The effect of artifacts resulting from probes in electromagnetic fields is assessed by comparing readings during power on/off cycles. Temperatures may be sampled along lines by positioning the thermistor bead at different points along the Teflon catheter. In thermal equilibrium states, the temperature gradients across the walls of the catheters are less than 0.1°C.

In the case of regional hyperthermia using magnetic induction coils, thermocouples are presently being used. Changing to use of non-perturbing probes such as the high resistance lead device of Bowman (110) or the fiber optic device of Christensen (111) or Cetas (112) will be particularly important in regional heating evaluation. Only patients having bulky tumors accessible for thermometry are accepted for regional heating. Catheters for probes are placed into at least one tumor site, into adjacent normal tissue, and into available natural orifices. Subcutaneous probes are positioned at sites of excessive superficial heating in the region (*e.g.*, xyphoid and coccyx areas). Radiographic localization of thermometer placement is performed in every case. Temperatures are recorded at multiple sites along the catheters by moving the thermocouples in and out. Both phantom and animal experiments are in progress to define power deposition patterns and to map temperatures achieved in multiple vital organ sites using circumferential magnetic induction electrodes.

In both local and regional heating using external applicators, it is found that power levels must be guided by the patient's perception of pain at superficial sites, rather than by observation of some limiting temperature at the specific sites chosen for probe placement. This reinforces the decision to use local and regional heating with external applicators only in patients not given general anesthesia. Patients treated with interstitial thermotherapy are necessarily given general anesthesia, so avoidance of hot spots in normal tissues must rely upon careful placement of needles into the tumor and extensive thermometry.

Clinical Results

HEAT ALONE

Much of the clinical work accomplished to date has used hyperthermia as an adjuvant to either radiation or chemotherapy. Several groups have used hyperthermia alone in limited trials in human cancer patients. These studies fall into groups consisting of hyperthermia produced by local, regional, or systemic techniques.

Published studies on the response of human patients treated with systemic hyperthermia alone have been presented by four major groups. These include Pettigrew and co-workers in Edinburgh, Scotland (97–99), Bull and co-workers at the National Cancer Institute (103), Larkin and co-workers from the University of New Mexico (101, 102), and Barlogie and co-workers at the M.D. Anderson Hospital and Tumor Institute (113). These groups have used a variety of techniques described in a preceeding section to induce systemic hyperthermia. All of these groups have been able to treat patients to a maximum of 41.8 to 42.0°C for times usually on the order of a few hours. In some cases, treatment times extended up to a maximum of 20 hours. Multiple heat treatments were given in each of the studies, and usually ranged from three to four individual treatments. Treatments were generally separated by times of at least 1 week. All authors concluded that whole body hyperthermia at maximum temperatures of 41.8 to 42.0°C was safe if carefully monitored. Major side effects noted included peripheral neuropathies and liver associated toxicities. Although these studies were designed as Phase I toxicity trials, the clinical results were unimpressive in terms of efficacy. Several responses were noted. These usually included initial tumor regression and subjective palliation. However, significant tumor control for extended periods of time was not noted.

A second group of patients has been treated with hyperthermia alone, using regional techniques. Storm and co-workers at U.C.L.A. Medical Center used magnetic induction techniques (93). In contrast to previous studies which were designed to employ temperatures usually less than 45°C for local and regional treatments and less than 42°C for systemic therapy, Storm's design purposefully attempted to achieve tumor temperatures in excess of 45°C and sometimes reached tumor temperatures exceeding 50°C. A variety of tumor types was treated. Toxicity from these treatments included several cases of skin burns and two cases of small localized areas of subcutaneous fibrosis occurring in obese patients when normal tissue temperatures were in the 42 to 45°C temperature range. The efficacy of this trial is somewhat unclear due to short follow-up times of patients treated. Again, this trial was designed as a Phase I toxicity trial and demonstrated safety when using regional heating techniques involving magnetic induction heating.

A third area of heat alone studies involves treatments designed to heat local areas only. One such study was conducted at Stanford University by Marmor and colleagues (90). This group used ultrasonic heating methods to treat tumor recurrences in previously irradiated sites. Sixteen patients were treated who had received radiation doses ranging from 4,400 to 11,000 rad. Attempts were made to cool normal tissues while elevating tumor temperatures to 43 to 45°C. Complications included several cases of minor burns at the site of temperature probe insertion. No other complications were observed. This group observed significant tumor responses in 11 of 16 patients treated with heat alone (partial plus complete responders). Studies at the University of Arizona (using a variety of techniques to produce localized heating) have yielded results similar to these previous studies (71). Temperatures in the 43 to 44°C range from 30 to 40 minutes per treatment have been used. Treatment number has ranged from 2 to 30 with the most frequent treatment number of 10. We have treated a variety of histologies (see Table 12.1). The results showed an objective response rate less than 30 percent in the total patient treatment group (see Table 12.2). Few long-term responses have been apparent.

There is some reason to believe that the mechanism of tumor damage by temperatures in the 43 to 44°C range is different than the mechanism of damage produced by the very high hyperthermic temperature used by Storm et al. (93). As has been reported by others, the authors observed rapid size changes and necrosis in tumors responding to heat therapy alone.

TABLE 12.1. *Summary of Responses to Hyperthermia Alone Therapy*[a,b]

Response	Number of Patients Treated (14 Total)	
	Number of Responses (% of Total)	Duration of Responses
No Response	10 (72%)	1 with stable disease for 1½ years
Partial	1 (7%)	1 month, regrowth
Complete	3 (21%)	1 month to 8 months, regrowth Retreatment unsuccessful

[a] Heat dose = 43 to 44°C for 40 minutes, 2 to 30 fractions separated by 72 hours; in two cases, tumor temperature did not exceed 40°C, followed by no response.

[b] Of the 10 non-responders, all had pain relief, 7 with temporary stabilization of disease. Central necrosis present in most.

TABLE 12.2. *Summary of Responses to External Heat Combined with External Beam (High-Dose-Rate) Radiation Therapy*[a]

Response	Number of Patients Treated (14 Total)	
	Number of Responses (% of Total)	Duration of Responses
No Response	9 (30%)	
Partial	12 (40%)	1 month to 6 months, no disease progression observed during follow-up
Complete	9 (30%)	2 months to 2½ years 4 patients alive without recurrence in treated volume 3 expired but controlled locally 2 patients have recurred at 1 month and 7 months

[a] Heat dose = 43 to 44°C for 40 minutes, sequence: heat followed by XRT within one hour, approximately 6 heat fractions/patient, radiation dose range 2,000 rads to 6,400 rads.

This effect was more frequent in initially bulky tumors. In contrast, Storm observed little change in tumor volume after treatment, but did observe significant necrosis in surgically removed tumor. This difference could be due, in part, to the possibility that the use of very high temperatures completely thromboses tumor blood vessels, thus destroying mechanisms for removal of non-viable, necrotic tumor cells.

In general, it can be summarized that heat alone is safe as a therapeutic modality, but lacks significant effectiveness based on limited clinical trials conducted to date. Some significant responses (complete or partial tumor disappearance) have been observed. However, tumor responses have been limited to a few months with regrowth of tumor in the treatment volume often observed.

HEAT PLUS RADIATION THERAPY

Approaches to combining heat and radiation in human clinical trials have generally focused on localized heating techniques combined with high dose rate external beam radiotherapy (71, 74–77, 79–84). Studies prior to 1976 have been reviewed previously (89). These results have primarily given Phase I toxicity information, and although they are anecdotal and uncontrolled, they suggest that the combination can be used safely. Furthermore, significant tumoricidal activity can be observed. Since 1977, five groups have reported on trials combining localized hyperthermia with external beam radiation therapy. Kim and co-workers from Memorial Sloan-Kettering have reported on a group of 36 patients treated with hyperthermia, produced either by water bath heating or by radiofrequency inductive heating (74–76). The major finding of the study was that the combination of heat and radiation produced normal tissue reactions which were not measurably greater than those produced by radiation alone. Heat doses were 43.5°C for times ranging from 30 to 60 minutes. Radiation doses ranged from 1,000 to 2,500 rad. Tumor regressions were noted with follow-up times approaching one year. Marmor and Hahn at Stanford treated five patients with combinations of ultrasound-induced hyperthermia and fractionated radiotherapy (90). Six tumor sites were treated in these five patients. Heat doses were again 43 to 45°C for 30 minutes with total radiation doses ranging from 1,200 to 2,400 rad. Three complete responses, two partial responses and one no-response were observed in these six irradiated sites. Johnson *et al.* from Roswell Park reported on a pilot study investigating the thermal enhancement ratio of 41.5 to 42°C hyperthermia in combination with radiation (114). These investigators treated cutaneous and subcutaneous tumor nodules, and assessed both normal skin as well as tumor regressions. Again, marked tumor responses were noted. The investigators commented on the difficulty in obtaining interpretable results regarding therapeutic ratio. A general conclusion from this study is that, as in the previous study, localized hyperthermia combined with radiotherapy is safe and can be quite effective.

A recent study by Bicher and co-workers at Henry Ford Hospital confirms the results of these previous trials (89). This group has employed a protocol with curative intent, consisting of four hyperthermia-alone treatments of 45°C for 90 minutes, with treatment intervals of 72 hours. Direct-contact microwave applicators were used. Patients were allowed to rest for 1 week to evaluate their response to heat alone, and were then given combined radiation therapy and hyperthermia treatments. This group of treatments consisted of four individual treatments with 400 rad radiation fractions followed by hyperthermia fractions of 42°C for 90 minutes. The combined fractions were separated again with 72 hour intervals. As in previous studies, no abnormal toxicity was observed using the combination of heat and radiation. Many of the tumors treated showed marked responses, with a number exhibiting total tumor disappearance. These investigators noted that melanoma and lymphomas were most sensitive to the treatment.

The authors' own results to date are summarized in Table 12.3. A variety of radiofrequency and microwave techiques to produce localized hyperthermia were used. Normal tissue toxicity was minimal. Overall tumor responses (partial plus complete remissions) approached 70 percent in this group of patients.

Another approach employed for combining heat and radiation is interstitial thermoradiotherapy (70, 71). As discussed previously, this technique used heating by localized radiofrequency current fields. Radiation doses were administered by low dose rate radiation sources. Unlike previous trials, only one heat treatment was used in combination with the radiation dose (excepting one patient who received two heat doses). Heat treatments were given immediately after placement either of radiation source guides or radium needles. Temperatures were 43 to 44°C for 30 to 40 minutes. Radioactive sources were usually placed within 1 to 3 hours after hyperthermia. This group of patients showed the most significant overall response of any clinical trial yet reported. Complete responses (complete tumor

TABLE 12.3. *Summary of Responses to Interstitial Thermoradiotherapy*[a]

Responses	Number of Patients Treated (14 Total)	
	Number of Responses (% of Total)	Duration of Responses
No Response	1 (3%)	Progressive disease
Partial	11 (33%)	1 to 9 months, no disease progression observed during follow-up, further response possible in recently treated patients
Complete	21 (64%)	1 to 15 months, 1 patient with regrowth in treated volume. Remainder having complete response without regrowth during follow-up or until death 6 patients alive without evidence of disease in treated volume

[a] Dose range 1,800 rads in 30 hours to 4,500 rads in 76 hours.

disappearance in the treated volume) presented in 64 percent of these 33 patients. Only 1 of these 33 patients showed less than a 50 pecent decrease in tumor volume following therapy, for an overall response rate of 97 percent. As in all previous trials employing heat in combination with radiation, normal tissue complications have been minimal and have not exceeded those expected for standard radiotherapy alone. No problem with normal tissue healing around areas of tumor destruction has been observed. Regrowth of tumor in a treated volume was observed to date in only 1 of the 33 patients treated. Responses have been maintained during follow-up periods of months to 1 to 2 years. Table 12.4 summarizes the response for the three treatment approaches as a function of tumor histology treated. As can be seen, all tumor types showed good responses to therapy. Interstitial thermoradiotherapy results were better than those with localized heat in combination with high dose rate radiotherapy alone. This is reflected not only in the overall response rates to treatment, but also in the distribution of partial and complete response rate.

HEAT PLUS CHEMOTHERAPY

The use of heat in combination with chemotherapy has received less study in human clinical trials than has the combination of heat and radiation. A major regional heat in combination with chemotherapy trial has been conducted by Stehlin and co-workers in Houston. These investigators have treated malignancies in limbs using regional perfusions since the late 1960's. While they have treated a variety of histologies, the major focus of their work has been to treat melanomas and sarcomas with regional perfusates of 43 to 46°C in combination with melphalan and Cytoxan. The responses reported by this group are indeed remarkable and far exceed those reported using any other form of therapy for the treatment of these diseases (64–68).

Several of the groups using systemic approaches to thermotherapy have also initiated Phase I studies of heat combined with chemotherapy. To date, the tumor responses, as for heat alone, have been unremarkable. The initial Phase I results again suggest that the methods are safe, but efficacy has been limited in the small number of patients treated. A major exception to this generalization is the work of Parks et al. (69). These investigators recently reported a large trial combining chemotherapy with systemic hyperthermia using extracorporeal heating methods. They treated a variety of tumor histologies and noted significant responses, especially in patients with lung carcinomas. Detailed investigations combining heat and chemotherapeutic drugs have yet to be conducted which address the known importance of sequencing of these agents, the pharmacological changes induced at elevated temperatures, and the thermal lability of various drugs.

TABLE 12.4. *Cumulative Summary of Response (PR + CR) Based on Histology*

Histology	Treatment			Totals
	Heat Alone	External Heat Then Radiation	Interstitial Thermoradiotherapy	
Squamous Cell Ca.	3/5	6/9	9/10	18/24 (75%)
Adenocarcinoma	1/4	4/6	17/17	22/27 (81%)
Melanoma	0/1	6/9	3/3	9/13 (69%)
Sarcoma (Soft Tissue and Bone)	0/4	5/6	3/3	8/13 (62%)
Totals	4/14 (28%)	21/30 (70%)	32/33 (97%)	57/77 (74%)

Future Directions in Cancer Hyperthermia

Hopefully from the preceding sections, the reader has received some flavor of accomplishments to date as well as of the vast areas of inadequate understanding of molecular, cellular, and environmental effects of heat, of heat delivery techniques, and of actual thermal distributions in patients. The biology of heat, drugs, and radiation given as combined modalities must be understood to develop schedules of therapy having therapeutic gain and curative potential.

Clinical trials to date employing local hyperthermia have been Phase I studies, in which establishment of toxicity patterns is a principal goal. The Phase I trial is also a therapeutic intent study that may provide evidence of anti-cancer activity. Although many of the indications of efficacy so far can be criticized as anecdotal evidence, the data certainly support extension of clinical activity into disease-oriented Phase II/III trials. Hyperthermia *alone* will probably play a very limited role as a curative modality. New studies will test the efficacy of combined modalities against historical controls as well as against concurrent controls not receiving hyperthermia. At the University of Arizona, Phase II trials of Stage IIIB and IVA squamous cell carcinoma of the cervix and of locally advanced malignant melanoma have been started. In the former case, conventional external radiation together with transperineal interstitial thermoradiotherapy is used. In the latter case, external heating and radiation techniques are used.

Regional heating is still being studied principally in Phase I, since the toxicity patterns of regional heating with chemotherapy or radiation are not clear. Regional inductive heating combined with radiation in large animal models and in patients with locally advanced tumors of the thorax, pelvis, or extremities having disease accessible for thermometry are being investigated. Phase I regional as well as local hyperthermia and chemotherapy studies are also planned. Hyperthermia studies are in progress at many other centers as well, as has been indicated in the clinical results section. The potential of systemic heating will probably lie in combining heat with drug therapy: combinations of systemic, local, and regional heating together with drug therapy and concurrent radiotherapy are also possibilities deserving extensive investigation in Phase I and II trials.

A variety of heating techniques has been discussed. None of them approaches the ideal of a non-invasive heat source resulting in *selective* heating of a tumor, *i.e.*, elevating the temperature of the tumor but not normal tissue. Most techniques to date can *preferentially* heat some tumors, however. Preferential heating implies relatively greater temperature elevation in tumor than normal tissue. One can speculate that combinations of radiosensitizing agents, radio- and chemo- protective agents, and systemic or regional blood cooling, together with local and regional heating, could increase the differential thermal effects between tumor and normal tissue;

controlled induction of thermotolerance in normal tissues may also be a mechanism for varying the thermal responsiveness of tissues. While new heating techniques will be welcomed, the potential of existing techniques remains to be delineated. A closely related area of interest will be in defining optimal sequencing, fractionation and duration of multi-modal therapy.

In the opposite direction from the ideal of a non-invasive heat source is the possibility of further developing and improving invasive approaches. One such approach being investigated at the University of Arizona is implanting ferromagnetic seeds, possibly radioactivated, into tumors as an open procedure: this is being considered as an approach to the treatment of brain tumors (115, 116). If the Curie temperature of the seeds is appropriately chosen near the desired maximum temperature, this may give a thermally self-regulating implant that can be heated with magnetic induction to significantly higher temperatures than surrounding tissue.

Another possibility is that of placing coaxial RF probes into tumor and heating interstitially (80, 88). This also is an approach for brain tumor heating, and in other sites is an alternative to interstitial thermotherapy via implanted needle electrodes as reported by Manning *et al.* (70, 71).

Considering future directions in thermometry, an ideal system can be specified. A non-invasive, non-perturbing means for determining volume *distributions* of temperature in real time at any desired site would be a physicist's delight. Short of the ideal are numerous areas for investigation.

Several optical probes are becoming available, as previously mentioned, that approach the ideal of a non-perturbing thermometer. Measured temperatures still characterize an average over some small volume ("point"); the *distribution* must be inferred from a matrix of point measurements. Invasive placement of a probe may itself traumatize tissues and alter the electromagnetic and thermal properties. Interpolating from a matrix of point measurements is possible in principle if the power deposition and heat dissipation parameters in the bioheat equation are known. Measurement of the thermal conductivity of tissues as well as electrical conductivity and dielectric permitivity is presently possible using specialized probes developed by Bowman, by Chato, and by others (117-129). Few measurements have been performed in humans to date, but these are being started in animal and human subjects at the University of Arizona. Also germane to these investigations is modeling of tumor and normal tissue vascularity. Whether accumulation of data in specific subjects will lead eventually to approaches useful for *predicting* temperature distributions in specific cases remains to be seen, but even retrospective reconstruction of temperatures may be useful.

Use of ultrasound as a non-invasive probe of tissue properties, from which temperatures can be inferred, is an appealing possibility. Measurement of microwave emission from deep tissues is a non-invasive radiometric technique that may also have potential for determining temperatures. Cetas has discussed these methods in Chapter 2 and has included pertinent references.

It is difficult to review future directions without some degree of speculation. The authors have tried to sketch state-of-the-art clinical hyperthermia as well as indicate areas of current experimental work that spreads across disciplines of biology, physiology, electrical engineering, biophysics, and clinical oncology, in which areas the present purview is limited. Further work on the biomolecular aspects of hyperthermia will be extremely important, especially so that laboratory results can be applied *predictively* to clinical situations. With so many variables, including heating methods, sequencing of combined modalities and duration of treatments, it seems unlikely that unmotivated empirical clinical schemes will optimize the promising role of hyperthermia in clinical cancer therapy. With a clearly developed rationale and an alliance of disciplines, however, the use of hyperthermia may significantly improve the curability of human cancer.

REFERENCES

1. NAUTS, H. C. Pyrogen Therapy of Cancer. A Historical Overview and Current Activities. *In: Proceedings of the International Symposium on Cancer Therapy by Hyperthermia and Radiation.* Robinson, J. E. and Wisenberg, M. J. (Eds). American College of Radiology, Bethesda, Maryland, pp. 239–250, 1976.
2. LAMBERT, R. A. Demonstration of the greater susceptibility to heat of sarcoma cells as compared with actively proliferating connective tissue cells. *J.A.M.A.*, 59: 2147–2148, 1912.
3. SCHREK, R. Sensitivity of normal and leukemic lymphocytes and leukemic myeloblasts to heat. *J. Nat. Cancer Inst.*, 37: 649–654, 1966.
4. CHEN, T. T. AND HEIDELBERGER, C. Quantitative studies on the malignant transformation of mouse prostate cells by carcinogenic hydrocarbons *in vitro. Int. J. Cancer*, 4: 166–178, 1969.
5. WARREN, S. Preliminary study of the effect of artificial fever upon hopeless tumor cases. *Am. J. Roentgenol.*, 33: 75–87, 1935.
6. CAVALIERE, R., CISCATTO, E. C., GIOVANELLA, B. C., HEIDELBERGER, C., JOHNSON, R. O., MARGOTTINI, M., MONDOVI, B., MORICCA, G., AND ROSSI-FANELLI, A. Selective heat sensitivity of cancer cells. Biochemical and clinical studies. *Cancer*, 20: 1351–1381, 1967.
7. HARTMAN, J. T. AND CRILE, G., JR. Heat treatment of osteogenic sarcoma. *Clin. Orthop.*, 61: 269–276, 1968.
8. SUTTON, C. H. Tumor hyperthermia in the treatment of malignant gliomas of the brain. *Trans. Am. Neurol. Assoc.*, 96: 195–199, 1971.
9. BELLI, J. A. AND BONTE, F. J. Influence of temperature on the radiation response of mammalian cells in tissue culture. *Radiat. Res.*, 18: 272–276, 1963.
10. WESTRA, A. AND DEWEY, W. C. Variation in sensitivity to heat shock during the cell-cycle of Chinese hamster cells *in vitro. Int. J. Radiat. Biol.*, 19: 467–477, 1971.
11. BEN-HUR, E., BRONK, B. V. AND ELKIND, M. M. Thermally enhanced radiosensitivity of cultured Chinese hamster cells. *Nature*, 238: 209–211, 1972.
12. BEN-HUR, E., ELKIND, M. M. AND BRONK, B. V. Thermally enhanced radio-response of cultured Chinese hamster cells: Inhibition of repair of sublethal damage and enhancement of lethal damage. *Radiat. Res.*, 58: 38–51, 1974.
13. ROBINSON, J. E., WIZENBERG, M. J., EDELSACK, E. A. AND MCCREADY, W. A. Radiation and hyperthermal response of normal tissue *in situ*—3 fraction studies. *Radiat. Res.*, 59: 141, 1974.

14. ROBINSON, J. E., WIZENBERG, M. J. AND MCCREADY, W. A. Radiation and hyperthermia response of normal tissue *in situ. Radiology, 113:* 195–198, 1974.
15. Robinson, J. E., Wizenberg, M. J., McCready, W. A. and Edelsack, E. A. Tumor response to a three-fraction regimen combining hyperthermia and X-radiation. *Radiat. Res., 59:* 185, 1974.
16. THRALL, D. E., GILLETTE, E. L. AND BAUMAN, C. Effect of heat on the C3H mouse mammary adenocarcinoma evaluated in terms of tumor growth. *Eur. J. Cancer, 9:* 871–875, 1973.
17. THRALL, D. E., GILLETTE, E. L. AND DEWEY, W. C. Effect of heat and ionizing radiation on normal and neoplastic tissue of the C3H mouse. *Radiat. Res., 63:* 363–377, 1975.
18. MONDOVI, B., ROTILLO, G., STROM, R., AGRO, A. F., FANELLI, A. R. AND CAVALIERE, R. The biochemical mechanism of selective heat sensitivity of cancer cells: I. Studies on cellular respiration. *Eur. J. Cancer, 5:* 129–236, 1969.
19. MONDOVI, B., AGRO, A. F., ROTILLO, G., STROM, R., MORICCA, G. AND FANELLI, A. R. The biochemical mechanism of selective heat sensitivity of cancer cells: II. Studies on nucleic acid and protein synthesis. *Eur. J. Cancer, 5:* 137–146, 1969.
20. TURANO, C., FERRARO, A., STROM, R., CAVALIERE, R. AND FANELLI, A. R. The biochemical mechanism of selective heat sensitivity of cancer cells: III. Studies of lysosomes. *Eur. J. Cancer, 6:* 67–72, 1970.
21. STROM, R., SANTORO, A. S., CRIFO, C., BOZZI, A., MONDOVI, B. AND FANELLI, A. R. The biochemical mechanism of selective heat sensitivity of cancer cells: IV. Inhibition of RNA synthesis. *Eur. J. Cancer, 9:* 103–112, 1973.
22. OVERGAARD, K. AND OVERGAARD, J. Investigations on the possibility of a thermic tumor therapy. I. (Short-wave treatment of a transplanted isologous mouse mammary carcinoma). *Eur. J. Cancer, 8:* 65–78, 1972.
23. HAHN, G. M. Metabolic aspects of the role of hyperthermia in mammalian cell inactivation and their possible relevance to cancer treatment. *Cancer Res., 34:* 3117–3123, 1974.
24. DEWEY, W. C., FREEMAN, M. L., RAAPHORST, G. P., CLARK, E. P., WONG, R. S. L., HIGHFIELD, D. P., SPIRO, I. J., TOMASOVIC, S. P., DENMAN, D. L. AND COSS, R. A. Cell biology of hyperthermia and radiation. *In:* Radiation Biology in Cancer Research. Meyn, R. W. and Withers, H. R. (Eds). Raven Press, N.Y., pp. 589–621, 1980.
25. MILLER, R. C., LEITH, J. T., VEOMETT, R. C. AND GERNER, E. W. Potentiation of radiation myelitis by hyperthermia treatment. *Br. J. Radiol., 49:* 895–896, 1976.
26. GOFFINET, D. R., CHOI, K. Y. AND BROWN, J. M. The combined effects of hyperthermia and ionizing radiation on the adult mouse spinal cord. *Radiat. Res., 72:* 238–245, 1977.
27. GILLETTE, E. L. Large animal studies of hyperthermia and radiation. *Cancer Res., 39:* 2242–2244, 1979.
28. HAHN, G. M. Potential for therapy of drugs and hyperthermia. *Cancer Res., 39:* 2264–2268, 1979.
29. DONALDSON, S., GORDON, L. AND HAHN, G. M. Protective effect of hyperthermia against the cytotoxicity of actionomycin D on Chinese hamster cells. *Cancer Treat. Rept., 62:* 1489–1495, 1978.
30. YATVIN, M. B., WEINSTEIN, J. N., DENNIS, W. H. AND BLUMENTHAL, R. Design of lipsomes for enhanced local release of drugs by hyperthermia. *Science, 202:* 1290–1293, 1978.
31. WEINSTEIN, J. N., MAGUN, R. L., YATVIN, M. B. AND FAHARKO, D. S. Liposomes and local hyperthermia: Selective delivery of methotrexate to heated tumors. *Science, 204:* 188–191, 1979.
32. ALBERTS, D. S., PENG, Y-M, CHEN, H-S, G., MOON, T. E., CETAS, T. C. AND HOESCHELE, J. Therapeutic synergism of hyperthermia/cis platinum in a mouse tumor model. *J. Nat. Cancer Inst., 65:* 177–180, 1980.
33. GIOVANELLA, B. C., STEHLIN, J. S. AND YIM, S. O. Correlation of the thermosensitivity of cells to their malignant potential. *Ann. N.Y. Acad. Sci., 335:* 206–214, 1980.

34. KASE, K. AND HAHN, G. M. Differential heat response of normal and transformed human cells in tissue culture. *Nature, 255:* 228–230, 1975.

35. HOFER, K. G., CHOPPIN, D. A. AND HOFER, M. G. Effect of hyperthermia on the radiosensitivity of normal and malignant cells in mice. *Cancer, 38:* 279, 1976.

36. CRESS, A. E. AND GERNER, E. W. Cholesterol content inversely reflects the thermal sensitivity of mammalian cells in culture. *Nature, 382:* 677–680, 1980.

37. DEWEY, W. C., HIGHFIELD, D. P., FREEMAN, M. L., COSS, R. A., WONG, R. S. L. AND BARRAU, M. D. Cell biology of hyperthermia and radiation. *In: Proceedings of the Sixth International Congress of Radiation Research.* Okada, S., Imamura, M., Terashima, T. and Yamaguchi, H. (Eds). Japanese Association for Radiation Research, Tokyo, Japan, pp. 832–840, 1979.

38. GERNER, E. W., CRESS, A. E., STICKNEY, D. G., HOLMES, D. K. AND CULVER, P. S. Factors regulating membrane permeability alter thermal resistance. *Ann. N.Y. Acad. Sci., 335:* 215–230, 1980.

39. GERNER, E. W., HOLMES, D. K., STICKNEY, D. G., NOTERMAN, J. A. AND FULLER, D. J. M. Enhancement of hyperthermia-induced cytotoxicity by the polyamines. *Cancer Res., 40:* 432–438, 1980.

40. GERNER, E. W. AND SCHNEIDER, M. J. Induced thermal resistance in HeLa cells. *Nature, 256:* 500–502, 1975.

41. GERNER, E. W., BOONE, R., CONNOR, W. G., HICKS, J. A. AND BOONE, M. L. M. A transient thermotolerant survival response produced by single thermal doses in HeLa cells. *Cancer Res., 36:* 1035–1040, 1976.

42. HENLE, K. J. AND LEEPER, D. B. Interaction of hyperthermia and radiation in CHO cells: Recovery kinetics. *Radiat. Res., 66:* 505–518, 1976.

43. HARISIADIS, L., SUNG, D. AND HALL, E. J. Thermal tolerance and repair of thermal damage by cultured cells. *Radiology, 123:* 505–509, 1977.

44. HENLE, K. J. AND DETHLEFSEN, L. A. Heat fractionation and thermotolerance: A review. *Cancer Res., 38:* 1843–1851, 1978.

45. HARRIS, M. Temperature-resistant variants in clonal populations of pig kidney cells. *Exp. Cell Res., 46:* 301–314, 1967.

46. REEVES, O. R. Mechanisms of acquired resistance to acute heat shock in cultured mammalian cells. *J. Cell. Physiol., 79:* 157–170, 1972.

47. ROTI ROTI, J. L. Heat induced cell death and radiosensitization: Molecular mechanisms. *J. Nat. Cancer Inst.,* (in press).

48. LANDRY, J. AND MARCEAU, N. Rate-limiting events in hyperthermic cell killing. *Radiat. Res., 75:* 573–585, 1978.

49. OVERGAARD, J. Effect of hyperthermia on malignant cells *in vivo.* A review and a hypothesis. *Cancer, 39:* 1–28, 1977.

50. HUME, S. P., ROGERS, M. A. AND FIELD, S. B. Two qualitatively different effects of hyperthermia on acid phosphatase staining in mouse spleen, dependent on the severity of the treatment. *Int. J. Radiat. Biol., 34:* 401–409, 1978.

51. HOFER, K. G., BRIZZARD, B. AND HOFER, M. G. Effect of lysosome modification on the heat potentiation of radiation damage and direct heat death of BP-8 sarcoma cells. *Eur. J. Cancer, 15:* 1449–1457, 1979.

52. MAGUN, B. E. AND FENNIE, C. W. Effects of hyperthermia on binding, internalization and degradation of epidermal growth factor. *Radiat. Res., 86:* 133–146, 1981.

53. ASHBURNER, M. AND BONNER, J. J. The induction of gene activity in drosophila by heat shock. *Cell, 17:* 241–254, 1979.

54. BOUCHE, G., AMALRIC, F., CAIZERGUES, M. AND ZALTA, J. P. Effects of heat shock on gene expression and subcellular protein distribution in Chinese hamster ovary cells. *Nuc. Acids Res., 7:* 1739–1747, 1979.

55. KELLY, P. M. AND SCHLESINGER, M. J. The effect of amino acid analogs and heat shock on gene expression in chicken embryo fibroblasts. *Cell, 15:* 1277–1286, 1978.

56. MCALISTER, L. AND FINKELSTEIN, D. B. Heat shock proteins and thermal resistance in yeast. *Biochem. Biophys. Res. Commun., 93:* 819–824, 1980.
57. REINHOLD, H. S., BLACHIEWICZ, B. AND BERG-BLOK, A. Decrease in tumor microcirculation during hyperthermia. *In: Cancer Therapy by Hyperthermia and Radiation.* Streffer, C., van Beuningen, D., Dietzel, F., Rottinger, E. Robinson, J. E., Scherer, E., Seeber, S., Trott, K.-R. (Eds). Urban and Schwarzenberg, Baltimore-Munich, p. 231–232 1978.
58. SONG, C. W. Physiological factors in hyperthermia. *J. Nat. Cancer Inst.,* (in press).
59. DEWHIRST, M. W., OZIMEK, E. J., GROSS, J. AND CETAS, T. C. Will hyperthermia conquer the elusive hypoxic cell? *Radiology, 137:* 811–817, 1980.
60. SONG, C. W., KANG, M. S. RHEE, J. G. AND LEVITT, S. H. Effect of hyperthermia on vascular function in normal and neoplastic tissue. *Ann. N.Y. Acad. Sci., 335:* 35–43, 1980.
61. DICKSON, J. A. AND CALDERWOOD, S. K. Temperature range and selective sensitivity of tumors to hyperthermia: A critical review. *Ann. N.Y. Acad. Sci., 335:* 180–201, 1980.
62. BRONK, B. V., WILKINS R. J. AND REGAN, J. D. Thermal enhancement of DNA damage by an alkylating agent in human cells. *Biochem. Biophys. Res. Commun., 52:* 1064–1070, 1973.
63. COLEY, W. B. The treatment of malignant tumors by repeated inoculations of erysipelas, with a report of ten original cases. *Am. J. Med. Sci., 105:* 487–511, 1893.
64. STEHLIN, J. S., JR., CLARK, R. L., VICKERS, W. E. AND MONGES, A. Perfusion for malignant melanoma of the extremities. *Am. J. Surg., 105:* 607–614, 1963.
65. STEHLIN, J. S., JR. Hyperthermic perfusion with chemotherapy for cancers of the extremities. *Surg. Gynecol. Obstet., 129:* 305–308, 1969.
66. STEHLIN, J. S., JR., GIOVANELLA, B. C., DEIPOLYI, P. D., MUENZ, L. R. AND ANDERSON, R. F. Results of hyperthermic perfusion for melanoma of the extremities. *Surg. Gynecol. Obstet., 140:* 339–348, 1975.
67. STEHLIN, J. S., JR., GIOVANELLA, B. C., DEIPOLYI, P. D. AND ANDERSON, R. F. Clinical and biological studies of localized hyperthermia. *Cancer Res., 39:* 2255–2257, 1979.
68. STEHLIN, J. S., JR. Hyperthermic perfusion for melanoma of the extremities: Experience with 165 patients, 1967–1979. *Ann. N.Y. Acad. Sci., 335:* 352–355, 1980.
69. PARKS, L. C., MINABERRY, R. N., SMITH, D. P. AND NEELY, W. A. Treatment of far-advanced bronchogenic carcinoma by extracorporeally induced systemic hyperthermia. *J. Thorac. Cardiovasc. Surg., 78:* 883–892, 1979.
70. MANNING, M. R. AND GERNER, E. W. Interstitial thermoradiotherapy. *In: Hyperthermia in Cancer Therapy,* Storm, F. K. Hall, G. K. (Eds). Boston, MA. (in press).
71. MANNING, M. R., CETAS, T. C., MILLER, R. C., OLESON, J. R., CONNOR, W. G. AND GERNER, E. W. Clinical hyperthermia: Results of a Phase I trial employing hyperthermia alone or in combination with external beam or interstitial radiotherapy. *Cancer,* (in press).
72. CARPENTER, C. M. AND PAGE, A. B. The production of fever in man by short radiowaves. *Science, 71:* 450–452, 1930.
73. GEYSER, A. C. Diathermia and the physiological treatment of cancer. *Fischer's Magazine,* December, pp. 6–9, 1924.
74. KIM, J. H., HAHN, E. W., TOKITA, N. AND NISCE, L. Z. Local tumor hyperthermia in combination with radiation therapy. *Cancer, 40:* 161–169, 1977.
75. KIM, J. H., HAHN, E. W. AND TOKITA, N. Clinical trial with hyperthermia and radiotherapy: Cutaneous cancers as a model system. *In: Cancer Therapy by Hyperthermia and Radiation.* Streffer, C. (Ed). Urgan and Schwarzenberg, Baltimore-Munich, pp. 335–336, 1978.
76. KIM, J. H. AND HOHN, E. W. Clinical and biological studies of localized hyperthermia. *Cancer Res., 39:* 2258–2261, 1979.
77. ANTICH, P. P., TOKITA, N., KIM, J. H. AND HAHN, E. W. Selective heating of cutaneous tumors at 27.12 MHz. *IEEE Trans. Microwave Theory Tech., MTT-26:* 569–572, 1978.
78. HAHN, E. W. AND KIM, J. H. Clinical observations on the selective heating of cutaneous

tumors with the radiofrequency inductive method. *Ann. N.Y. Acad. Sci., 335:* 347–351, 1980.

79. MENDECKI, J., FRIEDENTHAL, E., BOTSTEIN, C., STERZER, F., PAGLIONE, R., NOWOGRODZKI, M. AND BECK, E. Microwave-induced hyperthermia in cancer treatment: Apparatus and preliminary results. *Int. J. Radiat. Onc. Biol. Phys., 4:* 1095–1103, 1978.

80. MENDECKI, J., FRIEDENTHAL, E., AND BOTSTEIN, C. Induction of hyperthermia in deepseated tumors by a special microwave applicator. *In: Cancer Therapy by Hyperthermia and Radiation.* Streffer, C. (Ed). Urban and Schwarzenberg, Baltimore-Munich, pp. 125–127, 1978.

81. U, R., NOELL, K. T., WOODWARD, K. T., WORDE, B. T., FISHBURN, R. I. AND MILLER, L. S. Microwave-induced local hyperthermia in combination with radiotherapy of human malignant tumors. *Cancer, 45:* 638–646, 1980.

82. HORNBACK, N. B., SHUPE, R., SHIDNIA, H., JOE, B. T., SAYOC, E., GEORGE, R. AND MARSHALL, C. Radiation and microwave therapy in the treatment of advanced cancer. *Radiology, 130:* 459–464, 1979.

83. BICHER, H. K., SANDHER, T. S. AND HETZEL, F. W. Hyperthermia and radiation in combination: A clinical fractionation regime. *Int. J. Radiat. Onc. Biol. Phys., 6:* 867–870, 1980.

84. CETAS, T. C., CONNOR, W. G. AND MANNING, M. R. Monitoring of tissue temperature during hyperthermia therapy. *Ann. N.Y. Acad. Sci., 335:* 281–297, 1980.

85. LEVEEN, H. H., WAPNICK, S., PICCONE, V., FALK, G. AND AHMED, N. Tumor eradication by radiofrequency therapy: Response in 21 patients. *J.A.M.A., 235:* 2198–2200, 1976.

86. LEVEEN, H. H., AHMED, N., PICCONE, V. A., SHUGAAR, S. AND FALK, G. Radiofrequency therapy: Clinical experience. *Ann. N.Y. Acad. Sci., 335:* 362–371, 1980.

87. CETAS, T. C., CONNOR, W. G. AND BOONE, M. L. M. Thermal dosimetry: Some biophysical considerations. *In: Cancer Therapy by Hyperthermia and Radiation.* Streffer, C. (Ed). Urban and Schwarenberg, Baltimore-Munich, pp. 3–12, 1978.

88. LEBOURGEOIS, J. P., CONERT, G. AND DUFOUR, J. An interstitial device for microwave hyperthermia of human tumors. *In: Cancer Therapy by Hyperthermia and Radiation.* Streffer, C. (Ed). Urban and Schwarzenberg, Baltimore-Munich, pp. 122–124, 1978.

89. MILLER, R. C., CONNOR, W. G., HEUSINKVELD, R. S. AND BOONE, M. L. M. Prospects for hyperthermia in human cancer therapy. *Radiology, 123:* 489–495, 1977.

90. MARMOR, J. B. AND HAHN, G. M. Ultrasound heating in previously irradiated sites. *Int. J. Radiat. Onc. Biol. Phys., 4:* 1029–1032, 1978.

91. LELE, P. P. Hyperthermia by ultrasound. *In: Proceedings of the International Symposium on Cancer Therapy by Hyperthermia and Radiation.* Washington, American College of Radiology, p. 168, April, 1975.

92. HAHN, G. M., KERNAHAN, P., MARTINEZ, A., POUNDS, D., PRIONAS, S., ANDERSON, T. AND JUSTICE, G. Some heat transfer problems associated with heating by ultrasound, microwaves or radiofrequency. *Ann. N.Y. Acad. Sci., 335:* 327–346, 1980.

93. STORM, F. K., HARRISON, W. H., ELLIOTT, R. S. AND MORTON, D. L. Normal tissue and solid tumor effects of hyperthermia in animal models and clinical trials. *Cancer Res., 39:* 2245–2251, 1979.

94. OLESON, J. R., STAUFFER, P. R., CETAS, T. C., DEWHIRST, M. W., HEUSINKVELD, R. S. AND JONES R. C. Magnetic induction heating in heterogeneous material. Presented at the Third International Symposium: Cancer Therapy by Hyperthermia, Drugs and Radiation, held at Colorado State University, Fort Collins, CO., June 1980.

95. STORM, F. K., HARRISON, W. H., ELLIOTT, R. S. HATZITHEOFILOU, C., MORTON, D. L. Human hyperthermic therapy: Relation between tumor type and capacity to induce hyperthermia by radiofrequency. *Am. J. Surg., 138:* 170–174, 1979.

96. SHORT, J. G. AND TURNER, P. F. Physical hyperthermia and cancer therapy. *Proc. IEEE, 68:* 133–142, 1980.

97. PETTIGREW, R. T., GALT, J. M., LUDGATE, C. M. AND SMITH, A. N. Clinical effects of whole-body hyperthermia in advanced malignancy. *Br. Med. J.*, 4: 679–682, 1974.

98. PETTIGREW, R. T., GALT, J. M., LUDGATE, C. M., HORN D. B., AND SMITH, A. N. Circulatory and biochemical effects of whole-body hyperthermia. *Br. J. Surg.*, 61: 727–730, 1974.

99. PETTIGREW, R. T., LUDGATE, C. M., GEE, A. P. AND SMITH, A. N. Whole-body hyperthermia combined with chemotherapy in the treatment of advanced human cancer. *In: Cancer Therapy by Hyperthermia and Radiation.* Streffer, C. (Ed). Urban and Schwarzenberg, Baltimore-Munich, pp. 337–339, 1978.

100. LAW, H. T. AND PETTIGREW, R. T. Heat transfer in whole-body hyperthermia. *Ann. N.Y. Acad. Sci.*, 335: 298–310, 1980.

101. LARKIN, J. M., EDWARDS, W. S., SMITH, D. E. AND CLARK, P. J. *Systemic thermotherapy: Description of a method and physiologic tolerance in clinical subjects. Cancer*, 40: 3155–3159, 1977.

102. LARKIN, J. M. A clinical investigation of total-body hyperthermia as cancer therapy. *Cancer Res.*, 39: 2252–2254, 1979.

103. BULL, J. M., LEES, D., SCHUETTE, W., WHANG-PENG, J., SMITH, R., BYNUM, G., ATKINSON, E. R., GOTTDIENER, J. S., GRALNICK, H. R., SHAWKER, T. H. AND DEVITA, V. T., JR. Whole body hyperthermia: A Phase I trial of a potential adjuvant to chemotherapy. *Ann. Int. Med.*, 90: 317–323, 1979.

104. GUY, A. W. Physical aspects of the electromagnetic heating of tissue volume. *In: Proceedings of the International Symposium on Cancer Therapy by Hyperthermia and Radiation.* Washington, American College of Radiology, p. 179, April, 1975.

105. GUY, A. W. Analyses of electromagnetic fields induced in biological tissues by thermographic studies on equivalent phantom models. *IEEE Trans. Microwave Theory Tech.*, 19: 205–214, 1971.

106. GUY, A. W., LEHMANN, J. F., STONEBRIDGE, J. B. AND SORENSEN, C. C. Development of a 915-MHz direct-contact applicator for therapeutic heating of tissues. *IEEE Trans. Microwave Therapy Tech.*, 26: 550–555, 1978.

107. LEHMAN, J. F., GUY, A. W., STONEBRIDGE, J. B. AND DELATEUR, B. J. Evaluation of a therapeutic direct-contact 915-MHz microwave applicator for effective deep-tissue heating in humans. *IEEE Trans. Microwave Theory Tech.*, 26: 556–562,

108. KANTOR, G., WITTERS, D. M., JR. AND GREISER, J. W. The performance of a new direct contact applicator of microwave diathermy. *IEEE Trans. Microwave Theory Tech.*, 26: 563–568, 1978.

109. CETAS, T. C. AND CONNOR, W. G. Thermometry considerations in localized hyperthermia. *Med. Phys.*, 5: 79–91, 1978.

110. BOWMAN, R. R. A probe for measuring temperature in radiofrequency-heated material. *IEEE Trans. Biomed. Eng.*, MTT 24: 43–45, 1976.

111. CHRISTENSEN, D. A. A new nonperturbing temperature probe using semi-conductor band edge shift. *J. Bioeng.*, 1: 541–545, 1977.

112. CETAS, T. S. A birefringent crystal optical thermometer for measurements in electromagnetically induced heating. *In: Proceedings 1975 USNC/URSI Symposium.* Johnson, C. C. and Shore, J. L. (Eds). Bureau of Radiological Health, Rockville, MD, 1976.

113. BARLOGIE, B., CORRY, P. M., YIP, E., LIPPMAN, L., JOHNSTONE, D. A., KHALIL, K., TENCZYNSKI, T. F., REILLY, E., LAWSON, R., DOSIK, G., RIGOR, B., HANKENSON, R. AND FREIREICH, E. J. Total-body hyperthermia with and without chemotherapy for advanced human neoplasms. *Cancer Res.*, 39: 1481–1489, 1979.

114. JOHNSON, R. J. R., SANDU, T. S., HETZEL, F. W., SONG, S.-Y., BICHER, H. I., SUBJECK, J. R. AND KOWAL, H. S. A pilot study to investigate skin and tumor thermal enhancement ratios of 41.5–42°C hyperthermia with radiation. *Int. J. Radiat. Oncol. Biol. Phys.*, 5: 947–953, 1979.

115. STAUFFER, P. R. A magnetic induction system for inducing localized hyperthermia in brain tumors. Thesis, University of Arizona, Department of Electrical Engineering, 1979.
116. STAUFFER, P. R., CETAS, T. C., JONES, R. C. AND MANNING, M. R. A system for producing localized hyperthermia in brain tumors through magnetic induction heating of ferromagnetic implants. Abstract presented at the Bioelectromagnetics Symposium at the University of Washington, June 18–22, 1979.
117. CHATO, J. C. A method for the measurement of the thermal properties of biological material. *In: Thermal Problems in Biotechnology.* ASME Symposium Series, pp. 16–25, 1968.
118. BOWMAN, H. F., BALASUBRAMANIAN, T. A. AND WOODS, M. Determination of tissue perfusion from *in vivo* thermal conductivity measurements. ASME Paper 77-WA/HT-40, 1977.
119. BALASUBRAMANIAN, T. A. AND BOWMAN, H. F. Temperature field due to a time dependent heat source of spherical geometry in an infinite medium. *J. Heat Transfer, 96:* 296–299, 1974.
120. BALASUBRAMANIAN, T. A. AND BOWMAN, H. F. Thermal conductivity and thermal diffusivity of biomaterials: a simultaneous measurement technique. *J. Biomech. Eng.,* Transactions of the ASME 99, Series K, No. 3, 1977.

Index